USD 49

THE LONG-TERM CARE

STATE OPERATIONS MANUAL

HCPro

The Long-Term Care State Operations Manual is published by HCPro, Inc. No claim to original U.S. government work.

ISBN: 978-1-60146-128-5

HCPro, Inc., provides information resources for the healthcare industry.

HCPro, Inc., is not affiliated in any way with The Joint Commission, which owns the JCAHO and Joint Commission trademarks.

Noelle Shough, Executive Editor
Kerry Vegliando, Editorial Assistant
Emily Sheahan, Group Publisher
Mike Mirabello, Senior Graphic Artist
Jean St. Pierre, Director of Operations
Shane Katz, Cover Designer

Arrangements can be made for quantity discounts. For more information, contact:

HCPro, Inc.
P.O. Box 1168
Marblehead, MA 01945
Telephone: 800/650-6787 or 781/639-1872
Fax: 781/639-2982
E-mail: *customerservice@hcpro.com*

Visit HCPro at its World Wide Web sites:
www.hcpro.com* and *www.hcmarketplace.com

Revised 10/2007
21305

CONTENTS

PART 1

SURVEY PROTOCOL

State Operations Manual
Appendix P - Survey Protocol for Long Term Care Facilities - Part I

(Rev. 26, 08-17-07)

Transmittals for Appendix P

I. Introduction

Skilled nursing facilities (SNFs) and nursing facilities (NFs) are required to be in compliance with the requirements at 42 CFR Part 483, Subpart B, to receive payment under the Medicare or Medicaid programs. To certify a SNF or NF, complete at least a:

- Life Safety Code (LSC) survey; and
- Standard Survey. There are two types of Standard Surveys:
    - The Quality Indicators Survey (QIS), which uses the QIS procedures and forms as contained in the QIS Surveyor Training Manual. The QIS is only used by a State Survey Agency upon approval by CMS, and only by the surveyors who have received QIS training; and
    - The Traditional Survey, which uses Forms CMS-670, CMS-671, CMS-672, CMS-677, and CMS-801 through CMS-807 (see <u>Exhibits 85, 86, and 88 thru 95</u>).

NOTE: CMS is beginning the process of a staged implementation of a revised survey process, the Quality Indicators Survey (QIS) as a replacement for the current (Traditional) survey process. The QIS is a two-staged, computer-assisted survey process with Stage 1 consisting of both computer analysis of offsite data from the Minimum Data Set system as well as data collected by surveyors onsite from observations, interviews, and record reviews of large computer-selected resident samples. The information collected throughout Stage 1 is analyzed by computer to derive a set of approximately 160 Quality of Care Indicators (QCIs) that are used to compare the facility being surveyed to national norms. QCIs that score beyond a statistical threshold are computer-selected for Stage 2 review, and the relevant residents are also computer selected. Stage 2 consists of systematic surveyor investigations of triggered issues and residents using a set of detailed investigative tools known as critical elements protocols. In addition to the Stage 1 and Stage 2 sample-based investigations, the QIS also contains several facility-level tasks that are unstaged and are completed either on every survey or when triggered as areas of concern.

During this period, as CMS conducts pilot implementation, CMS deems both the QIS and Traditional Survey as surveys-of-record to evaluate compliance of nursing homes with the requirements at 42 CFR 483.5-483.75.

Do not announce SNF/NF surveys to the facility. Conduct standard surveys and complete them on consecutive workdays, whenever possible. They may be conducted at any time including weekends, 24 hours a day. When standard surveys begin at times beyond the business hours of 8:00 a.m. to 6:00 p.m., or begin on a Saturday or Sunday, the entrance conference and initial tour should be modified in recognition of the residents' activity (e.g., sleep, religious services) and types and numbers of staff available upon entry.

Use the standard survey procedure discussed in this section for all standard surveys of SNFs and NFs, whether freestanding, distinct parts, or dually participating. For surveys of facilities predominantly serving short stay residents, modifications of offsite survey preparation and sampling procedures will be necessary.

NOTE: Do not use this process for surveys of intermediate care facilities for the mentally retarded (ICFs/MR), swing-bed hospitals, or skilled nursing sections of hospitals that are not separately certified as SNF distinct parts. Survey Protocols and Interpretive Guidelines for these surveys are found in Appendix J (ICFs/MR) and Appendix T (swing-bed hospitals and hospitals with non-distinct part SNFs).

When the survey team suspects substandard quality of care (SQC), expand the standard (or abbreviated) survey sample as necessary to determine scope. If the existence of SQC is verified, then inform the Administrator that the facility has SQC and an extended (or partial extended) survey will be conducted.

Surveys

If a possible noncompliant situation related to any requirement is identified while conducting the information gathering tasks of the survey, investigate the situation to determine whether the facility is in compliance with the requirements.

Standard Survey

The QIS Standard Survey is composed of Tasks 1 – 9 and the Traditional Standard Survey is composed of Tasks 1 – 7. Both versions of the survey process are resident-centered, outcome-oriented inspections that rely on a case-mix stratified sample of residents to gather information about the facility's compliance with participation requirements. Outcomes include both actual and potential negative outcomes, as well as failure of a facility to help residents achieve their highest practicable level of well-being. Based on the specific procedures detailed in this Appendix, a standard survey assesses:

- Compliance with residents' rights and quality of life requirements;
- The accuracy of residents' comprehensive assessments and the adequacy of care plans based on these assessments;
- The quality of care and services furnished, as measured by indicators of medical, nursing, rehabilitative care and drug therapy, dietary and nutrition services, activities and social participation, sanitation and infection control; and
- The effectiveness of the physical environment to empower residents, accommodate resident needs, and maintain resident safety, including whether requested room variances meet health, safety, and quality of life needs for the affected residents.

Extended Survey

The extended survey is conducted after substandard quality of care is determined during a standard survey. If, based on performing the resident-centered tasks of the standard survey it is determined that the facility has provided substandard quality of care in 42 CFR 483.13, Resident Behavior and Facility Practices; 42 CFR 483.15, Quality of Life; and/or 42 CFR 483.25, Quality of Care, conduct an extended survey within 14 days after completion of the standard survey. (See Sction II.A.2. for further information about the QIS extended survey and Section III for further information about the Traditional Extended Survey.

Abbreviated Standard Survey

This survey focuses on particular tasks that relate, for example, to complaints received or a change of ownership, management or director of nursing. The abbreviated standard survey does not cover all aspects covered in the standard survey, but rather concentrates on a particular area of concern(s). For example, an abbreviated standard survey may be conducted to substantiate a complaint. The survey team can expand the abbreviated standard survey to cover additional areas, or to a Traditional Standard Survey if, during the Abbreviated Standard Survey, evidence is found that warrants a more extensive review. (See also Chapter 5 of this manual for additional administrative procedures related to complaints.) At this time, the QIS is not used to conduct an abbreviated standard survey. See §II.A.4. below for investigation of complaints during the QIS standard survey.

Partial Extended Survey

A partial extended survey is always conducted after substandard quality of care is found during an abbreviated standard survey or during a revisit, when substandard quality of care was not previously identified. If, based on performing the abbreviated standard survey or revisit it is determined that the facility has provided substandard quality of care in 42 CFR 483.13, Resident Behavior and Facility Practices; 42 CFR 483.15, Quality of Life; and/or 42 CFR 483.25, Quality of Care, conduct a partial extended survey. (See Section III for further information about the partial extended survey. At this time, the QIS is not used for partial extended surveys.)

Post-Survey Revisit (Follow-Up)

The post-survey revisit is an onsite visit intended to verify correction of deficiencies cited in a prior survey. See §2732 and Appendix P, Part I, Section VI, "Writing the Statement of Deficiencies." (See Section II.A.3. for further information about the QIS revisit and Section VI. for further information about the Traditional revisit.) If substandard quality of care is determined during a revisit, complete a partial extended survey, if a partial extended or extended survey had not been conducted as the result of the prior standard or abbreviated standard survey.

Initial Certification Survey

In a survey for initial certification of SNFs or NFs, perform the tasks of both the Traditional Standard and Extended Surveys. During the initial survey, focus both on residents and the structural requirements that relate to qualification standards and resident rights notification, whether or not problems are identified during the information gathering tasks. Gather additional information to verify compliance with every tag number. For example, during an initial survey, verify the qualifications of the social worker, dietitian, and activities professional. Also, review the rights notification statements on admissions contracts. Complete the "Statement of Deficiencies and Plan of Correction" (Form CMS-2567) in Exhibit 7.

Specialty Surveyors

All members of a survey team need not be onsite for the entire survey. Specialty surveyors participating in surveys (e.g., a pharmacist, physician, or registered dietitian) must be onsite during that portion of the survey dealing with their area of expertise.

However, they must conduct that portion while the rest of the team is present. All members of the survey team should enter the facility at the same time, if possible. Before leaving the facility, at the completion of his/her portion of the survey, the specialty surveyor must meet with the team or team coordinator to discuss his/her findings and to provide supporting documentation. The specialty surveyor should also share any information he/she obtained that may be useful to other team members. If he/she is not present at the information analysis for deficiency determination, the specialty surveyor should be available by telephone at that time and during the exit conference.

Team Communication

Throughout the survey process, the team (including specialty surveyors onsite at the time) should discuss among themselves, on a daily basis, observations made and information obtained in order to focus on the concerns of each team member, to facilitate information gathering and to facilitate decision making at the completion of the standard survey.

II. The Survey Process

II.A. - The Quality Indicators Survey (QIS)

The QIS survey is used as the survey-of-record only for states that have received CMS approval, and only by surveyors who have completed QIS training. Sections II.A.1.-4. below describe the use of the QIS for standard surveys, extended surveys, post-survey revisits, and complaint investigations.

1. The QIS Standard Survey

The QIS standard survey consists of the following Tasks (details are contained in the QIS Surveyor Training Manual, which is incorporated by reference):

Introduction

Task 1: Offsite Survey Preparation:

- Offsite Survey Preparation and Initial Sampling

Task 2: Onsite Preparatory Activities and Entrance Conference

- Prior to the Entrance Conference
- Entrance Conference
- Possible Off Hours Activities

Task 3: Initial Tour

- Tour

Task 4: Stage I Survey Tasks

- Finalize Sample Selection
  - Stage I Sample Selection Procedures
- Stage I Team Meetings (first meeting)
- Stage I Information Gathering
- Stage I Admission Sample Review
  - Medical Record Review
- Stage I Census Sample Review
  - Resident Interviews
  - Resident Unavailable for Interviews
  - Resident Observations
  - Staff Interviews
  - Medical Record Review
  - Family Interviews

Task 5: Non-Staged Survey Tasks

- Resident Council President/Representative Interview
- Dining Observation
- Kitchen/Food Service Observation
- Infection Control Policies and Practices
- Demand Billing Review
- Abuse Prohibition Review
- Quality Assessment and Assurance (QA&A Review)

Task 6: Transition From Stage I to Stage II

- Update the Resident Pool
- Review Completion of Stage I
- Review Surveyor-Initiated Residents and/or Care Areas
- Import All Data into the Primary Laptop
- Review the Relevant Findings Report

- Review the QCI Results Report

Task 7: Stage II Survey Tasks

- Introduction
- Team Meetings
- Stage II Sample Selection
    - Substituting Residents
    - Supplementing the Sample
- Staff Assignments
- Stage II Information Gathering
    - Stage II Critical Element Pathways
    - Medication Administration Observation and Unnecessary Drug Review
- Facility-Level Investigations
    - Environmental Observation
    - Resident Funds
    - Admission, Transfer, and Discharge Review
    - Sufficient Staff

Task 8: Analysis and Decision-Making: Integration of Information

- Integration of Facility-Level Information
- Integration of Critical Element Pathways
- Analysis of Information Gained
- Analysis of Scope and Severity and Team Decision-Making

Task 9: Exit Conference

- Exit Conference

2. The QIS Extended Survey

When the survey team is conducting a QIS standard survey and they have determined there is substandard quality of care, they will conduct QIS extended survey procedures. Substandard quality of care is defined as one or more deficiencies with scope/severity levels of F, H, I, J, K, or L in any of the following regulatory groupings:

- 42 CFR 483.13, Resident Behavior and Facility Practices;

- 42 CFR 483.15, Quality of Life; and/or
- 42 CFR 483.25, Quality of Care.

The purpose of the QIS extended survey is to gather further information (unless already gathered during the standard survey) concerning the facility's nursing and medical services and administration, in order to evaluate systemic issues with the facility's provision of services and management that may be non-complaint with the long term care requirements, and may have contributed to problems cited in the substandard quality of care deficiency(ies). When conducting the QIS extended survey, the survey team coordinator will surveyor-initiate all Tags within the following regulatory groupings into the QIS survey software: 42 CFR 483.30, Nursing Services; 42 CFR 483.40, Physician Services; and 42 CFR 483.75, Administration. There are no specific QIS forms to assist this review. The survey team shall document their findings about these Tags on Surveyor Notes Worksheets (Form CMS-807) and shall input their findings into the QIS software. If the QIS Staffing Review protocol was not already completed during the standard survey, the survey team will complete this protocol.

At the discretion of the State Survey Agency, the QIS extended survey can be conducted either:

- Prior to the exit conference, in which case the facility will be provided with findings from the standard and extended survey; or

- Subsequent to the standard survey, but no longer than 2 weeks after the completion of the standard survey, if the survey team is unable to complete the extended survey prior to the exit conference.

3. The QIS Post-Survey Revisit (Follow-up)

A QIS post-survey revisit is conducted in accordance with §7317 to confirm that the facility is in compliance and has the ability to remain in compliance. The purpose of the revisit is to reevaluate the specific care and services that were cited as noncompliant during the QIS standard and/or extended survey. The specific procedures for each revisit depend on the deficiencies that were cited during the QIS standard survey. Detailed procedures are found in the QIS Surveyor Training Manual. For each QIS revisit, the surveyor(s) will use portions of the QIS standard survey, only as applicable to their need to evaluate the facility's return to compliance for requirements cited as deficiencies. For all QIS revisits, the surveyor(s) will review offsite the Statement of Deficiencies and conduct a focused review of the summary information from the QIS standard survey. Once onsite, the surveyor(s) will ask the facility to provide a roster of residents. The surveyor(s) will use the QIS software as well as information from the QIS standard survey (such as residents investigated) to surveyor-initiate the Care Areas and/or Tags and residents to be investigated. The surveyor(s) will use Stage 2 Critical Element Pathways (CEs) protocols as applicable to the Tags that have been cited, or the general CE for aspects of care not covered by the other CEs. For example, if deficiencies were cited for pressure ulcers and medication errors, the surveyor(s) would use the pressure ulcer CE and the QIS Medication Administration and Unnecessary Drug Review form to conduct these investigations. The surveyor(s) will input findings into the QIS software and proceed through QIS deficiency decision making, and scoring of scope and severity for any deficiencies that are cited.

4. The QIS Complaint Survey Procedures

The QIS is used for investigation of complaints during a QIS standard survey. The survey team coordinator will surveyor-select the complaint area(s) of concern and the resident(s) involved in the complaint and add them to the list of issues and residents evaluated during the QIS standard survey. The QIS Surveyor Training Manual contains further details concerning the manner in which these surveyor-selected concerns and issues are added to the standard survey for investigation, determination of whether they are substantiated or unsubstantiated, and conveying of findings into the CMS ASPEN data system.

At this time, the QIS is not used for investigation of complaints during an abbreviated standard survey. Surveyors should use the procedures contained in §VII.A. below for these investigations.

II.B. - The Traditional Survey

II.B.1 - Traditional Standard Survey Tasks

Task 1 - Offsite Survey Preparation

A. General Objectives

The objectives of offsite survey preparation are to analyze various sources of information available about the facility in order to:

- Identify and pre-select concerns for Phase 1 of the survey, based on the Facility Quality Measure/Indicator Report (see description below at B.3.a.). This pre-selection is subject to amendment based on the results of the tour;

- Pre-select potential residents for Phase I of the survey based on the Resident Level Quality Measure/Indicator Reports (see description below at B.3.a.) This pre-selection is subject to amendment based on the results gathered during the tour, entrance conference, and facility Roster/Sample Matrix;

- Note concerns based on other sources of information listed below and note other potential residents who could be selected for the sample; and

- Determine if the areas of potential concerns or special features of the facility require the addition to the team of any specialty surveyors.

B. Information Sources for Offsite Survey Preparation

The following sources of information (1-8) are used during the offsite team meeting to focus the survey.

1. Quality Measure/Indicator Reports

QM/QIs are to be used as indicators of potential problems or concerns that warrant further investigation. They are not determinations of facility compliance with the long term care requirements. There are three QM/QI reports which should be downloaded from the State database:

- Facility Characteristics Report (Exhibit 268)

  This report provides demographic information about the resident population (in percentages) for a selected facility compared to all the facilities in the State. It includes information in the following domains: Gender, age, payment source, diagnostic characteristics, type of assessment, stability of conditions, and discharge potential.

- Facility Quality Measure/Indicator Report (Exhibit 269)

  This report provides facility status for each of the MDS-based QM/QIs (quality measures and quality indicators) as compared to State and national averages. Listed are the individual QM/QIs (grouped by domains). This report begins with a set of 12 domains and a total of 31 QM/QIs for the chronic (long stay) resident population, followed by three additional QM/QIs for the post-acute care (PAC) resident population. For each QM/QI, (reading across a row from left to right) are:

  - The numerator - the number of residents in the facility who have the condition;
  - The denominator - the number of residents in the facility who could have the condition;
  - The facility observed percentage of residents who have the condition;
  - The facility adjusted percentage of residents who have the condition;
  - The State average percentage of residents who have the condition;
  - The national average percentage of residents who have the condition; and

- The State percentile ranking of the facility on the QM/QI - a descriptor of how the facility compares (ranks) with other facilities in the state. The higher the percentile rank, the greater potential there is for a care concern in the facility.

- An asterisk is present in any row in which the facility flagged on a QM/QI, which means that the facility is at or above the 90th percentile; and any of the three sentinel event rows if any resident has the condition (see D. below for more information on sentinel events).

- Resident Level Quality Measure/Indicator Reports (Exhibit 270)

  The resident level reports are divided into Chronic Care and PAC samples, to correspond to the division of residents in the Facility Quality Measure/Indicator Report described above. Both reports provide resident-specific information generated using current records from the CMS Minimum Data Set (MDS) data base. An X appears in a QM/QI column for a resident who has that condition. If a QM/QI is risk adjusted, this X is in either the high or low risk subcolumn, indicating whether this resident was at high or low risk to develop the condition. The Chronic Care version contains the following columns for each long-stay resident, reading from left to right:

  - Resident identification number;
  - Resident name in alphabetical order;
  - MDS type of assessment (1 = admission, 2 = annual, 3 = significant change, 4 = significant correction, and 5 = quarterly);
  - Columns for each QM/QI for the chronic care resident in the same order and under the same domains as on the Facility Quality Measure/Indicator Report; and
  - A column that counts how many QM/QIs the resident triggered.

The PAC version contains the following columns for each PAC resident, reading from left to right:

- Resident identification number;
- Resident name in alphabetical order;
- Columns for the three PAC QM/QIs; and
- A column that counts how many QM/QIs the resident triggered.

NOTE: Resident-specific information in the Resident Level reports must be kept confidential in accordance with the Privacy Act. These reports are only for the use of the State agency, CMS representatives, and the facility.

2. Statements of Deficiencies (CMS-2567) and Statements of Isolated Deficiencies Which Cause No Actual Harm With Only Potential For Minimal Harm (Form A)

   Statements of deficiencies from the previous survey should be reviewed, along with the sample resident identifiers list. Review the specific information under each deficiency and note any special areas of concern. For example, a deficiency was cited for comprehensive care planning last year. Share with the team the specific care planning problems that were listed as the reasons for this deficiency. For resident-centered requirements, determine if any residents identified in the deficiency might be good candidates for the sample. For example, a deficiency was cited for abuse partly based on surveyor observation of a staff member striking a resident who was combative. Identify this resident by name and add the name to the Offsite Preparation Worksheet. During the Initial Tour, evaluate this resident for inclusion in the sample.

3. OSCAR Report 3, History Facility Profile, and OSCAR Report 4, Full Facility Profile from CMS' OSCAR Computer System

   (Refer to Exhibit 96 for sample copies of Reports 3 and 4.) Report 3 contains the compliance history of the facility over the past 4 surveys. Use it to determine if the facility has patterns of repeat deficiencies in particular tags or related tags. This report also lists the dates of any complaint investigations and Federal monitoring surveys during the 4-year time period.

   Report 4 contains information provided by the facility during the previous survey on the Resident Census (Form CMS-672). This report compares facility population characteristics with State, CMS region, and national averages.

4. Results of Complaint Investigations

   Review information from both complaints investigated since the previous standard survey and complaints filed with the survey agency, but not yet investigated. Note resident and staff names related to the complaints and note patterns of problems relating to specific wings or shifts.

5. Information about Waivers or Variances

   If the facility has, or has requested any staffing waiver or room variances, note these for onsite review. The team will determine onsite if these should be granted, continued, or revoked due to a negative effect on resident care or quality of life.

6. Information from the State Ombudsman Office

   Note any potential areas of concern reported by the ombudsman office and note resident names reported as potential sample residents, residents for closed record review, or family members for family interviews and the reasons for their recommendation by the ombudsman.

7. Preadmission Screening and Resident Review Reports (PASRR)

   Some States may have formal mechanisms to share with the survey agency the results of PASRR screens for residents with mental illness or mental retardation. If this information is available, evaluate if there are any potential concerns and note names of residents for possible inclusion in the sample.

8. Other Pertinent Information

   At times, the survey agency may be aware of special potential areas of concern that were reported in the news media or through other sources. Evaluate this information to determine if there are potential areas of concern that should be investigated onsite.

C. Team Coordinator Responsibilities

The team coordinator and/or designee is responsible for completing the following tasks:

1. Contact the ombudsman office in accordance with the policy developed between the State survey agency and State ombudsman agency. The purposes of this contact are to notify the ombudsman of the proposed day of entrance into the facility and to obtain any information the ombudsman wishes to share with the survey team. Ascertain whether the ombudsman will be available if residents participating in the group or individual interviews wish her/him to be present.

2. Obtain all information sources listed in B. above for presentation at the offsite team meeting. (See Section B. for descriptive information about these reports.) They are as follows:

   - Specified QI/QM Reports:

     - Facility Characteristics Report;

     - Facility Quality Measure/Indicator Report; and

     - The two resident level reports:

- Resident Level Quality Measure/Indicator Report: Chronic Care Sample; and
- Resident Level Quality Measure/Indicator Report: Post Acute Care Sample

NOTE: It is important that the QM/QI reports be generated as close to the date of survey as possible, preferably no more than a few days prior to the survey.

- Form CMS-2567 and Statement of Isolated Deficiencies Which Cause No Actual Harm With Only Potential For Minimal Harm;
- Standard OSCAR Report 3 and 4;
- Results of complaint investigations;
- Information about waivers or variances;
- Information from the State Ombudsman office;
- Preadmission Screening and Resident Review Reports; and
- Other pertinent information.

3. Complete the following additional duties:

   - Copy and distribute to the team the facility's floor plan if the team is unfamiliar with the facility's layout;
   - Make extra copies of the OSCAR Reports 3 and 4, and the QM/QI reports to be given to the facility's administrator;
   - Obtain an extra copy of the group interview worksheet (see Form CMS-806B, Exhibit 94) to give to the council president.

D. Offsite Survey Preparation Team Meeting

Present copies of the information obtained to the survey team members for review at a team meeting offsite. The team must prepare for the survey offsite, so that they are ready to begin the Entrance Conference and Initial Tour immediately after they enter the facility. The team should:

1. Review the Facility Characteristics Report to note the facility's demographics. This report can be used to identify whether the facility's population is unusual, e.g., high prevalence of young or male residents, high prevalence of residents

with psychiatric diagnosis, high percentage of significant change assessments, etc.;

2. Use a copy of the Roster/Sample Matrix (Form CMS-802, Exhibit 90) to highlight concerns the team identifies for Phase 1 of the survey, and to list residents pre-selected and the QM/QI conditions for which each was selected. Mark the offsite block on this form to distinguish it from the Phase 1 version that will be completed in Task 4, "Sample Selection;"

   The Facility Quality Measure/Indicator Report divides the QM/QIs into a set for the chronic care residents, followed by three post acute measures, which are based on MDS information for short-stay residents. The three PAC QM/QI items include two that are the same topics as the chronic care residents (13.2, Short-stay residents who had moderate to severe pain, and 13.3, Short-stay residents with pressure ulcers) and one unique item (13.1, Short-stay residents with delirium). Use this report to select concerns based on the following:

   - Any sentinel health event QM/QI that is flagged. For the chronic care sample, a "sentinel health event" is a QM/QI that represents a significant occurrence that should be selected as a concern, even if it applies to only one or a few residents. The sentinel event QM/QIs are 5.4, Prevalence of fecal impaction, 7.3, Prevalence of dehydration, and 12.2, Low-risk residents with pressure ulcers. This means that even if one resident has any of these conditions, this QM/QI will flag and the care area must be selected as a concern and the resident with the problem must be selected for the sample. If there are multiple residents who flag on a sentinel event QM/QI, it is not necessary to select all of them;

   - Any other QM/QI that is flagged at the 90th percentile; and

   - Any unflagged QM/QI in which the facility is at the 75th percentile or greater.

   For the items that are duplicated between the chronic care and PAC residents (pain and pressure ulcers), note whether the area of concern was selected based on only chronic or PAC samples, or both. The survey team may also wish to select as concerns any other QM/QIs that are of interest to them because they are related to QM/QIs that have been selected.

3. Begin selection of potential residents for the Phase 1 survey sample with the chronic care sample residents to represent the concerns that have been selected, including selecting residents who have sentinel event QM/QI conditions; if multiple residents have a sentinel event QM/QI condition, it is not necessary to select all of them. Use Table 1 in this section and the number of the total resident census to determine the sample size for the Phase 1 sample. Pre-select a few more residents (3-5) than the actual number that will be required for Phase 1

sample since some selected residents may no longer be available. Most if not all residents from the PAC sample are likely to have been discharged. The survey team may use this sample of residents from which to select potential closed records for review. (If some PAC residents that triggered a selected QM/QI are still at the facility, the team may select some of these residents in order to investigate issues of concern).

- In any facility in which the team has noted concerns with weight loss, dehydration, and/or pressure sores, select approximately one-half of the pre-selected sample as residents who have one or more of these conditions.

  For the condition of hydration, select a resident who has flagged for the sentinel event QM/QI 7.3 (Prevalence of dehydration) and residents may be selected who have any of the following related QM/QI conditions: 5.4 – Prevalence of fecal impaction; 6.1, - Residents with a urinary tract infection; 7.1 – Residents who lose too much weight; 7.2 – Prevalence of tube feeding; and 9.1 – Residents whose need for help with daily activities has increased. The best residents to select will be those who also have multiple care areas that have been selected as concerns. For any facility in which these concerns were not identified, the team should still select some residents who have these QM/QI conditions, if any, on the Resident Level Quality Measure/Indicator Reports, but this need not be 50% of the Phase 1 sample size.

- For the remaining half of the Phase 1 preliminary sample, select residents to represent the remaining areas of concern.

NOTE: If there are no other QM/QIs that have been selected as concerns, the team may select residents based on other sources of information, e.g., complaints or a report from the ombudsman, or may wait to select the remaining Phase 1 residents based on Initial Tour findings.

If the average length of stay for the facility's population is less than 14 days, there may be little information available. Pre-selection of QM/QI-based concerns and/or the full sample may not be possible. Selection of some or all concerns and residents may need to be totally conducted onsite.

- The survey team should be alert to inconsistencies on the Facility Quality Measure/Indicator Report that may indicate facility error in completing and/or transmitting its Minimum Data Set (MDS) records, or a problem with State's software or CMS' database. The following are some possible indicators of data quality problems:

  - The denominator for QM/QIs that use "all residents" substantially exceeds or is substantially smaller than the facility bed size;

- o The number of residents with a QM/QI condition, i.e., the numerator, exceeds the resident population; or,

- o The numerator for a particular QM/QI is zero although other information sources indicate otherwise. For example, the QM/QI report shows zero residents in restraints, but the ombudsman notified the team that she/he verified complaints about restraints. The most common reason for this type of inconsistency is incorrect MDS coding by the facility.

If these or other potential accuracy concerns are noted, the team should add resident assessment accuracy as a concern for the survey.

NOTE: This review need not be done for "short-stay" facilities, which will often have unusual values in the numerator and denominator due to rapid turnover of residents.

The Facility Quality Measure/Indicator Report is generated using the current MDS records in the State database at the time the report was generated. However, it excludes residents who have only an initial MDS record in the system. This was done so that the report reflects the care residents have received while residing in the facility, as opposed to the conditions of residents at the time of admission to the facility. The Resident Level reports are calculated using the most recently transmitted MDS record, e.g., annual, significant change, quarterly, or initial MDS record. Differences could be seen between the Facility Quality Measure/Indicator Report and the Resident Level reports since the former does not use the admission MDS data. For example, a Resident Level report may indicate a resident had a catheter but the Facility Quality Measure/Indicator Report might show a "0." This is not an accuracy problem, it only reflects the use of different data to generate each report.

4. Review the OSCAR reports after the review of the QM/QI reports to add corroborative information to the QM/QI information, e.g., a pattern of repeat deficiencies in a requirement related to a flagged QM/QI, and/or to point out areas of large discrepancies between the QM/QI numerators and the OSCAR Reports, e.g., the OSCAR 4 report lists the facility as having triple the average number of residents in restraints, but the QM/QI for restraints shows the facility has less restraints than most facilities). The team coordinator may wish to discuss such discrepancies with the administrator on entrance to determine the reason for them.

   Relate information between Reports 3 and 4 such as a pattern of repeat deficiencies in range of motion and a lower than average percentage of residents receiving rehabilitative services. Also, note any special resident characteristics not contained in the QM/QI reports.

NOTE: Both the OSCAR reports and the QM/QI reports can alert surveyors to the acuity and characteristics of the facility's residents at the time the information for these reports was determined. This information may not represent the current condition of residents in the facility at the time of the survey. Keep in mind that the OSCAR information is approximately 1 year old, and the QM/QI information may be from 2-6 months old. Resident characteristics that were reported by the facility during the last survey may have changed significantly and may be the source of some discrepancies between OSCAR and QM/QI information.

5. Review all other sources of information and record additional information on the Offsite Preparation Worksheet (Form CMS-801, Exhibit 89), for example, residents' names for possible inclusion in the Phase 2 sample based on non-QM/QI sources of information (B. 2 through 8 above), special features of the facility, or special resident populations. Identify any outstanding complaints needing investigation. At this meeting, establish preliminary surveyor assignments and projections of which days team members will enter early and/or stay late to make observations of resident care and quality of life.

Task 2 - Entrance Conference/Onsite Preparatory Activities

(Rev. 26; Issued: 08-17-07; Effective/Implementation Dates: 08-17-07)

A. Entrance Conference

1. The team coordinator informs the facility's administrator about the survey and introduces team members.

2. After the introduction to the administrator, the other team members should proceed to the initial tour (Task 3), while the team coordinator conducts the entrance conference.

3. The team coordinator should:

   - Request a copy of the actual working schedules for licensed and registered nursing staff for this time period by the end of the tour or earlier if possible.

   - Inform facility staff that the survey team will be communicating with them throughout the survey and will ask for facility assistance when needed. (See §2713.A for further information about facility staff accompanying surveyors.) Advise them that they have the opportunity to provide the team with any information that would clarify an issue brought to their attention.

   - Explain the survey process and answer any questions from facility staff.

   - Give the Administrator copies of the QM/QI reports and the OSCAR 3 and 4 reports that are being used for the survey. Briefly explain these reports and how they were used by the survey team in Task 1. If there are discrepancies between the OSCAR information and the QM/QI Facility Characteristics report, ask the administrator, or person designated by the administrator, to explain the discrepancies.

- Ask the administrator to describe any special features of the facility's care and treatment programs, organization, and resident case-mix. For example, does the facility have a special care unit for residents with dementia? Are residents with heavy care needs placed in particular units? If so, which ones?

- *Ask the administrator if the facility utilizes paid feeding assistants. If yes, request further information about how and where the paid feeding assistants receive their training. Determine whether the training for the paid feeding assistant was provided through a State-approved training program by qualified professionals as defined by State law, with a minimum of 8 hours of training.*

- *Request the names of staff (including agency staff) who have successfully completed training for paid feeding assistants, and who are currently assisting selected residents with eating meals and/or snacks;*

  NOTE: *Paid feeding assistants must work under the supervision of a registered nurse (RN) or licensed practical nurse (LPN). Therefore, if a facility has a nursing waiver, that facility cannot use paid feeding assistants when a licensed nurse is not available.*

- Inform the administrator that there will be interviews with individual residents, groups of residents, family members, friends, and legal representatives, and that these interviews are conducted privately, unless the interviewees request the presence of a staff member. Ask the administrator to ensure that there are times during the survey when residents can contact the survey team without facility staff present and without having to ask facility staff to leave or to allow access to the team.

- Determine through interview with the administrator if the facility has a functioning QA&A committee. Determine:

  - Which staff participate on the committee;

  - Who leads the committee;

  - How often the committee meets; and

  - With whom should the survey team discuss QA&A concerns.

- Ask the administrator to provide the following information within 1 hour of the conclusion of the entrance conference (or later at the survey team's option):

    1. List of key facility personnel and their locations, e.g., the Administrator; directors of finance, nursing services, social services, and activities; dietitian or food supervisor; rehabilitation services staff; charge nurses; pharmacy consultant; plant engineer; housekeeping supervisor; persons responsible for infection control and quality assurance; health information management professional; and the medical director;

    2. A copy of the written information that is provided to residents regarding their rights;

    3. Meal times, dining locations, copies of all menus, including therapeutic menus that will be served for the duration of the survey;

    4. Medication pass times (by unit, if variable);

    5. List of admissions during the past month, and a list of residents transferred or discharged during the past 3 months with destinations;

    6. A copy of the facility's layout, indicating the location of nurses' stations, individual resident rooms, and common areas, if not obtained in Task 1;

    7. A copy of the facility admission contract(s) for all residents, i.e., Medicare, Medicaid, other payment sources;

    8. Facility policies and procedures to prohibit and investigate allegations of abuse and the name of a person the administrator designates to answer questions about what the facility does to prevent abuse. (See Task 5G, Abuse Prohibition Review, for further information);

    9. Evidence that the facility, on a routine basis, monitors accidents and other incidents, records these in the clinical or other record; and has in place a system to prevent and/or minimize further accidents and incidents;

        NOTE: At the discretion of the facility, this evidence could include or be a record of accident and incident reports.

    10. The names of any residents age 55 and under; and

11. The names of any residents who communicate with non-oral communication devices, sign language, or who speak a language other than the dominant language of the facility.

- Ask the facility to complete, to the best of their ability, the Roster/Sample Matrix (Form CMS-802), including all residents on bed-hold, by the end of the initial tour, or to provide this information in some other format, e.g., computer-generated list.

NOTE: This is an important source of resident information, which is crucial for the team to have for their sample selection meetings. Stress to the facility that this form should be completed first and given to the team coordinator by the end of the initial tour. After the Roster/Sample Matrix is delivered to the team, the facility may make modifications for accuracy or add additional information within 24 hours.

- Ask the facility to provide the following within 24 hours of the Entrance Conference:

1. A completed Long Term Care Facility Application for Medicare and Medicaid (Form CMS-671), (see Exhibit 85) and a Resident Census and Conditions of Residents (Form CMS-672), (See Exhibit 86); and

2. A list of Medicare residents who requested demand bills in the last 6 months (SNFs or dually-participating SNF/NFs only).

- Also, ask the administrator the following questions:

1. Which, if any, rooms have less square footage than required? Do you have a variance in effect and are you prepared to continue to request a variance for any such rooms? (F458)

2. Which, if any, rooms are occupied by more than four residents? Do you have a variance in effect and are you prepared to continue to request a variance for any such rooms? (F457)

3. Is there at least one window to the outside in each room? (F461)

4. Which, if any, bedrooms are not at or above ground level? (F461)

5. Do all bedrooms have access to an exit corridor? (F459)

6. What are the procedures to ensure water is available to essential areas when there is a loss of normal supply? (F466)

NOTE: If the survey is commencing at times beyond the business hours of 8:00 a.m. to 6:00 p.m., or on a Saturday or Sunday, once onsite, announce the survey, ascertain who is in charge, ask the person to notify the administrator that a survey has begun. Modify the entrance conference in accordance with staff available and complete the task and the onsite preparatory activity as appropriate within the context of the survey.

4. For any survey conducted outside of the influenza season (October 1-March 31), obtain the name of the staff person who is responsible for coordinating and implementing the facility's immunization program to request a list of current residents who were in the facility during the previous influenza season, October 1 to March 31.

B. Onsite Preparatory Activities

1. In areas easily observable by residents and visitors, post, or ask the facility to post, signs announcing that a survey is being performed and that surveyors are available to meet with residents in private.

2. The team coordinator or designee should contact the resident council president after the Entrance Conference to introduce her/himself and to announce the survey. Provide the president with a copy of the group interview questions. Request the assistance of the president for arranging the group interview and to solicit any comments or concerns. Ask the council president for permission to review council minutes for the past 3 months (see Task 5D, Section 3B, for further information). If there is not an active resident council, or if the council does not have officers, ask for a list of residents who attend group meetings, if any, and select a resident representative to assist in arranging the group interview. If the ombudsman has indicated interest in attending the group interview, ask the president if that is acceptable to the group; if it is, notify the ombudsman of the time/place of the meeting.

3. The team coordinator, the surveyor assigned to conduct the group interview, or a designee should arrange for date, time and private meeting space for the interview. Advise the facility staff that non-interviewable residents are not part of this meeting. (See Task 5D for further guidance.)

Task 3 - Initial Tour

A. General Objectives

The Initial Tour is designed to:

- Provide an initial review of the facility, the residents, and the staff;

- Obtain an initial evaluation of the environment of the facility, including the facility kitchen; and
- Confirm or invalidate the pre-selected concerns, if any, and add concerns discovered onsite.

B. General Procedures

The initial tour is used to gather information about concerns which have been pre-selected; new concerns discovered onsite; and whether residents pre-selected for the Phase 1 sample offsite are still present in the facility. In addition, attempt to meet and talk with as many residents as possible during the tour in order to identify other candidates for the sample, to get an initial overview of facility care and services, to observe staff/resident interactions; and to evaluate the impact of the facility environment on the residents. The tour also includes a first brief look at the facility's kitchen.

Document tour information, on either the Roster/Sample Matrix (Form CMS-802 or the Surveyor Notes Worksheet (Form CMS-807). Document any concerns regarding the general environment on the General Observations of the Facility Worksheet, (Form CMS-803) or Surveyor Notes Worksheets, (Form CMS-807). (See Task 5A for further information.) Surveyors may also document notes on the facility's Roster/Sample Matrix or other list of residents provided by the facility. Document any concerns noted in the brief tour of the facility kitchen on the Kitchen/Food Service Observation worksheet (Form CMS-804, Exhibit 92). (See Task 5B for information regarding observations to make during this brief tour.)

C. Protocol

Surveyors should tour individually as assigned by the team coordinator. It is desirable for team members to have a facility staff person who is familiar with the residents accompany them during the tour to answer questions and provide introductions to residents or family. However, do not delay the beginning of the Initial Tour if facility staff are not available. Begin the tour as soon as possible after entering the facility.

NOTE: When standard surveys begin at times beyond the business hours of 8:00 a.m. to 6:00 p.m., or begin on a Saturday or Sunday, the initial tour will need to be modified in recognition of the residents' activity, e.g., sleep, religious services, and types and numbers of staff available upon entry. The tour may focus on specific care and quality of life issues, e.g., restraint use, meal service, use of foam or paper meal service products rather than regular dinnerware, adherence to the planned menu; sufficiency of staff; whether enteral/parenteral fluids are being administered as ordered; whether incontinent residents are being checked, toileted, changed; etc., as appropriate. The tour should not be delayed for lack of staff to accompany the surveyor and/or survey team.

Phase 1-- Pre-selected Concerns and Potential Residents:

During the tour, determine whether each resident pre-selected offsite for the Phase 1 sample is still there. Determine which, if any, of the pre-selected Phase 1 sample residents are interviewable residents who can be selected to participate in a Quality of Life Assessment Resident Interview or Group Interview. (See Task 5D.) This can be accomplished by talking with residents and asking questions. Examples of questions that can be asked are: What is your name? What are you planning to do today?

NOTE: Do not rely solely on the information that the facility provides concerning which residents are interviewable. The survey team should determine the residents who are able to participate in a Quality of Life Assessment interview.

If possible, determine if there are family members of non-interviewable residents in the pre-selected Phase 1 sample who can be selected for a Quality of Life Assessment family interview. Also note other non-interviewable residents among the facility population whose family members could be selected for interviews;

Observations of All Residents During the Tour

Ask staff to identify those residents who have no family or significant others. The team may include one or more of these residents in the Phase 2 sample for investigation of quality of life issues.

Have staff identify newly admitted residents, i.e., who have been admitted within the past 14 days, for possible inclusion in the sample for investigation of decline or deterioration that may have occurred before all MDS, other resident assessment information, and care planning is completed.

Have staff identify any residents for whom transfer or discharge is planned within the next 30 days.

Note residents who are interviewable or who have special factors, as listed in Task 4. When on the Initial Tour, observe and document possible quality of care and quality of life concerns in addition to those pre-selected offsite. If observed concerns involve specific residents, note the resident's name and room number on the worksheet, and the date/time when describing the observed concern. Include the details of the observation in documentation, including any effects on the residents involved.

Conduct a brief initial observation of the kitchen. (See Task 5B for further information).

While on tour, identify the licensed and registered nursing staff who are currently on duty. At the end of the tour, compare the observed staff with the duty roster the facility is to provide. If there are discrepancies between the duty roster and the staff observed onsite, ask the person in charge to explain the discrepancies. This information will be used in Task 6 to determine if the facility is compliant with the requirements for licensed and registered nursing staff at 42 CFR 483.30(a)(2), F353 and 42 CFR 483.30(b)(1), F354.

During the tour focus on the following:

- Quality of Life

    1. Resident grooming and dress, including appropriate footwear;

    2. Staff - resident interaction related to residents' dignity; privacy and care needs, including staff availability and responsiveness to residents' requests for assistance;

    3. The way staff talk to residents, the nature and manner of interactions, and whether residents are spoken to when care is given; and

    4. Scheduled activities taking place and appropriateness to the residents.

- Emotional and behavioral conduct of the residents and the reactions and interventions by the staff:

    1. Resident behaviors such as crying out, disrobing, agitation, rocking, pacing; and

    2. The manner in which these behaviors are being addressed by staff, including nature and manner of staff interactions, response time, staff availability, and staff means of dealing with residents who are experiencing catastrophic reactions. (See "Abuse Prohibition Investigative Protocol" in Task 5G for a definition of catastrophic reaction.)

- Care issues, how care is provided, and prevalence of special care needs

    1. Skin conditions, e.g., excessive dryness, wetness;

    2. Skin tears, bruising, or evidence of fractures that warrant investigation;

    3. Dehydration risk factors including availability of water for most residents, and other indicators or factors, e.g., the amount and color of urine in tubing and collection bags, dependence on staff, the presence of strong urinary odors, and resident complaints of dry mouth and lips;

    4. Clinical signs such as edema, emaciation and contractures;

    5. Functional risk factors such as poor positioning and use of physical restraints;

6. Side effects of antipsychotic drug use such as tardive dyskinesia, e.g., lip, tongue or other involuntary abnormal movements;

7. Presence or prevalence (numbers) of infections including antibiotic resistant strains of bacteria (e.g., Methicillin Resistant Staphylococcus Aureus (MRSA), Vancomycin Resistant Enterococcus (VRE), Clostridium Difficile (C-Diff) or other infections: Urinary tract infections, draining wounds, eye infections, skin rashes (especially if spreading, undiagnosed, and/or not responding to treatment), respiratory infections, gastroenteritis including diarrhea, etc.

8. Pressure sores, old scars from pressure sores or evidence of surgical repair of pressure sores;

9. Amputation;

10. Significant weight loss;

11. Feeding tubes and/or improper positioning while feeding is infusing; and

12. Ventilators, oxygen, or intravenous therapies.

- Impact of the facility environment and safety issues:

1. Infection control practices, e.g., handwashing, glove use, and isolation procedures);

2. Functional and clean equipment, including kitchen equipment;

3. Presentation and maintenance of a homelike and clean environment; and

4. Availability, use, and maintenance of assistive devices.

NOTE: If the initial tour is being conducted during a mealtime, include an initial brief observation of the dining areas. Note if there are any concerns with meal service, quality of life, positioning, sufficient space, etc.

Task 4 - Sample Selection

A. General Objective

The objective of this task is to select a case-mix stratified sample (see Special Factors to Consider in Sample Selection below for further information) of facility residents based on QM/QIs and other offsite and onsite sources of information in order to assess compliance with the resident-centered long term care requirements.

B. General Procedures

- The Phase 1 sample is pre-selected during Task 1, "Offsite Survey Preparation," based on QM/QIs and other areas of concern. The pre-selected sample is reviewed during the sample selection meeting and residents are retained for the sample unless they are discharged, or the survey team has another reason to substitute, e.g., to select interviewable residents. Each team member is assigned a certain number of residents, completing all facets of review that have been selected including any quality of life assessment protocols selected for these residents.

- The Phase 2 sample is selected onsite, part way through the survey when surveyors have collected enough information to determine the focus of the remainder of the survey. The Phase 2 sample residents are selected to represent new concerns and/or to continue further investigation of Phase 1 concerns when Phase 1 reviews proved inconclusive or when necessary to determine scope of a problem. It is statutorily required that the sample in each facility be case-mix stratified in order to capture both interviewable and non-interviewable residents as well as residents from both heavy and light care categories.

NOTE: If the team is conducting sample selection during meal time, delay or interrupt this task to conduct brief observations of the dining areas. Note if there are any concerns with meal service, quality of life, positioning, sufficient space, etc.

C. Definitions

- Interviewable Resident --This is a resident who has sufficient memory and comprehension to be able to answer coherently the majority of questions contained in the Resident Interview. These residents can make day-to-day decisions in a fairly consistent and organized manner.

- Comprehensive Review -- For Task 5C, "Resident Review," this includes observations, interviews, and record reviews for all care areas for the sampled residents, as applicable.

- Focused Review -- For Task 5C, "Resident Review," this includes the following:

  - For Phase 1: Observations, interviews and record reviews concerning all highlighted areas of concern and all unhighlighted areas pertinent to the resident; and

  - For Phase 2: Observations, interviews and record review for all highlighted areas of concern pertinent to the resident.

- Closed Record Review -- For Task 5C, "Resident Review," this includes a record review of residents' care issues and transfer and discharge.

- Roster/Sample Matrix -- This worksheet, (Exhibit 265, Form CMS-802), is used by the survey team during Offsite Survey Preparation, and at the Phase 1 and Phase 2 Sample Selection meetings to note areas of concern for the survey, and to select residents for the sample. There are separate sets of instructions for the use of this form by the survey team and the facility. (See these instructions at Exhibits 266 and 267.

D. Protocol

1. Phase 1 - Sample Selection

The Phase 1 sample is pre-selected during Task 1, Offsite Survey Preparation, based on the facility's QM/QIs of concern. (See Task 1 for further information.) Final Phase 1 sample selection occurs after the tour is completed and the facility has provided the completed Roster/Sample Matrix (Form CMS-802, Exhibit 265), or provided this information in some other format, e.g., computer-generated list. However, do not delay Phase 1 sample selection if the facility's Roster/Sample Matrix has not arrived. The team will complete the sample selection for Phase 1 by performing the following tasks:

NOTE: For facilities with a population of "short-stay" residents, the team may not have been able to pre-select concerns or potential sampled residents. In that instance, Phase 1 sample selection will occur during this task.

- First determine if any pre-selected concerns should be dropped due to the QM/QI data not representing the conditions of current residents. For example, there was a pre-selected QM/QI concern with residents with tube feedings, but the tour has verified there are no residents in the facility who are receiving tube feedings. Note new concerns and determine if some pre-selected residents can be evaluated for the new concerns as well as those originally selected.

- Review the Roster/Sample Matrix provided by the facility and compare it to the findings from the tour to determine if there is a reason to substitute another resident for any of the residents from the Offsite sample. A pre-selected resident who is no longer in the facility can be considered for the closed record review. The team may substitute other residents for those pre-selected, if necessary. They can select either from the QM/QI reports, the tour, or the facility's Roster/Sample Matrix.

If any resident is substituted for a pre-selected resident, record a short explanation on the Offsite Roster/Sample Matrix next to that person's name, e.g., "discharged."

- Check "Phase 1" on the copy of the Roster/Sample Matrix that will be used to denote the resident sample for Phase 1 of the survey.
    - Highlight the column for each identified concern for Phase 1.

- Use Table 1 in this section and the number of the total resident census to determine the number of comprehensive and focused reviews, number of closed records, number of resident and family interviews, and the minimum number of residents who have conditions of weight loss, hydration risk and/or pressure sores, i.e., the WHP group. The number in the WHP column represents the minimum total of residents who must be selected for the Phase 1 sample to represent any or all of these conditions. For example, in a facility with 96 residents, out of 12 residents selected for the Phase 1 sample, a minimum of 6 will be those who have any of the conditions mentioned above, if any of these 3 QM/QIs were selected as concerns.

- Use the unnumbered blocks to the right of Resident Name to fill in the total number of residents in each sub-sample for the entire survey as listed in Table 1. For example, in a facility with a census of 100, the total number of individual interviews is 5. Enter that number in the small block below that title.

- All residents selected for comprehensive reviews are selected by the team during the Phase 1 sample selection. Residents selected for focused reviews, closed record reviews, individual and family interviews may be selected during Phase 1 or Phase 2 sample selection.

- Each resident the team selects is entered on the worksheet. Note the following about each resident:

    - Resident number and room number;

    - Surveyor assigned to complete the resident review and any quality of life assessment protocols (Resident Interview or Family Interview) that are selected for the resident;

    - Check any columns that pertain to this resident, whether or not they are highlighted as concerns for Phase 1. Each resident will be reviewed for each checked area, not just those that are highlighted; and

    - If there is anything about this resident that the team decides to investigate that is not one of the numbered columns on the worksheet, use a blank column at the far right to write the item that will be assessed and check that column for that resident. For example, if the team wants to assess ventilator use for a particular resident, write "ventilator" in one of the blank columns and make a check mark in that column for that resident.

2. Phase 2 Sample Selection

Part way through the survey, after the team has obtained enough information to decide what concerns need further investigation, the team meets to determine the areas of concern, if any, for Phase 2 of the survey and to select the remaining sample. It is not necessary to complete all the reviews of all residents in Phase 1 before this meeting. Determine which Phase 1 concerns are ruled out as these do not need to be carried over into Phase 2 sample selection.

- Select concerns for Phase 2 based on the following:
    - Initial concerns noted during Offsite Survey Preparation or the Initial Tour that have not yet been reviewed;
    - Currently un-reviewed concerns that are related to those under investigation, e.g., adding residents who have had falls based on results of the Phase 1 discovery of a problem with use of psychoactive drugs; and
    - Current concerns for which the information gathered is inconclusive.
- Select residents for the Phase 2 sample based on the following:
    - The statute requires selection of a "case mix stratified" sample (but not for each phase of the sample selection, just for the total sample). This stratification is defined by CMS as including residents who are interviewable and non-interviewable, and as including residents who require heavy and light care. It is important that at least one resident in the sample represent each of these categories. The requirements of the sample selection procedures make it necessary for survey teams to select interviewable and non-interviewable residents in order to complete the Task 5D, Quality of Life Assessment Interviews, so those categories of case-mix stratification will be automatically filled by complying with the sample selection procedures. At the beginning of the Phase 2 sample selection meeting, the team should review the Phase 1 sample to determine if at least one heavy care and one light care resident has been selected to fulfill this portion of the case mix stratification requirement. If not, it is a priority to ensure that if either heavy or light care residents are missing from the Phase 1 sample, that at least one is selected from the missing category in Phase 2.
    - Select residents who represent one or more of the areas of concern the team has selected for Phase 2 of the survey.
    - If no residents have been selected for the Phase 1 sample for hydration, and if any residents are seen during Phase 1 of the survey who appear to have risk factors for dehydration, e.g., such as residents who are

dependent on staff for activities of daily living, are immobile, receive tube feedings, or have dementias in which the resident no longer recognizes thirst, select at least one of these residents at risk and review the care area of dehydration.

- During Phase 2 sample selection, a clean copy of the Sample/Matrix worksheet is used as follows:

    - Check "Phase 2" on the copy of the Roster/Sample Matrix that will be used to denote the resident sample for Phase 2 of the survey;

    - Highlight the column for each identified concern for Phase 2;

    - Each resident the team selects is entered on the worksheet. Note the following about each resident:

        - Resident number and room number;

        - Surveyor assigned to complete the resident review and any quality of life assessment protocols (Resident Interview, or Family Interview) that are selected for the resident;

        - Checkmarks are made only in the highlighted columns and these residents will be reviewed for these concerns, and any other concerns that are discovered during this review;

        - Be sure that residents are selected to complete the required number of resident interviews, family interviews, and closed record reviews.

- If there are no outstanding areas of concern and the team has already selected interviewable, non-interviewable, heavy care and light care residents, then select remaining residents to represent any of the following, in no particular order:

    - An area of concern on the worksheet that has not been highlighted, but which the team has determined should be assessed;

    - Living units that are unrepresented; and

    - Special factors below that have not been reviewed.

NOTE: When selecting the sample in a facility in which there are no outstanding areas of concern, each resident will be reviewed for at least one area on the Roster/Sample Matrix that has not yet been reviewed.

3. Special Factors to Consider in Sample Selection

Residents must be selected for both the Phase 1 and Phase 2 samples as representatives of concerns to be investigated and to fulfill the case mix stratified sample requirement. If during sample selection, many more residents are identified than can be selected to represent the concerns of interest, consider the factors below in determining which residents to select:

- New admissions, especially if admitted during the previous 14 days. Even though the Resident Assessment Instrument (RAI) is not required to be completed for these residents, the facility must plan care from the first day of each resident's admission;

- Residents most at risk of neglect and abuse, i.e., residents who have dementia; no or infrequent visitors, psychosocial, interactive, and/or behavioral dysfunction; or residents who are bedfast and totally dependent on care;

- Residents in rooms in which variances have been granted for room size or number of beds in room;

- Residents receiving hospice services;

- Residents with end-stage renal disease;

- Residents under the age of 55;

- Residents with mental illness or mental retardation; and

- Residents who communicate with non-oral communication devices, sign language, or who speak a language other than the dominant language of the facility.

4. Other Phase 2 Tasks

- If there are any concerns about residents' funds, check that the amount of the surety bond is at least equal to the amount of residents' funds the facility is managing as of the most recent quarter.

- If concerns have been identified in the area of infection control, review policies and procedures including a focus on what preventative infection control practices the facility has in place. For example, does the facility administer the influenza vaccine yearly to its residents, and administer pneumococcal vaccine to new residents as appropriate (does facility evaluate whether new residents have received the pneumococcal vaccine within the last 5 years)?

- Complete Task 5F Quality Assessment Assurance Review.

- If the group interview has not yet occurred, discuss what special concerns to ask of the group.

- If the facility has or has requested a nurse staffing waiver, review the requirements at 42 CFR 483.30.

- Review the Resident Census and Condition of Residents (Form CMS-672) that the facility has completed. Note any new areas of concern and determine if there appears to be large discrepancies between what is recorded by the facility and what the team has observed. For example, the team has noted 13 residents with pressure sores and the facility has listed 3. If there are large discrepancies, ask the facility to verify their totals. Answer questions F146 - F148 on the Resident Census.

- If the team has identified quality of care problems during Phase 1 of the survey, use the investigative protocol at Task 5C: Nursing Services, Sufficient Staffing to gather information and (at Task 6) to determine compliance with the following requirement: 42 CFR 483.30(a), F353 Nursing services, Sufficient Staff. If problems with staffing have been discovered early in Phase 1, this protocol can begin in Phase 1.

5. Substituting Residents

If the team has found it necessary during the survey to remove a resident from the sample, e.g., a resident refused to complete the interview, replace this resident with another who best fulfills the reasons the first person was selected. For example, the resident who was removed had been selected because he/she was in restraints and had a pressure sore. Attempt to select another resident who meets both of these criteria. In Phase 1, the substituted resident should be selected from the pre-selected list of residents which was determined offsite, if possible, or from other information gained during the survey. Make the substitution as early in the survey as feasible. Note on the Roster/Sample Matrix that the new resident was substituted for resident #___, and briefly give the reason the first resident was dropped.

6. Supplementary Sample

If sampled residents are found not to provide enough information to make deficiency determinations concerning specific requirements under review, or to determine if there is "substandard quality of care" (see Task 6 for further information), supplement the sample with residents who represent the areas of concern under investigation. Focus review for these residents only on the concern under investigation and any other concerns that are discovered during this review. Add the names of these residents to the Phase 2 Sample Matrix worksheet, checking the relevant categories. Use the Resident Review Worksheet to complete these investigations.

Table 1 - Survey Procedures for Long Term Care Facilities - Resident Sample Selection

Survey Procedures for Long Term Care Facilities
Resident Sample Selection

Resident Census	Phase 1/ Phase 2	Compre-hensive Reviews *	Focused Reviews *	Closed Rec. Reviews *	Res./ Family Interviews	W, H, P Group **
1 - 4	All / 0	2	2	0	1/1	All
5 - 10	3 / 2	2	2	1	1 / 1	2
11 - 20	5 / 3	2	5	1	2 / 2	3
21 - 40	6 / 4	2	7	1	3 / 2	3
41 - 44	7 / 4	2	8	1	3 / 2	4
45 - 48	7 / 5	2	9	1	3 / 2	4
49 - 52	8 / 5	3	9	1	4 / 2	4
53 - 56	8 / 6	3	9	2	4 / 2	4
57 - 75	9 / 6	4	9	2	4 / 2	5
76 / 80	10 / 6	4	9	3	4 / 2	5
81 - 85	10 / 7	4	10	3	4 / 2	5
86 - 90	11 / 7	4	11	3	4 / 2	6
91 - 95	11 / 8	4	12	3	4 / 2	6
96 - 100	12 / 8	5	12	3	5 / 2	6
101 - 105	13 / 8	5	13	3	5 / 2	7
106 - 110	13 / 9	5	14	3	5 / 2	7
111 - 115	14 / 9	5	15	3	5 / 2	7
116 - 160	14 / 10	5	16	3	5 / 2	7
161 - 166	15 / 10	5	17	3	5 / 2	8
167 - 173	16 / 10	5	18	3	5 / 2	8
174 - 180	16 / 11	5	19	3	5 / 2	8
181 - 186	17 / 11	5	20	3	5 / 2	9
187 - 193	17 / 12	5	21	3	5 / 2	9
194 - 299	18 / 12	5	22	3	5 / 2	9
300 - 400	18 / 12	5	22	3	6 / 3	9
401 -	18 / 12	5	22	3	7 / 3	9

* Comprehensive reviews plus focused reviews plus closed record reviews added together equals the total sample size (Phase 1 plus Phase 2).

** For any survey in which there are identified concerns in the areas of (W) unintended weight loss, (H) hydration, and/or (P) pressure sores, this is the minimum total of residents who must be selected for the Phase 1 sample to represent any or all of these conditions.

Task 5 - Information Gathering

(Rev. 22, Issued: 12-15-06, Effective/Implementation: 12-18-06)

Task 5 provides an organized, systematic, and consistent method of gathering information necessary to make decisions concerning whether the facility has met the requirements reviewed during the Standard Survey.

Task 5 includes the following sub-tasks:

5A General Observations of the Facility: Assessment of the environment of the facility affecting the resident's life, health and safety;

5B Kitchen/Food Service Observations: Assessment of the facility's food storage, preparation and service;

5C Resident Review: An integrated, holistic assessment of the sampled residents which includes the assessment of: drug therapies, the quality of life of the resident as affected by his/her room environment and daily interactions with staff, and assessment of those pertinent care concerns identified for each sampled resident by the survey team. Closed record reviews and dining observations are integrated into the resident review;

5D Quality of Life Assessment: Assessment of residents' quality of life through individual interviews, a group interview, family interviews, and observations of residents who are non-interviewable;

5E Medication Pass and Pharmacy Services: An assessment of the pharmaceutical services provided in the facility, including the provision of the medication pass observation; the application of the medication error detection methodology; the provision of services by a licensed pharmacist; and facility procedures and processes in place regarding the acquiring, receiving, dispensing and administering medications, use of controlled medications, and medication access and storage.

5F Quality Assessment and Assurance Review: An assessment of the facility's Quality Assessment and Assurance program to determine if the facility identifies and addresses specific care and quality issues and implements a program to resolve those issues; and

5G Abuse Prohibition Review: A determination of whether the facility has developed and operationalized policies and procedures designed to protect residents from abuse, neglect, involuntary seclusion, and misappropriation of their property. This includes policies and procedures for hiring practices, training and ongoing supervision for employees and volunteers who provide services, and the reporting and investigation of allegations and occurrences that may indicate abuse.

Use survey worksheets and Guidance to Surveyors, also known as the Interpretive Guidelines, for each of the sub-tasks and requirements reviewed in Task 5. While these sub-tasks are discrete information gathering activities, there are a number of things to take into consideration during Task 5.

A. General Procedures

As appropriate, use the interpretations, definitions, probes, and procedures provided in the Guidance to Surveyors to guide the investigation and to help determine whether, based on the investigation and findings, the facility has met the requirements.

Worksheet documentation should be resident-centered, as appropriate. For example, if the lack of a reading light near the resident's bedroom chair is being documented, also note that this resident has said he/she prefers to read in his/her chair, and that the light over the chair is inadequate.

Relate to the requirements and provide clear evidence, as appropriate, of the facility's failure to meet a requirement. As information is collected, keep in mind that the information written on the worksheet will be used by the team to determine if there are any deficiencies, and, if so, the degree of severity and scope. Make documentation specific enough so that these decisions can be made. Include information about how the faulty facility practice affected residents, the number of residents affected, and the number of residents at risk. This documentation will be used both to make deficiency determinations and to categorize deficiencies for severity and scope. The Guidance to Surveyors assists in gathering information in order to determine whether the facility has met the requirements. For example, the facility has care plan objectives which are measurable. If the resident does not meet her/his goals, does the documentation reflect how the lack of implementation of the care plan and/or lack of quarterly assessments prevents the resident from reaching her/his goals?

In conducting the survey, use the worksheets in conjunction with the survey procedures and Guidance to Surveyors. When investigating a concern, note the tag number listed on the worksheet for that requirement and use the Guidance to Surveyors for that tag to direct the investigation.

Devote as much time as possible during the survey to performing observations and conducting formal and informal interviews. Limit record reviews to obtaining specific information, i.e., look at what is needed, not the whole record.

The information gathering tasks are interrelated. Information acquired while doing observations and interviews will direct the record review. Likewise, information obtained while doing the record review may help direct what observations or interviews are needed. Acquire the information that is necessary to make deficiency decisions in Task 6 using the survey worksheets and corresponding Guidance to Surveyors for each of the sub-tasks in Task 5.

Regardless of the task, be alert at all times to the surrounding care environment and activities. For example, while conducting the dining observations of sampled residents and the medication pass observation, observe the environment and residents, e.g., care being given, staff interactions with residents, and infection control practices.

The team should meet on a daily basis to share information, e.g., findings to date, areas of concern, any changes needed in the focus of the survey. These meetings include discussions of concerns observed, possible requirements to which those problems relate, and strategies for gathering additional information to determine whether the facility is meeting the requirements.

Throughout the survey, discuss observations, as appropriate, with team members, facility staff, residents, family members, and the ombudsman. Maintain an open and ongoing dialogue with the facility throughout the survey process. This gives the facility the opportunity to provide additional information in considering any alternative explanations before making deficiency decisions. This, however, does not mean that every negative observation is reported on a daily basis, e.g., at a nightly conference. Moreover, if the negative observation relates to a routine that needs to be monitored over time to determine whether a deficiency exists, wait until a trend has been established before notifying the facility of the problem. If it has been verified through observation and record review that a resident's condition has declined, start the investigation to determine if this decline was avoidable or unavoidable by asking a knowledgeable facility staff member, such as the nurse or other professional staff member charged with responsibility for the resident's care, to provide documentation in the resident's chart that provides the reasons for why they believe this decline occurred. Use this information to guide the investigation, but use professional judgment and team approach to determine if a deficient practice has occurred.

In conducting the tasks of the Standard Survey, situations may be identified to indicate that the facility may not be meeting a requirement not routinely reviewed in the Standard Survey.

Investigate this further. For example, residents at the council meeting say that they have not had a visit from a physician (or extender) for several months. This would lead to an investigation of facility compliance with the requirements for frequency of physician visits.

Verify information and observations in terms of credibility and reliability. If the credibility or reliability of information is doubted, validate that information or gather additional information before using it to make a compliance decision.

B. Observations

The objectives of the observational portion of information gathering are to gather resident-specific information for the residents included in the sample, and also, to be alert to the provision of care, staff-resident interactions, and quality of life for all residents.

C. Informal and Formal Interviews

The objectives of interviews are to:

- Collect information;
- Verify and validate information obtained from other survey procedures; and
- Provide the opportunity for all interested parties to provide what they believe is pertinent information.

Interview residents, staff, family, ombudsman, family council representatives, and other appropriate persons. Informal interviews are conducted throughout the duration of the information gathering tasks of the survey. Formal structured interviews are also done as part of the Quality of Life Assessment protocols. Use the information obtained from interviews to assist in deciding what additional observations and record review information is necessary. Avoid asking leading questions, but use the Guidance to Surveyors for specific requirements to focus questions and determine the significance of the answers.

In general, the individual who provides information during an interview will not be identified as providing that information. However, it is possible that their identity may be revealed if a deficiency is cited based in whole or part on their information, and that deficiency citation is appealed.

If residents appear reticent in providing information or express concern about retaliation:

- Verify that residents have information on whom to contact in the event they become the objects of retaliation by the facility; and
- With the resident's permission, notify the ombudsman of the resident's concerns.

D. Record Review

The objectives of the record review are to:

- Acquire information to direct initial and/or additional observations and interviews;

- Provide a picture of the current status of the resident as assessed by the facility; and

- Evaluate assessments, plans of care, and outcomes of care interventions for residents included in the sample. Record review of RAI information, care planning, implementation of the care plan, and evaluation of care is one facet of the resident review which determines if there has been a decline, improvement, or maintenance in identified focus areas.

NOTE: Do not spend excessive time gathering and recording information from the record. Use the record review to obtain information necessary to validate and/or clarify information obtained through observation and interviews. Ask facility staff to assist in finding any information that has not been found or that requires validation.

E. Determining Citations of Past Noncompliance at the Time of the Current Survey

During information gathering, findings of past noncompliance may be identified. Before considering a citation of past noncompliance with a specific regulatory tag, surveyors must determine if current compliance with the specific regulatory tag exists. Similar to verifying correction of current noncompliance on a revisit, surveyors should use a variety of methods to determine whether correction of the past noncompliance occurred and continues. This may include, but is not limited to, the following:

- Interviews with facility staff, such as the administrator, nursing staff, social services staff, medical director, quality assessment and assurance committee members, and/or other facility staff, as indicated, to determine what procedures, systems, structures, and processes have been changed.

- Reviewing through observation, interview, and record review, how the facility identified and implemented interventions to address the noncompliance. Examples of interventions may include, but are not limited to:

  - The facility's review, revision, or development of policies and/or procedures to address the areas of concerns;

  - The provision and use of new equipment, as necessary;

  - The provision of staff training required to assure ongoing compliance for the implementation and use of new and/or revised policies, procedures, and/or equipment, especially with new and/or temporary staff;

  - The provision of additional staffing, changes in assignments or deployment of staff, as needed; and

- The provision of a monitoring mechanism to assure that the changes made are being supervised, evaluated, and reinforced by responsible facility staff.

- Evaluating whether the facility has a functioning quality assessment and assurance committee, whose responsibilities include the identification of quality issues; providing timely response to ascertain the cause; implementing corrective action; implementing monitoring mechanisms in place to assure continued correction and revision of approaches as necessary to eliminate the potential risk of occurrence to other residents and to assure continued compliance.

A citation of past noncompliance must meet all of the criteria described in section H of Task 6 below.

Sub-Task 5A - General Observations of the Facility

(Rev. 22, Issued: 12-15-06, Effective/Implementation: 12-18-06)

A. General Objective

The general objective of this task is to observe physical features in the facility's environment that affect residents' quality of life, health, and safety. Use the General Observations of the Facility worksheet (Form CMS-803, Exhibit 91) to complete this task.

B. General Procedures

During the Initial Tour, each surveyor should note and document any concerns in resident rooms and the general environment. Any concerns should be investigated and followed up either through the resident review for sampled residents or during the General Observation task. During the remainder of the survey, one surveyor is assigned to complete the General Observation of the Facility worksheet (Form CMS-803). This surveyor assures that all items on this worksheet are completed. Each surveyor who completes a medication pass observation should review medication storage on the assigned units and provide information regarding that review to the assigned surveyor responsible for the completion of Form CMS-803. All surveyors should share any additional concerns regarding the environment with the surveyor assigned to complete the worksheet. Begin observations as soon as possible after entering the facility, normally after introductions at the entrance conference.

During Task 5A, review the condition of the environment, e.g., cleanliness, sanitation, presence or absence of pests, accident hazards, functioning of equipment, and the proper and safe storage of drugs, biologicals, housekeeping compounds and equipment. (See Form CMS-803 worksheet for specific areas to review.)

C. Making Observations

The focus in Task 5A is on quality of life and environmental health and safety indicators in areas of the facility that would be visited or used by residents. However, some non-resident areas should also be reviewed due to their potential negative effect on residents, e.g., utility rooms.

Document thoroughly at the time of observations. If additional documentation space is needed, use the Surveyor Notes Worksheet Form CMS-807.

Plan to observe the facility's environment at different times during the survey, e.g., first and second shift, common areas when in use by residents.

Share any concerns with the team coordinator and other team members to determine the possible need to gather additional information.

Sub-Task 5B - Kitchen/Food Service Observation

A. General Objective

The general objective of the Kitchen/Food Service Observation is to determine if the facility is storing, preparing, distributing, and serving food according to 42 CFR 483.35(h)(2) to prevent food borne illness.

B. General Procedures

One surveyor is assigned to conduct the Kitchen/Food service observation.

> **NOTE**: The surveyor assigned to complete this task should begin the task with a brief visit to the kitchen as part of the initial tour, in order to observe the sanitation practices and cleanliness of the kitchen. Observe whether potentially hazardous foods have been left on counter tops or steam table and/or being prepared, the manner in which foods are being thawed, the cleanliness, sanitary practices, and appearance of kitchen staff, e.g., appropriate attire, hair restraints.

Use the Kitchen/Food Service Observation worksheet to direct observations of food storage, food preparation, and food service/sanitation. (See Kitchen/Food Service Observation worksheet (Form CMS-804, Exhibit 92) for specific areas to review).

In addition to completion of the Form CMS-804, also evaluate:

- The availability of food in relation to the number of residents; and
- Whether food being prepared is consistent with the written, planned menu.

NOTE: During team meetings, if surveyors, during the Dining Observation portion of the Resident Review, identified any concerns, such as the provision of meals that are not consistent in quality (such as color and texture of vegetables or meats, the preparation and presentation of mechanically altered foods); complaints regarding taste or texture of food and foods with an "off" or bad odor; or residents being at nutritional risk, including high prevalence of residents with unintended weight loss; then the surveyor assigned to Task 5(b) should review the following as appropriate.

Direct observations to the tray line and kitchen to determine:

- If recipes are available and consistent with the menu and followed by employees;
- If appropriate equipment is available and used to prepare and serve foods;
- If the food is being held for more than 30 minutes prior to food service, e.g., in the steam table, oven, refrigerator rather than freezer for frozen foods, etc.; and
- If cooked leftovers used during food preparation were stored and used within the appropriate time frames, and reheated to at least 165 degrees F.

Sub-Task 5C - Resident Review

(Rev. 26; Issued: 08-17-07; Effective/Implementation Dates: 08-17-07)

A. General Objectives

The general objectives of the Resident Review are to determine:

- How resident outcomes and the resident's quality of life are related to the provision of care by the facility;
- If the care provided by the facility has enabled residents to reach or maintain their highest practicable physical, mental, and psychosocial well-being;
- If residents are assisted to have the best quality of life that is possible. The review will include aspects of the environment, staff interactions, and provision of services that affect sampled residents in their daily lives;
- If the facility has properly assessed its residents through the completion of the Resident Assessment Instrument (RAI), including accurate coding and transmitting of the Minimum Data Set (MDS) and has properly assessed care needs, conducted proper care planning, implemented the plan and evaluated care provided to the residents; and

- If there are additional areas of concern that need to be investigated in Phase II of the survey.

B. General Procedures

The team coordinator assigns specific residents in the sample to surveyors.

One surveyor should conduct the entire Resident Review for an assigned resident. If the resident has been chosen for a Quality of Life Assessment protocol (Task 5D), this same surveyor should also complete that protocol. If a surveyor has not passed the Surveyor Minimum Qualifications Test (SMQT) or if the complexity of a resident's care requires expertise of more than one discipline, surveyors should work jointly to complete the review. A surveyor must successfully complete the SMQT to survey independently.

To facilitate the Resident Review, ask the charge nurse for schedules of the following, as appropriate:

1. Meals;
2. Medications;
3. Activities;
4. Tube feedings and special treatments;
5. Specialized rehabilitation therapies; and
6. Physician visits or visits of other health professionals such as dentists, podiatrists, or nurse practitioners.

For all sampled residents except closed records, parts A, B, and C (Resident Room Review, Daily Life Review, and Assessment of Drug Therapies) on the Resident Review Worksheet (Exhibit 93) are completed. The difference between the two reviews is that the focus of the part D Care Review is more extensive for Comprehensive Reviews. Determine, as appropriate, if there has been a decline, maintenance or improvement of the resident in the identified focused care areas and/or Activities of Daily Living (ADL) functioning. If there has been a lack of improvement or a decline, determine if the decline or lack of improvement was avoidable or unavoidable.

C. Comprehensive Care Review

A Comprehensive Review includes observations, interviews, and a record review. After observing and talking with the resident, the surveyor conducts a comprehensive review, which includes the following:

- A check of specific items on the MDS for accurate coding of the resident's condition. The specific items to be checked will be based on QM/QIs identified for the resident on the Resident Level Summary. At least 2 of the QM/QIs identified for the resident must be matched against the QM/QI definitions (see Exhibit 270) and against evidence other than the MDS to verify that the resident's condition is accurately recorded in the MDS. What is being verified is that the resident's condition was accurately assessed at the time the MDS was completed;

- An overall review of the facility's completion of the RAI process including their:
    - Use of the Resident Assessment Protocols (RAPs);
    - Evaluation of assessment information not covered by the RAPs;
    - Identification of risks and causes of resident conditions;
    - Completion of the RAP Summary;
    - Development of a care plan that meets the identified needs of the resident;
- A review of the implementation of the care plan and resident response;
- A review of the relationship of the resident's drug regimen to the resident's condition (see the description of procedures for completing part C below);
- A thorough review of any of the following conditions that apply to the resident: weight loss, dehydration, pressure sores. This review is completed using the investigative protocols found below as a guide. (NOTE: All the residents selected for comprehensive reviews should have one or more of these concerns checked on the QM/QI reports [unless there are no residents with these concerns in the facility]); and
- An evaluation of the resident's dining experience (see Dining Observation Protocol below).

D. Focused Care Review Phase 1

This focused review includes observations, interviews, and a record review. This review focuses on care areas that were checked for the resident on the Resident Level Summary and any additional care items checked by the team as pertinent to the resident, e.g., all areas that are checked on the Roster/Sample Matrix by the team for the resident are reviewed, whether or not they have been highlighted as concerns for the survey. The dining observation is done for a resident if the resident has any checkmarks related to dining or the investigating team member has any concerns about the resident related to dining, e.g., such as weight loss.

The Phase 1 focused care review includes all care areas the team has checked for the resident: a review of the MDS, the facility's use of the RAPs, care planning, implementation of the care plan, and the resident's response to the care provided.

E. Focused Care Review Phase 2

This focused review includes observations, interviews and a record review, which concentrates only on those areas of concern for which the team requires additional information. For example, if the team needs additional information concerning facility compliance with the requirements for tube feeding, review only those RAI areas related to tube feeding; make observations of nutritional status, complications, and techniques of tube feeding, and interview residents, family and staff concerning related areas.

F. Closed Record Review

This includes a record review of the resident's care issues and transfer and discharge requirements. It may be possible to select some or all of the closed records from the preselected list of residents for the Phase 1 sample, if any of these preselected residents were noted onsite to be discharged or deceased.

Assess quality of care and quality of life requirements that relate to the identified care areas for the sampled resident. While assessing these, note and investigate concerns with any other requirements.

G. Conducting the Resident Review

The Resident Review consists of 4 main sections: Resident Room Review, Daily Life Review, Assessment of Drug Therapies, and Care Review. See Resident Review Worksheet and instructions (Form CMS-805, Exhibit 93) for specific areas to review.

1. Section A - The Resident Room Review assesses aspects of accommodation of needs, environmental quality, and quality of life in the resident's room. Through observations and interviews, evaluate how the resident's environment affects his/her quality of life.

2. Section B - The Daily Life Review is a review of the resident's daily quality of life, especially in the areas of staff responsiveness to resident grooming and other needs, staff interactions, choices, and activities. Through ongoing observations and interviews, evaluate the resident's daily life routines and interactions with staff.

3. Section C - The Assessment of Drug Therapies is a review of the medications the resident is receiving to evaluate whether the effectiveness of the therapeutic regimen, including all drugs that may play a significant role in the resident's everyday life, is being monitored and assessed. Record the information on the Resident Review Worksheet, Form CMS-805. Review and record, as pertinent, all non-prescription and prescription medications taken by the resident during the past 7 days. In addition follow the guidance in Appendix PP, Tag F329 for the determination of unnecessary medications.

4. Section D -- The care review is an assessment of those quality of care areas (see 42 CFR 483.25) that are pertinent to the sampled resident. The survey team, through use of the Roster/Sample Matrix, determines what care areas will be reviewed for each sampled resident. Additional areas for evaluation may be identified during the review.

   There are a designated number of comprehensive, focused and closed record care reviews completed, depending on the size of the sample.

H. Care Observations and Interviews -- Make resident observations and conduct interviews, which include those factors or care areas as determined by the Roster/Sample Matrix. For example, if the resident was chosen because he/she is receiving tube feedings, observe the care and the outcomes of the interventions, facility monitoring and assessment, and nutritional needs/adequacy related to tube feeding.

Complete the following tasks:

- Observe the resident and caregivers during care and treatments, at meals, and various times of the day, including early morning and evening, over the entire survey period. Observe residents in both informal and structured settings, e.g., receiving specialized rehabilitation services, participating in formal and informal activities. Also, observe staff-resident interactions;

- Gather resident-specific information, including information on the resident's functional ability, potential for increasing ability, and any complications concerning special care needs;

- Evaluate implementation of the care plan. Determine if the care plan is consistently implemented by all personnel at all times of the day, and if the care plan is working for the resident. If the care plan is not working, look for evidence that the facility has identified this and acted on it even if the care plan has not formally been revised;

- Determine if there is a significant difference between the facility's assessment of the resident and observations; and

- Evaluate the adequacy of care provided to the resident using the Guidance to Surveyors.

Do not continue to follow residents once enough information has been accrued to determine whether the resident has received care in accordance with the regulatory requirements.

If there are indicators to suggest the presence of a quality of care problem that is not readily observable, e.g., a leg ulcer covered with a dressing, or a sacral pressure sore, ask facility staff to assist in making observations by removing, for example, a dressing or bedclothes.

Resident care observations should be made by those persons who have the clinical knowledge and skills to evaluate compliance.

When observing residents, respect their right to privacy, including the privacy of their bodies. If the resident's genital or rectal area or female breast area must be observed in order to document and confirm suspicions of a care problem, a member of the nursing staff must be present at this observation, and the resident must give clear consent.
If the resident is unable to give consent, e.g., is unresponsive, incompetent, and a legal surrogate (family member who can act on the resident's behalf or legal representative as provided by State law) is present, ask this individual to give consent.

An observation of a resident's rectal or genital area (and for females, the breast area) may be made without a resident's or legal surrogate's consent, under the following conditions:

1. It is determined that there is a strong possibility that the resident is receiving less than adequate care, which can only be confirmed by direct observation;

2. The resident is unable to give clear consent; and
3. A legal surrogate is not present in the facility.

Only a surveyor who is a licensed nurse, a physician's assistant or a physician may make an observation of a resident's genitals, rectal area, or, for females, the breast area.

I. Record Review

Conduct a record review to provide a picture of the current status of the resident as assessed by the facility; information on changes in the resident's status over the last 12 months for those areas identified for review; and information on planned care, resident goals, and expected outcomes.

Use the record review to help determine whether the assessments accurately reflect the resident's status and are internally consistent. An example of inconsistency may be that the facility assessed the resident's ADLs as being independently performed yet had indicated that the resident requires task segmentation for performing ADLs.

For sampled residents selected for either a comprehensive or a focused review, conduct a review of the RAI information including:

- The face sheet of the MDS for background information including customary routines and demographic information to provide an understanding of the resident prior to admission. This assists in assessing the quality of life of the resident.

- The latest MDS to determine which RAPS were triggered. For a sampled resident receiving a comprehensive review, note all triggered areas. Also, review the facility's assessment of the resident's level of functioning and note particularly drug therapy and cognitive, behavior, and ADL function. For a resident receiving a focused review in Phase I of the survey, review both the areas of concern specific to the resident and the other care areas that have been identified with the Roster/Sample Matrix. For Phase 2 residents, review only those areas that have been identified by the team as areas of concern.

If the RAI is less than 9 months old, review and compare with the previous RAI and the most recent quarterly review. If the RAI is 9 months or older, compare the current RAI with the most recent quarterly review. Review the following:

- The RAP summary sheet to see where the assessment documentation is located for any RAP triggered;

- The information summarizing the assessments (RAPS) and decision to proceed or not to proceed to care planning. Determine if the assessments indicate that the facility used the RAPs and considered the nature of the problem, the causal and risk factors, the need for referrals, complications, and decisions for care planning. If this is a reassessment, review whether the facility determined if the care plan required revision or was effective in moving the resident toward his/her goals;
- The care plan to identify whether the facility used the RAI to make sound care planning decisions. Determine whether the facility identified resident strengths, needs, and problems which needed to be addressed to assist the resident to maintain or improve his/her current functional status. Determine whether the facility identified resident-centered, measurable goals and specific interventions to achieve those goals. With observations, interviews, and record review, determine if the facility implemented the interventions defined; and

- Determine whether the facility documentation and resident status as observed indicate the decision to proceed or not to proceed to care planning was appropriate. This information will assist in determining whether a resident's decline or failure to improve was avoidable or unavoidable.

- It is not necessary to review the entire resident record. Review only those sections that are necessary to verify and clarify the information necessary to make compliance decisions. These sections may include, for example, laboratory reports, progress notes, and drug regimen review reports.

- In any care area in which it is determined that there has been a lack of improvement, a decline, or failure to reach highest practicable well being, assess if the change for the resident was avoidable or unavoidable. Note both the faulty facility practice and its effect on resident(s). Determine if a reassessment based on significant change should have been conducted, and if the absence of reassessment contributed to the resident's decline or lack of improvement.

- Verify that the information needed has been obtained to determine if the facility fulfilled its obligation to provide care that allowed the resident to attain or maintain the highest practicable physical, mental, and psychosocial well-being.

NOTE: When conducting either a focused or comprehensive review, if there are areas of concern which fall outside the care areas identified, investigate these, as necessary.

The following are special investigative protocols which should be used in Task 5C to gather information and in Task 6, to determine facility compliance in the care areas of pressure sore/ulcer(s), hydration, unintended weight loss, sufficient nursing staffing, and dining and food services.

NOTE: "Although the RAI assessments discussed in the following [investigative protocols] must occur at specific times, by Federal regulation, a facility's obligation to meet each resident's needs through ongoing assessment is not neatly confined to these mandated time frames. Likewise, completion of the RAI in the prescribed time frame does not necessarily fulfill a facility's obligation to perform a comprehensive assessment. Facility's are responsible for assessing areas that are relevant to individual residents regardless of whether these areas are included in the RAI." ("CMS Long-Term Care Facility Resident Assessment Instrument User's Manual," Version 2.0.)

Investigative Protocol

Hydration

Objectives:

- To determine if the facility identified risk factors which lead to dehydration and developed an appropriate preventative care plan; and

- To determine if the facility provided the resident with sufficient fluid intake to maintain proper hydration and health.

Task 5C: Use:

Use this protocol for the following situations:

- A sampled resident who flagged for the sentinel event of dehydration (QM/QI 7.3);
- A sampled resident who has one or more of the following QM/QI conditions:
    - 5.4 – Prevalence of fecal impaction;

  - 6.1 – Residents with a urinary tract infection;
  - 7.1 – Residents who lose too much weight;
  - 7.2 – Prevalence of tube feeding;
  - 9.1 – Residents whose need for help with daily activities has increased; and
  - Any of the three pressure ulcer QM/QIs: 12.1, 12.2, or 13.3.

- A sampled resident who was discovered to have any of the following risk factors: vomiting/diarrhea resulting in fluid loss, elevated temperatures and/or infectious processes, dependence on staff for the provision of fluid intake, use of medications including diuretics, laxatives, and cardiovascular agents, renal disease, dysphagia, a history of refusing fluids, limited fluid intake or lacking the sensation of thirst.

Procedures:

- Observations/interviews conducted as part of this procedure should be recorded on the Forms CMS-805 and/or the Form CMS-807.

- Determine if the resident was assessed to identify risk factors that can lead to dehydration, such as those listed above and whether there were abnormal laboratory test values which may be an indicator of dehydration.

  NOTE: A general guideline for determining baseline daily fluid needs is to multiply the resident's body weight in kilograms (kg) x 30ml (2.2 lbs = 1 kg), except for residents with renal or cardiac distress, or other restrictions based on physician orders. An excess of fluids can be detrimental for these residents.

- Determine if an interdisciplinary care plan was developed utilizing the clinical conditions and risk factors identified, taking into account the amount of fluid that the resident requires. If the resident is receiving enteral nutritional support, determine if the tube feeding orders included a sufficient amount of free water, and whether the water and feeding are being administered in accordance with physician orders?

- Observe the care delivery to determine if the interventions identified in the care plan have been implemented as described.

  - What is the resident's response to the interventions? Does staff provide the necessary fluids as described in the plan? Do the fluids provided contribute to dehydration, e.g., caffeinated beverages, alcohol? Was the correct type of fluid provided with a resident with dysphagia?

- o Is the resident able to reach, pour and drink fluids without assistance and is the resident consuming sufficient fluids? If not, are staff providing the fluids according to the care plan?

- o Is the resident's room temperature (heating mechanism) contributing to dehydration? If so, how is the facility addressing this issue?
- o If the resident refuses water, are alternative fluids offered that are tolerable to the resident?

- o Are the resident's beverage preferences identified and honored at meals?

- o Does staff encourage the resident to drink? Are they aware of the resident's fluid needs? Are staff providing fluids during and between meals?

- o Determine how the facility monitors to assure that the resident maintains fluid parameters as planned. If the facility is monitoring the intake and output of the resident, review the record to determine if the fluid goals or calculated fluid needs were met consistently.

- Review all related information and documentation to look for evidence of identified causes of the condition or problem. This inquiry should include interviews with appropriate facility staff and health care practitioners, who by level of training and knowledge of the resident, should know of, or be able to provide information about the causes of a resident's condition or problem.

  NOTE: If a resident is at an end of life stage and has an advance directive, according to State law, (or a decision has been made by the resident's surrogate or representative, in accordance with State law) or the resident has reached an end of life stage in which minimal amounts of fluids are being consumed or intake has ceased, and all appropriate efforts have been made to encourage and provide intake, then dehydration may be an expected outcome and does not constitute noncompliance with the requirement for hydration. Conduct observations to verify that palliative interventions, as described in the plan of care, are being implemented and revised as necessary, to meet the needs/choices of the resident in order to maintain the resident's comfort and quality of life. If the facility has failed to provide the palliative care, cite noncompliance with 42 CFR 483.25, F309, Quality of Care.

- Determine if the care plan is evaluated and revised based on the response, outcomes, and needs of the resident.

Task 6: Determination of Compliance:

- Compliance with 42 CFR 483.25(j), F327, Hydration:
    - For this resident, the facility is compliant with this requirement to maintain proper hydration if they properly assessed, care planned, implemented the care plan, evaluated the resident outcome, and revised the care plan as needed. If not, cite at F327.
- Compliance with 42 CFR 483.20(b)(1) & (2), F272, Comprehensive Assessments:
    - For this resident in the area of hydration, the facility is compliant with this requirement if they assessed factors that put the resident at risk for dehydration, whether chronic or acute. If not, cite at F272.
- Compliance with 42 CFR 483.20(k)(1), F279, Comprehensive Care Plans:
    - For this resident in the area of hydration, the facility is compliant with this requirement if they developed a care plan that includes measurable objectives and timetables to meet the resident's needs as identified in the resident's assessment. If not, cite at F279.
- Compliance with 42 CFR 483.20(k)(3)(ii), F 282, Provision of care in accordance with the care plan:
    - For this resident in the area of hydration, the facility is compliant with this requirement if qualified persons implemented the resident's care plan. If not, cite at F282.

Investigative Protocol

Unintended Weight Loss

Objectives:

- To determine if the identified weight loss is avoidable or unavoidable; and
- To determine the adequacy of the facility's response to the weight loss.

Task 5C: Use:

Utilize this protocol for a sampled resident with unintended weight loss.

Procedures:

- Observations/interviews conducted as part of this procedure should be recorded on the Form CMS-805 if they pertain to a specific sampled resident and on the Form CMS-807 if they relate to general observations of the dining service/dining room.

- Determine if the resident was assessed for conditions that may have put the resident at risk for unintended weight loss such as the following:

  - Cancer, renal disease, diabetes, depression, chronic obstructive pulmonary disease, Parkinson's disease, Alzheimer's disease, malnutrition, infection, dehydration, constipation, diarrhea, Body Mass Index (BMI) below 19, dysphagia, chewing and swallowing problems, edentulous, ill fitting dentures, mouth pain, taste/sensory changes, bedfast, totally dependent for eating, pressure ulcer, abnormal laboratory values (review in accordance with the facility's laboratory norms) associated with malnutrition (serum albumin, plasma transferrin, magnesium, hct/hgb, BUN/creatinine ratio, potassium, cholesterol), and use of medications such as diuretics, laxatives, and cardiovascular agents.

  NOTE: Amputation of a body part will contribute to a significant decrease in previously targeted weight range. Once the new weight goals are established, the resident should be assessed within the parameters of the unintended weight loss investigative protocol.

  NOTE: Body Mass Index (BMI) estimates total body mass and is highly correlated with the amount of body fat. It provides important information about body composition, making it a useful indicator of nutritional status. BMI is easy to calculate because only information about height and weight are needed.

  $$\text{BMI} = \text{weight (Kg)/height (M}^2\text{) or}$$

  $$\text{BMI} = \text{weight (lbs.)/height (inches}^2\text{) X 705}$$

- Determine if the facility has assessed the resident's nutritive and fluid requirements, dining assistance needs, such as assistive devices, food cultural/religious preferences, food allergies, and frequency of meals.

- Review all related information and documentation to look for evidence of identified causes of the condition or problem. This inquiry should include interviews with appropriate facility staff and health care practitioners, who by level of training and knowledge of the resident should know of, or be able to provide information about the causes of a resident's condition or problem.

- Determine if the care plan was developed utilizing the clinical conditions and risk factors identified in the assessment for unintended weight loss. Were the care plan interventions, such as oral supplements, enteral feeding, alternative eating schedule, liberalized diet, nutrient supplements, adaptive utensils, assistance and/or increased time to eat developed to provide an aggressive program of consistent intervention by all appropriate staff?

- Determine if the care plan was evaluated and revised based on the response, outcomes, and needs of the resident.

  NOTE: If a resident is at an end of life stage and has an advance directive according to State law, (or a decision has been made by the resident's surrogate or representative in accordance with State law) or the resident has reached an end of life stage in which minimal amounts of nutrients are being consumed or intake has ceased, and all appropriate efforts have been made to encourage and provide intake, then the weight loss may be an expected outcome and may not constitute noncompliance with the requirement for maintaining nutritional parameters. Conduct observations to verify that palliative interventions, as described in the plan of care, are being implemented and revised as necessary, to meet the needs/choices of the resident in order to maintain the resident's comfort and quality of life. If the facility has failed to provide the palliative care, cite noncompliance with 42 CFR 483.25, F309, Quality of Care.

- Observe the delivery of care as described in the care plan, e.g., staff providing assistance and/or encouragement during dining; serving food as planned with attention to portion sizes, preferences, nutritional supplements, and/or between-meal snacks, to determine if the interventions identified in the care plan have been implemented. Use the Dining and Food Service Investigative Protocol to make this determination.

Task 6: Determination of Compliance:

- Compliance with 42 CFR 483.25(I), F325, Nutrition

  - For this resident, the unintended weight loss is unavoidable if the facility properly assessed, care planned, implemented the care plan, evaluated the resident outcome, and revised the care plan as needed. If not, the weight loss is avoidable; cite at F325.

- Compliance with 42 CFR 483.25, F309, Quality of Care:

  - For the resident who is in an end-of-life stage and palliative interventions, as described in the plan of care, are being implemented and revised as necessary, to meet the needs/choices of the resident in order to maintain the resident's comfort and quality of life, then for this resident, in the area of palliative care, the facility is compliant with this requirement. If not, cite F309.

- Compliance with 42 CFR 483.20(b)(1) and (2), F272, Comprehensive Assessments:

    - For this resident in the area of unintended weight loss, the facility is compliant with this requirement if they assessed the factors that put the resident at risk for weight loss. If not, cite at F272.

- Compliance with 42 CFR 483.20(k)(1), F279, Comprehensive Care Plans:

    - For this resident in the area of unintended weight loss, the facility is compliant with this requirement if they developed a care plan that includes measurable objectives and timetables to meet the resident's needs as identified in the resident's assessment. If not, cite at F279.

- Compliance with 42 CFR 483.20(k)(3)(ii), F 282, Provision of care in accordance with the care plan:

    - For this resident in the area of unintended weight loss, the facility is compliant with this requirement if qualified persons implemented the resident's care plan. If not, cite at F282.

Investigative Protocol

Dining and Food Service

Objectives:

- To determine if each resident is provided with nourishing, palatable, attractive meals that meet the resident's daily nutritional and special dietary needs;

- To determine if each resident is provided services to maintain or improve eating skills; and

- To determine if the dining experience enhances the resident's quality of life and is supportive of the resident's needs, including food service and staff support during dining.

Task 5C: Use

This protocol will be used for:

- All sampled residents identified with malnutrition, unintended weight loss, mechanically altered diet, pressure sores/ulcers, and hydration concerns; and

- Food complaints received from residents, families and others.

General Considerations:

- Use this protocol at two meals during the survey, preferably the noon and evening meals.

- Record information on the Form CMS-805 if it pertains to a specific sampled resident, or on the Form CMS-807 if it relates to the general observations of the dining service/dining room.

    - o Discretely observe all residents, including sampled residents, during meals keeping questions to a minimum to prevent disruption in the meal service.

- For each sampled resident being observed, identify any special needs and the interventions planned to meet their needs. Using the facility's menu, record in writing what is planned in writing to be served to the resident at the meal observed.

- Conduct observations of food preparation and quality of meals.

Procedures:

1. During the meal service, observe the dining room and/or resident's room for the following:

    - Comfortable sound levels;

    - Adequate illumination, furnishings, ventilation; absence of odors; and sufficient space;

    - Tables adjusted to accommodate wheelchairs, etc.; and

    - Appropriate hygiene provided prior to meals.

2. Observe whether each resident is properly prepared for meals. For example:

    - Resident's eyeglasses, dentures, and/or hearing aids are in place;

    - Proper positioning in chair, wheelchair, gerichair, etc., at an appropriate distance from the table (tray table and bed at appropriate height and position); and

    - Assistive devices/utensils identified in care plans provided and used as planned.

3. Observe the food service for:

- Appropriateness of dishes and flatware for each resident. Single use disposable dining ware is not used except in an emergency and, other appropriate dining activities. Except those with fluid restriction, each resident has an appropriate place setting with water and napkin;

- Whether meals are attractive, palatable, served at appropriate temperatures and are delivered to residents in a timely fashion.

    - Did the meals arrive 30 minutes or more past the scheduled mealtime?

    - If a substitute was needed, did it arrive more than 15 minutes after the request for a substitute?

- Are diet cards, portion sizes, preferences, and condiment requests being honored?

4. Determine whether residents are being promptly assisted to eat or provided necessary assistance/cueing in a timely manner after their meal is served.
    - Note whether residents at the same table or in resident rooms, are being served and assisted concurrently.

- *If you observe a resident who is being assisted by a staff member to eat or drink, and the resident is having problems with eating or drinking, inquire if the staff member who is assisting them is a paid feeding assistant. If so, follow the procedures at tag F373.*

5. Determine if the meals served were palatable, attractive, nutritious and met the needs of the resident. Note the following:

    - Whether the resident voiced concerns regarding the taste, temperature, quality, quantity and appearance of the meal served;

    - Whether mechanically altered diets, such as pureed, were prepared and served as separate entree items (except when combined food, e.g., stews, casseroles, etc.);

    - Whether attempts to determine the reason(s) for the refusal and a substitute of equal nutritive value was provided, if the resident refused/rejected food served; and

    - Whether food placement, colors, and textures were in keeping with the resident's needs or deficits, e.g., residents with vision or swallowing deficits.

Sample Tray Procedure

If residents complain about the palatability/temperature of food served, the survey team coordinator may request a test meal to obtain quantitative data to assess the complaints. Send the meal to the unit that is the greatest distance from the kitchen or to the affected unit or dining room. Check food temperature and palatability of the test meal at about the time the last resident on the unit is served and begins eating.

6. Observe for institutional medication pass practices that interfere with the quality of the residents' dining experience. This does not prohibit the administration of medications during meal service for medications that are necessary to be given at a meal, nor does this prohibit a medication to be given during a meal upon request of a resident who is accustomed to taking the medication with the meal, as long as it has been determined that this practice does not interfere with the effectiveness of the medication.

   - Has the facility attempted to provide medications at times and in a manner to support the dining experience of the resident, such as:

     - Pain medications being given prior to meals so that meals could be eaten in comfort;

     - Foods served are not routinely or unnecessarily used as a vehicle to administer medications (mixing the medications with potatoes or other entrees).

7. Determine if the sampled resident consumed adequate amounts of food as planned.

   - Determine if the facility is monitoring the foods/fluids consumed. Procedures used by the facility may be used to determine percentage of food consumed, if available; otherwise, determine the percentage of food consumed using the following point system:

     - Each food item served except for water, coffee, tea, or condiments equals one point. Example: Breakfast: juice, cereal, milk, bread and butter, coffee (no points) equals four points. If the resident consumes all four items in the amount served, the resident consumes 100% of breakfast. If the resident consumes two of the four food items served, then 50% of the breakfast would have been consumed. If three-quarters of a food item is consumed, give one point; for one-half consumed, give .5 points; for one-fourth or less, give no points. Total the points consumed x 100 and divide by the number of points given for that meal to give the percentage of meal consumed. Use these measurements when determining the amount of liquids consumed: Liquid measurements: 8 oz. cup = 240 cc, 6 oz. cup = 180 cc, 4 oz. cup = 120 cc, 1 oz. cup = 30 cc.

- Compare these findings with the facility's documentation to determine if the facility has accurately recorded the intake. Ask the staff if these findings are consistent with the resident's usual intake; and

- Note whether plates are being returned to the kitchen with 75% or more of food not eaten.

8. If concerns are noted with meal service, preparation, quality of meals, etc., interview the person(s) responsible for dietary services to determine how the staff are assigned and monitored to assure meals are prepared according to the menu, that the meals are delivered to residents in a timely fashion, and at proper temperature, both in the dining rooms/areas and in resident rooms.

NOTE: If concerns are identified in providing monitoring by supervisory staff during dining or concerns with assistance for residents to eat, evaluate nursing staffing in accord with 42 CFR 483.30(a), F353, and quality of care at 42 CFR 483.25(a)(2) and (3).

Task 6: Determination of Compliance:

- Compliance with 42 CFR 483.35(d)(1)(2), F364, Food

  - The facility is compliant with this requirement when each resident receives food prepared by methods that conserve nutritive value, palatable, attractive and at the proper temperatures. If not, cite F364.

- Compliance with 42 CFR 483.35(b), F362, Dietary services, sufficient staff

  - The facility is compliant with this requirement if they have sufficient staff to prepare and serve palatable and attractive, nutritionally adequate meals at proper temperatures. If not, cite F362.

  NOTE: If serving food is a function of the nursing service rather than dietary, refer to 42 CFR 483.30(a), F353.

- Compliance with 42 CFR 483.15(h)(1), F252, Environment

  - The facility is compliant with this requirement if they provide a homelike environment during the dining services that enhances the resident's quality of life. If not, cite F252.

- Compliance with 42 CFR 483.70(g)(1)(2)(3)(4), F464, Dining and Resident Activities

- The facility is compliant with this requirement if they provide adequate lighting, ventilation, furnishings and space during the dining services. If not, cite F464.

Investigative Protocol

Nursing Services, Sufficient Staffing

Objectives:

- To determine if the facility has sufficient nursing staff available to meet the residents' needs.

- To determine if the facility has licensed registered nurses and licensed nursing staff available to provide and monitor the delivery of resident care.

Task 5C: Use:

NOTE: This protocol is not required during the standard survey, unless it is triggered in the event of care concerns/problems which may be associated with sufficiency of nursing staff. It is required to be completed for an extended survey.

This protocol is to be used when:

- Quality of care problems have been identified, e.g., residents not receiving the care and services to prevent pressure sore/ulcer(s), unintended weight loss and dehydration, and to prevent declines in their condition as described in their comprehensive plans of care, such as bathing, dressing, grooming, transferring, ambulation, toileting, and eating; and

- Complaints have been received from residents, families or other resident representatives concerning services, e.g., care not being provided, call lights not being answered in a timely fashion, and residents not being assisted to eat.

Procedures:

- Determine if the registered/licensed nursing staff are available to:
    - Supervise and monitor the delivery of care by nursing assistants according to residents' care plans;
    - Assess resident condition changes;
    - Monitor dining activities to identify concerns or changes in residents' needs;

- o Respond to nursing assistants' requests for assistance;
- o Correct inappropriate or unsafe nursing assistants techniques; and
- o Identify training needs for the nursing assistants.

- If problems were identified with care plans/services not provided as needed by the resident, focus the discussion with supervisory staff on the situations which led to using the protocol: how do they assure that there are adequate staff to meet the needs of the residents; how do they assure that staff are knowledgeable about the needs of the residents and are capable of delivering the care as planned; how do they assure that staff are appropriately deployed to meet the needs of the residents; how do they provide orientation for new or temporary staff regarding the resident needs and the interventions to meet those needs; and how do they assure that staff are advised of changes in the care plan?

- Determine if nursing assistants and other nursing staff are knowledgeable regarding the residents' care needs, e.g., the provision of fluids and foods for residents who are unable to provide these services for themselves; the provision of turning, positioning and skin care for those residents identified at risk for pressure sore/ulcers; and the provision of incontinence care as needed;

- If necessary, review nursing assistant assignments in relation to the care and or services the resident requires to meet his/her needs;

- In interviews with residents, families and/or other resident representatives, inquire about the staff's response to requests for assistance, and the timeliness of call lights being answered; and

- Determine if the problems are facility-wide, cover all shifts or if they are limited to certain units or shifts, or days of the week. This can be based on information already gathered by the team with additional interviews of residents, families, and staff, as necessary.

Task 6: Determination of Compliance:

NOTE: Meeting the State-mandated staffing ratio, if any, does not preclude a deficiency of insufficient staff if the facility is not providing needed care and services to residents.

- Compliance with 42 CFR 483.30(a), F353, Sufficient Staff:
    - o The facility is compliant with this requirement if the facility has provided a sufficient number of licensed nurses and other nursing personnel to meet the needs of the residents on a 24-hour basis. If not, cite F353.

J. Closed Record Reviews

Closed records are included in the total resident sample. If possible, select closed records of residents who have been identified through the use of offsite information concerning a particular care issue. If there is a care area that is an identified concern, try to obtain the closed records of residents who had the same care needs before death, discharge, or transfer. Document information on the Form CMS-805, Sections C and D, as appropriate.

Look for information to determine compliance with quality of care and other requirements such as:

- Assessment and care of infections;
- Pressure sores;
- Significant weight loss;
- Restraints;
- Multiple falls or injuries;
- Discharge planning; and
- Transfer and discharge requirements.

Unless there is a reason to review the entire record, focus the review on the appropriateness of care and treatment surrounding the resident's discharge or transfer, and the events leading up to that discharge or transfer. For example, if the survey team has identified a concern with inadequate identification and care of residents with infections, and several residents have recently been hospitalized with serious infections, the review would be a focused review on the care and assessment these residents received before they were hospitalized. In addition:

- Look for documentation related to transfer, discharge, and bed-hold, including facility's discharge planning, notices, and reasons for facility-initiated moves, e.g., proper planning and transferring subsequent to a change in payor or care needs; and
- Determine if within 30 days of the death of a resident, the facility conveyed the deceased resident's personal funds and a final accounting to the individual or probate jurisdiction administering the individual's estate as provided by State law (see 42 CFR 483.10(c)(6), F160).

K. Review of a Resident Receiving Hospice Care

When a facility resident has also elected the Medicare hospice benefit, the hospice and the nursing home must communicate, establish, and agree upon a coordinated plan of care for both providers which reflects the hospice philosophy, and is based on an assessment of the individual's needs and unique living situation in the facility. The plan of care must include directives for managing pain and other uncomfortable symptoms and be revised and updated as necessary to reflect the individual's current status.

The hospice must designate a registered nurse from the hospice to coordinate the implementation of the plan of care.

This coordinated plan of care must identify the care and services which the SNF/NF and hospice will provide in order to be responsive to the unique needs of the patient/resident and his/her expressed desire for hospice care.

The SNF/NF and the hospice are responsible for performing each of their respective functions that have been agreed upon and included in the plan of care. The hospice retains overall professional management responsibility for directing the implementation of the plan of care related to the terminal illness.
For residents receiving Hospice benefit care, evaluate if:

- The plan of care reflects the participation of the hospice, the facility, and the patient to the extent possible;

- The plan of care includes directives for managing pain and other uncomfortable symptoms and is revised and updated as necessary to reflect the individual's current status;

- Drugs and medical supplies are provided as needed for the palliation and management of the terminal illness and related conditions;

- The hospice and the facility communicate with each other when any changes are indicated to the plan of care;

- The hospice and the facility are aware of the other's responsibilities in implementing the plan of care;

- The facility's services are consistent with the plan of care developed in coordination with the hospice, (the hospice patient residing in a SNF/NF should not experience any lack of SNF/NF services or personal care because of his/her status as a hospice patient); and

- The SNF/NF offers the same services to its residents who have elected the hospice benefit as it furnishes to its residents who have not elected the hospice benefit. The patient/resident has the right to refuse any services.

NOTE: If there are concerns about the resident in relation to care provided by the hospice agency, refer the issue to the State Agency responsible for surveying hospices.

L. Review of a Resident Receiving Dialysis Services

When dialysis is provided in the facility by an outside entity, or the resident leaves the facility to obtain dialysis, the nursing home must have an agreement or arrangement with the entity in accordance with 42 CFR 483.75 (h). This agreement/arrangement should include all aspects of how the resident's care is to be managed, including:

- Medical and non-medical emergencies;
- Development and implementation of the resident's care plan;
- Interchange of information useful/necessary for the care of the resident; and
- Responsibility for waste handling, sterilization, and disinfection of equipment.

If there is a sampled resident who is receiving dialysis care, evaluate the following, in addition to the standard Resident Review protocol:

- Whether medication is given at times for maximum effect;
- Whether staff know how to manage emergencies and complications, including equipment failure and alarm systems (if any), bleeding/hemorrhaging, and infection/bacteremia/septic shock;
- Whether facility staff are aware of the care of shunts/fistulas, infection control, waste handling, nature and management of end stage renal disease (including nutritional needs, emotional and social well-being, and aspects to monitor); and
- Whether the treatment for this (these) resident(s), affects the quality of life, rights or quality of care for other residents, e.g., restricting access to their own space, risk of infections.

M. Review of Influenza and Pneumococcal Immunizations

o Use the Investigative Protocol contained at Tag F334 to complete a review of the implementation of the facility's immunization policies and procedures.

Sub-Task 5D - Quality of Life Assessment

A. Introduction

The assessment of the quality of life and rights of residents incorporates review of selected tags within the following requirements:

- 42 CFR 483.10, Resident Rights;
- 42 CFR 483.12, Admission, Transfer and Discharge Rights;
- 42 CFR 483.13, Resident Behavior and Facility Practices;
- 42 CFR 483.15, Quality of Life; and
- 42 CFR 483.70, Physical Environment.

Since quality of life and quality of care are closely interrelated concepts, the survey process holistically integrates the quality of life assessment into the following tasks or sub-tasks:

- Task 5A, General Observations of the Facility (see <u>Task 5A</u> for further description);
- Task 5C, Resident Review, Sections A and B (see <u>Task 5C</u> for further description); and
- Task 5D, Quality of Life Assessment.

B. General Objectives

The general objectives of the quality of life assessment are:

- To determine if the facility protects and promotes the rights of residents;
- To assess the impact of the facility's environment, facility schedules and policies, and staff interactions with residents on the quality of residents' lives;
- To determine if the facility is assisting residents to achieve and maintain their highest practicable well-being; and
- To determine if the facility provides equal access to quality care for all residents, regardless of payment source.

5D. Quality of Life Protocols

Task 5D includes the following sub-tasks: interviews of interviewable residents, a meeting with the resident group or council, family interviews of residents who are not interviewable, and observations of these same non-interviewable residents. These are each described below.

1. Resident Interview

These interviews are conducted with a subsample of interviewable residents from the resident sample. Refer to Table 1 in Task 4 to determine how many residents to interview. For example, in a facility with a census of 100, Table 1 directs the team to select 5 residents to interview.

It is helpful to divide the interview into two or more short segments. Seeing the resident more than once helps to establish rapport and gives the resident a chance to think over the questions and provide more information later. Surveyors are encouraged to have several short conversations with interviewable residents during the course of the survey.

Locate a private place for the interview, and arrange interview times at the resident's convenience. Resident interviews should be conducted privately unless the resident expresses a preference to have a family member, staff member or the ombudsman present.

Prior to the interview, complete question 11 by writing any concerns that have been discovered about this resident or about the facility that you would like to discuss with the resident. Issues that are already covered in the other questions of the interview need not be listed.

For example, during Offsite Survey Preparation, the team has noted that the facility has had repeated deficiencies for pest control of roaches. On the Initial Tour, it may have been noticed the resident and her roommate were speaking angrily to each other. During the survey, the team has discovered disagreeable smells in this resident's unit, low levels of lighting in the dining room and some residents who go into others' rooms and rummage through drawers. Also, add items discovered in the Resident Review about any of this resident's special needs and preferences that the facility should be taking into account. For example, a preference for a shower instead of a bath, or a need to have extra strong lighting because of a vision deficit. Add all these items to Question 11.

At the beginning of the first interview segment, use the probes on the first page of the interview to guide the explanation to the resident of the purpose of the interview. Discuss with the resident that some of his/her answers may be written down, and ask if that is all right. Then take a few minutes to establish rapport by letting the resident direct the conversation. For residents who are uncommunicative at first, use cues from their surroundings or from what is known about this resident to begin the conversation. Try to seek some commonality that will allow the resident to develop some ease in talking. For example, remark on family pictures and other personal items seen in the resident's room, or bring up a past occupation or hobby or a current activity preference of the resident that is of mutual interest. Share a little about yourself, as appropriate.

Use the resident interview protocol to guide the conversation with the resident, but bring up topics in an order that is sensible to the conversation. Probe for further information if the answer the resident is giving is incomplete or unclear. After the interview, follow-up on the concerns the resident has raised. Include in the documentation both the facility practice in question and its effect on the resident. Share these concerns with team members so that they can pursue them during the remainder of the survey. (See the tag numbers in parentheses after particular questions for interpretive guidance on following up on resident comments.)

NOTE: There are some problems that a resident will express that are not within the scope of the long-term care requirements. For example, a resident is complaining during an interview that he/she is displeased that he/she does not have a private room. This facility does not have private rooms, nor do the requirements mandate private rooms. If there is no issue related to one of the requirements, further investigation is not needed.

2. Group Interview

This interview is conducted with members of the resident council if one exists, or with an informal group of residents if there is no council. Staff members and residents' family members are not to be present at this interview unless the group specifically requests a certain person's presence. The group need not be restricted to officers of the resident council. The survey team members should feel free to invite other residents they encounter who are able to converse and provide information. The resident council should also be encouraged to invite other residents at their discretion. It is preferable to keep the group size manageable, e.g., usually no more than 12, to facilitate communication. Residents who are not able to participate should not be included in this interview.

Prior to the meeting, review council minutes if they were provided by the council. Determine if there are any particular concerns you would like to discuss. Write in Question 13 these concerns and any other special concerns the team has learned about this facility during Offsite Survey Preparation, the Initial Tour, or during other observations and interviews. Concerns that are already covered in other questions of the interview need not be written.)

During the meeting, it may be helpful to have one surveyor conduct the interview while another takes notes. At the beginning of the meeting, use the probes on the first page of the protocol to guide introductions and describing the purpose of the interview. Spend a few minutes establishing rapport with the group by letting them direct the conversation. If residents have nothing to say at this time, use a general question such as, "Tell me what life is like in this facility," or "What makes a good day for you here?" Then continue with the protocol questions, probing for more information where necessary and presenting questions in an order that is sensible to the conversation. Get residents to talk in terms of actual situations or examples, using open-ended probes such as: "Can you tell me more about that? Can you give me an example?" or "How does that work here?"

After the meeting, follow-up on any concerns the residents have raised that are within the scope of the long-term care requirements. Share these concerns with the team to focus their investigations.

3. Interview With Family Member or Friend of Non-Interviewable Resident

The family interview is the first part of a two-part protocol. The purpose of this interview is to obtain information about the prior and current preferences of a subsample of non-interviewable residents to help assess whether the facility is individualizing daily life activities, care and services to the highest practicable level. The information gained through the interview will be used to complete Part D. below, the Observation of Non-Interviewable Resident. Follow-up on any concerns raised by the family member about the resident's treatment by the facility.

Use Table 1 in Task 4, to determine how many residents will receive the family interview and resident observation. For example, in a facility with a census of 100, 2 residents are selected.

Prior to the interview, review the relevant sections of the Minimum Data Set about past activities and preferences, and the resident's social history and activities assessment, if any. Begin completing this worksheet with information from the chart, and then use the interview to fill in missing information.

Information about a resident's past lifestyle and preferences may be more or less relevant, depending on the resident's condition and on the length of time spent in the nursing home. However, even after years of institutionalization, some features of a resident's prior life may still be relevant, even if the resident is now debilitated and uncommunicative. Collect information about how the resident's current cognitive status and physical condition have changed his/her past preferences.

Family members do not always know the prior history of a nursing home resident. Therefore, Question 1 of this interview serves to obtain information about the family member's knowledge of the resident. If the family member's answers to Question 1 show that he/she has little or no knowledge of the resident's past history, this interview may be discontinued. If discontinued, end the interview with a general question such as, "What would you like to tell me about this facility and how your relative is treated?" This resident can still remain as part of the survey sample. Select another non-interviewable resident from the sample for a family interview and observation of non-interviewable resident protocol.

If the family member has partial knowledge, the interview may be partially completed with whatever information is obtained in answer to the protocol questions.

Be aware that family members may have strong emotions about their relative's decline and institutionalization. Allow them to express their feelings, but gently direct them back to the questions of the protocol.

The interview may be conducted in person with a family member who was met on tour or by telephone, if necessary.

The second part of this protocol is the Observation of Non-Interviewable Resident. The purpose of this protocol is to obtain information through direct observation about the quality of life of the non-interviewable residents who have received family interviews.

Combine the information gained during the interview with what has been learned about the resident during the Resident Review to write any special items to observe in item 1. What special needs and preferences does this resident have that the nursing home should be taking into account? For example, a resident is ambulatory with Alzheimer's Disease. Her prior life included meeting the school bus at 3 p.m. every day to pick up her children. Now she attempts to leave the facility around that time. What is the facility doing to accommodate this agenda of the resident? Another resident enjoyed being outdoors, and the family member stated she believes this resident would still like the opportunity to go outdoors. Is the facility responding to this preference? Another resident preferred tea to coffee. Is this preference taken into account? A resident preferred to be addressed as Mrs. Hernandez. How does staff address this resident? A resident liked to ski, but can no longer do so due to her condition. However, she may like to see a movie on skiing, have a skiing picture in her room, or go outside in the snow. Has the facility noted this preference? A resident always watched a certain soap opera every day. The family member says that even though she is now confused, this show may still attract her interest. Is this show being made available to the resident?

Use this protocol to complete approximately 1 hour of observations per resident, divided into short segments in at least three settings, at different times of the day. This need not be dedicated time -- surveyors can complete other tasks while conducting this observation. Part of the time should be spent in a location in which what is happening as staff interact with the resident in his/her room can be observed. The remainder of the time should be divided among other locations frequented by the resident, including the dining room, activities rooms, other common areas, and therapy rooms. Some observations of this resident may have already been completed prior to the interview, as part of the Resident Review. Continue making observations until all probes on the worksheet are covered, including the special items noted for observation. When making observations of the resident in particular settings, e.g., an activity or physical therapy, observations need not be for the entire duration of the activity or therapy session.

Use the probes in this protocol to guide observations. Note the areas of concern on the Resident Review Worksheet. For each concern, be specific in noting time, location, and exact observations. Record what is seen and heard, rather than a judgment of the situation. Instead of writing that the resident's dignity was violated by some interaction, simply record the interaction.

NOTE: During the individual, group and family interviews, ask questions regarding their awareness of to whom and how to report allegations, incidents and/or complaints. Share this information with the surveyor assigned to complete Task 5G.

Follow-up on areas of concern observed. For example, at lunch it was observed that the resident was given only one food item at a time. The resident was reaching out for other food and his/her drink. Determine through staff interview and chart review if this method of feeding this resident has a therapeutic purpose or if it is an unnecessary restriction on his/her freedom to select the food he/she wishes to eat.

Share observations with the team to assist them in their investigations of quality of life of other residents.

D. Follow-Up on Concerns Raised Through Interviews

Whenever information is obtained about areas of concern through resident interviews, attempt to investigate these areas through whatever means are appropriate. These might include interviews with other residents, staff, and families, and reviews of written facility information such as policies and procedures, and the admission rights information given to residents.

Sometimes these other sources will provide no other corroborating information. If that is the case, the team will determine during decision-making if the requirement is met or not met through the information obtained in resident interviews.

E. Confidentiality

If residents or family members have stated during interviews that they do not want certain information they have shared in confidence to be shared with the facility, respect their wishes. However, the issue can still be investigated. During the survey, discuss the issue with the team and make the topic the subject of other interviews and observations. For example, a resident has said that certain staff "make fun" of him/her, but he/she asks you to keep that in confidence. The resident's comment may not be referred to in the statement of deficiencies. However, discuss this with the team and decide how best to pursue the matter while respecting the resident's wishes. Team members may want to address this topic with other residents, family members or the resident group. When aware of which staff are involved, attempt to observe these staff interacting with residents.

If other residents have complained about the same problem, their comments may be referred to generally as a group. For example, "Three out of five residents interviewed reported that..." Use judgment to determine if the statement would compromise the resident's confidentiality

Sub-Task 5E - Medication Pass and Pharmacy Services

(Rev. 22, Issued: 12-15-06, Effective/Implementation: 12-18-06)

A. Objectives

- To determine whether the facility safely administers medications including:
    - Accuracy of medication administration (including preparation and technique);
    - Labeling that contains at least the name and strength/concentration of the medication, as well as expiration date when applicable, and
    - Security of medications;
- To determine whether medications are stored and handled in accordance with manufacturers' recommendations and/or state or federal requirements;
- To determine whether the facility reconciles controlled medications, as appropriate;
- To determine whether the facility obtains the services of a licensed pharmacist; and
- To determine whether the facility provides or obtains pharmaceutical services, including routine and emergency medications, to meet the needs of each resident.

B. Use

- The medication pass (C.1) and a review of storage and access to medications (C.2) must be conducted on every Initial and Standard survey; and on Partial Extended, Abbreviated Standard and Revisit, as necessary;
- Review for the provision of licensed pharmacist consultation (C.5) on the initial survey and on any other survey type, if the survey team has identified concerns that indicate:
    - That the facility does not have a licensed pharmacist; and/or
    - That the licensed pharmacist may not have performed his/her functions related to the provision of pharmaceutical services;
- Review for the development and implementation of pharmaceutical procedures (C.4) if, during the course of the survey, concerns have been identified regarding

the availability of medications; accurate and timely medication acquisition; receiving, dispensing, administering, labeling, and storage of medications; reconciliation of controlled medications (C.3); and the use of qualified, authorized personnel to handle and dispense medications.

C. General Procedures

1. Medication Pass (includes labeling)

See Guidance to Surveyors at 483.25(m) for information on conducting the medication pass and for the identification of medication errors. Use the Medication Pass Worksheet (Form CMS-677, Exhibit 88) to record observations. On Form CMS-677, the column marked "Record" is for the purpose of recording the prescriber's actual order if different than what was observed as administered.

When observing the medication pass:

- Be as neutral and unobtrusive as possible;

- Observe different routes and/or forms of medications such as intravenous (IV), intramuscular (IM), or subcutaneous (SQ) injections; transdermal patches; inhaler medications; eye drops; and medications provided through enteral tubes;

- Initially observe the administration at least 20-25 medications, observing as many staff administering medications as possible to facilitate a review of the facility's entire medication distribution system;

- Record, from the medication label, the name and dose/concentration of each medication administered. Also record the route of administration (if other than oral) and the expiration date, if expired;

- Record all multiples, such as 2 drops or 2 tablets. For liquids, record actual volume, or in the case of items such as psyllium, record number of "rounded teaspoonfuls" and the amount of liquid. In the absence of a number, it is assumed to be one;

- Observe whether staff confirmed the resident's identity prior to giving medications and whether the medications were identified up to the point of administration. Note any concerns;

- Record the techniques and procedures that staff used to handle and administer medications, such as proper hand hygiene, checking pulses, flushing gastric tubes, crushing medications, route and location of administration (e.g., sub-Q or IM injection, eye, ear, inhalation, or skin patch), shaking and/or rotating medication, giving medications with or between food or meals, whether medications are under the direct control/observation of the authorized staff; and

- Observe whether staff immediately documented the administration and/or refusal of the medication after the administration or the attempt. Note any concerns.

After the medication pass, compare your observations with the prescriber's orders. Review to assure that medication records, including prescriber's orders and the Medication Administration Record (MAR) are accurate and complete. Determine whether there was an error(s) in medication administration. A medication error is the preparation or administration of medications or biologicals that is not in accordance with any of the following:

- The prescriber's order (whether given incorrectly or omitting an ordered dosage);

- Manufacturer's specifications (not recommendations) regarding the preparation and administration of the medication or biological;

- Accepted professional standards and principles that apply to professionals providing services;

  NOTE: If no errors are found after reconciliation of the pass with the prescriber's orders, the medication pass observation is complete.

- If one or more errors are found, observe the administration of another 20-25 medications.

After completion of the observations and reconciliations, calculate the facility's medication error rate, if one or more errors are found. Add the number of significant and non-significant errors (see guidance at F332/333) and divide by the opportunities for error (doses given plus the doses ordered but not given). Multiply this by 100.

If it is determined that the facility's overall error rate (including significant and non-significant errors) is 5 percent or more, a medication error deficiency exists at F332.

If one or more significant errors were identified, a medication error deficiency exists at F333.

NOTE: If a **significant** medication error has been identified during the course of a Resident Review, including a complaint investigation, it is not necessary to have observed a medication pass in order to cite a deficiency at F333.

2. **Medication Storage (includes labeling)**

Review medication storage (Use CMS Form 803 for documentation) in order to determine whether:

- Medications and biologicals are accessible only to authorized staff and are locked when not under the direct observation of the authorized staff;
- Controlled medications are stored in a manner to limit access and to facilitate reconciliation in accordance with the facility policies;
- Medications are stored to maintain their integrity and to support safe administration of the correct medication to the correct resident, by the correct route and in the correct dose, such as:
    - Temperature, light, and humidity controls meet specifications for the medication;
    - Medications available for use are not expired, contaminated, or unusable;
    - Medication labels are legible; intact; contain the name and dose/concentration of the medication, appropriate cautionary/accessory instructions such as "do not crush," expiration date when applicable; and support the safe administration of the medication; and
    - Multi-dose vials are labeled per facility policy and manufacturer's specifications once use of the vial has been initiated.

3. Controlled Medications

If a concern regarding controlled medications was identified during the survey process or during the medication pass, interview facility staff, such as the director of nursing, and the licensed pharmacist regarding the concern. If a potential problem has been identified regarding lack of reconciliation or loss of controlled medications:

- Determine whether Scheduled II controlled medications are in separately locked, permanently affixed compartments (or are a minimal amount of unit dose packages);
- Review the facility procedure and a sample of the reconciliation records, and compare the amount of medication available with the amount the records indicate should be available; and
- Interview the director of nursing and/or licensed pharmacist regarding:

- Actual frequency of the reconciliation;

- How the facility investigates loss or inability to reconcile controlled medications; and

- How the licensed pharmacist has been involved in recognizing the situation and collaborating with the facility to review and update its practices and procedures.

4. Pharmaceutical Services

If concerns have been identified regarding pharmaceutical services (such as: any of the required components related to safe medication use, storage, labeling; the use of authorized staff to administer medications; emergency medication issues; licensed pharmacist consultation), review the facility's evidence (e.g., licensed pharmacist's reports to the facility) that they have been receiving ongoing pharmacy consultation regarding all aspects of the provision of pharmaceutical services in the facility, including identification of problems and recommendations for corrective actions. Determine whether the licensed pharmacist is available during the survey or identify how to contact the licensed pharmacist in order to respond to surveyor questions about pharmaceutical services. Review procedures and interview staff and/or the licensed pharmacist regarding the areas of concern.

For example, the following steps might be used, if a concern has been identified regarding medications not being administered in a timely manner:

- Identify the types of medications (such as antibiotics, pain medications) that are not being passed on a timely basis,

- Interview the director of nursing and/or the staff responsible for passing medications regarding:

    - A delay in obtaining or administering a medication(s);

    - The potential causes of the delay; and

    - Facility procedures for scheduled times of administration;

- Interview the licensed pharmacist to determine if he/she identified the concern regarding timely medication administration and had made recommendations to facility staff in order to address the concern;

- Interview facility staff regarding the response to recommendations made by the licensed pharmacist; and

- As necessary, if concerns are identified regarding sufficient authorized staff to pass medications, interview the director of nursing regarding staff assignments and work allocation in relation to medication passes in order to meet the needs of the residents.

5. Provision of a Licensed Pharmacist

If there is no licensed pharmacist providing services in the facility, interview the administrator and others, as appropriate, regarding:

- The length of time the facility has been without the services of a licensed pharmacist; and

- Current efforts underway to obtain the services of a licensed pharmacist.

If the facility has a licensed pharmacist, and concerns have been identified regarding the provision of services related to his/her functions, interview the licensed pharmacist, administrator, and, as necessary, the director of nurses and/or medical director regarding the processes to provide and oversee pharmaceutical services consultation.

Sub-Task 5F - Quality Assessment and Assurance **(QA&A)** Review

A. General Objectives—The QA&A review protocol is designed to determine if:

- A QA&A committee exists and meets in accordance with the regulatory requirements of 42 CFR 483.75 (o); and

- The QA&A committee is functional, i.e., it identifies, develops, plans, implements, monitors, and ensures correction of deviations from quality.

B. General Procedures—to complete Sub-Task 5F, follow the Investigative Protocol contained in the Guidance to Surveyors at F520.

NOTE: The surveyor(s) completing Sub-Task 5F should not conduct a review of the minutes of the QA&A committee, as the regulation does not require the facility to disclose the records of the QA&A committee.

Sub-Task 5G - Abuse Prohibition Review

A. General Objective

To determine if the facility has developed and operationalized policies and procedures that prohibit abuse, neglect, involuntary seclusion and misappropriation of property for all residents. The review includes components of the facility's policies and procedures as contained in the Guidance to Surveyors at 42 CFR 483.13(c), F226. (See Guidance to Surveyors for further information.)

These include policies and procedures for the following:

- Screening of potential hirees;
- Training of employees (both for new employees, and ongoing training for all employees);
- Prevention policies and procedures;
- Identification of possible incidents or allegations which need investigation;
- Investigation of incidents and allegations;
- Protection of residents during investigations; and
- Reporting of incidents, investigations, and facility response to the results of their investigations.

B. General Procedures:

- Utilize the Abuse Prohibition Investigative Protocol to complete this task.

Investigative Protocol

Abuse Prohibition

Objective:

To determine if the facility has developed and operationalized policies and procedures that prohibit abuse, neglect, involuntary seclusion and misappropriation of property for all residents.

Use:

Use this protocol on every standard survey.

Task 5G Procedures:

- Obtain and review the facility's abuse prohibition policies and procedures to determine that they include the key components, i.e. screening, training, prevention, identification, investigation, protection and reporting/response. (See

Guidance to Surveyors at F226.) It is not necessary for these items to be collected in one document or manual.

- Interview the individual(s) identified by the facility as responsible for coordinating the policies and procedures to evaluate how each component of the policies and procedures is operationalized, if not obvious from the policies. How do you monitor the staff providing and/or supervising the delivery of resident care and services to assure that care service is provided as needed to assure that neglect of care does not occur? How do you determine which injuries of unknown origin should be investigated as alleged occurrences of abuse? How are you ensuring that residents, families, and staff feel free to communicate concerns without fear of reprisal?

- Request written evidence of how the facility has handled alleged violations. Select 2-3 alleged violations (if the facility has this many) since the previous standard survey or the previous time this review has been done by the State.

  - Determine if the facility implemented adequate procedures:

    - For reporting and investigating;

    - For protection of the resident during the investigation;

    - For the provision of corrective action;

  NOTE: The reporting requirements at 483.13(c) specify both a report of the alleged violation and a report of the results of the investigation to the State survey agency.

  - Determine if the facility reevaluated and revised applicable procedures as necessary.

- Interview several residents and families regarding their awareness of to whom and how to report allegations, incidents and/or complaints. This information can be obtained through the resident, group, and family interviews at Task 5D.

- Interview at least five direct care staff, representing all three shifts, including activity staff and nursing assistants, to determine the following:

  - If staff are trained in and are knowledgeable about how to appropriately intervene in situations involving residents who have aggressive or catastrophic reactions.

    NOTE: Catastrophic reactions are extraordinary reactions of residents to ordinary stimuli, such as the attempt to provide care. One definition in current literature is: ". . . catastrophic reactions

[are] defined as reactions or mood changes of the resident in response to what may seem to be minimal stimuli (e.g., bathing, dressing, having to go to the bathroom, a question asked of the person) that can be characterized by weeping, blushing, anger, agitation, or stubbornness. "Catastrophic reactions and other behaviors of Alzheimer residents: Special unit compared to traditional units." Elizabeth A Swanson, Meridean L. Maas, and Cathleen Buckwalter. Archives of Psychiatric Nursing. Vol. VII No. 5 (October 1993). Pp. 292-299.

- o If staff are knowledgeable regarding what, when and to whom to report according to the facility policies.

- Interview at least three front line supervisors of staff who interact with residents (Nursing, Dietary, Housekeeping, Activities, Social Services). Determine how they monitor the provision of care/services, the staff/resident interactions, deployment of staff to meet the residents' needs, and the potential for staff burnout which could lead to resident abuse.

- Obtain a list of all employees hired within the previous 4 months, and select five from this list. Ask the facility to provide written evidence that the facility conducted pre-screening based on the regulatory requirements at 42 CFR 483.13(c).

Task 6 Determination of Compliance:

Take account of all the information gained during this review as well as all other information gained during the survey. When a deficiency exists, determine if F225 or F226 provides the best regulatory support for the deficiency.

- 483.13(c), F226, Staff Treatment of Residents:
  - o The facility is compliant with this requirement if they have developed and implemented written policies and procedures that prohibit mistreatment, neglect, and abuse of residents and misappropriation of resident property. If not, cite at F226.

- 483.13(c)(1)(2)(3)and (4), F225, Staff Treatment of Residents:
  - o The facility is compliant with this requirement if they took appropriate actions in the areas of screening, reporting, protecting, investigating and taking appropriate corrective actions. If not, cite at F225.

Task 6 - Information Analysis for Deficiency Determination

A. General Objectives

The objectives of information analysis for deficiency determination are:

- To review and analyze all information collected and to determine whether or not the facility has failed to meet one or more of the regulatory requirements; and

- To determine whether to conduct an extended survey.

B. Overview

The worksheets and procedures are designed to assist the surveyor in gathering, investigating, organizing, and analyzing information about the quality of services provided by the facility in order to determine whether the facility has failed to meet long-term care requirements.
The information gathering portions of the survey have focused on the resident and the delivery of services by the facility using observation, interview and record review as sources of information. The information analysis and decision-making portion of the survey focuses on making determinations about whether the facility meets requirements.

Information analysis and decision Making builds on discussions of the daily team meetings, which should include discussions of observed problems, areas of concern, and possible failure to meet requirements.

Decisions about deficiencies are to be team decisions with each member of the team, including specialty surveyors (see Section I.C.), having input into the decisions. The team coordinator or designee should document the deficiency decisions and the substance of the evidence on the Form CMS- 807.

For initial surveys, a determination must be made regarding whether the facility meets every long-term care requirement.

C. Decision-Making Process

Each member of the team should review his/her worksheets to identify concerns and specific evidence relating to requirements that the facility has potentially failed to meet. In order to identify the facility's deficient practices and to enable collating and evaluating the evidence, worksheets should reflect the source of the evidence and should summarize the concerns on relevant data tags.

- Begin the decision-making task by taking into account the daily discussions, the findings documented on the worksheets, discussions with the facility, observations over the course of the survey, and the discussions regarding definitions of deficiencies in the following section. At a minimum, focus on the regulatory groupings 42 CFR 483.10, Resident Rights; 42 CFR 483.13, Resident Behavior and Facility Practice; 42 CFR 483.15, Quality of Life; 42 CFR 483.20, Resident Assessment' and 42 CFR 483.25, Quality of Care. Gather information from all worksheets pertinent to the particular requirements being reviewed (e.g., documentation from all worksheets concerning resident rights). In general, what is the facility's performance in meeting these requirements? Does the facility protect and promote resident rights? Discuss results of the information-gathering phase in the context of facility conformance with these resident-centered requirements and the examples of resident-facility interactions that cause you to believe there may be deficiencies.

- Prioritize the review of worksheets so that the first information the team discusses relates to those requirements that the facility has potentially failed to meet. For example, what documentation on the Quality of Life Assessment worksheet supports the belief that the facility does not protect and promote resident rights? What information on other worksheets supports or does not support the team's assessment of Resident Rights? Evaluate the specifics of the regulatory language and the specific data collected (e.g., observation, resident, family and staff interview information) with respect to the facility's performance in each requirement. Review the worksheets on an individual tag-by-tag basis. If data indicate that the facility has not met a specific requirement (see Task 6, Section D), document that deficiency.

- In order to ensure that no requirements are missed, proceed through the requirements sequentially as they appear in the interpretive guidelines, preferably section by section. Findings/evidence within each section should be shared by each team member during this discussion. Consider all aspects of the requirements within the tag/section being discussed and evaluate how the information gathered relates to the specifics of the regulatory language and to the facility's performance in each requirement. The team should come to consensus on each requirement for which problems have been raised by any member. If no problems are identified for a particular tag number during the information gathering process, then no deficiency exists for that tag number.

- The team coordinator, or a designee, collates all information and records the substance of the decision-making discussion on the Form CMS-807. (See Exhibit 95.)

- Determine if there is substandard quality of care.

- If substandard quality of care exists, conduct an extended survey.

D. Deficiency Criteria

To determine if a deficiency exists, use the following definitions and guidance:

- A "deficiency" is defined as a facility's failure to meet a participation requirement specified in the Social Security Act or in Part 483, Subpart B (i.e., 42 CFR 483.5 - 42 CFR 483.75).

- To help determine if a deficiency exists, look at the language of the requirement. Some requirements need to be met for each resident. Any violation of these requirements, even for one resident, is a deficiency.

- Other requirements focus on facility systems.

For some requirements, especially those in the regulatory grouping of Quality of Life (42 CFR 483.15), the team will evaluate the sum of the staff actions and/or decisions for an individual resident to determine if the requirement is met for that individual. Quality of Life requirements are best evaluated comprehensively, rather than in terms of a single incident. However, a single incident which is considered severe enough may result in a deficiency.

Certain facility systems requirements must be met in an absolute sense, e.g., a facility must have a RN on duty 7 days a week unless it has received a waiver. Other facility system requirements are best evaluated comprehensively, rather than in terms of a single incident. In evaluating these requirements, the team will examine both the individual parts of the system, e.g., the adequacy of the infection control protocol, the adequacy of facility policy on hand washing, as well as the actual implementation of that system.

E. Evidence Evaluation

The survey team must evaluate the evidence documented during the survey to determine if a deficiency exists due to a failure to meet a requirement and if there are any negative resident outcomes due to the failure. Failure to meet requirements related to quality of care, resident rights, and quality of life generally fall into two categories:

1. Potential or Actual Physical, Mental or Psychosocial Injury or Deterioration to A Resident Including Violation of Residents' Rights

   Some situations which illustrate this level of harm could be:

   a. Development of, or worsening of, a pressure sore;

   b. Loss of dignity due to lying in a urine-saturated bed for a prolonged period; and

c. Social isolation caused by staff failure to assist the resident in participating in scheduled activities.

This category of negative outcome may be identified when an identified facility practice is so divergent from accepted principles of practice that harm has occurred or a future negative outcome or harm is probable. An example would be nurse aides in a facility who often fail to wash their hands between caring for residents. In this example, there is a strong potential for harm although there has been no evidence of a high facility infection rate, or of infections spreading from one resident to another. Should a resident contract an infection or become colonized with a highly contagious bacteria, there is a high potential for a major outbreak of nosocomial infection.

2. Lack of (or the Potential for Lack of) Reaching the Highest Practicable Level of Physical, Mental or Psychosocial Well-Being

No deterioration occurred, but the facility failed to provide necessary care for resident improvement. For example:

a. The facility identified the resident's desire to reach a higher level of ability, e.g., improvement in ambulation, and care was planned accordingly. However, the facility failed to implement, or failed to consistently implement the plan of care, and the resident failed to improve, i.e., did not reach his/her highest practicable well-being;

b. The facility identified a need in the comprehensive assessment, e.g., the resident was withdrawn/depressed, but the facility did not develop a care plan or prioritize this need of the resident, planning to address it at a later time. The resident received no care or treatment to address the need and did not improve, i.e., remained withdrawn/depressed. Therefore, the resident was not given the opportunity to reach his/her highest practicable well-being;

c. The facility failed to identify the resident's need/problem/ability to improve, e.g., the ability to eat independently if given assistive devices, and, therefore, did not plan care appropriately. As a result, the resident failed to reach his/her highest practicable well-being, i.e., eat independently.

d. A facility's written procedures or oral explanations do not provide information about which residents are supposed to be fully informed, e.g., the resident is provided treatment which they may have wished to refuse.

If the resident is the primary source of information, the team should conduct further information gathering and analysis. This may include additional interviews with family and staff or record reviews to supplement or corroborate the resident's report. If additional sources of information are not available, determine if the interviewees are reliable sources of information and if the information received is accurate. If so, citation of a deficiency may be based on resident information alone.

In cases where residents are unable to speak for themselves, the survey team should assess how most people would react to the situation in question. For example, a female resident who is unable to express herself is wheeled down the hall in a wheelchair on the way to her shower with only a towel partially covering her body. The team will decide if this incident is inappropriate because the resident is unable to express herself. Quality of life and Residents' Rights requirements are most often evaluated using this type of analysis.

F. Determination of Substandard Quality of Care

The team must determine if substandard quality of care exists. Substandard quality of care is defined as one or more deficiencies related to participation requirements under 42 CFR 483.13, Resident Behavior and Facility Practices, 42 CFR 483.15, Quality of Life, or 42 CFR 483.25, Quality of Care which, constitute either immediate jeopardy to resident health or safety, pattern or widespread deficiencies at severity level 3, or widespread deficiencies at severity level 2. (See Section V., Deficiency Categorization.)

G. Special Circumstances

Substandard quality of care and immediate jeopardy determinations trigger additional survey tasks and must be determined during the information gathering tasks of the survey and/or during information analysis and decision-making.

Immediate jeopardy is defined as a situation in which the facility's failure to meet one or more requirements of participation has caused, or is likely to cause, serious injury, harm, impairment, or death to a resident. At any time during the survey, if one or more team members identifies possible immediate jeopardy, the team should meet immediately to confer. The guiding principles to determine immediate jeopardy and serious threat make it clear that the threat can be related to mental, as well as physical well-being, and that the situation in question need not be a widespread problem. If the team concurs, the team coordinator must consult immediately with his/her supervisor. If the supervisor concurs that the situation constitutes immediate jeopardy, the team coordinator informs the facility Administrator or designee that the immediate jeopardy termination procedures are being invoked. The team coordinator should explain the nature of the immediate jeopardy to the Administrator or designee. The survey team should complete the entire survey. See Appendix Q for guidance regarding determination of immediate jeopardy, and §3010 for procedures to follow if the immediate jeopardy termination procedures are invoked.

When surveyors suspect substandard quality of care (SQC), they expand the standard (or abbreviated) survey sample as necessary to determine scope (Refer to Task 4,

Supplementary Sample for further information). If there is no deficiency(ies) classified as substandard quality of care and there is a deficiency under the regulatory Groupings of 42 CFR 483.13, 42 CFR 483.15 and/or 42 CFR 483.25, that are classified as an isolated incident of severity level 3, or, as a pattern of severity level 2, then determine if there is sufficient evidence to make the decision that there is not substandard quality of care.

If the evidence is not adequate and the number of observations only allowed for isolated scope when there is a severity level 3, or pattern for scope when there is a severity level 2, then expand the sample to include additional reviews of that requirement. For example, if residents in the facility are receiving care for a colostomy, and for the one resident with a colostomy in the sample, it is determined that care provided caused actual harm to the resident, there would be a deficiency of isolated actual harm, but there would not be sufficient evidence to determine that there was substandard quality of care. Thus, the sample would need to be expanded before determining that substandard quality of care did or did not exist. On the other hand, if the number of individuals with a colostomy in the facility was the same (6), and 4 residents with colostomies were included in the sample and only one had deficient care, there would be no need to expand the sample. If the team verifies the existence of SQC, the Administrator should be informed that the facility is in SQC and an extended (or partial extended) survey will be conducted. If expanding the sample determines that SQC does not exist, no extended or partial extended survey will be conducted.

H. Determining Citations of Past Noncompliance at the Time of the Current Survey

Past noncompliance may be identified during any survey of a nursing home. To cite past noncompliance with a specific survey data tag (F-tag or K-tag), all of the following three criteria must be met:

1. The facility was not in compliance with the specific regulatory requirement(s) (as referenced by the specific F-tag or K-tag) at the time the situation occurred;
2. The noncompliance occurred after the exit date of the last standard recertification survey and before the survey (standard, complaint, or revisit) currently being conducted; and
3. There is sufficient evidence that the facility corrected the noncompliance and is in substantial compliance at the time of the current survey for the specific regulatory requirement(s), as referenced by the specific F-tag or K-tag.

Task 7 - Exit Conference

A. General Objective

The general objective of the exit conference is to inform the facility of the survey team's observations and preliminary findings.

B. Conduct of Exit Conference

Conduct the exit conference with facility personnel. Invite the ombudsman and an officer of the organized residents group, if one exists, to the exit conference. Also, invite one or two residents to attend. The team may provide an abbreviated exit conference specifically for residents after completion of the normal facility exit conference. If two exit conferences are held, notify the ombudsman and invite the ombudsman to attend either or both conferences.

Do not discuss survey results in a manner that reveals the identity of an individual resident. Provide information in a manner that is understandable to those present, e.g., say the deficiency "relates to development of pressure sores," not "Tag F314."

Describe the team's preliminary deficiency findings to the facility and let them know they will receive a report of the survey which will contain any deficiencies that have been cited (Form CMS-2567). If requested, provide the facility with a list of residents included in the standard survey sample. Do not give the team's Roster/Sample Matrixes to the facility, because they contain confidential information.

If an extended survey is required and the survey team cannot complete all or part of the extended survey prior to the exit conference, inform the Administrator that the deficiencies, as discussed in the conference, may be amended upon completion of the extended survey. (See §2724 for additional information concerning exit conferences.)

During the exit conference, provide the facility with the opportunity to discuss and supply additional information that they believe is pertinent to the identified findings. Because of the ongoing dialogue between surveyors and facility staff during the survey, there should be few instances where the facility is not aware of surveyor concerns or has not had an opportunity to present additional information prior to the exit conference.

II.B – The Traditional Survey (Continued)

II.B.2. - The Traditional Extended and/or Partial Extended Survey

Conduct an extended survey subsequent to a standard survey and conduct a partial extended survey subsequent to an abbreviated survey when you have determined that there is a substandard quality of care in:

- 42 CFR 483.13, Resident behavior and facility practices;
- 42 CFR 483.15, Quality of life; and/or
- 42 CFR 483.25, Quality of care.

When conducting the extended/partial extended survey, at a minimum, fully review and verify compliance with each tag number within 42 CFR 483.30, Nursing Services; 42 CFR 483.40, Physician Services; and 42 CFR 483.75, Administration. Focus on the facility's policies and procedures that may have produced the substandard quality of care. As appropriate, include a review of staffing, inservice training and the infection control program. An extended/partial extended survey explores the extent to which structure and process factors such as written policies and procedures, staff qualifications and functional responsibilities, and specific agreements and contracts of the facility may have contributed to the outcomes. If the extended/partial extended survey was triggered by a deficiency in quality of care, conduct a detailed review of the accuracy of resident assessment. During the partial extended survey, consider expanding the scope of the review to include a more comprehensive evaluation of the requirements at 42 CFR 483.13, 42 CFR 483.15, and/or 42 CFR 483.25 in which substandard quality of care was found.
Document the observations from the extended or partial extended survey on the Form CMS-805, (see Exhibit 93) or the Form CMS-807 (see Exhibit 95).

Review of the Accuracy of Resident Assessments During an Extended/Partial Extended Survey

The objective of this review is to determine if resident assessments are accurate.

If an extended/partial extended survey is conducted based on substandard quality of care in Quality of Care (42 CFR 483.25), review the accuracy of resident assessments by:

- Reviewing a sample of comprehensive resident assessments completed no more than 30 days prior to conducting the survey;

- Comparing observations of the resident with the facility's assessment;

- Conducting the number of assessment reviews needed to make a decision concerning the accuracy of the facility's resident assessments; and

- Determining if observations of the resident, and interviews with resident/staff/family, "match" the facility's assessment (or specific portions of the assessment) of the resident. If observations and interviews do not "match," investigate further.

Record the indepth review of the accuracy of resident assessments on page 3 of the Form CMS-805. (See Exhibit 93.)

Timing for Conducting the Extended Survey and Partial Extended Survey

Conduct the extended or partial extended survey:

- Prior to the exit conference, in which case the facility will be provided with information from the standard, abbreviated standard, partial extended or extended surveys; or,

- Not later than 2 weeks after the standard/abbreviated survey is completed, if the team is unable to conduct the extended survey or partial extended survey concurrent with the standard survey or the abbreviated survey. Advise the facility's Administrator that there will be an extended or partial extended survey conducted and that an exit conference will be held at the completion of the survey.

II.B. – The Traditional Survey (Continued)

II.B.3 - The Traditional Post Survey Revisit (Follow-Up)

In accordance with §7317, the State agency conducts a revisit, as applicable, to confirm that the facility is in compliance and has the ability to remain in compliance. The purpose of the post-survey revisit (follow-up) is to re-evaluate the specific care and services that were cited as noncompliant during the original standard, abbreviated standard, extended or partial extended survey(s). Ascertain the status of corrective actions being taken on all requirements not in substantial compliance. Section 7304 contains the 5 elements a facility must address in developing an acceptable plan of correction. One of these elements is what continuous quality improvement system(s) a facility has in place to monitor its performance in identifying the deficient practice/care and assuring that it does not recur.

Because this survey process focuses on the care of the resident, revisits are generally necessary to ascertain whether the deficient practices have been corrected. The nature of the noncompliance dictates the scope of the revisit. For example, do not perform another drug pass if no drug distribution related deficiencies were cited on the initial survey. Do interviews and closed record reviews, as appropriate. Prior to the revisit, review appropriate documents, including the plan of correction, to focus the revisit review.

Conduct as many survey tasks as needed to determine compliance status. Always conduct Sub-Task 5F. However, the team is not prohibited from gathering information related to any requirement during a post-survey revisit.

When selecting the resident sample for the revisit survey, determine the sample size using 60% of the sample size for a standard survey as described in Table 1, Resident Sample Selection. (Phase 1 sample size is 60%.) The follow-up survey does not require a 2 Phase sample selection.

Focus on selecting residents who are most likely to have those conditions/needs/problems cited in the original survey. If possible, include some residents identified as receiving substandard quality of care during the prior survey. If, after completing the revisit activities, you determine that the cited incidence(s) of noncompliance was not corrected, initiate enforcement action, as appropriate. (See §7400 for specific guidance concerning initiation of enforcement action.)

Use appropriate CMS forms during this survey. However, if the need for documentation is minimal, use the Surveyor Notes Worksheet (Form CMS-808). (See Exhibit 95 to record the results of the revisit.)

II.B. – The Traditional Survey (Continued)

II.B.4 - The Traditional Abbreviated Standard Survey

A. Complaint Investigations

(See also Chapter 5)

B. Substantial Changes in a Facility's Organization and Management

If a facility notifies the survey agency of a change in organization or management, review the change to ensure compliance with the regulations. Request copies of the appropriate documents, e.g., written policies and procedures, personnel qualifications and agreements. If changes in a facility's organization and management are significant and raise questions of its continued compliance, determine, through a survey, whether certain changes have caused a decline in quality of care furnished by a SNF or NF.

III. Writing the Statement of Deficiencies

A. General Objective

The general objective of this section is to write the statement of deficiencies in terms specific enough to allow a reasonably knowledgeable person to understand the aspect(s) of the requirement(s) that is (are) not met. For findings of past noncompliance and or current noncompliance indicate the data prefix tag and regulatory citation, followed by a summary of the evidence and supporting observations using resident identifiers. This documentation must be written in language specific enough to use to identify levels of severity and scope at the completion of the survey. If information was identified during confidential resident interviews, do not include a resident identifier when recording the source of the evidence. List the data tags in the order specified in the Code of Federal Regulations.

When a citation of past noncompliance is written, a nursing home does not provide a plan of correction as the deficiency is already corrected; however, the survey team documents the facility's corrective actions on Form CMS-2567. (Additional information about citations of past noncompliance is found at Chapter 7.)

When a facility is in substantial compliance, but has deficiencies which are isolated with no actual harm and potential for only minimal harm, the deficiencies are recorded on the "Notice of Isolated Deficiencies" instead of on the Form CMS-2567. A plan of correction is not required but a facility is expected to correct all deficiencies.

The statement of deficiencies should:

- Specifically reflect the content of each requirement that is not met;
- Clearly identify the specific deficient entity practices and the objective evidence concerning these practices;
- Identify the extent of the deficient practice, including systemic practices, where appropriate; and
- Identify the source(s) of the evidence, e.g., interview, observation, or record review.

Following deficiency categorization (Section V), enter on Form CMS-2567L the letter corresponding to the box of the scope and severity grid (Chapter 7, §7400.E.) for at least any deficiency which constitutes substandard quality of care and any deficiency which drives the choice of a required remedy category. Enter these letters in ID prefix tag column immediately below the tag number of the Form CMS-2567L.

IV. Deficiency Categorization

A. General Objective

After the survey team determines that a deficiency (ies) exists, assess the effect on resident outcome (severity level) and determine the number of residents potentially or actually affected (scope level). Use the results of this assessment to determine whether or not the facility is in substantial compliance or is noncompliant. When a facility is noncompliant, consider how the deficient practice is classified according to severity and scope levels in selecting an appropriate remedy. (See §7400 for discussion of remedies.)

Scope and severity determinations are also applicable to deficiencies at §483.70(a), Life Safety from Fire.

B. Guidance on Severity Levels

There are four severity levels. Level 1, no actual harm with potential for minimal harm; Level 2, no actual harm with potential for more than minimal harm that is not immediate jeopardy; Level 3, actual harm that is not immediate jeopardy; Level 4, immediate jeopardy to resident health or safety. These four levels are defined accordingly:

1. Level 1 is a deficiency that has the potential for causing no more than a minor negative impact on the resident(s).

2. Level 2 is noncompliance that results in no more than minimal physical, mental and/or psychosocial discomfort to the resident and/or has the potential (not yet realized) to compromise the resident's ability to maintain and/or reach his/her highest practicable physical, mental and/or psychosocial well-being as defined by an accurate and comprehensive resident assessment, plan of care, and provision of services.

3. Level 3 is noncompliance that results in a negative outcome that has compromised the resident's ability to maintain and/or reach his/her highest practicable physical, mental and psychosocial well-being as defined by an accurate and comprehensive resident assessment, plan of care, and provision of services. This does not include a deficient practice that only could or has caused limited consequence to the resident.

4. Level 4 is immediate jeopardy, a situation in which immediate corrective action is necessary because the facility's noncompliance with one or more requirements of participation has caused, or is likely to cause, serious injury, harm, impairment, or death to a resident receiving care in a facility. (See Appendix Q.)

C. Guidance on Scope Levels

Scope has three levels: isolated; pattern; and widespread. The scope levels are defined accordingly:

III. Scope is isolated when one or a very limited number of residents are affected and/or one or a very limited number of staff are involved, and/or the situation has occurred only occasionally or in a very limited number of locations.

IV. Scope is a pattern when more than a very limited number of residents are affected, and/or more than a very limited number of staff are involved, and/or the situation has occurred in several locations, and/or the same resident(s) have been affected by repeated occurrences of the same deficient practice. The effect of the deficient practice is not found to be pervasive throughout the facility.

3. Scope is widespread when the problems causing the deficiencies are pervasive in the facility and/or represent systemic failure that affected or has the potential to affect a large portion or all of the facility's residents. Widespread scope refers to the entire facility population, not a subset of residents or one unit of a facility. In addition, widespread scope may be identified if a systemic failure in the facility (e.g., failure to maintain food at safe temperatures) would be likely to affect a large number of residents and is, therefore, pervasive in the facility.

D. General Procedures

After the team makes a decision to cite a deficiency(ies), evaluate the deficient practice's impact on the resident(s) and the prevalence of the deficient practice. Review deficiency statements, worksheets, and results of team discussions for evidence on which to base these determinations. The team may base evidence of the impact or prevalence for residents of the deficient practices on record reviews, interviews and/or observations. Whatever the source, the evidence must be credible.

After determining the severity level of a deficient practice, determine scope. When determining scope, evaluate the cause of the deficiency. If the facility lacks a system/policy (or has an inadequate system) to meet the requirements and this failure has the potential to affect a large number of residents in the facility, then the deficient practice is likely to be widespread. If an adequate system/policy is in place but is being inadequately implemented in certain instances, or if there is an inadequate system with the potential to impact only a subset of the facility's population, then the deficient practice is likely to be pattern. If the deficiency affects or has the potential to affect one or a very limited number of residents, then the scope is isolated.

If the evidence gathered during the survey for a particular requirement includes examples of various severity or scope levels, surveyors should generally classify the deficiency at the highest level of severity, even if most of the evidence corresponds to a lower severity level. For example, if there is a deficiency in which one resident suffered a severity 3 while there were widespread findings of the same deficiency at severity 2, then the deficiency would be generally classified as severity 3, isolated.

E. Psychosocial Outcome Severity Guide

Purpose

The purpose of the Psychosocial Outcome Severity Guide is to help surveyors determine the severity of psychosocial outcomes resulting from the identified noncompliance at a specific F tag. The Guide is used to determine the severity of a deficiency in any regulatory grouping (e.g., Quality of Care, Quality of Life) that resulted in a negative psychosocial outcome.

This Guide is not intended to replace the current scope and severity grid. It is to be used in conjunction with the scope and severity grid to determine the severity of outcomes to each resident involved in a deficiency that has resulted in a psychosocial outcome. The team should select the level of severity for the deficiency based on the highest level of physical or psychosocial outcome. For example, a resident who was slapped by a staff member may experience only a minor physical outcome from the slap but suffer a greater psychosocial outcome. In this case the severity level based on the psychosocial outcome would be used as the level of severity for the deficiency.

Overview

Psychosocial outcomes (i.e., mood and behavior) may result from a facility's noncompliance with any regulatory requirement. Although a resident may experience either a negative physical outcome or a negative psychosocial outcome, some may experience or have the potential to experience both types of negative outcomes. Psychosocial outcomes and physical outcomes are equally important in determining the severity of noncompliance, and both need to be considered before assigning a severity level. The severity level assigned should reflect the most significant negative outcome or highest level of harm/potential harm.

The presence of a given affect (i.e., behavioral manifestation of mood demonstrated by the resident) does not necessarily indicate a psychosocial outcome that is the direct result of noncompliance. A resident's reactions and responses (or lack thereof) also may be affected by pre-existing psychosocial issues, illnesses, medication side effects, and/or other factors. Because many nursing home residents have sadness, anger, loss of self-esteem, etc. in reaction to normal life experiences, the survey team must have determined that the psychosocial outcome is a result of the noncompliance.

Psychosocial outcomes of interest to surveyors are those caused by the facility's noncompliance with any regulation. This also includes psychosocial outcomes resulting from facility failure to assess and develop an adequate care plan to address a resident's pre-existing psychosocial issues, which led to continuation or worsening of the condition.

Instructions

This Guide is designed to be used separately for each resident included in the deficiency.

Each resident's psychosocial response to the noncompliance is the basis for determining psychosocial severity of a deficiency. To determine severity, use the information gathered through the investigative process (Task 5). Compare the resident's behavior (e.g., their routine, activity, and responses to staff or to everyday situations) and mood before and after the noncompliance.

If the survey team determines that a facility's noncompliance has resulted in a negative psychosocial outcome to one or more residents, the team should use this Guide to evaluate the severity of the outcome for each resident identified in the deficiency (in accordance with the instructions at Task 6). The team should determine severity based on the resident's response in the following circumstances:

- If the resident can communicate a psychosocial reaction to the deficient practice, compare this response to the Guide; or

- If the resident is unable to express her/himself verbally but shows a noticeable non-verbal response that is related to the deficient practice, compare the non-verbal response to the Guide.

Application of the Reasonable Person Concept

There are circumstances in which the survey team may apply the "reasonable person concept" to determine severity of the deficiency. To apply the reasonable person concept, the survey team should determine the severity of the psychosocial outcome or potential outcome the deficiency may have had on a reasonable person in the resident's position (i.e., what degree of actual or potential harm would one expect a reasonable person in a similar situation to suffer as a result of the noncompliance).

NOTE: The reasonable person concept described in this Guide is merely a tool to assist the survey team's assessment of the severity level of negative psychosocial outcomes. Although the reasonable person concept is used in many areas of the law, the application of common law defenses to the assessment of severity pursuant to this Guide would be inappropriate and is expressly precluded.

The survey team should use the reasonable person concept when the resident's psychosocial outcome may not be readily determined through the investigative process:

- When there is no discernable response or when circumstances obstruct the direct evaluation of the resident's psychosocial outcome. Such circumstances may include, but are not limited to, the resident's death, subsequent injury, cognitive impairments, physical impairments, or insufficient documentation by the facility. In this situation, the survey team may use the reasonable person concept to evaluate the severity (Level 2, Level 3, or Level 4) of the deficient practice; or

- When the resident's reaction to a deficient practice is markedly incongruent with the level of reaction the reasonable person would have to the deficient practice. In this situation, the survey team may use the reasonable person concept to evaluate the potential severity (Level 2 or Level 4) of the deficient practice.

Clarification Of Terms

"Anger" refers to an emotion caused by the frustrated attempts to attain a goal, or in response to hostile or disturbing actions such as insults, injuries, or threats that do not come from a feared source.[1]

"Apathy" refers to a marked indifference to the environment; lack of a response to a situation; lack of interest in or concern for things that others find moving or exciting; absence or suppression of passion, emotion, or excitement.[2]

"Anxiety" refers to the apprehensive anticipation of future danger or misfortune accompanied by a feeling of distress, sadness, or somatic symptoms of tension. Somatic symptoms of tension may include, but are not limited to, restlessness, irritability, hyper-vigilance, an exaggerated startle response, increased muscle tone, and teeth grinding. The focus of anticipated danger may be internal or external.[3]

"Dehumanization" refers to the deprivation of human qualities or attributes such as individuality, compassion, or civility.[4] Dehumanization is the outcome resulting from having been treated as an inanimate object or as having no emotions, feelings, or sensations.

"Depressed mood" (which does not necessarily constitute clinical depression) is indicated by negative statements; self-deprecation; sad facial expressions; crying and tearfulness; withdrawal from activities of interest; and/or reduced social interactions.[5] Some residents such as those with moderate or severe cognitive impairment may be more likely to demonstrate nonverbal symptoms of depression.

"Humiliation" refers to a feeling of shame due to being embarrassed, disgraced, or depreciated. Some individuals lose so much self-esteem through humiliation that they become depressed.[6]

PSYCHOSOCIAL OUTCOME SEVERITY GUIDE

The following are levels of negative psychosocial outcomes that developed, continued, or worsened as a result of the facility's noncompliance. This Guide is only to be used once the survey team has determined noncompliance at a regulatory requirement. The survey team must have established a connection between the noncompliance and a negative psychosocial outcome to the resident as evidenced by observations, record review, and/or interviews with residents, their representatives, and/or staff.

Severity Level 4 Considerations: Immediate Jeopardy to Resident Health or Safety

Immediate Jeopardy is a situation in which the facility's noncompliance with one or more requirements of participation:

- Has allowed/caused/resulted in, or is likely to allow/cause /result in serious injury, harm, impairment, or death to a resident; and

- Requires immediate correction, as the facility either created the situation or allowed the situation to continue by failing to implement preventative or corrective measures.

Examples of negative psychosocial outcomes as a result of the facility's noncompliance may include but are not limited to:

- Suicidal ideation/thoughts and preoccupation (with a plan) or suicidal attempt (active or passive) such as trying to jump from a high place, throwing oneself down a flight of stairs, refusing to eat or drink in order to kill oneself.

- Engaging in self-injurious behavior that is likely to cause serious injury, harm, impairment, or death to the resident (e.g., banging head against wall).
- Sustained and intense crying, moaning, screaming, or combative behavior.

- Expressions (verbal and/or non-verbal) of severe, unrelenting, excruciating, and unrelieved pain; pain has become all-consuming and overwhelms the resident.

- Recurrent (i.e., more than isolated or fleeting) debilitating fear/anxiety that may be manifested as panic, immobilization, screaming, and/or extremely aggressive or agitated behavior(s) (e.g., trembling, cowering) in response to an identifiable situation (e.g., approach of a specific staff member).

- Ongoing, persistent expression of dehumanization or humiliation in response to an identifiable situation, that persists regardless of whether the precipitating event(s) has ceased and has resulted in a potentially life-threatening consequence.

- Expressions of anger at an intense and sustained level that has caused or is likely to cause serious injury, harm, impairment, or death to self or others.

Severity Level 3 Considerations: Actual Harm that is not Immediate Jeopardy

Severity Level 3 indicates noncompliance that results in actual harm, and can include but may not be limited to clinical compromise, decline, or the resident's inability to maintain and/or reach his/her highest practicable well-being.

Examples of negative psychosocial outcomes as a result of the facility's noncompliance may include but are not limited to:

- Significant decline in former social patterns that does not rise to a level of immediate jeopardy.

- Persistent depressed mood[7,8,9] that may be manifested by verbal and nonverbal symptoms such as:

  - Social withdrawal; irritability; anxiety; hopelessness; tearfulness; crying; moaning;

  - Loss of interest or ability to experience or feel pleasure nearly every day for much of the day;

  - Psychomotor agitation[10] (e.g., inability to sit still, pacing, hand-wringing, or pulling or rubbing of the skin, clothing, or other objects), accompanied by a bothered or sad expression;

  - Psychomotor retardation (e.g., slowed speech, thinking, and body movements; increased pauses before answering);

  - Verbal agitation[11] (e.g., repeated requests for help, groaning, sighing, or other repeated verbalizations), accompanied by sad facial expressions;

  - Expressions of feelings of worthlessness or excessive guilt nearly every day (not merely self-reproach or guilt about being sick or needing care);

  - Markedly diminished ability to think or concentrate;

  - Recurrent thoughts of death (not just fear of dying) or statements without an intent to act (e.g., "I wish I were dead" or "my family would be better off without me").

- Expressions (verbal and/or non-verbal) of persistent pain or physical distress (e.g., itching, thirst) that has compromised the resident's functioning such as diminished level of participation in social interactions and/or ADLs, intermittent crying and moaning, weight loss and/or diminished appetite. Pain or physical distress has become a central focus of the resident's attention, but it is not all-consuming or overwhelming (as in Severity Level 4).

- Chronic or recurrent fear/anxiety that has compromised the resident's well-being and that may be manifested as avoidance of the fear-inducing situation(s) or person(s); preoccupation with fear; resistance to care and/or social interaction; moderate aggressive or agitated behavior(s) related to fear; sleeplessness due to fear; and/or verbal expressions of fear. Expressions of fear/anxiety are not to the level of panic and immobilization (as in Severity Level 4).

- Ongoing, persistent feeling and/or expression of dehumanization or humiliation that persists regardless of whether the precipitating, dehumanizing event(s) or situation(s) has ceased. The feelings of dehumanization and humiliation have not resulted in a life-threatening consequence.

- Apathy and social disengagement such as listlessness; slowness of response and thought (psychomotor retardation); lack of interest or concern especially in matters of general importance and appeal, resulting from facility noncompliance.
- Sustained distress (e.g., agitation indicative of understimulation as manifested by fidgeting; restlessness; repetitive verbalization of not knowing what to do, needing to go to work, and/or needing to find something).

- Anger that has caused aggression that could lead to injuring self or others. Verbal aggression can be manifested by threatening, screaming, or cursing; physical aggression can be manifested by self-directed responses or hitting, shoving, biting, and scratching others.

Severity Level 2 Considerations: No Actual Harm with Potential for More Than Minimal Harm that is Not Immediate Jeopardy

Severity Level 2 indicates noncompliance that results in a resident outcome of no more than minimal discomfort and/or has the potential to compromise the resident's ability to maintain or reach his or her highest practicable level of well being. The potential exists for greater harm to occur if interventions are not provided.

Examples of negative psychosocial outcomes as a result of the facility's noncompliance may include but are not limited to:

- Intermittent sadness, as reflected in facial expression and/or demeanor, tearfulness, crying, or verbal/vocal agitation (e.g., repeated requests for help, moaning, and sighing).

- Feelings and/or complaints of discomfort or moderate pain. The resident may be irritable and/or express discomfort.

- Fear/anxiety that may be manifested as expressions or signs of minimal discomfort (e.g., verbal expressions of fear/anxiety; pulling away from a feared object or situation) or has the potential, not yet realized, to compromise the resident's well-being.

- Feeling of shame or embarrassment without a loss of interest in the environment and the self.

- Complaints of boredom and/or reports that there is nothing to do, accompanied by expressions of periodic distress that do not result in maladaptive behaviors (e.g., verbal or physical aggression).

- Verbal or nonverbal expressions of anger that did not lead to harm to self or others.

Severity Level 1 Considerations: No Actual Harm with Potential for Minimal Harm

Severity Level 1 is not an option because any facility practice that results in a reduction of psychosocial well-being diminishes the resident's quality of life. The deficiency is, therefore, at least a Severity Level 2 because it has the potential for more than minimal harm.

ENDNOTES

[1] Gall, S., Beins, B., & Feldman, J. (1996). The Gale Encyclopedia of Psychology. Detroit, MI: Gale Research.

[2] Random House. (1981). The Random House Dictionary of the English Language. New York: Author.

[3] American Psychiatric Association (1994). Diagnostic and statistical manual of mental disorders (Fourth Edition). Washington, DC: Author.

[4] Random House. (1981).

[5] Minimum Data Set Version 2.0, Section E.
[6] Corsini, R. (1999). The Dictionary of Psychology. Ann Arbor, MI: Taylor and Francis.

[7] Alexopolous, G., Abrams, R., Young, R., & Shamoian, C. (1988). Cornell scale for depression in dementia. Biological Psychiatry, 23, 271-284.

[8] Brink, T.L., Yesavage, J.A., Lum, O., Heersema, P., Adey, M., & Rose, T.L. (1982). Screening tools for geriatric depression. Clinical Gerontologist, 1, 37-43.

[9] Warren, W.L. (1994). Revised Hamilton Rating Scale for Depression (RHRSD). Los Angeles, CA: Western Psychological Services.

[10] Cohen-Mansfield, J. (2003). Agitation in the elderly: Definitional and theoretical conceptualizations. In D.P. Hay, D. Klein, L. Hay, G. Grossberg, & J.S. Kennedy (Eds.) Agitation in Patients with Dementia: A Practical Guide to Diagnosis and Management (pp. 1-22). Washington, DC: American Psychiatric Publishing Inc.

[11] Cohen-Mansfield, J. (2003). Agitation in the elderly: Definitional and theoretical conceptualizations.

V. Confidentiality and Respect for Resident Privacy

Conduct the survey in a manner that allows for the greatest degree of confidentiality for residents, particularly regarding the information gathered during the in-depth interviews. Use the resident identifier (e.g., a code number the survey team has assigned to each resident in the sample) on the Form CMS-2567 in place of the resident's name, which should never be used on the Form CMS-2567.

When communicating to the facility about substandard quality of care, fully identify the resident(s) by name if the situation was identified through observation or record review. Improperly applied restraints, medication error, cold food, gloves not worn for a sterile procedure, and diet inconsistent with order are examples of practices that can be identified to the facility by resident name. Information about injuries due to broken equipment, prolonged use of restraints, and opened mail is more likely to be obtained through resident and family interviews. Do not identify residents or family members providing this information without their permission.

Notes and worksheets contain pre-decisional information and are, therefore, not required to be disclosed to the facility at the time of the survey. However, once the Form CMS-2567 has been written, portions of the worksheets explaining the findings reported on the Form CMS-2567 may become subject to release under the Freedom of Information Act (FOIA). Information on the worksheets that was not subsequently used as a basis for writing a deficiency remains pre-decisional and is exempt from disclosure. That information would have to be deleted, according to FOIA guidelines, before the worksheets could be released.

The requirements of the FOIA apply only to those documents held by the Federal government. They do not apply to State or local governments. Therefore, surveyor worksheets held by the State are subject to State disclosure laws only.

VI. Information Transfer

In conjunction with conducting surveys, the State should provide information to the facility about care and regulatory topics that would be useful to the facility for understanding and applying best practices in the care and treatment of long term care residents.

This information exchange is not a consultation with the facility, but is a means of disseminating information that may be of assistance to the facility in meeting long term care requirements. States are not liable, nor are they to be held accountable if training which occurs during information transfer does not "correct" problems at the facility.

Performance of the function is at the discretion of the State and can be performed at various times, including during the standard survey, during follow-up or complaint surveys, during other conferences or workshops or at another time mutually agreeable to the survey agency and the facility. The time allotted for this information transfer should not usually exceed one hour. In no instance should the information transfer delay the survey process.

The Centers for Medicare & Medicaid Services, in cooperation with State survey agencies and consumer and provider groups, will develop and provide packages of training materials suitable for use in this activity.

VII. Additional Procedures for Medicare Participating Long Term Care Facilities

Medicare-participating long term care facilities are obligated to inform Medicare beneficiaries about specific rights related to billing, and to submit bills to the Medicare intermediary when requested by the beneficiary. In a Medicare-participating long term care facility, verify compliance with these requirements. Listed below are the requirements and the survey process to follow:

- If a Medicare SNF provider believes, on admission, or during a resident's stay, that Medicare will not pay for skilled nursing or specialized rehabilitative services, the facility must inform the resident or his/her legal representative in writing why these specific services may not be covered. The facility must use the mandatory denial notice found in §358 of the Skilled Nursing Facility Manual, and keep a copy of this uniform denial notice on file. Failure to give notice using the uniform facility denial notice or to submit the bill, if requested by a resident, may constitute a violation of the facility's provider agreement to submit information to the intermediary. (See 42 CFR 489.21(b).)

- The facility is also required to inform each Medicare resident of his/her right to request that the facility submit the bill to the Medicare payor (demand bill). If the resident requests that the bill be submitted to the intermediary or carrier for a Medicare decision, then evidence that the submission has occurred should also appear in the resident's record. The facility must not charge the resident while the demand bill is under review by the Medicare payor.

- During the entrance conference, obtain a list of Medicare residents who requested demand bills in the past 6 months. From this list, randomly select one resident's file to determine if the bill was properly submitted to the intermediary. In addition, draw a sample of all residents in the facility.

The number sampled for this procedure must be equal to the sample size selected for quality of life resident interviews. Use the sample selection table, Table 1, to obtain the correct sample size. Check to determine that the denial letters included appropriate notice information and that bills were submitted upon request. Review billing records for the last 6 months for each resident selected. During resident interviews use the following probes:

- [Individual] Do you know what things or services you pay for out of your own pocket? Who handles the payment for these items?

- [Individual] How do you find out how much these services or things cost?
- [Individual] Tell me how you find out what you have to pay for here?
- [Individual] When you receive a bill to pay for services out-of-pocket, does the facility explain why it believes Medicare will not pay for the services? Does the facility let you know that, if you disagree, you can have a bill submitted to Medicare?
- [Individual] Have you received a bill which you asked to have submitted to Medicare or your insurance company? How has the facility helped you or discouraged you from submitting the bill?
- [Group] Have there been any changes in the charges since you've been here? How do you find out about these changes?
- [Group] How does the facility give you information about your Medicare or Medicaid benefits?
- [Group] Did you or your family receive an explanation of any charges or monthly bills?

If residents are not clear about the scope of services they are entitled to, or the additional services provided by the facility and the cost of these services, or their right to have bills submitted to Medicare, and/or problems are identified during the review of resident records, either in the uniform notice or the bill submittal process, interview administrative staff to determine how the facility informs residents about their Medicare and Medicaid benefits, the non-covered services the facility provides, and the facility's charges for these services. Review additional resident records to assure the facility is using the uniform facility denial notice.

If the facility is in violation of the provider agreement with respect to resident billing requirements, cite tag F492, 42 CFR 483.75(b), Compliance with Federal, State and local laws and professional standards. If the facility is in violation of notice requirements, cite tag F156.

When reviewing facility plans of correction, if a deficiency is noted with respect to billing procedures, it may be appropriate to expect submission of past claims.

Transmittals Issued for this Appendix

Rev #	Issue Date	Subject	Impl Date	CR#
R26SOM	08/17/2007	Revised Appendix P and Appendix PP-New Tag F373	08/17/2007	N/A
R22SOM	12/15/2006	Revisions to Appendix P and Appendix PP	12/18/2006	N/A
R21SOM	10/20/2006	Revised Appendix P & Appendix PP-New Tag F334	10/15/2006	N/A
R20SOM	06/09/2006	Revisions to Appendix P	06/08/2006	N/A
R09SOM	08/05/2005	Revision to Appendix P and Certain Exhibits	08/05/2005	N/A
R05SOM	11/19/2004	Revisions to Appendix P and Appendix PP	11/19/2004	N/A
R01SOM	05/21/2004	Initial Release of pub 100-07	N/A	N/A

PART 2

SURVEYOR GUIDANCE

State Operations Manual
Appendix PP - Guidance to Surveyors for Long Term Care Facilities

Table of Contents

(Rev. 26, 08-17-07)

Transmittals for Appendix PP

INDEX

§483.13 Resident Behavior and Facility Practices

§483.13(a) Restraints

§483.13(b) Abuse

§483.13(c) Staff Treatment of Residents (F224* and F226**)

§483.15 Quality of Life

§483.15(a) Dignity

§483.15(b) Self-Determination and Participation

§483.15(c) Participation in Resident and Family Groups

§483.15(d) Participation in Other Activities

§483.15(e) Accommodation of Needs

§483.15(f) Activities

§483.15(g) Social Services

§483.15(h) Environment

§483.20 Resident Assessment

§483.20(a) Admission Orders

§483.20(b) Comprehensive Assessments

§483.20(c) Quality Review Assessment

§483.20(d) Use

§483.20(e) Coordination

§483.20(f) Automated Data Processing Requirement

§483.20(g) Accuracy of Assessment

§483.20(h) Coordination

§483.20(i) Certification

§483.20(j) Penalty for Falsification

§483.20(k) Comprehensive Care Plans

§483.20(l) Discharge Summary

§483.20(m) Preadmission Screening for Mentally Ill Individuals and Individuals With Mental Retardation.

§483.25 Quality of Care

§483.25(a) Activities of Daily Living

§483.25(b) Vision and hearing

§483.25(c) Pressure Sores

§483.25(d) Urinary Incontinence

§483.25(e) Range of motion.

§483.25(f) Mental and Psychosocial Functioning

§483.25(g) Naso-Gastric Tubes

§483.25(h) Accidents

§483.25(i) Nutrition

§483.25(j) Hydration

§483.25(k) Special Needs

§483.25(l) Unnecessary Drugs

§483.25(m) Medication Errors

§483.25(n) Influenza and Pneumococcal Immunizations

§483.30 Nursing Services

§483.30(a) Sufficient Staff

§483.30(b) Registered Nurse

§483.30(c) Nursing facilities

§483.30(d) SNFs

§483.30(e) Nurse Staffing Information

§483.35 Dietary Services

§483.35(a) Staffing

§483.35 (b) Standard Sufficient Staff

§483.35(c) Standard Menus and Nutritional Adequacy

§483.35(d) Food

§483.35(e) Therapeutic Diets

§483.35(f) Frequency of Meals

§483.35(g) Assistive Devices

§483.35(h) Paid Feeding Assistants

§483.35(i) Sanitary Conditions

§483.40 Physician Services

§483.40(a) Physician Supervision

§483.40(b) Physician Visits

§483.40(c) Frequency of Physician Visits

§483.40(d) Availability of Physicians for Emergency Care

§483.40(e) Physician Delegation of Tasks in SNFs

§483.40(f) Performance of Physician Tasks in NFs

§483.45 Specialized Rehabilitative Services

§483.45(a) Provision of Services

§483.45(b) Qualifications

§483.55 Dental Services

§483.55(a) Skilled Nursing Facilities

§483.55(b) Nursing Facilities

§483.60 Pharmacy Services

§483.60(a) Procedures

§483.60(b) Service Consultation

§483.60(c) Drug Regimen Review

§483.60(d) Labeling of Drugs and Biologicals

§483.60(e) Storage of Drugs and Biologicals

§483.65 Infection Control

§483.65(a) Infection Control Program

§483.65(b) Preventing Spread of Infection

§483.65(c) Linens

§483.70 Physical Environment

§483.70(a) Life Safety From Fire

§483.70(b) Emergency Power

§483.70(c) Space and equipment

§483.70(d) Resident Rooms

§483.70(e) Toilet Facilities

§483.70(f) Resident Call System

§483.70(g) Dining and Resident Activities

§483.70(h) Other Environmental Conditions

§483.75 Administration

§483.75(a) Licensure

§483.75(b) Compliance With Federal, State, and Local Laws and Professional Standards

§483.75(c) Relationship to Other HHS Regulations

§483.75(d) Governing Body

§483.75(e) Required Training of Nursing Aides

§483.75(f) Proficiency of Nurse Aides

§483.75(g) Staff Qualifications

§483.75(h) Use of Outside Resources

§483.75(i) Medical Director

§483.75(j) Laboratory Services

§483.75(k) Radiology and Other Diagnostic Services

§483.75(l) Clinical Records

§483.75(m) Disaster and Emergency Preparedness

§483.75(n) Transfer Agreement

§483.75(o) Quality Assessment and Assurance

§483.75(p) Disclosure of Ownership

F150

§483.5 Definitions

(a) Facility defined. For purposes of this subpart "facility" means, a skilled nursing facility (SNF) or a nursing facility (NF) which meets the requirements of §§1819 or 1919(a), (b), (c), and (d) of the Social Security Act, the Act. "Facility" may include a distinct part of an institution specified in §440.40 of this chapter, but does not include an institution for the mentally retarded or persons with related conditions described in §440.150 of this chapter. For Medicare and Medicaid purposes (including eligibility, coverage, certification, and payment), the "facility" is always the entity which participates in the program, whether that entity is comprised of all of, or a distinct part of a larger institution. For Medicare, a SNF (see §1819(a)(1)), and for Medicaid, a NF (see §1919(a)(1)) may not be an institution for mental diseases as defined in §435.1009.

Interpretive Guidelines §483.5

The following are the statutory definitions at §§1819(a) and 1919(a) of the Act for a SNF and a NF:

"Skilled nursing facility" is defined as an institution (or a distinct part of an institution) which is primarily engaged in providing skilled nursing care and related services for residents who require medical or nursing care, or rehabilitation services for the rehabilitation of injured, disabled, or sick persons, and is not primarily for the care and treatment of mental diseases; has in effect a transfer agreement (meeting the requirements of §1861(l)) with one or more hospitals having agreements in effect under §1866; and meets the requirements for a SNF described in subsections (b), (c), and (d) of this section.

"Nursing facility" is defined as an institution (or a distinct part of an institution) which is primarily engaged in providing skilled nursing care and related services for residents who require medical or nursing care, rehabilitation services for the rehabilitation of injured, disabled, or sick persons, or on a regular basis, health-related care and services to individuals who because of their mental or physical condition require care and services (above the level of room and board) which can be made available to them only through institutional facilities, and is not primarily for the care and treatment of mental diseases; has in effect a transfer agreement (meeting the requirements of §1861(1)) with one or more hospitals having agreements in effect under §1866; and meets the requirements for a NF described in subsections (b), (c), and (d) of this section.

If a provider does not meet one of these definitions, it cannot be certified for participation in the Medicare and/or Medicaid programs.

NOTE: If the survey team finds substandard care in §§483.13, 483.15, or 483.25, follow the instructions for partial extended or extended surveys.

---

§483.10 Resident Rights

The resident has a right to a dignified existence, self-determination, and communication with and access to persons and services inside and outside the facility. A facility must protect and promote the rights of each resident, including each of the following rights

Interpretive Guidelines §483.10

All residents in long term care facilities have rights guaranteed to them under Federal and State law. Requirements concerning resident rights are specified in §§483.10, 483.12, 483.13, and 483.15. Section 483.10 is intended to lay the foundation for the remaining resident's rights requirements which cover more specific areas. These rights include the resident's right to:

- Exercise his or her rights (§483.10(a));
- Be informed about what rights and responsibilities he or she has (§483.10(b));
- If he or she wishes, have the facility manage his personal funds (§483.10(c));
- Choose a physician and treatment and participate in decisions and care planning (§483.10(d));
- Privacy and confidentiality (§483.10(e));

- Voice grievances and have the facility respond to those grievances (§483.10(f));
- Examine survey results (§483.10(g));
- Work or not work (§483.10(h));
- Privacy in sending and receiving mail (§483.10(i));
- Visit and be visited by others from outside the facility (§483.10(j));
- Use a telephone in privacy (§483.10(k));
- Retain and use personal possessions (§483.10(1)) to the maximum extent that space and safety permit;
- Share a room with a spouse, if that is mutually agreeable (§483.10(m));
- Self-administer medication, if the interdisciplinary care planning team determines it is safe (§483.10(n)); and
- Refuse a transfer from a distinct part, within the institution (§483.10(o)).

A facility must promote the exercise of rights for each resident, including any who face barriers (such as communication problems, hearing problems and cognition limits) in the exercise of these rights. A resident, even though determined to be incompetent, should be able to assert these rights based on his or her degree of capability.

F151

§483.10(a) Exercise of Rights

§483.10(a)(1) The resident has the right to exercise his or her rights as a resident of the facility and as a citizen or resident of the United States.

§483.10(a)(2) The resident has the right to be free of interference, coercion, discrimination, and reprisal from the facility in exercising his or her rights.

Interpretive Guidelines §483.10(a)(1)

Exercising rights means that residents have autonomy and choice, to the maximum extent possible, about how they wish to live their everyday lives and receive care, subject to the facility's rules, as long as those rules do not violate a regulatory requirement.

Intent §483.10(a)(2)

This regulation is intended to protect each resident in the exercise of his or her rights.

Interpretive Guidelines §483.10(a)(2)

The facility must not hamper, compel, treat differentially, or retaliate against a resident for exercising his/her rights. Facility behaviors designed to support and encourage resident participation in meeting care planning goals as documented in the resident assessment and care plan are not interference or coercion.

Examples of facility practices that may limit autonomy or choice in exercising rights include reducing the group activity time of a resident trying to organize a residents' group; requiring residents to seek prior approval to distribute information about the facility; discouraging a resident from hanging a religious ornament above his or her bed; singling out residents for prejudicial treatment such as isolating residents in activities; or purposefully assigning inexperienced aides to a resident with heavy care needs because the resident and/or his/her representative, exercised his/her rights.

Procedures §483.10(a)(2)

Pay close attention to resident or staff remarks and staff behavior that may represent deliberate actions to promote or to limit a resident's autonomy or choice, particularly in ways that affect independent functioning. Because reprisals may indicate abuse, if the team determines that a facility has violated this requirement through reprisals taken against residents, then further determine if the facility has an effective system to prevent the neglect and abuse of residents. (§483.13(c), F224-F225.)

F152

§483.10(a)(3) -- In the case of a resident adjudged incompetent under the laws of a State by a court of competent jurisdiction, the rights of the resident are exercised by the person appointed under State law to act on the resident's behalf.

§483.10(a)(4) -- In the case of a resident who has not been adjudged incompetent by the State court, any legal-surrogate designated in accordance with State law may exercise the resident's rights to the extent provided by State law.

Interpretive Guidelines §483.10(a)(3) and (4)

When reference is made to "resident" in the Guidelines, it also refers to any person who may, under State law, act on the resident's behalf when the resident is unable to act for himself or herself. That person is referred to as the resident's surrogate or representative. If the resident has been formally declared incompetent by a court, the surrogate or representative is whoever was appointed by the court - a guardian, conservator, or committee. The facility should verify that a surrogate or representative has the necessary authority. For example, a court-appointed conservator might have the power to make financial decisions, but not health care decisions.

A resident may wish to delegate decision-making to specific persons, or the resident and family may have agreed among themselves on a decision-making process. To the degree permitted by State law, and to the maximum extent practicable, the facility must respect the resident's wishes and follow that process.

The rights of the resident that may be exercised by the surrogate or representative include the right to make health care decisions. However, the facility may seek a health care decision (or any other decision or authorization) from a surrogate or representative only when the resident is unable to make the decision. If there is a question as to whether the resident is able to make a health care decision, staff should discuss the matter with the resident at a suitable time and judge how well the resident understands the information. In the case of a resident who has been formally declared incompetent by a court, lack of capacity is presumed. Notwithstanding the above, if such a resident can understand the situation and express a preference, the resident should be informed and his/her wishes respected to the degree practicable. Any violations with respect to the resident's exercise of rights should be cited under the applicable tag number.

The involvement of a surrogate or representative does not automatically relieve a facility of its duty to protect and promote the resident's interests. For example, a surrogate or representative does not have the right to insist that a treatment be performed that is not medically appropriate, and the right of a surrogate or representative to reject treatment may be subject to State law limits.

Procedures §483.10(a)(3) and (4)

Determine as appropriate if the rights of a resident who has been adjudged incompetent or who has a representative acting on his/her behalf to help exercise his/her rights are exercised by the legally appointed individual.

F153

§483.10(b)(2) -- The resident or his or her legal representative has the right--

> **(i) Upon an oral or written request, to access all records pertaining to himself or herself including current clinical records within 24 hours (excluding weekends and holidays); and**
>
> **(ii) After receipt of his or her records for inspection, to purchase at a cost not to exceed the community standard photocopies of the records or any portions of them upon request and 2 working days advance notice to the facility.**

Interpretive Guidelines §483.10(b)(2)

An oral request is sufficient to produce the current record for review.

In addition to clinical records, the term "records" includes all records pertaining to the resident, such as trust fund ledgers pertinent to the resident and contracts between the resident and the facility.

"Purchase" is defined as a charge to the resident for photocopying. If State statute has defined the "community standard" rate, facilities should follow that rate. In the absence of State statute, the "cost not to exceed the community standard" is that rate charged per copy by organizations such as the public library, the Post Office or a commercial copy center, which would be selected by a prudent buyer in addition to the cost of the clerical time needed to photocopy the records. Additional fees for locating the records or typing forms/envelopes may not be assessed.

F154

§483.10(b)(3) -- The resident has the right to be fully informed in language that he or she can understand of his or her total health status, including but not limited to, his or her medical condition;

Interpretive Guidelines §483.10(b)(3)

"Total health status" includes functional status, medical care, nursing care, nutritional status, rehabilitation and restorative potential, activities potential, cognitive status, oral health status, psychosocial status, and sensory and physical impairments. Information on health status must be presented in language that the resident can understand. This includes minimizing use of technical jargon in communicating with the resident, having the ability to communicate in a foreign language and the use of sign language or other aids, as necessary. (See §483.10(d)(3), F175, for the right of the resident to plan care and treatment.)

Procedures §483.10(b)(3)

Look, particularly during observations and record reviews, for on-going efforts on the part of facility staff to keep residents informed. Look for evidence that information is communicated in a manner that is understandable to residents and communicated at times it could be most useful to residents, such as when they are expressing concerns, or raising questions, as well as on an on-going basis.

§483.10(d)(2) – The resident has the right to be fully informed in advance about care and treatment and of any changes in that care or treatment that may affect the resident's well-being;

Interpretive Guidelines §483.10(d)(2)

"Informed in advance" means that the resident receives information necessary to make a health care decision, including information about his/her medical condition and changes in medical condition, about the benefits and reasonable risks of the treatment, and about reasonable available alternatives.

F155

§483.10(b)(4) -- The resident has the right to refuse treatment, to refuse to participate in experimental research, and to formulate an advance directive as specified in paragraph (8) of this section; and

Interpretive Guidelines §483.10(b)(4)

"Treatment" is defined as care provided for purposes of maintaining/restoring health, improving functional level, or relieving symptoms.

"Experimental research" is defined as development and testing of clinical treatments, such as an investigational drug or therapy, that involve treatment and/or control groups. For example, a clinical trial of an investigational drug would be experimental research.

"Advance directive" means a written instruction, such as a living will or durable power of attorney for health care, recognized under State law relating to the provision of health care when the individual is incapacitated.

As provided under State law, a resident who has the capacity to make a health care decision and who withholds consent to treatment or makes an explicit refusal of treatment either directly or through an advance directive, may not be treated against his/her wishes.

A facility may not transfer or discharge a resident for refusing treatment unless the criteria for transfer or discharge are met. (See §483.12(a)(1) and (2).)

If the resident is unable to make a health care decision, a decision by the resident's surrogate or representative to forego treatment may, subject to State law, be equally binding on the facility. The facility should determine exactly what the resident is refusing and why. To the extent the facility is able, it should address the resident's concern. For example, a resident requires physical therapy to learn to walk again after sustaining a fractured hip. The resident refuses therapy. The facility is expected to assess the reasons for this resident's refusal, clarify and educate the resident as to the consequences of refusal, offer alternative treatments, and continue to provide all other services.

If a resident's refusal of treatment brings about a significant change, the facility should reassess the resident and institute care planning changes. A resident's refusal of treatment does not absolve a facility from providing a resident with care that allows him/her to attain or maintain his/her highest practicable physical, mental and psychosocial well-being in the context of making that refusal.

The resident has the right to refuse to participate in experimental research. A resident being considered for participation in experimental research must be fully informed of the nature of the experiment (e.g., medication, treatment) and understand the possible consequences of participating. The opportunity to refuse to participate in experimental research must occur prior to the start of the research. Aggregated resident statistics that do not identify individual residents may be used for studies without obtaining residents' permission.

Procedures §483.10(b)(4)

If the facility participates in any experimental research involving residents, does it have an Institutional Review Board or other committee that reviews and approves research protocols? In this regard, §483.75(c), Relationship to Other HHS Regulations applies (i.e., the facility must adhere to 45 CFR Part 46, Protection of Human Subjects of Research).

See §483.10(b)(8), F156 with respect to the advance directive requirement.

F156

§483.10(b)(1) -- The facility must inform the resident both orally and in writing in a language that the resident understands of his or her rights and all rules and regulations governing resident conduct and responsibilities during the stay in the facility. The facility must also provide the resident with the notice (if any) of the State developed under §1919(e)(6) of the Act. Such notification must be made prior to or upon admission and during the resident's stay. Receipt of such information, and any amendments to it, must be acknowledged in writing;

Intent §483.10(b)(1)

This requirement is intended to assure that each resident know his or her rights and responsibilities and that the facility communicates this information prior to or upon admission, as appropriate during the resident's stay, and when the facility's rules change.

Interpretive Guidelines §483.10(b)(1)

"In a language that the resident understands" is defined as communication of information concerning rights and responsibilities that is clear and understandable to each resident, to the extent possible considering impediments which may be created by the resident's health and mental status. If the resident's knowledge of English or the predominant language of the facility is inadequate for comprehension, a means to communicate the information concerning rights and responsibilities in a language familiar to the resident must be available and implemented. For foreign languages commonly encountered in the facility locale, the facility should have written translations of its statements of rights and responsibilities, and should make the services of an interpreter available. In the case of less commonly encountered foreign languages, however, a representative of the resident may sign that he or she has explained the statement of rights to the resident prior to his/her acknowledgement of receipt. For hearing impaired residents who communicate by signing, the facility is expected to provide an interpreter. Large print texts of the facility's statement of resident rights and responsibilities should also be available.

"Both orally and in writing" means if a resident can read and understand written materials without assistance, an oral summary, along with the written document, is acceptable.

Any time State or Federal laws relating to resident rights or facility rules change during the resident's stay in the facility, he/she must promptly be informed of these changes.

"All rules and regulations" relates to facility policies governing resident conduct. A facility cannot reasonably expect a resident to abide by rules he or she has never been told about. Whatever rules the facility has formalized, and by which it expects residents to abide, should be included in the statement of rights and responsibilities.

§483.10(b)(5) -- The facility must--

(i) Inform each resident who is entitled to Medicaid benefits, in writing, at the time of admission to the nursing facility or, when the resident becomes eligible for Medicaid of--

(A) The items and services that are included in nursing facility services under the State plan and for which the resident may not be charged;

(B) Those other items and services that the facility offers and for which the resident may be charged, and the amount of charges for those services; and

(ii) Inform each resident when changes are made to the items and services specified in paragraphs (5)(i)(A) and (B) of this section.

§483.10(b)(6) -- The facility must inform each resident before, or at the time of admission, and periodically during the resident's stay, of services available in the facility and of charges for those services, including any charges for services not covered under Medicare or by the facility's per diem rate.

Interpretive Guidelines §483.10(b)(5) and (6)

Residents should be told in advance when changes will occur in their bills. Providers must fully inform the resident of services and related changes.

"Periodically" means that whenever changes are being introduced that will affect the residents liability and whenever there are changes in services.

A Medicare beneficiary who requires services upon admission that are not covered under Medicare may be required to submit a deposit provided the notice provisions of §483.10(b)(6), if applicable, are met.

Procedures §483.10(b)(5) and (6)

See §483.10(c)(8) for those items and services that must be included in payment under skilled nursing and nursing facility benefits.

§483.10(b)(7) -- The facility must furnish a written description of legal rights which includes--

(i) A description of the manner of protecting personal funds, under paragraph (c) of this section;

(ii) A description of the requirements and procedures for establishing eligibility for Medicaid, including the right to request an assessment under section 1924(c) which determines the extent of a couple's non-exempt resources at the time of institutionalization and attributes to the community spouse an equitable share of resources which cannot be considered available for payment toward the cost of the institutionalized spouse's medical care in his or her process of spending down to Medicaid eligibility levels;

(iii) A posting of names, addresses, and telephone numbers of all pertinent State client advocacy groups such as the State survey and certification agency, the State licensure office, the State ombudsman program, the protection and advocacy network, and the Medicaid fraud control unit; and

(iv) A statement that the resident may file a complaint with the State survey and certification agency concerning resident abuse, neglect, and misappropriation of resident property in the facility, and non-compliance with the advance directives requirements.

Interpretive Guidelines §483.10(b)(7)

"The protection and advocacy network" refers to the system established to protect and advocate the rights of individuals with developmental disabilities specified in the

Developmental Disabilities Assistance and Bill of Rights Act, and the protection and advocacy system established under the Protection and Advocacy for Mentally Ill Individuals Act.

Procedures §483.10(b)(7)

At the Entrance Conference, request a copy of the written information that is provided to residents regarding their rights and review it to determine if it addresses the specified requirements. Additional requirements that address the implementation of these rights are cross-referenced below.

§483.10(b)(8) -- The facility must comply with the requirements specified in subpart I of part 489 of this chapter relating to maintaining written policies and procedures regarding advance directives. These requirements include provisions to inform and provide written information to all adult residents concerning the right to accept or refuse medical or surgical treatment and, at the individual's option, formulate an advance directive. This includes a written description of the facility's policies to implement advance directives and applicable State law

Interpretive Guidelines §483.10(b)(8)

This provision applies to residents admitted on or after December 1, 1991. 42 CFR 489.102 specifies that at the time of admission of an adult resident, the facility must:

- Provide written information concerning his/her rights under State law (whether or not statutory or recognized by the courts of the State) to make decisions concerning medical care, including the right to accept or refuse medical or surgical treatment, and the right to formulate advance directives;

- Document in the resident's medical record whether or not the individual has executed an advance directive;

- Not condition the provision of care or discriminate against an individual based on whether or not the individual has executed an advance directive;

- Ensure compliance with requirements of State law regarding advance directives;

- Provide for educating staff regarding the facility's policies and procedures on advance directives; and

- Provide for community education regarding the right under State law (whether or not recognized by the courts of the State) to formulate an advance directive and the facility's written policies and procedures regarding the implementation of these rights, including any limitations the facility may have with respect to implementing this right on the basis of conscience.

The facility is not required to provide care that conflicts with an advance directive. In addition, the facility is not required to implement an advance directive if, as a matter of conscience, the provider cannot implement an advance directive and State law allows the provider to conscientiously object. (See §483.10(b)(4), F155.)

The sum total of the community education efforts must include a summary of the State law, the rights of residents to formulate advance directives, and the facility's implementation policies regarding advance directives. Video and audio tapes may be used in conducting the community education effort. Individual education programs do not have to address all the requirements if it would be inappropriate for a particular audience.

Procedures §483.10(b)(8)

During Resident Review, review the records of two selected sampled residents admitted on or after December 1, 1991, for facility compliance with advance directive notice requirements.

- Determine to what extent the facility educates its staff regarding advance directives.
- Determine to what extent the facility provides education for the community regarding one's rights under State law to formulate advance directives.

§483.10(b)(9) -- The facility must inform each resident of the name, specialty, and way of contacting the physician responsible for his or her care.

Interpretive Guidelines §483.10(b)(9)

"Physician responsible for his or her care" is defined as the attending or primary physician or clinic, whichever is responsible for managing the resident's medical care, and excludes other physicians whom the resident may see from time to time. When a resident has selected an attending physician, it is appropriate for the facility to confirm that choice when complying with this requirement. When a resident has no attending physician, it is appropriate for the facility to assist residents to obtain one in consultation with the resident and subject to the resident's right to choose. (See §483.10(d)(1), F163.)

If a facility uses the services of a clinic or similar arrangement, it may be sufficient for residents to have the name and contact information for the primary physician and/or a central number for the clinic itself.

§483.10(b)(10) -- The facility must prominently display in the facility written information, and provide to residents and applicants for admission oral and written information about how to apply for and use Medicare and Medicaid benefits, and how to receive refunds for previous payments covered by such benefits.

Interpretive Guidelines §483.10(b)(10)

To fulfill this requirement, the facility may use written materials issued by the State Medicaid agency and the Federal government relating to these benefits. Facilities may fulfill their obligation to orally inform residents or applicants for admission about how to apply for Medicaid or Medicare by assisting them in contacting the local Social Security Office or the local unit of the State Medicaid agency. Nursing facilities are not responsible for orally providing detailed information about Medicare and Medicaid eligibility rules.

"Refunds for previous payments" refers to refunds due as a result of Medicaid and Medicare payments when eligibility has been determined retroactively.

As part of determining Medicaid eligibility, at the time of admission, a married couple has the right to request and have the appropriate State agency assess the couple's resources.

F157

§483.10(b)(11) -- Notification of changes.

(i) A facility must immediately inform the resident; consult with the resident's physician; and if known, notify the resident's legal representative or an interested family member when there is--

(A) An accident involving the resident which results in injury and has the potential for requiring physician intervention;

(B) A significant change in the resident's physical, mental, or psychosocial status (i.e., a deterioration in health, mental, or psychosocial status in either life-threatening conditions or clinical complications);

(C) A need to alter treatment significantly (i.e., a need to discontinue an existing form of treatment due to adverse consequences, or to commence a new form of treatment); or

(D) A decision to transfer or discharge the resident from the facility as specified in <u>§483.12(a)</u>.

(ii) The facility must also promptly notify the resident and, if known, the resident's legal representative or interested family member when there is--

(A) A change in room or roommate assignment as specified in §483.15(e)(2); or

(B) A change in resident rights under Federal or State law or regulations as specified in paragraph (b)(1) of this section.

(iii) The facility must record and periodically update the address and phone number of the resident's legal representative or interested family member.

Interpretive Guidelines §483.10(b)(11)

For purposes of §483.10(b)(11)(i)(B), life-threatening conditions are such things as a heart attack or stroke. Clinical complications are such things as development of a stage II pressure sore, onset or recurrent periods of delirium, recurrent urinary tract infection, or onset of depression. A need to alter treatment "significantly" means a need to stop a form of treatment because of adverse consequences (e.g., an adverse drug reaction), or commence a new form of treatment to deal with a problem (e.g., the use of any medical procedure, or therapy that has not been used on that resident before).

In the case of a competent individual, the facility must still contact the resident's physician and notify interested family members, if known. That is, a family that wishes to be informed would designate a member to receive calls. Even when a resident is mentally competent, such a designated family member should be notified of significant changes in the resident's health status because the resident may not be able to notify them personally, especially in the case of sudden illness or accident.

The requirements at §483.10(b)(1) require the facility to inform the resident of his/her rights upon admission and during the resident's stay. This includes the resident's right to privacy (§483.10(e), F164). If, after being informed of the right to privacy, a resident specifies that he/she wishes to exercise this right and not notify family members in the event of a significant change as specified at this requirement, the facility should respect this request, which would obviate the need to notify the resident's interested family member or legal representative, if known. If a resident specifies that he/she does not wish to exercise the right to privacy, then the facility is required to comply with the notice of change requirements.

In the case of a resident who is incapable of making decisions, the representative would make any decisions that have to be made, but the resident should still be told what is happening to him or her.

In the case of the death of a resident, the resident's physician is to be notified immediately in accordance with State law.

The failure to provide notice of room changes could result in an avoidable decline in physical, mental, or psychosocial well-being.

---

§483.10(c) Protection of Resident Funds

F158

§483.10(c)(1) Protection of Resident Funds

The resident has the right to manage his or her financial affairs, and the facility may not require residents to deposit their personal funds with the facility.

F159

§483.10(c)(2) Management of Personal Funds

Upon written authorization of a resident, the facility must hold, safeguard, manage, and account for the personal funds of the resident deposited with the facility, as specified in paragraphs (c)(3)-(8) of this section.

§483.10(c)(3) Deposit of Funds

(i) Funds in excess of $50. The facility must deposit any residents' personal funds in excess of $50 in an interest bearing account (or accounts) that is separate from any of the facility's operating accounts, and that credits all interest earned on resident's funds to that account. (In pooled accounts, there must be a separate accounting for each resident's share.)

(ii) Funds less than $50. The facility must maintain a resident's personal funds that do not exceed $50 in a non-interest bearing account, interest-bearing account, or petty cash fund.

NOTE: The Social Security Amendments of 1994 amended §1819(c)(6)(B)(i) to raise the limit from $50.00 to $100.00 for the minimum amount of resident funds that facilities must entrust to an interest bearing account. This increase applies only to Medicare SNF residents. While a facility may continue to follow a minimum of $50.00, the regulations do not require it.

Interpretive Guidelines §483.10(c)(1) through (3)

This requirement is intended to assure that residents who have authorized the facility in writing to manage any personal funds have ready and reasonable access to those funds. If residents choose to have the facility manage their funds, the facility may not refuse to handle these funds, but is not responsible for knowing about assets not on deposit with it.

Placement of residents' personal funds of less than $50.00 ($100.00 for Medicare residents) in an interest bearing account **is** permitted. Thus, a facility may place the total amount of a resident's funds, including funds of $50.00 ($100.00 for Medicare residents) or less, into an interest-bearing account. The law and regulations are intended to assure that residents have access to $50.00 ($100.00 for Medicare residents) in cash within a reasonable period of time, when requested. Requests for less than $50.00 ($100.00 for Medicare residents) should be honored within the same day. Requests for $50.00 ($100.00 for Medicare residents) or more should be honored within three banking days. Although the facility need not maintain $50.00 ($100.00 for Medicare residents) per resident on its premises, it is expected to maintain amounts of petty cash on hand that may be required by residents.

If pooled accounts are used, interest must be prorated per individual on the basis of actual earnings or end-of quarter balance.

Residents should have access to petty cash on an ongoing basis and be able to arrange for access to larger funds.

"Hold, safeguard, manage and account for" means that the facility must act as fiduciary of the resident's funds and report at least quarterly on the status of these funds in a clear and understandable manner. Managing the resident's financial affairs includes money that an individual gives to the facility for the sake of providing a resident with a noncovered service (such as a permanent wave). It is expected that in these instances, the facility will provide a receipt to the gift giver and retain a copy.

"Interest bearing" means a rate of return equal to or above the passbook savings rate at local banking institutions in the area.

Although the requirements are silent about oral requests by residents to have a facility hold personal funds, under the provisions regarding personal property (§483.10(l)), and misappropriation of property (§483.13(c)), residents may make oral requests that the facility temporarily place their funds in a safe place, without authorizing the facility to manage those funds. The facility has the responsibility to implement written procedures to prevent the misappropriation of these funds.

If you determine potential problems with funds through interviews, follow-up using the following procedures as appropriate:

If the facility does not have written authorization to handle resident's funds, but is holding funds for more than a few days, determine if the facility is managing these funds without written authorization. There must be written authorization for the facility to be in compliance with this requirement.

To assure that facilities are not using oral requests by residents as a way to avoid obtaining written authorization to hold, manage, safeguard and account for resident's funds, make sure that:

- There is a written declaration by the resident that the funds are being held for no more than a few days by the facility at the resident's request;
- These funds are not held for more than a few days; and
- The facility provides the resident a receipt for these funds and retains a copy for its records.

Review the administrative or business file and the bookkeeping accounts of residents selected for a comprehensive review who have authorized the facility to handle their personal funds.

- Are residents' funds over $50.00 ($100.00 for Medicare residents) or, at the facility's option, all resident funds, in an interest bearing account(s)?
- What procedure was followed when residents requested their funds?
- How long does it take for residents to receive: (a) petty cash allotments; (b) funds needing to be withdrawn from bank accounts?
- Were limits placed on amounts that could be withdrawn? If yes, was the reason based on resident care needs or facility convenience?
- Are funds records treated with privacy as required at F164?

NOTE: Banks may charge the resident a fee for handling their funds. Facilities may not charge residents for managing residents' funds because the services are covered by Medicare or Medicaid.

If problems are identified, review also §483.10(b)(7), Tag F156.

Monies due residents should be credited to their respective bank accounts within a few business days.

§483.10(c)(4) Accounting and Records

The facility must establish and maintain a system that assures a full and complete and separate accounting, according to generally accepted accounting principles, of each resident's personal funds entrusted to the facility on the resident's behalf.

(i) The system must preclude any commingling of resident funds with facility funds or with the funds of any person other than another resident.

(ii) The individual financial record must be available through quarterly statements and on request to the resident or his or her legal representative.

Interpretive Guidelines §483.10(c)(4)

This requirement constitutes the overall response of the facility to the resident's right to have the facility manage the resident's funds.

"Generally accepted accounting principles" means that the facility employs proper bookkeeping techniques, by which it can determine, upon request, the amount of individual resident funds and, in the case of an interest bearing account, how much interest these funds have earned for each resident, as last reported by the banking institution to the facility.

Proper bookkeeping techniques would include an individual ledger card, ledger sheet or equivalent established for each resident on which only those transactions involving his or her personal funds are recorded and maintained. The record should have information on when transactions occurred, what they were, as well as maintain the ongoing balance for every resident.

Anytime there is a transaction the resident should be given a receipt and the facility retains a copy.

Monies due residents should be credited to their respective bank accounts within a few business days.

"Quarterly statements" are to be provided in writing to the resident or the resident's representative within 30 days after the end of the quarter.

§483.10(c)(5) Notice of Certain Balances

The facility must notify each resident that receives Medicaid benefits--

> **(i) When the amount in the resident's account reaches $200 less than the SSI resource limit for one person, specified in section <u>1611(a)(3)(B)</u> of the Act; and**
>
> **(ii) That, if the amount in the account, in addition to the value of the resident's other nonexempt resources, reaches the SSI resource limit for one person, the resident may lose eligibility for Medicaid or SSI.**

Interpretive Guidelines §483.10(c)(5)

The Social Security District Office can provide you with information concerning current SSI resource limits.

Procedures §483.10(c)(5)

If problems are identified for sampled residents who are Medicaid recipients, review financial records to determine if their accounts are within $200.00 of the SSI limit. If there are sampled residents in this situation, ask them or their representatives if they have received notice.

F160

483.10(c)(6) Conveyance upon death

Upon the death of a resident with a personal fund deposited with the facility, the facility must convey within 30 days the resident's funds, and a final accounting of those funds, to the individual or probate jurisdiction administering the resident's estate.

Procedures §483.10(c)(6)

As part of closed records review, determine if within 30 days of death, the facility conveyed the deceased resident's personal funds and a final accounting to the individual or probate jurisdiction administering the individual's estate as provided by State law.

F161

483.10(c)(7) Assurance of Financial Security

The facility must purchase a surety bond, or otherwise provide assurance satisfactory to the Secretary, to assure the security of all personal funds of residents deposited with the facility.

Interpretive Guidelines §483.10(c)(7)

A surety bond is an agreement between the principal (the facility), the surety (the insurance company), and the obligee (depending on State law, either the resident or the State acting on behalf of the resident), wherein the facility and the insurance company agree to compensate the resident (or the State on behalf of the resident) for any loss of residents' funds that the facility holds, safeguards, manages, and accounts for.

The purpose of the surety bond is to guarantee that the facility will pay the resident (or the State on behalf of the resident) for losses occurring from any failure by the facility to hold, safeguard, manage, and account for the residents' funds, i.e., losses occurring as a result of acts or errors of negligence, incompetence or dishonesty.

Unlike other types of insurance, the surety bond protects the obligee (the resident or the State), not the principal (the facility), from loss. The surety bond differs from a fidelity bond, which covers no acts or errors of negligence, incompetence or dishonesty.

The surety bond is the commitment of the facility in an objective manner to meet the standard of conduct specified in §483.10(c)(2), that the facility will hold, safeguard, manage and account for the funds residents have entrusted to the facility. The facility assumes the responsibility to compensate the obligee for the amount of the loss up to the entire amount of the surety bond.

Reasonable alternatives to a surety bond must:

- Designate the obligee (depending on State law, the resident individually or in aggregate, or the State on behalf of each resident) who can collect in case of a loss;

- Specify that the obligee may collect due to any failure by the facility, whether by commission, bankruptcy, or omission, to hold, safeguard, manage, and account for the residents' funds; and

- Be managed by a third party unrelated in any way to the facility or its management.

The facility cannot be named as a beneficiary.

Self-insurance is not an acceptable alternative to a surety bond. Likewise, funds deposited in bank accounts protected by the Federal Deposit Insurance Corporation, or similar entity, also are not acceptable alternatives.

Procedures §483.10(c)(7)

As part of Phase 2, if your team has any concerns about residents' funds, check the amount of the surety bond to make sure it is at least equal to the total amount of residents' funds, as of the most recent quarter.

If the State survey agency determines that individual circumstances associated with a facility's surety bond or its alternative are such that the survey agency cannot determine whether or not the facility is in compliance with the requirements at §483.10(c)(7), then it would be appropriate to make the referral to the State's fiscal department.

If a corporation has a surety bond that covers all of its facilities, there should be a separate review of the corporation's surety bond by the appropriate State agency, such as the State's fiscal department, to ensure that all the residents in the corporation's facilities within the State are covered against any losses due to acts or errors by the corporation or any of its facilities. The focus of the review should be to ensure that if the corporation were to go bankrupt or otherwise cease to operate, the funds of the residents in the corporation's facilities would be protected.

F162

§483.10(c)(8) Limitation on Charges to Personal Funds

The facility may not impose a charge against the personal funds of a resident for any item or services for which payment is made under Medicaid or Medicare (except for applicable deductible and coinsurance amounts).

The facility may charge the resident for requested services that are more expensive than or in excess of covered services in accordance with §489.32 of this chapter. (This does not affect the prohibition on facility charges for items and services for which Medicaid has paid. See §447.15, which limits participation in the Medicaid program to providers who accept, as payment in full, Medicaid payment plus any deductible, coinsurance, or copayment required by the plan to be paid by the individual.)

(i) Services included in Medicare or Medicaid payment. During the course of a covered Medicare or Medicaid stay, facilities may not charge a resident for the following categories of items and services:

(A) Nursing services as required at §483.30 of this subpart.

(B) Dietary services as required at §483.35 of this subpart.

(C) An activities program as required at §483.15(f) of this subpart.

(D) Room/bed maintenance services.

(E) Routine personal hygiene items and services as required to meet the needs of residents, including, but not limited to, hair hygiene supplies, comb, brush, bath soap, disinfecting soaps or specialized cleansing agents when indicated to treat special skin problems or to fight infection, razor, shaving cream, toothbrush, toothpaste, denture adhesive, denture cleaner, dental floss, moisturizing lotion, tissues, cotton balls, cotton swabs, deodorant, incontinence care and supplies, sanitary napkins and related supplies, towels, washcloths, hospital gowns, over the counter drugs, hair and nail hygiene services, bathing, and basic personal laundry.

(F) Medically-related social services as required at §483.15(g) of this subpart.

(ii) Items and services that may be charged to residents' funds. Listed below are general categories and examples of items and services that the facility may charge to residents' funds if they are requested by a resident, if the facility informs the resident that there will be a charge, and if payment is not made by Medicare or Medicaid:

(A) Telephone;

(B) Television/radio for personal use;

(C) Personal comfort items, including smoking materials, notions and novelties, and confections;

(D) Cosmetic and grooming items and services in excess of those for which payment is made under Medicaid or Medicare;

(E) Personal clothing;

(F) Personal reading matter;

(G) Gifts purchased on behalf of a resident;

(H) Flowers and plants; and

(I) Social events and entertainment offered outside the scope of the activities program, provided under §483.15(f) of this subpart.

(J) Noncovered special care services such as privately hired nurses or aides.

(K) Private room, except when therapeutically required (for example, isolation for infection control).

(L) Specially prepared or alternative food requested instead of the food generally prepared by the facility, as required by §483.35 of this subpart.

Intent §483.10(c)(8)

The intent of this requirement is to specify that facilities not charge residents for items and services for which payment is made under Medicare or Medicaid.

Interpretive Guidelines §483.10(c)(8)

The facility may charge the resident the difference for requested services that are more expensive than or in excess of covered services in accordance with §489.32 of this chapter. (This does not affect the prohibition on facility charges for items and services for which Medicaid has paid. See §447.15, which limits participation in the Medicaid program to providers who accept, as payment in full, Medicaid payment plus any deductible, coinsurance, or co-payment required by the plan to be paid by the individual.) If a State plan does not cover an item or service, such as eyeglasses, the resident may purchase that item or service out of his/her funds. See §483.15(g), F250 for the facility's responsibility to assist the resident in obtaining those services.

Procedures §483.10(c)(8)

As appropriate during Phase 2 of the survey, review the written information given to Medicare/Medicaid eligible residents and family members on admission that notifies them of the items and services that are covered under Medicare or the State plan. Review a sample of residents' monthly statements to ensure that personal funds are not used to pay for covered services. If charges found on monthly statements indicate that residents may have paid for covered items or services, determine if these items or services are over and above what is paid by Medicare or Medicaid.

If, through observations or interviews of residents selected for comprehensive or focused review, the team determines that families or residents hire sitters, and/or that a large number of residents or families are paying for outside food, determine if these practices reflect inadequate staffing and/or food.

Interpretive Guidelines §483.10(c)(8)(i)(E)

Prescription drugs are part of the pharmaceutical services that facilities are required to provide. (See §483.25(l) and (m), and §483.60.) However, at times, a resident needs a medical service that is recognized by State law, but not covered by the State plan. Such a medical service includes a prescription drug that is not on the State's formulary or that exceeds the number of medications covered by Medicaid. It may also include prescription eyeglasses or dentures. If a resident needs a recognized medical service over what is allowed by the State plan, the resident has the right under the Medicaid statute to spend his/her income on that service. If the service is more than what Medicaid pays, the resident may deduct the actual cost of the service from the Medicaid share of the cost. The facility must assist the resident in exercising his or her right to the uncovered medical expense deduction and may not charge the resident for such services.

"Hair hygiene supplies" refers to comb, brush, shampoos, trims and simple hair cuts provided by facility staff as part of routine grooming care. Hair cuts, permanent waves, hair coloring, and relaxing performed by barbers and beauticians not employed by a facility are chargeable.

"Nail hygiene services" refers to routine trimming, cleaning, filing, but not polishing of undamaged nails, and on an individual basis, care for ingrown or damaged nails.

"Basic personal laundry" does not include dry cleaning, mending, washing by hand, or other specialty services that need not be provided. A resident may be charged for these specialty services if he or she requests and receives them.

Interpretive Guidelines §483.10(c)(8)(ii)(I) Social Events

Facilities are required by §483.15(f) to provide an ongoing program of activities designed to meet, in accordance with the comprehensive assessment, the interests and physical, mental, and psychosocial well-being of each resident, and cannot charge residents for these services, whether they occur at the facility or off-site. Resident funds should not be charged for universal items such as bookmobile services or local newspaper subscriptions intended for use by more than one resident. However, if a resident requests and attends a social event or entertainment that is not part of the activities assessment and care plan for that resident, a facility may charge that resident's account only for actual expenses. Further, because of expenses associated with transportation, escorts and other related costs, a resident may be charged for actual expenses for an event or entertainment he or she requests and attends that may be free to the public.

Interpretive Guidelines §483.10(c)(8)(ii)(L) Specially Prepared Foods

A resident may refuse food usually prepared and food substitutions of similar nutritive value because of personal, religious, cultural, or ethnic preference. If the resident requests and receives food that is either not commonly purchased by the facility or easily prepared, then the facility may charge the resident. For example, the facility may charge the resident's account for specially prepared food if the facility has a restricted diet policy and notified the resident on admission of the fact, in accordance with §483.10(b). The facility may not charge the resident's account for specially prepared foods that are required by the physician's order of a therapeutic diet. If a facility changes its menu so that the menu no longer reflects the food preferences of residents, see F165, F242, and F243 to determine compliance with these requirements.

(iii) Requests for items and services.

(A) The facility must not charge a resident (or his or her representative) for any item or service not requested by the resident.

(B) The facility must not require a resident (or his or her representative) to request any item or service as a condition of admission or continued stay.

(C) The facility must inform the resident (or his or her representative) requesting an item or service for which a charge will be made that there will be a charge for the item or service and what the charge will be.

Interpretive Guidelines §483.10(c)(8)(iii) Requests for Items and Services

A facility may not charge a resident or the resident's representative for items and services that are not requested by the resident or representative, whether or not the item or services is requested by a physician. The item or service ordered by the physician should fit in with the resident's care plan.

---

§483.10(d) Free Choice

The resident has the right to--

F163

§483.10(d)(1) -- Choose a personal attending physician

Interpretive Guidelines §483.10(d)(1)

The right to choose a personal physician does not mean that the physician must or will serve the resident, or that a resident must designate a personal physician. If a physician of the resident's choosing fails to fulfill a given requirement, such as §483.25(l)(1), Unnecessary drugs; §483.25(l)(2), Antipsychotic drugs; or §483.40, frequency of physician visits, the facility will have the right, after informing the resident, to seek alternate physician participation to assure provision of appropriate and adequate care and treatment. A facility may not place barriers in the way of residents choosing their own physicians. For example, if a resident does not have a physician, or if the resident's physician becomes unable or unwilling to continue providing care to the resident, the facility must assist the resident in exercising his or her choice in finding another physician.

Before consulting an alternate physician, one mechanism to alleviate a possible problem could involve the facility's utilization of a peer review process for cases which cannot be satisfactorily resolved by discussion between the medical director and the attending physician. Only after a failed attempt to work with the attending physician or mediate differences in delivery of care should the facility request an alternate physician when requested to do so by the resident or when the physician will not adhere to the regulations.

If it is a condition for admission to a continuing care retirement center, the requirement for free choice is met if a resident is allowed to choose a personal physician from among those who have practice privileges at the retirement center.

A resident in a distinct part of a general acute care hospital can choose his/her own physician, unless the hospital requires that physicians with residents in the distinct part have hospital admitting privileges. If this is so, the resident can choose his/her own physician, but cannot have a physician who does not have hospital admitting privileges.

If residents appear to have problems in choosing physicians, determine how the facility makes physician services available to residents.

F164

§483.10(e) Privacy and Confidentiality

The resident has the right to personal privacy and confidentiality of his or her personal and clinical records.

(1) Personal privacy includes accommodations, medical treatment, written and telephone communications, personal care, visits, and meetings of family and resident groups, but this does not require the facility to provide a private room for each resident;

(2) Except as provided in paragraph (e)(3) of this section, the resident may approve or refuse the release of personal and clinical records to any individual outside the facility;

(3) The resident's right to refuse release of personal and clinical records does not apply when--

> **(i) The resident is transferred to another health care institution; or**
>
> **(ii) Record release is required by law**

Interpretive Guidelines §483.10(e)

"**Right to privacy**" means that the resident has the right to privacy with whomever the resident wishes to be private and that this privacy should include full visual, and, to the extent desired, for visits or other activities, auditory privacy. Private space may be created flexibly and need not be dedicated solely for visitation purposes.

For example, privacy for visitation or meetings might be arranged by using a dining area between meals, a vacant chapel, office or room; or an activities area when activities are not in progress. Arrangements for private space could be accomplished through cooperation between the facility's administration and resident or family groups so that private space is provided for those requesting it without infringement on the rights of other residents.

With the exception of the explicit requirement for privacy curtains in all initially certified facilities (see §483.70(d)(1)(v)), the facility is free to innovate to provide privacy for its residents, as exemplified in the preceding paragraph. This may, but need not, be through the provision of a private room.

Facility staff must examine and treat residents in a manner that maintains the privacy of their bodies. A resident must be granted privacy when going to the bathroom and in other activities of personal hygiene. If an individual requires assistance, authorized staff should respect the individual's need for privacy. Only authorized staff directly involved in treatment should be present when treatments are given. People not involved in the care of the individual should not be present without the individual's consent while he/she is being examined or treated. Staff should pull privacy curtains, close doors, or otherwise remove residents from public view and provide clothing or draping to prevent unnecessary exposure of body parts during the provision of personal care and services.

Personal and clinical records include all types of records the facility might keep on a resident, whether they are medical, social, fund accounts, automated or other.

Additional guidelines on mail, visitation rights and telephone communication are addressed in §483.10(i), (j) and (k). See §483.70(d)(1)(iv) for full visual privacy around beds.

Procedures §483.10(e)(1) - (3)

Document **any** instances where you **observe** a resident's privacy being violated. Completely document how the resident's privacy was violated (e.g., Resident #12 left without gown or bed covers and unattended), and where and when this occurred (e.g., 2B Corridor, 3:30 pm, February 25). If possible, identify the responsible party.

§483.75(l)(4) The facility must keep confidential all information contained in the resident's records, regardless of the form or storage method of the records, except when release is required by--

(i) Transfer to another health care institution;

(ii) Law;

(iii) Third party payment contract; or

(iv) The resident.

Interpretive Guidelines §483.75(l)(4)

"Keep confidential" is defined as safeguarding the content of information including video, audio, or other computer stored information from unauthorized disclosure without the consent of the individual and/or the individual's surrogate or representative.

If there is information considered too confidential to place in the record used by all staff, such as the family's financial assets or sensitive medical data, it may be retained in a secure place in the facility, such as a locked cabinet in the administrator's office. The record should show the location of this confidential information.

---

§483.10(f) Grievances

A resident has the right to--

F165

A resident has the right to –

§483.10(f)(1) --Voice grievances without discrimination or reprisal. Such grievances include those with respect to treatment which has been furnished as well as that which has not been furnished; and

(SEE TAG 166 FOR GUIDANCE)

F166

A resident has the right to--

§483.10(f)(2) -- Prompt efforts by the facility to resolve grievances the resident may have, including those with respect to the behavior of other residents.

Intent §483.10(f)

The intent of the regulation is to support each resident's right to voice grievances (e.g., those about treatment, care, management of funds, lost clothing, or violation of rights) and to assure that after receiving a complaint/grievance, the facility actively seeks a resolution and keeps the resident appropriately apprised of its progress toward resolution

Interpretive Guidelines §483.10(f)

"Voice grievances" is not limited to a formal, written grievance process but may include a resident's verbalized complaint to facility staff.

"Prompt efforts...to resolve" include facility acknowledgment of complaint/grievances and actively working toward resolution of that complaint/grievance.

If residents' responses indicate problems in voicing grievances and getting grievances resolved, determine how the facility deals with and makes prompt efforts to resolve resident complaints and grievances.

- With permission, review resident council minutes.
- Interview staff about how grievances are handled.
- Interview staff about communication (to resident) of progress toward resolution of complaint/grievance.

If problems are identified, also investigate compliance with §483.10(b)(7)(iii).

---

§483.10(g) Examination of Survey Results

F167

A resident has the right to--

(1) Examine the results of the most recent survey of the facility conducted by Federal or State surveyors and any plan of correction in effect with respect to the facility. The facility must make the results available for examination in a place readily accessible to residents and must post a notice of their availability; and

SEE GUIDANCE UNDER TAG 168

F168

A resident has the right to:

§483.10(g)(2) -- Receive information from agencies acting as client advocates, and be afforded the opportunity to contact these agencies.

Interpretive Guidelines §483.10(g)(1)-(2)

"Results of the most recent survey" means the Statement of Deficiencies (Form CMS-2567) and the Statement of Isolated Deficiencies generated by the most recent standard survey and any subsequent extended surveys, and any deficiencies resulting from any subsequent complaint investigation(s).

"Made available for examination" means that survey results and approved plan of correction, if applicable, are available in a readable form, such as a binder, large print, or are provided with a magnifying glass, have not been altered by the facility unless authorized by the State agency, and are available to residents without having to ask a staff person.

"Place readily accessible to residents" is a place (such as a lobby or other area frequented by most residents) where individuals wishing to examine survey results do not have to ask to see them.

F169

§483.10(h) Work

The resident has the right to--

(1) Refuse to perform services for the facility;

(2) Perform services for the facility, if he or she chooses, when--

(i) The facility has documented the need or desire for work in the plan of care;

(ii) The plan specifies the nature of the services performed and whether the services are voluntary or paid;

(iii) Compensation for paid services is at or above prevailing rates; and

(iv) The resident agrees to the work arrangement described in the plan of care

Interpretive Guidelines §483.10(h)(1)-(2)

"Prevailing rate" is the wage paid to workers in the community surrounding the facility for essentially the same type, quality, and quantity of work requiring comparable skills.

All resident work, whether of a voluntary or paid nature, must be part of the plan of care. A resident's desire for work is subject to discussion of medical appropriateness. As part of the plan of care, a therapeutic work assignment must be agreed to by the resident. The resident also has the right to refuse such treatment at any time that he or she wishes. At the time of development or review of the plan, voluntary or paid work can be negotiated.

Procedures §483.10(h)(1)-(2)

Are residents engaged in what may be paid or volunteer work (e.g., doing housekeeping, doing laundry, preparing meals)? Pay special attention to the possible work activities of residents with mental retardation or mental illness. If you observe such a situation, determine if the resident is in fact performing work and, if so, is this work, whether voluntary or paid, described in the plan of care?

§483.10(i) Mail

The resident has the right to privacy in written communications, including the right to--

F170

§483.10(i)(1) Send and promptly receive mail that is unopened; and

SEE GUIDANCE UNDER TAG 171

F171

§483.10(i)(2) Have access to stationery, postage, and writing implements at the resident's own expense.

Interpretive Guidelines §483.10(i)(1)-(2)

"Promptly" means delivery of mail or other materials to the resident within 24 hours of delivery by the postal service (including a post office box) and delivery of outgoing mail to the postal service within 24 hours, except when there is no regularly scheduled postal delivery and pick-up service.

F172

§483.10(j) Access and Visitation Rights

§483.10(j)(1) The resident has the right and the facility must provide immediate access to any resident by the following:

(i) Any representative of the Secretary;

(ii) Any representative of the State;

(iii) The resident's individual physician;

(iv) The State long term care ombudsman (established under section 307 (a)(12) of the Older Americans Act of 1965);

(v) The agency responsible for the protection and advocacy system for developmentally disabled individuals (established under part C of the Developmental Disabilities Assistance and Bill of Rights Act);

(vi) The agency responsible for the protection and advocacy system for mentally ill individuals (established under the Protection and Advocacy for Mentally Ill Individuals Act);

(vii) Subject to the resident's right to deny or withdraw consent at any time, immediate family or other relatives of the resident; and

(viii) Subject to reasonable restrictions and the resident's right to deny or withdraw consent at any time, others who are visiting with the consent of the resident.

§483.10(j)(2) The facility must provide reasonable access to any resident by any entity or individual that provides health, social, legal, or other services to the resident, subject to the resident's right to deny or withdraw consent at any time.

Interpretive Guidelines: §483.10(j)(1) and (2)

The facility must provide immediate access to any representative of the Secretary of the Department of Health and Human Services, the State, the resident's individual physician, the State long term care ombudsman, or the agencies responsible for the protection and advocacy of developmentally disabled or mentally ill individuals. The facility cannot refuse to permit residents to talk with surveyors. Representatives of the Department of Health and Human Services, the State, the State ombudsman system, and protection and advocacy agencies for mentally ill and mentally retarded individuals are not subject to visiting hour limitations.

Immediate family or other relatives are not subject to visiting hour limitations or other restrictions not imposed by the resident. However, the facility may try to change the location of visits to assist care giving or protect the privacy of other residents, if these visitation rights infringe upon the rights of other residents in the facility. For example, a resident's family visits in the late evening, which prevents the resident's roommate from sleeping.

Non-family visitors must also be granted "immediate access" to the resident. The facility may place reasonable restrictions upon the exercise of this right such as reasonable visitation hours to facilitate care giving for the resident or to protect the privacy of other residents, such as requiring that visits not take place in the resident's room if the roommate is asleep or receiving care.

An individual or representative of an agency that provides health, social, legal, or other services to the resident has the right of "reasonable access" to the resident, which means that the facility may establish guidelines regarding the timing or other circumstances of the visit, such as location. These guidelines must allow for ready access of residents to these services.

Procedures §483.10(j)(1) and (2)

If you identify problems during interviews, determine how the facility ensures access to:

- Representatives of the State;
- Representatives of the U.S. Department of Health and Human Services;
- The resident's individual physician;
- Representatives of the State long-term care ombudsman;
- Representatives of agencies responsible for protecting and advocating rights of persons with mental illness or developmental disabilities;
- Family or relatives; and
- Other visitors.

F173

§483.10(j)(3) -- The facility must allow representatives of the State Ombudsman, described in paragraph (j)(1)(iv) of this section, to examine a resident's clinical records with the permission of the resident or the resident's legal representative, and consistent with State law.

Procedures §483.10(j)(3)

Ask the ombudsman if the facility allows him/her to examine residents' clinical records with the permission of the resident, and to the extent allowed by State law.

F174

§483.10(k) Telephone

The resident has the right to have reasonable access to the use of a telephone where calls can be made without being overheard.

Interpretive Guidelines §483.10(k)

Telephones in staff offices or at nurses' stations do not meet the provisions of this requirement. Examples of facility accommodations to provide reasonable access to the use of a telephone without being overheard include providing cordless telephones or having telephone jacks in residents' rooms.

"Reasonable access" includes placing telephones at a height accessible to residents who use wheelchairs and adapting telephones for use by the residents with impaired hearing.

---

§483.10(l) Personal Property

The resident has the right to retain and use personal possessions, including some furnishings, and appropriate clothing, as space permits, unless to do so would infringe upon the rights or health and safety of other residents.

Intent §483.10(l)

The intent of this regulation is to encourage residents to bring personal possessions into the facility, as space, safety considerations and fire code permits.

Interpretive Guidelines §483.10(l)

All residents' possessions, regardless of their apparent value to others, must be treated with respect, for what they are and for what they may represent to the resident. The right to retain and use personal possessions assures that the residents' environment be as homelike as possible and that residents retain as much control over their lives as possible. The facility has the right to limit the resident's exercise of this right on grounds of space and health or safety.

Procedures §483.10(l)

If residents' rooms have few personal possessions, ask residents, families and the local ombudsman if:

- Residents are encouraged to have and to use them;
- The facility informs residents not to bring in certain items and for what reason; and
- Personal property is safe in the facility.

Ask staff if the facility sets limits on the value of the property that residents may have in their possession or requires that residents put personal property in the facility's safe.

F175

§483.10(m) Married Couples

The resident has the right to share a room with his or her spouse when married residents live in the same facility and both spouses consent to the arrangement.

Interpretive Guidelines §483.10(m)

The right of residents who are married to each other to share a room does not give a resident the right, or the facility the responsibility, to compel another resident to relocate to accommodate a spouse. The requirement means that when a room is available for a married couple to share, the facility must permit them to share it if they choose. If a married resident's spouse is admitted to the facility later and the couple want to share a room, the facility must provide a shared room as quickly as possible. However, a couple is not able to share a room if one of the spouses has a different payment source for which the facility is not certified (if the room is in a distinct part, unless one of the spouses elects to pay for his or her care).

F176

§483.10(n) Self-Administration of Drugs

An individual resident may self-administer drugs if the interdisciplinary team, as defined by §483.20(d)(2)(ii), has determined that this practice is safe.

Interpretive Guidelines §483.10(n)

If a resident requests to self-administer drugs, it is the responsibility of the interdisciplinary team to determine that it is safe for the resident to self-administer drugs before the resident may exercise that right. The interdisciplinary team must also determine who will be responsible (the resident or the nursing staff) for storage and documentation of the administration of drugs, as well as the location of the drug administration (e.g., resident's room, nurses' station, or activities room). Appropriate notation of these determinations should be placed in the resident's care plan.

The decision that a resident has the ability to self-administer medication(s) is subject to periodic re-evaluation based on change in the resident's status. The facility may require that drugs be administered by the nurse or medication aide, if allowed by State law, until the care planning team has the opportunity to obtain information necessary to make an assessment of the resident's ability to safely self-administer medications. If the resident chooses to self-administer drugs, this decision should be made at least by the time the care plan is completed within seven days after completion of the comprehensive assessment.

Medication errors occurring with residents who self-administer drugs should not be counted in the facility's medication error rate (see Guidelines for §483.25(m)), but should call into question the judgment made by the facility in allowing self-administration for those residents.

Probes: §483.10(n)

For residents selected for a comprehensive review or a focused review, as appropriate:

- Does resident self-administer drugs? Which ones? How much? How often?
- Does the care plan reflect self-administration?

F177

§483.10(o) Refusal of Certain Transfers

(1) An individual has the right to refuse a transfer to another room within the institution, if the purpose of the transfer is to relocate--

(i) A resident of a SNF, from the distinct part of the institution that is a SNF to a part of the institution that is not a SNF, or

(ii) A resident of a NF, from the distinct part of the institution that is a NF to a distinct part of the institution that is a SNF.

(2) A resident's exercise of the right to refuse transfer under paragraph (o)(1) of this section does not affect the individual's eligibility or entitlement to Medicare or Medicaid benefits.

Interpretive Guidelines §483.10(o)

This requirement applies to transfer within a physical plant.

These provisions allow a resident to refuse transfer from a room in one distinct part of an institution to a room in another distinct part of the institution for purposes of obtaining Medicare or Medicaid eligibility. If a resident refuses to transfer from a portion of the institution that is not Medicare certified, the resident forgoes the possibility of Medicare coverage for the care received there. If that portion of the institution is Medicaid certified and the resident is Medicaid-eligible, then Medicaid covered services would be paid by Medicaid. If the resident is Medicaid-eligible, but that portion of the institution is not Medicaid certified, then the resident would assume responsibility for payment for the services. If the resident is unable to pay for those services, then the facility may, after giving the resident a 30-day notice, transfer the resident under the provisions of §483.12(a).

When a resident occupies a bed in a distinct part NF that participates in Medicaid and not in Medicare, he or she may not be moved involuntarily to another part of the institution by the facility (or required to be moved by the State) solely for the purpose of assuring Medicare eligibility for payment. Such moves are only appropriate when they occur at the request of a resident (for example, when a privately paying Medicare beneficiary believes that admission to a bed in a Medicare-participating distinct part of the institution may result in Medicare payment).

See Guidelines, §483.12 for further discussion regarding transfers.

For transfers of residents between Medicare or Medicaid approved distinct parts:

- Is there a documented medical reason for the transfer?
- Was the resident transferred because of a change in payment source?
- If a Medicare or Medicaid resident is notified that he/she is no longer eligible, does the facility transfer the resident? Did the facility give the resident the opportunity to refuse the transfer? How? What happened?
- Ask the local ombudsman about facility compliance with transfer requirements. See also §483.12, Criteria for Transfer.

§483.12 Admission, Transfer, and Discharge Rights

§483.12(a) Transfer, and Discharge

(1) Definition

Transfer and discharge includes movement of a resident to a bed outside of the certified facility whether that bed is in the same physical plant or not. Transfer and discharge does not refer to movement of a resident to a bed within the same certified facility.

Guidelines §483.12

This requirement applies to transfers or discharges that are initiated by the facility, not by the resident. Whether or not a resident agrees to the facility's decision, these requirements apply whenever a facility initiates the transfer or discharge. "Transfer" is moving the resident from the facility to another legally responsible institutional setting, while "discharge" is moving the resident to a non-institutional setting when the releasing facility ceases to be responsible for the resident's care.

If a resident is living in an institution participating in both Medicare and Medicaid (SNF/NF) under separate provider agreements, a move from either the SNF or NF would constitute a transfer.

Transfer and discharge provisions significantly restrict a facility's ability to transfer or discharge a resident once that resident has been admitted to the facility. The facility may not transfer or discharge the resident unless:

1. The transfer or discharge is necessary to meet the resident's welfare and the resident's welfare cannot be met in the facility;
2. The transfer or discharge is appropriate because the resident's health has improved sufficiently so the resident no longer needs the services provided by the facility;
3. The safety of individuals in the facility is endangered;
4. The health of individuals in the facility would otherwise be endangered;
5. The resident has failed, after reasonable and appropriate notice, to pay for a stay at the facility; or
6. The facility ceases to operate.

To demonstrate that any of the events specified in 1 - 5 have occurred, the law requires documentation in the resident's clinical record. To demonstrate situations 1 and 2, the **resident's** physician must provide the documentation. In situation 4, the documentation must be provided by **any** physician. (See §483.12(a)(2).)

Moreover, before the transfer or discharge occurs, the law requires that the facility notify the resident and, if known, the family member, surrogate, or representative of the transfer and the reasons for the transfer, and record the reasons in the clinical record. The facility's notice must include an explanation of the right to appeal the transfer to the State as well as the name, address, and phone number of the State long-term care ombudsman. In the case of a developmentally disabled individual, the notice must include the name, address and phone number of the agency responsible for advocating for the developmentally disabled, and in the case of a mentally ill individual, the name, address and phone number of the agency responsible for advocating for mentally ill individuals. (See §483.12(a)(3) and (5).)

Generally, this notice must be provided at least 30 days prior to the transfer. Exceptions to the 30-day requirement apply when the transfer is effected because of:

- Endangerment to the health or safety of others in the facility;
- When a resident's health has improved to allow a more immediate transfer or discharge;
- When a resident's urgent medical needs require more immediate transfer; and

- When a resident has not resided in the facility for 30 days.

In these cases, the notice must be provided as soon as practicable before the discharge. (See §483.12(a)(4).)

Finally, the facility is required to provide sufficient preparation and orientation to residents to ensure safe and orderly discharge from the facility. (See §483.12(a)(6).)

Under Medicaid, a participating facility is also required to provide notice to its residents of the facility's bed-hold policies and readmission policies prior to transfer of a resident for hospitalization or therapeutic leave. Upon such transfer, the facility must provide written notice to the resident and an immediate family member, surrogate or representative of the duration of any bed-hold. With respect to readmission in a Medicaid participating facility, the facility must develop policies that permit residents eligible for Medicaid, who were transferred for hospitalization or therapeutic leave, and whose absence exceeds the bed-hold period as defined by the State plan, to return to the facility in the first available bed. (See §483.12(b).)

A resident cannot be transferred for non-payment if he or she has submitted to a third party payor all the paperwork necessary for the bill to be paid. Non-payment would occur if a third party payor, including Medicare or Medicaid, denies the claim and the resident refused to pay for his or her stay.

§483.10(o), Tag F177, addresses the right of residents to refuse certain transfers within an institution on the basis of payment status.

F201

§483.12(a)(2) Transfer and Discharge Requirements

The facility must permit each resident to remain in the facility, and not transfer or discharge the resident from the facility unless--

(i) The transfer or discharge is necessary for the resident's welfare and the resident's needs cannot be met in the facility;

(ii) The transfer or discharge is appropriate because the resident's health has improved sufficiently so the resident no longer needs the services provided by the facility;

(iii) The safety of individuals in the facility is endangered;

(iv)The health of individuals in the facility would otherwise be endangered;

(v) The resident has failed, after reasonable and appropriate notice, to pay for (or to have paid under Medicare or Medicaid) a stay at the facility. For a resident who becomes eligible for Medicaid after admission to a nursing facility, the nursing facility may charge a resident only allowable charges under Medicaid; or

(vi) The facility ceases to operate.

SEE GUIDANCE UNDER TAG 202

F202

§483.12(a)(3) Documentation

When the facility transfers or discharges a resident under any of the circumstances specified in paragraphs (a)(2)(i) through (v) of this section, the resident's clinical record must be documented. The documentation must be made by--

(i) The resident's physician when transfer or discharge is necessary under paragraph (a)(2)(i) or paragraph (a)(2)(ii) of this section; and

(ii) A physician when transfer or discharge is necessary under paragraph (a)(2)(iv) of this section.

Interpretive Guidelines §483.12(a)(2) and (3)

If transfer is due to a significant change in the resident's condition, but not an emergency requiring an immediate transfer, then prior to any action, the facility must conduct the appropriate assessment to determine if a new care plan would allow the facility to meet the resident's needs. (See <u>§483.20(b)(4)(iv), F274</u>, for information concerning assessment upon significant change.)

Conversion from a private pay rate to payment at the Medicaid rate does not constitute non-payment.

Refusal of treatment would not constitute grounds for transfer, unless the facility is unable to meet the needs of the resident or protect the health and safety of others.

Documentation of the transfer/discharge may be completed by a physician extender unless prohibited by State law or facility policy.

Procedures §483.12(a)(2) and (3)

During closed record review, determine the reasons for transfer/discharge.

- Do records document accurate assessments and attempts through care planning to address resident's needs through multi-disciplinary interventions, accommodation of individual needs and attention to the resident's customary routines?

- Did the resident's physician document the record if:

    - The resident was transferred/discharged for the sake of the resident's welfare and the resident's needs could not be met in the facility (e.g., a resident develops an acute condition requiring hospitalization)? or

    - The resident's health improved to the extent that the transferred/discharged resident no longer needed the services of the facility.

- Did a physician document the record if residents were transferred because the health of individuals in the facility is endangered?

- Do the records of residents transferred/discharged due to safety reasons reflect the process by which the facility concluded that in each instance transfer or discharge was necessary? Did the survey team observe residents with similar safety concerns in the facility? If so, determine differences between these residents and those who were transferred or discharged.

- Look for changes in source of payment coinciding with transfer. If you find such transfer, determine if the transfers were triggered by one of the criteria specified in §483.12(a)(2).

- Ask the ombudsman if there were any complaints regarding transfer and/or discharge. If there were, what was the result of the ombudsman's investigation?

- If the entity to which the resident was discharged is another long term care facility, evaluate the extent to which the discharge summary and the resident's physician justify why the facility could not meet the needs of this resident.

F203

§483.12(a)(4) Notice Before Transfer

Before a facility transfers or discharges a resident, the facility must--

(i) Notify the resident and, if known, a family member or legal representative of the resident of the transfer or discharge and the reasons for the move in writing and in a language and manner they understand.

(ii) Record the reasons in the resident's clinical record; and

(iii) Include in the notice the items described in paragraph (a)(6) of this section.

§483.12(a)(5) Timing of the notice.

(i) Except when specified in paragraph (a)(5)(ii) of this section, the notice of transfer or discharge required under paragraph (a)(4) of this section must be made by the facility at least 30 days before the resident is transferred or discharged.

(ii) Notice may be made as soon as practicable before transfer or discharge when--

(A) The safety of the individuals in the facility would be endangered under paragraph (a)(2)(iii) of this section;

(B) The health of individuals in the facility would be endangered, under (a)(2)(iv) of this section;

(C) The resident's health improves sufficiently to allow a more immediate transfer or discharge, under paragraph (a)(2)(ii) of this section;

(D) An immediate transfer or discharge is required by the resident's urgent medical needs, under paragraph (a)(2)(i) of this section; or

(E) A resident has not resided in the facility for 30 days.

§483.12(a)(6) Contents of the notice

The written notice specified in paragraph (a)(4) of this section must include the following:

(i) The reason for transfer or discharge;

(ii) The effective date of transfer or discharge;

(iii) The location to which the resident is transferred or discharged;

(iv) A statement that the resident has the right to appeal the action to the State;

(v) The name, address and telephone number of the State long term care ombudsman;

(vi) For nursing facility residents with developmental disabilities, the mailing address and telephone number of the agency responsible for the protection and

advocacy of developmentally disabled individuals established under Part C of the Developmental Disabilities Assistance and Bill of Rights Act; and

(vii) For nursing facility residents who are mentally ill, the mailing address and telephone number of the agency responsible for the protection and advocacy of mentally ill individuals established under the Protection and Advocacy for Mentally Ill Individuals Act.

Procedures §483.12(a)(4)-(6)

If the team determines that there are concerns about the facility's transfer and discharge actions, during closed record review, look at notices to determine if the notice requirements are met, including:

- Advance notice (either 30 days or, as soon as practicable, depending on the reason for transfer/discharge);
- Reason for transfer/discharge;
- The effective date of the transfer or discharge;
- The location to which the resident was transferred or discharged;
- Right of appeal;
- How to notify the ombudsman (name, address, and telephone number); and
- How to notify the appropriate protection and advocacy agency for residents with mental illness or mental retardation (mailing address and telephone numbers).
- Determine whether the facility notified a family member or legal representative of the proposed transfer or discharge.

F204

§483.12(a)(7) Orientation for Transfer or Discharge

A facility must provide sufficient preparation and orientation to residents to ensure safe and orderly transfer or discharge from the facility.

Interpretive Guidelines §483.12(a)(7)

"Sufficient preparation" means the facility informs the resident where he or she is going and takes steps under its control to assure safe transportation. The facility should actively involve, to the extent possible, the resident and the resident's family in selecting the new residence. Some examples of orientation may include trial visits, if possible, by the resident to a new location; working with family to ask their assistance in assuring the resident that valued possessions are not left behind or lost; orienting staff in the receiving facility to resident's daily patterns; and reviewing with staff routines for handling transfers and discharges in a manner that minimizes unnecessary and avoidable anxiety or depression and recognizes characteristic resident reactions identified by the resident assessment and care plan.

Procedures §483.12(a)(7)

During Resident Review, check social service notes to see if appropriate referrals have been made and, if necessary, if resident counseling has occurred.

F205

§483.12(b) Notice of Bed-Hold Policy and Readmission

§483.12(b)(1) Notice before transfer. Before a nursing facility transfers a resident to a hospital or allows a resident to go on therapeutic leave, the nursing facility must provide written information to the resident and a family member or legal representative that specifies--

> **(i) The duration of the bed-hold policy under the State plan, if any, during which the resident is permitted to return and resume residence in the nursing facility; and**
>
> **(ii) The nursing facility's policies regarding bed-hold periods, which must be consistent with paragraph (b)(3) of this section, permitting a resident to return.**

§483.12(b)(2) Bed-hold notice upon transfer. At the time of transfer of a resident for hospitalization or therapeutic leave, a nursing facility must provide to the resident and a family member or legal representative written notice which specifies the duration of the bed-hold policy described in paragraph (b)(1) of this section.

Interpretive Guidelines §483.12(b)(1) and (2)

The nursing facility's bed-hold policies apply to all residents.

These sections require two notices related to the facility's bed-hold policies to be issued. The first notice of bed-hold policies could be given well in advance of any transfer. However, reissuance of the first notice would be required if the bed-hold policy under the State plan or the facility's policy were to change. The second notice, which specifies the duration of the bed-hold policy, must be issued at the time of transfer

In cases of emergency transfer, notice "at the time of transfer" means that the family, surrogate, or representative are provided with written notification within 24 hours of the transfer. The requirement is met if the resident's copy of the notice is sent with other papers accompanying the resident to the hospital.

Bed-hold for days of absence in excess of the State's bed-hold limit are considered non-covered services which means that the resident could use his/her own income to pay for the bed-hold. However, if such a resident does not elect to pay to hold the bed, readmission rights to the next available bed are specified at §483.12(b)(3). Non-Medicaid residents may be requested to pay for all days of bed-hold.

If residents (or their representatives in the case of residents who are unable to understand their rights) are unsure or unclear about their bed-hold rights, **review** facility bed-hold policies.

- Do policies specify the duration of the bed-hold?
- Is this time period consistent with that specified in the State plan?
- During closed record review, look at records of residents transferred to a hospital or on therapeutic leave to determine if bed-hold requirements were followed. Was notice given before and at the time of transfer?
- During closed record review, look at records of residents transferred to a hospital or on therapeutic leave to determine if bed-hold requirements were followed. Was notice given before and at the time of transfer?

F206

§483.12(b)(3) Permitting Resident to Return to Facility

A nursing facility must establish and follow a written policy under which a resident whose hospitalization or therapeutic leave exceeds the bed-hold period under the State plan, is readmitted to the facility immediately upon the first availability of a bed in a semi-private room if the resident--

(i) Requires the services provided by the facility; and

(ii) Is eligible for Medicaid nursing facility services.

Interpretive Guidelines §483.12(b)(3)

"First available bed in a semi-private room" means a bed in a room shared with another resident of the same sex. (see §483.10(m) for the right of spouses to share a room.)

Medicaid-eligible residents who are on therapeutic leave or are hospitalized beyond the State's bed-hold policy must be readmitted to the first available bed even if the residents have outstanding Medicaid balances. Once readmitted, however, these residents may be transferred if the facility can demonstrate that non-payment of charges exists and documentation and notice requirements are followed. The right to readmission is applicable to individuals seeking to return from a transfer or discharge as long as all of the specific qualifications set out in §483.12(b)(3) are met.

Procedures §483.12(b)(3)

For Medicaid recipients whose hospitalization or therapeutic leave exceeds the bed-hold period, do facility policies specify readmission rights?

Refer to the Minimum Data Set (MDS), section A.10, Discharge Planned; MDS 2.0, section Q, Discharge Potential and Overall Status.

Review the facility's written bed-hold policy to determine if it specifies legal readmission rights. Ask the local ombudsman if there are any problems with residents being readmitted to the facility following hospitalization. In closed record review, determine why the resident did not return to the facility.

Ask the social worker or other appropriate staff what he/she tells Medicaid-eligible residents about the facility's bed-hold policies and the right to return and how Medicaid-eligible residents are assisted in returning to the facility.

If potential problems are identified, talk to discharge planners at the hospital to which residents are transferred to determine their experience with residents returning to the facility.

F207

§483.12(c) Equal Access to Quality Care

§483.12(c)(1) A facility must establish and maintain identical policies and practices regarding transfer, discharge, and the provision of services under the State plan for all individuals regardless of source of payment;

§483.12(c)(2) The facility may charge any amount for services furnished to non-Medicaid residents consistent with the notice requirement in §483.10(b)(5)(i) and (b)(6) describing the charges; and

§483.12(c)(3) The State is not required to offer additional services on behalf of a resident other than services provided in the State plan.

Interpretive Guidelines §483.12(c)

Facilities must treat all residents alike when making transfer and discharge decisions. "Identical policies and practices" concerning services means that facilities must not distinguish between residents based on their source of payment when providing services that are required to be provided under the law. All nursing services, specialized rehabilitative services, social services, dietary services, pharmaceutical services, or activities that are mandated by the law must be provided to residents according to residents' individual needs, as determined by assessments and care plans.

Procedures §483.12(c)

Determine if residents are grouped in separate wings or floors for reasons other than care needs.

F208

§483.12(d) Admissions Policy

(1) The facility must--

(i) Not require residents or potential residents to waive their rights to Medicare or Medicaid; and

(ii) Not require oral or written assurance that residents or potential residents are not eligible for, or will not apply for, Medicare or Medicaid benefits.

Interpretive Guidelines §483.12(d)(1)

This provision prohibits both direct and indirect request for waiver of rights to Medicare or Medicaid. A direct request for waiver, for example, requires residents to sign admissions documents explicitly promising or agreeing not to apply for Medicare or Medicaid. An indirect request for waiver includes requiring the resident to pay private rates for a specified period of time, such as two years ("private pay duration of stay contract") before Medicaid will be accepted as a payment source for the resident. Facilities must not seek or receive any kind of assurances that residents are not eligible for, or will not apply for, Medicare or Medicaid benefits.

Procedures §483.12(d)(1)

If concerns regarding admissions procedures arise during interviews, review admissions packages and contracts to determine if they contain prohibited requirements (e.g., "side agreements" for the resident to be private pay or to supplement the Medicaid rate).

Ask staff what factors lead to decisions to place residents in different wings or floors. Note if factors other than medical and nursing needs affect these decisions. Do staff know the source of payment for the residents they take care of?

Ask the ombudsman if the facility treats residents differently in transfer, discharge and covered services based on source of payment.

With respect to transfer and discharge, if the facility appears to be sending residents to hospitals at the time (or shortly before) their payment source changes from private-pay or Medicare to Medicaid, call the hospitals and ask their discharge planners if they have detected any pattern of dumping. Also, ask discharge planners if the facility readmits Medicaid recipients who are ready to return to the facility. During the tour, observe possible differences in services

- Observe if there are separate dining rooms. If so, are different foods served in these dining rooms? For what reasons? Are residents excluded from some dining rooms because of source of payment?

- Observe the placement of residents in rooms in the facility. If residents are segregated on floors or wings by source of payment, determine if the facility is providing different services based on source of payment. Be particularly alert to differences in treatment and services. For example, determine whether less experienced aides and nursing staff are assigned to Medicaid portions of the facility. Notice the condition of the rooms (e.g., carpeted in private-pay wings, tile in Medicaid wings, proximity to the nurses' station, quality of food served as evening snacks).

As part of closed record review, determine if residents have been treated differently in transfers or discharges because of payment status. For example, determine if the facility is sending residents to acute care hospitals shortly before they become eligible for Medicaid as a way of getting rid of Medicaid recipients.

Ask social services staff to describe the facility's policy and practice on providing services, such as rehabilitative services. Determine if services are provided based on source of payment, rather than on need for services to attain or maintain functioning.

§483.12(d)(2) The facility must not require a third party guarantee of payment to the facility as a condition of admission or expedited admission, or continued stay in the facility. However, the facility may require an individual who has legal access to a resident's income or resources available to pay for facility care to sign a contract, without incurring personal financial liability, to provide facility payment from the resident's income or resources.

Interpretive Guidelines §483.12(d)(2)

The facility may not require a third person to accept personal responsibility for paying the facility bill out of his or her own funds. However, he or she may use the resident's money to pay for care. A third party guarantee is not the same as a third party payor, e.g., an insurance company; and this provision does not preclude the facility from obtaining information about Medicare or Medicaid eligibility or the availability of private insurance. The prohibition against third-party guarantees applies to all residents and prospective residents in all certified long term care facilities, regardless of payment source.

§483.12(d)(3) In the case of a person eligible for Medicaid, a nursing facility must not charge, solicit, accept, or receive, in addition to any amount otherwise required to be paid under the State plan, any gift, money, donation, or other consideration as a precondition of admission, expedited admission or continued stay in the facility. However,--

(i) A nursing facility may charge a resident who is eligible for Medicaid for items and services the resident has requested and received, and that are not specified in the State plan as included in the term "nursing facility services" so long as the facility gives proper notice of the availability and cost of these services to residents and does not condition the resident's admission or continued stay on the request for and receipt of such additional services; and

(ii) A nursing facility may solicit, accept, or receive a charitable, religious, or philanthropic contribution from an organization or from a person unrelated to a Medicaid eligible resident or potential resident, but only to the extent that the contribution is not a condition of admission, expedited admission, or continued stay in the facility for a Medicaid eligible resident.

Interpretive Guidelines §483.12(d)(3)

This requirement applies only to Medicaid certified nursing facilities.

Facilities may not charge for any service that is included in the definition of "nursing facility services" and, therefore, required to be provided as part of the daily rate. Facilities may not accept additional payment from residents or their families as a prerequisite to admission or to continued stay in the facility. Additional payment includes deposits from Medicaid-eligible residents or their families, or any promise to pay private rates for a specified period of time.

A nursing facility may charge a Medicaid beneficiary for a service the beneficiary has requested and received, **only** if:

- That service is not defined in the State plan as a "nursing facility" service;

- The facility informs the resident and the resident's representative in advance that this is not a covered service to allow them to make an informed choice regarding the fee; and

- The resident's admission or continued stay is not conditioned on the resident's requesting and receiving that service.

Procedures §483.12(d)(3)

Review State covered services. Compare with the list of items for which the facility charges to determine if the facility is charging for covered services.

Determine if the facility requires deposits from residents. If you identify potential problems with discrimination, review the files of one or more residents selected for a focused or comprehensive review to determine if the facility requires residents to submit deposits as a precondition of admission besides what may be paid under the State plan.

If interviews with residents suggest that the facility may have required deposits from Medicaid recipients at admission, except those admitted when Medicaid eligibility is pending, corroborate by, for example, reviewing the facility's admissions documents or interviewing family members.

§483.12(d)(4) States or political subdivisions may apply stricter admissions standards under State or local laws than are specified in this section, to prohibit discrimination against individuals entitled to Medicaid.

§483.13 Resident Behavior and Facility Practices

F221

Use Tag F221 for deficiencies concerning **physical** restraints.

USE GUIDANCE UNDER TAG F222

F222

Use Tag F222 for deficiencies concerning **chemical** restraints.

§483.13(a) Restraints

The resident has the right to be free from any physical or chemical restraints imposed for purposes of discipline or convenience, and not required to treat the resident's medical symptoms.

Intent §483.13(a)

The intent of this requirement is for each person to attain and maintain his/her highest practicable well-being in an environment that prohibits the use of restraints for discipline or convenience and limits restraint use to circumstances in which the resident has medical symptoms that warrant the use of restraints.

Interpretive Guidelines §483.13(a)

Definitions of Terms

"Physical Restraints" are defined as any manual method or physical or mechanical device, material, or equipment attached or adjacent to the resident's body that the individual cannot remove easily which restricts freedom of movement or normal access to one's body.

"Chemical Restraints" is defined as any drug that is used for discipline or convenience and not required to treat medical symptoms.

"Discipline" is defined as any action taken by the facility for the purpose of punishing or penalizing residents.

"Convenience" is defined as any action taken by the facility to control a resident's behavior or manage a resident's behavior with a lesser amount of effort by the facility and not in the resident's best interest.

"Medical Symptom" is defined as an indication or characteristic of a physical or psychological condition.

"Convenience" is defined as any action taken by the facility to control a resident's behavior or manage a resident's behavior with a lesser amount of effort by the facility and not in the resident's best interest.

Restraints may not be used for staff convenience. However, if the resident needs emergency care, restraints may be used for brief periods to permit medical treatment to proceed unless the facility has a notice indicating that the resident has previously made a valid refusal of the treatment in question. If a resident's unanticipated violent or aggressive behavior places him/her or others in imminent danger, the resident does not have the right to refuse the use of restraints. In this situation, the use of restraints is a measure of last resort to protect the safety of the resident or others and must not extend beyond the immediate episode. The resident's right to participate in care planning and the right to refuse treatment are addressed at §§483.20(k)(2)(ii) and 483.10(b)(4), respectively, and include the right to accept or refuse restraints.

Physical Restraints are defined as any manual method or physical or mechanical device, material, or equipment attached or adjacent to the resident's body that the individual cannot remove easily which restricts freedom of movement or normal access to one's body.

"Physical restraints" include, but are not limited to, leg restraints, arm restraints, hand mitts, soft ties or vests, lap cushions, and lap trays the resident cannot remove easily. Also included as restraints are facility practices that meet the definition of a restraint, such as:

- Using side rails that keep a resident from voluntarily getting out of bed;
- Tucking in or using velcro to hold a sheet, fabric, or clothing tightly so that a resident's movement is restricted;
- Using devices in conjunction with a chair, such as trays, tables, bars or belts, that the resident can not remove easily, that prevent the resident from rising;
- Placing a resident in a chair that prevents a resident from rising; and
- Placing a chair or bed so close to a wall that the wall prevents the resident from rising out of the chair or voluntarily getting out of bed.

Side rails sometimes restrain residents. The use of side rails as restraints is prohibited unless they are necessary to treat a resident's medical symptoms. Residents who attempt to exit a bed through, between, over or around side rails are at risk of injury or death. The potential for serious injury is more likely from a fall from a bed with raised side rails than from a fall from a bed where side rails are not used. They also potentially increase the likelihood that the resident will spend more time in bed and fall when attempting to transfer from the bed.

As with other restraints, for residents who are restrained by side rails, it is expected that the process facilities employ to reduce the use of side rails as restraints is systematic and gradual to ensure the resident's safety while treating the resident's medical symptom.

The same device may have the effect of restraining one individual but not another, depending on the individual resident's condition and circumstances. For example, partial rails may assist one resident to enter and exit the bed independently while acting as a restraint for another.

Orthotic body devices may be used solely for therapeutic purposes to improve the overall functional capacity of the resident.

An enclosed framed wheeled walker, with or without a posterior seat, would not meet the definition of a restraint if the resident could easily open the front gate and exit the device.

If the resident cannot open the front gate (due to cognitive or physical limitations that prevent him or her from exiting the device or because the device has been altered to prevent the resident from exiting the device), the enclosed framed wheeled walker would meet the definition of a restraint since the device would restrict the resident's freedom of movement (e.g. transferring to another chair, to the commode, or into the bed). The decision on whether framed wheeled walkers are a restraint must be made on an individual basis.

"Medical Symptom" is defined as an indication or characteristic of a physical or psychological condition.

The resident's medical symptoms should not be viewed in isolation, rather the symptoms should be viewed in the context of the resident's condition, circumstances and environment. Objective findings derived from clinical evaluation and the resident's subjective symptoms should be considered to determine the presence of the medical symptom. The resident's subjective symptoms may not be used as the sole basis for using a restraint. Before a resident is restrained, the facility must determine the presence of a specific medical symptom that would require the use of restraints, and how the use of restraints would treat the medical symptom, protect the resident's safety, and assist the resident in attaining or maintaining his or her highest practicable level of physical and psychosocial well-being.

Medical symptoms that warrant the use of restraints must be documented in the resident's medical record, ongoing assessments, and care plans. While there must be a physician's order reflecting the presence of a medical symptom, CMS will hold the facility ultimately accountable for the appropriateness of that determination. The physician's order alone is not sufficient to warrant the use of the restraint. It is further expected, for those residents whose care plans indicate the need for restraints, that the facility engage in a systematic and gradual process toward reducing restraints (e.g., gradually increasing the time for ambulation and muscle strengthening activities). This systematic process would also apply to recently admitted residents for whom restraints were used in the previous setting.

Consideration of Treatment Plan

In order for the resident to be fully informed, the facility must explain, in the context of the individual resident's condition and circumstances, the potential risks and benefits of all options under consideration including using a restraint, not using a restraint, and alternatives to restraint use. Whenever restraint use is considered, the facility must explain to the resident how the use of restraints would treat the resident's medical symptoms and assist the resident in attaining or maintaining his/her highest practicable level of physical or psychological well-being. In addition, the facility must also explain the potential negative outcomes of restraint use which include, but are not limited to, declines in the resident's physical functioning (e.g., ability to ambulate) and muscle condition, contractures, increased incidence of infections and development of pressure sores/ulcers, delirium, agitation, and incontinence. Moreover, restraint use may constitute an accident hazard. Restraints have been found in some cases to increase the incidence of falls or head trauma due to falls and other accidents (e.g., strangulation, entrapment). Finally, residents who are restrained may face a loss of autonomy, dignity and self respect, and may show symptoms of withdrawal, depression, or reduced social contact. In effect, restraint use can reduce independence, functional capacity, and quality of life. Alternatives to restraint use should be considered and discussed with the resident. Alternatives to restraint use might include modifying the resident's environment and/or routine.

In the case of a resident who is incapable of making a decision, the legal surrogate or representative may exercise this right based on the same information that would have been provided to the resident. (See §483.10(a)(3) and (4).) However, the legal surrogate or representative cannot give permission to use restraints for the sake of discipline or staff convenience or when the restraint is not necessary to treat the resident's medical symptoms. That is, the facility may not use restraints in violation of the regulation solely based on a legal surrogate or representative's request or approval.

Assessment and Care Planning for Restraint Use

There are instances where, after assessment and care planning, a least restrictive restraint may be deemed appropriate for an individual resident to attain or maintain his or her highest practicable physical and psychosocial well-being. This does not alter the facility's responsibility to assess and care plan restraint use on an ongoing basis.

Before using a device for mobility or transfer, assessment should include a review of the resident's:

- Bed mobility (e.g., would the use of a device assist the resident to turn from side to side? Is the resident totally immobile and unable to change position without assistance?); and

- Ability to transfer between positions, to and from bed or chair, to stand and toilet (e.g., does the raised side rail add risk to the resident's ability to transfer?).

The facility must design its interventions not only to minimize or eliminate the medical symptom, but also to identify and address any underlying problems causing the medical symptom.

- Interventions that the facility might incorporate in care planning include:

  - Providing restorative care to enhance abilities to stand, transfer, and walk safely;

  - Providing a device such as a trapeze to increase a resident's mobility in bed;

- Placing the bed lower to the floor and surrounding the bed with a soft mat;
- Equipping the resident with a device that monitors his/her attempts to arise;
- Providing frequent monitoring by staff with periodic assisted toileting for residents who attempt to arise to use the bathroom;
- Furnishing visual and verbal reminders to use the call bell for residents who are able to comprehend this information and are able to use the call bell device; and/or
- Providing exercise and therapeutic interventions, based on individual assessment and care planning, that may assist the resident in achieving proper body position, balance and alignment, without the potential negative effects associated with restraint use.

Procedures: §483.13(a)

Determine if the facility follows a systematic process of evaluation and care planning prior to using restraints. Since continued restraint use is associated with a potential for a decline in functioning if the risk is not addressed, determine if the interdisciplinary team addressed the risk of decline at the time restraint use was initiated and that the care plan reflected measures to minimize a decline. Also determine if the plan of care was consistently implemented. Determine whether the decline can be attributed to a disease progression or inappropriate use of restraints.

For sampled residents observed as physically restrained during the survey or whose clinical records show the use of physical restraints within 30 days of the survey, determine whether the facility used the restraint for convenience or discipline, or a therapeutic intervention for specific periods to attain and maintain the resident's highest practicable physical, mental, or psychosocial well-being.

Probes: §483.13(a)

This systematic approach should answer these questions:

1. What are the medical symptoms that led to the consideration of the use of restraints?
2. Are these symptoms caused by failure to:
    a. Meet individual needs in accordance with the resident assessments including, but not limited to, section III of the MDS, Customary Daily Routines (MDS Version 2.0, section AC), in the context of relevant

information in sections I and II of the MDS (MDS Version 2.0, sections AA and AB)?

b. Use rehabilitative/restorative care?

c. Provide meaningful activities?

d. Manipulate the resident's environment, including seating?

3. Can the cause(s) of the medical symptoms be eliminated or reduced?

4. If the cause(s) cannot be eliminated or reduced, then has the facility attempted to use alternatives in order to avoid a decline in physical functioning associated with restraint use? (See Physical Restraints Resident Assessment Protocol (RAP), paragraph I).

5. If alternatives have been tried and deemed unsuccessful, does the facility use the least restrictive restraint for the least amount of time? Does the facility monitor and adjust care to reduce the potential for negative outcomes while continually trying to find and use less restrictive alternatives?

6. Did the resident or legal surrogate make an informed choice about the use of restraints? Were risks, benefits, and alternatives explained?

7. Does the facility use the Physical Restraints RAP to evaluate the appropriateness of restraint use?

8. Has the facility re-evaluated the need for the restraint, made efforts to eliminate its use and maintained residents' strength and mobility?

F223

§483.13(b) Abuse

The resident has the right to be free from verbal, sexual, physical, and mental abuse, corporal punishment, and involuntary seclusion.

Intent §483.13(b)

Each resident has the right to be free from abuse, corporal punishment, and involuntary seclusion. Residents must not be subjected to abuse by anyone, including, but not limited to, facility staff, other residents, consultants or volunteers, staff of other agencies serving the resident, family members or legal guardians, friends, or other individuals.

Interpretive Guidelines §483.13(b) and (c)

"Abuse" means the willful infliction of injury, unreasonable confinement, intimidation, or punishment with resulting physical harm, pain or mental anguish." (42 CFR §488.301)

This also includes the deprivation by an individual, including a caretaker, of goods or services that are necessary to attain or maintain physical, mental, and psychosocial well-being. This presumes that instances of abuse of all residents, even those in a coma, cause physical harm, or pain or mental anguish.

"Verbal abuse" is defined as the use of oral, written or gestured language that willfully includes disparaging and derogatory terms to residents or their families, or within their hearing distance, regardless of their age, ability to comprehend, or disability. Examples of verbal abuse include, but are not limited to: threats of harm; saying things to frighten a resident, such as telling a resident that he/she will never be able to see his/her family again.

"Sexual abuse" includes, but is not limited to, sexual harassment, sexual coercion, or sexual assault.

"Physical abuse" includes hitting, slapping, pinching and kicking. It also includes controlling behavior through corporal punishment.

"Mental abuse" includes, but is not limited to, humiliation, harassment, threats of punishment or deprivation.

"Involuntary seclusion" is defined as separation of a resident from other residents or from her/his room or confinement to her/his room (with or without roommates) against the resident's will, or the will of the resident's legal representative. Emergency or short term monitored separation from other Residents will not be considered involuntary seclusion and may be permitted if used for a limited period of time as a therapeutic intervention to reduce agitation until professional staff can develop a plan of care to meet the resident's needs.

Investigation of possible involuntary seclusion, may involve one of two types of situations: that in which residents are living in an area of the facility that restricts their freedom of movement throughout the facility, or that in which a resident is temporarily separated from other residents.

- If the stated purpose of a unit which prevents residents from free movement throughout the facility is to provide specialized care for residents who are cognitively impaired, then placement in the unit is not considered involuntary seclusion, as long as care and services are provided in accordance with each resident's individual needs and preferences rather than for staff convenience, and as long as the resident, surrogate, or representative (if any) participates in the placement decision, and is involved in continuing care planning to assure placement continues to meet resident needs and preferences.

- If a resident is receiving emergency short-term monitored separation due to temporary behavioral symptoms (such as brief catastrophic reactions or combative or aggressive behaviors which pose a threat to the resident, other residents, staff or others in the facility), this is not considered involuntary seclusion as long as this is the least restrictive approach for the minimum amount of time, and is being done according to resident needs and not for staff convenience.

If a resident is being temporarily separated from other residents, i.e., for less than 24 hours, as an emergency short-term intervention, answer these questions:

1. What are the symptoms that led to the consideration of the separation?

2. Are these symptoms caused by failure to:

    a. Meet individual needs?

    b. Provide meaningful activities?

    c. Manipulate the resident's environment?

3. Can the cause(s) be removed?

4. If the cause(s) cannot be removed, has the facility attempted to use alternatives short of separation?

5. If these alternatives have been tried and found ineffective, does the facility use separation for the least amount of time?

6. To what extent has the resident, surrogate or representative (if any) participated in care planning and made an informed choice about separation?

7. Does the facility monitor and adjust care to reduce negative outcomes, while continually trying to find and use less restrictive alternatives?

If, during the course of the survey, you identify the possibility of abuse according to the definitions above, investigate through interviews, observations, and record review. (For investigative options, refer to the Guidelines for Complaint Investigation which outlines the steps of investigations for various types of suspected abuse and misappropriation of property.)

Report and record any instances where the survey team observes an abusive incident. Completely document who committed the abusive act, the nature of the abuse and where and when it occurred. Ensure that the facility addresses the incident immediately.

Properly trained staff should be able to respond appropriately to resident behavior. The CMS does not consider striking a combative resident an appropriate response in any situation. Retaliation by staff is abuse and should be cited as such.

---

§483.13(c) Staff Treatment of Residents (F224* and F226**)

The facility must develop and implement written policies and procedures that prohibit mistreatment, neglect, and abuse of residents and misappropriation of resident property.

§483.13(c)(1)(i) Staff Treatment of Residents

(1) The facility must--

(i) Not use verbal, mental, sexual, or physical abuse, corporal punishment, or involuntary seclusion;

F224 *

*** Intent §483.13(c) (F224)**

Each resident has the right to be free from mistreatment, neglect and misappropriation of property. This includes the facility's identification of residents whose personal histories render them at risk for abusing other residents, and development of intervention strategies to prevent occurrences, monitoring for changes that would trigger abusive behavior, and reassessment of the interventions on a regular basis.

* Use tag F224 for deficiencies concerning mistreatment, neglect, or misappropriation of resident property.

*** Guidelines §483.13(c) (F224)**

"Neglect" means failure to provide goods and services necessary to avoid physical harm, mental anguish, or mental illness. (42 CFR 488.301)

"Misappropriation of resident property" means the deliberate misplacement, exploitation, or wrongful, temporary or permanent use of a resident's belongings or money without the resident's consent. (42 CFR 488.301)

F226 **

** Intent §483.13(c), F226

The facility must develop and operationalize policies and procedures for screening and training employees, protection of residents and for the prevention, identification, investigation, and reporting of abuse, neglect, mistreatment, and misappropriation of property. The purpose is to assure that the facility is doing all that is within its control to prevent occurrences.

** Use tag F226 for deficiencies concerning the facility's development and implementation of policies and procedures.

** Guidelines §483.13(c), F226

The facility must develop and implement policies and procedures that include the seven components: screening, training, prevention, identification, investigation, protection and reporting/response. The items under each component listed below are examples of ways in which the facility could operationalize each component.

I. Screening (483.13(c)(1)(ii)(A)&(B): Have procedures to:

- Screen potential employees for a history of abuse, neglect or mistreating residents as defined by the applicable requirements at 483.13(c)(1)(ii)(A) and (B). This includes attempting to obtain information from previous employers and/or current employers, and checking with the appropriate licensing boards and registries.

II. Training (42 CFR 483.74(e)): Have procedures to:

- Train employees, through orientation and on-going sessions on issues related to abuse prohibition practices such as:
    - o Appropriate interventions to deal with aggressive and/or catastrophic reactions of residents;
    - o How staff should report their knowledge related to allegations without fear of reprisal;
    - o How to recognize signs of burnout, frustration and stress that may lead to abuse; and

- o What constitutes abuse, neglect and misappropriation of resident property.

III. Prevention (483.13(b) and 483.13(c)): Have procedures to:

- Provide residents, families and staff information on how and to whom they may report concerns, incidents and grievances without the fear of retribution; and provide feedback regarding the concerns that have been expressed. (See 483.10(f) for further information regarding grievances.)

- Identify, correct and intervene in situations in which abuse, neglect and/or misappropriation of resident property is more likely to occur.

- This includes an analysis of:

  - o Features of the physical environment that may make abuse and/or neglect more likely to occur, such as secluded areas of the facility;

  - o The deployment of staff on each shift in sufficient numbers to meet the needs of the residents, and assure that the staff assigned have knowledge of the individual residents' care needs;

  - o The supervision of staff to identify inappropriate behaviors, such as using derogatory language, rough handling, ignoring residents while giving care, directing residents who need toileting assistance to urinate or defecate in their beds; and

  - o The assessment, care planning, and monitoring of residents with needs and behaviors which might lead to conflict or neglect, such as residents with a history of aggressive behaviors, residents who have behaviors such as entering other residents' rooms, residents with self-injurious behaviors, residents with communication disorders, those that require heavy nursing care and/or are totally dependent on staff.

IV. Identification (483.13(c)(2)): Have procedures to:

- Identify events, such as suspicious bruising of residents, occurrences, patterns, and trends that may constitute abuse; and to determine the direction of the investigation.

V. Investigation (483.13(c)(3)): Have procedures to:

- Investigate different types of incidents; and

- Identify the staff member responsible for the initial reporting, investigation of alleged violations and reporting of results to the proper authorities. (See §483.13 (c)(2), (3), and (4).)

VI. Protection (483.13(c)(3): Have procedures to:

- Protect residents from harm during an investigation.

VII. Reporting/Response (483.13(c)(1)(iii), 483.13(c)(2) and 483.13(c)(4)): Have procedures to:

- Report all alleged violations and all substantiated incidents to the state agency and to all other agencies as required, and take all necessary corrective actions depending on the results of the investigation;

- Report to the State nurse aide registry or licensing authorities any knowledge it has of any actions by a court of law which would indicate an employee is unfit for service; and

- Analyze the occurrences to determine what changes are needed, if any, to policies and procedures to prevent further occurrences.

F225

The facility must—

§483.13(c)(1)(ii) Not employ individuals who have been--

(A) Found guilty of abusing, neglecting, or mistreating residents by a court of law; or

(B) Have had a finding entered into the State nurse aide registry concerning abuse, neglect, mistreatment of residents or misappropriation of their property; and

(iii) Report any knowledge it has of actions by a court of law against an employee, which would indicate unfitness for service as a nurse aide or other facility staff to the State nurse aide registry or licensing authorities

§483.13(c)(2) The facility must ensure that all alleged violations involving mistreatment, neglect, or abuse, including injuries of unknown source and misappropriation of resident property are reported immediately to the administrator of the facility and to other officials in accordance with State law through established procedures (including to the State survey and certification agency).

§483.13(c)(3) The facility must have evidence that all alleged violations are thoroughly investigated, and must prevent further potential abuse while the investigation is in progress.

§483.13(c)(4) The results of all investigations must be reported to the administrator or his designated representative and to other officials in accordance with State law (including to the State survey and certification agency) within 5 working days of the incident, and if the alleged violation is verified appropriate corrective action must be taken.

Intent §483.13(c)(1)(ii) and (iii)

The facility must not hire a potential employee with a history of abuse, if that information is known to the facility. The facility must report knowledge of actions by a court of law against an employee that indicates the employee is unfit for duty. The facility must report alleged violations, conduct an investigation of all alleged violations, report the results to proper authorities, and take necessary corrective actions.

Interpretive Guidelines §483.13(c)(1)(ii) and (iii)

Facilities must be thorough in their investigations of the past histories of individuals they are considering hiring. In addition to inquiry of the State nurse aide registry or licensing authorities, the facility should check information from previous and/or current employers and make reasonable efforts to uncover information about any past criminal prosecutions.

"**Found guilty** … **by a court of law**" applies to situations where the defendant pleads guilty, is found guilty, or pleads nolo contendere.

"**Finding**" is defined as a determination made by the State that validates allegations of abuse, neglect, mistreatment of residents, or misappropriation of their property.

A certified nurse aide found guilty of neglect, abuse, or mistreating residents or misappropriation of property by a court of law, must have her/his name entered into the nurse aide registry. A licensed staff member found guilty of the above must be reported to their licensing board. Further, if a facility determines that actions by a court of law against an employee are such that they indicate that the individual is unsuited to work in a nursing home (e.g., felony conviction of child abuse, sexual assault, or assault with a deadly weapon), then the facility must report that individual to the nurse aide registry (if a nurse aide) or to the State licensing authorities (if a licensed staff member). Such a determination by the facility is not limited to mistreatment, neglect and abuse of residents and misappropriation of their property, but to any treatment of residents or others inside or outside the facility which the facility determines to be such that the individual should not work in a nursing home environment.

A State must not make a finding that an individual has neglected a resident if the individual demonstrates that such neglect was caused by factors beyond the control of the individual.

Interpretive Guidelines §483.13(c)(2) and (4)

The facility's reporting requirements under 483.13(c)(2) and (4) include reporting both alleged violations and the results of investigations to the State survey agency.

"Injuries of unknown source" – An injury should be classified as an "injury of unknown source" when both of the following conditions are met:

- The source of the injury was not observed by any person **or** the source of the injury could not be explained by the resident; **and**

- The injury is suspicious because of the extent of the injury **or** the location of the injury (e.g., the injury is located in an area not generally vulnerable to trauma) **or** the number of injuries observed at one particular point in time **or** the incidence of injuries over time.

"Immediately" means as soon as possible, but ought not exceed 24 hours after discovery of the incident, in the absence of a shorter State time frame requirement. Conformance with this definition requires that each State has a means to collect reports, even on off-duty hours (e.g., answering machine, voice mail, fax).

The phrase **"in accordance with State law"** modifies the word "officials" only. As such, State law may stipulate that alleged violations and the results of the investigations be reported to additional State officials beyond those specified in Federal regulations. This phrase does not modify what **types** of alleged violations must be reported or the time frames in which the reports are to be made. As such, States may not eliminate the obligation for any of the alleged violations (i.e., mistreatment, neglect, abuse, injuries of unknown source, and misappropriation of resident property) to be reported, not can the State extablish longer time frames for reporting than mandated in the regulations at §§483.13(c)(2) and (4). No State can override the obligation of the nursing home to fulfill the requirements under §483.13(c), so long as the Medicare/Medicaid certification is in place.

F240

§483.15 Quality of Life

A facility must care for its residents in a manner and in an environment that promotes maintenance or enhancement of each resident's quality of life.

Interpretive Guidelines §483.15

The intention of the quality of life requirements is to specify the facility's responsibilities toward creating and sustaining an environment that humanizes and individualizes each resident. Compliance decisions here are driven by the quality of life each resident experiences.

F241

§483.15(a) Dignity

The facility must promote care for residents in a manner and in an environment that maintains or enhances each resident's dignity and respect in full recognition of his or her individuality.

Interpretive Guidelines §483.15(a)

"Dignity" means that in their interactions with residents, staff carries out activities that assist the resident to maintain and enhance his/her self-esteem and self-worth. For example:

- Grooming residents as they wish to be groomed (e.g., hair combed and styled, beards shaved/trimmed, nails clean and clipped);
- Assisting residents to dress in their own clothes appropriate to the time of day and individual preferences;
- Assisting residents to attend activities of their own choosing;
- Labeling each resident's clothing in a way that respects his or her dignity;
- Promoting resident independence and dignity in dining (such as avoidance of day-to-day use of plastic cutlery and paper/plastic dishware, bibs instead of napkins, dining room conducive to pleasant dining, aides not yelling);
- Respecting resident's private space and property (e.g., not changing radio or television station without resident's permission, knocking on doors and requesting permission to enter, closing doors as requested by the resident, not moving or inspecting resident's personal possessions without permission);
- Respecting resident's social status, speaking respectfully, listening carefully, treating residents with respect (e.g., addressing the resident with a name of the resident's choice, not excluding residents from conversations or discussing residents in community setting); and

- Focusing on residents as individuals when they talk to them and addressing residents as individuals when providing care and services.

Procedures §483.15(a)

For sampled residents, use the Resident Assessment Instrument (RAI) and comprehensive care plan to consider the resident's former life style and personal choices made while in the facility to obtain a picture of characteristic resident behaviors. As part of the team's information gathering and decision-making, look at the actions and omissions of staff and the uniqueness of the individual sampled resident and on the needs and preferences of the resident, not on the actions and omissions themselves.

Throughout the survey, observe: Do staff show respect for residents? When staff interact with a resident, do staff pay attention to the resident as an individual? Do staff respond in a timely manner to the resident's requests for assistance? In group activities, do staff focus attention on the group of residents? Or, do staff appear distracted when they interact with residents? For example, do staff continue to talk with each other while doing a "task" for a resident(s) as if she/he were not present?

If the survey team identifies potential compliance issues regarding the privacy of residents during treatment, refer to §483.10(e), F164.

F242

§483.15(b) Self-Determination and Participation

The resident has the right to--

(1) Choose activities, schedules, and health care consistent with his or her interests, assessments, and plans of care;

(2) Interact with members of the community both inside and outside the facility; and

(3) Make choices about aspects of his or her life in the facility that are significant to the resident.

Procedures §483.15(b)

Observe how well staff know each resident and what aspects of life are important to him/her. Determine if staff make adjustments to allow residents to exercise choice and self-determination.

Review MDS Background Information III (MDS version 2.0 section AC) for customary routines. For sampled residents, review MDS to determine level of participation in assessment and care planning by resident and family members. Review MDS, section G (MDS version 2.0 section F) for Psychosocial Well-Being and Care Planning.

If the facility has failed to reasonably accommodate the preferences of the resident consistent with interests, assessments and plan of care, see §483.15(e), F246.

Interpretive Guidelines §483.15(b)(3)

The intent of this requirement is to specify that the facility must create an environment that is respectful of the right of each resident to exercise his or her autonomy regarding what the resident considers to be important facets of his or her life. For example, if a facility changes its policy and prohibits smoking, it must allow current residents who smoke to continue smoking in an area that maintains the quality of life for these residents. Weather permitting, this may be an outside area. Residents admitted after the facility changes its policy must be informed of this policy at admission. (See §483.10(b)(1)). Or, if a resident mentions that her therapy is scheduled at the time of her favorite television program, the facility should accommodate the resident to the extent that it can.

F243

§483.15(c) Participation in Resident and Family Groups

(1) A resident has the right to organize and participate in resident groups in the facility;

(2) A resident's family has the right to meet in the facility with the families of other residents in the facility;

(3) The facility must provide a resident or family group, if one exists, with private space;

(4) Staff or visitors may attend meetings at the group's invitation;

(5) The facility must provide a designated staff person responsible for providing assistance and responding to written requests that result form group meetings;

SEE INTEPRETIVE GUIDANCE FOR §483.15(c) AT TAG F244

F244

§483.15(c)(6) When a resident or family group exists, the facility must listen to the views and act upon the grievances and recommendations of residents and families concerning proposed policy and operational decisions affecting resident care and life in the facility.

Interpretive Guidelines §483.15(c)

This requirement does not require that residents' organize a residents or family group. However, whenever residents or their families wish to organize, facilities must allow them to do so without interference. The facility must provide the group with space, privacy for meetings, and staff support. Normally, the designated staff person responsible for assistance and liaison between the group and the facility's administration and any other staff members attend the meeting only if requested.

- "A resident's or family group" is defined as a group that meets regularly to:
  - Discuss and offer suggestions about facility policies and procedures affecting residents' care, treatment, and quality of life;
  - Support each other;
  - Plan resident and family activities;
  - Participate in educational activities; or
  - For any other purpose.

The facility is required to listen to resident and family group recommendations and grievances. Acting upon these issues does not mean that the facility must accede to all group recommendations, but the facility must seriously consider the group's recommendations and must attempt to accommodate those recommendations, to the extent practicable, in developing and changing facility policies affecting resident care and life in the facility. The facility should communicate its decisions to the resident and/or family group.

Procedures §483.15(c)

If no organized group exists, determine if residents have attempted to form one and have been unsuccessful, and, if so, why.

F245

§483.15(d) Participation in Other Activities

A resident has the right to participate in social, religious, and community activities that do not interfere with the rights of other residents in the facility.

Interpretive Guidelines §483.15(d)

The facility, to the extent possible, should accommodate an individual's needs and choices for how he/she spends time, both inside and outside the facility.

Ask the social worker or other appropriate staff how they help residents pursue activities outside the facility.

F246

§483.15(e) Accommodation of Needs

A resident has a right to --

> **§483.15(e)(1) Reside and receive services in the facility with reasonable accommodations of individual needs and preferences, except when the health or safety of the individual or other residents would be endangered; and**

ALSO SEE INTERPRETIVE GUIDANCE AT TAG F247

F247

A resident has a right to—

§483.15(e)(2) Receive notice before the resident's room or roommate in the facility is changed.

Interpretive Guidelines §483.15(e)

"Reasonable accommodations of individual needs and preferences," is defined as the facility's efforts to individualize the resident's environment. The facility's physical environment and staff behaviors should be directed toward assisting the resident in maintaining and/or achieving independent functioning, dignity, and well-being to the extent possible in accordance with the resident's own preferences, assessment and care plans. The facility should attempt to adapt such things as schedules, call systems, and room arrangements to accommodate residents' preferences, desires, and unique needs.

This requirement applies to areas and environment in accordance with needs and preferences NOT addresses at: §§483.10(k), Telephone; 483.10(1), Personal Property; 483.10(m), Married Couples; 483.15(b), Self-Determination and Participation; 483.15(f)(1), Activities; 483.15(g)(1), Social Services; 483.15(h)(1), Homelike Environment; 483.25(a)(2) and (3), Activities of Daily Living;483.25(f)(1), Psychosocial functioning; 483.25(h)(2), Accidents, Prevention-Assistive devices; 483.35(d)(3), Food prepared in a form designed to meet individual needs.

The facility must demonstrate that it accommodates residents' needs. For example, if the resident refuses a bath because he or she prefers a shower, prefers it at a different time of day or on a different day, does not feel well that day, is uneasy about the aide assigned to help or is worried about falling, the staff should make the necessary adjustments realizing the resident is not refusing to be clean but refusing the bath under the circumstance provided. The facility staff should meet with the resident to make adjustments in the care plan to accommodate his or her needs.

This includes learning the residents preferences and taking them into account when discussing changes of rooms or roommates and the timing of such changes. In addition, this also includes making necessary adjustments to ensure that residents are able to reach call cords, buttons or other communication mechanisms, as well as accommodating food activities or room choices.

Procedures §483.15(e)

Observe resident-staff interaction and determine to what extent staff attempt to accommodate residents' preferences. For those areas not addressed in other regulations, determine what happens when a resident states a preference in the form of a refusal. How does the staff attempt to learn what the resident is refusing, and why, and make adjustments to an extent practicable to meet the resident's needs?

Probes: §483.15(e)

- Are rooms arranged such that residents in wheel chairs can easily access personal items and transfer in and out of bed?
- Does the facility respond to residents' stated needs and preferences?
- If the resident is unable to express needs and preferences that would individualize care, has the family expressed the resident's routine and has the facility responded?

Interpretive Guidelines §483.15(e)(1)

Review the extent to which the facility adapts the physical environment to enable residents to maintain unassisted functioning. These adaptations include, but are not limited to:

1. Furniture and adaptive equipment that enable residents to:
    a. Stand independently;
    b. Transfer without assistance (e.g., arm supports, correct chair height, firm support);

c. Maintain body symmetry; and

d. Participate in resident-preferred activities.

2. Measures that:

a. Enable residents with dementia to walk freely;

b. Reorient and remotivate residents with restorative potential (e.g., displaying easily readable calendars and clocks, wall hangings evocative of the lives of residents);

c. Promote conversation and socialization (pictures and decorations that speak to the resident's age cohort); and

d. Promote mobility and independence for disabled residents in going to the bathroom (e.g., grab bars, elevated toilet seats).

Determine if staff use appropriate measures to facilitate communication with residents who have difficulty communicating. For example, if necessary, does staff get at eye level, allow them to remove a resident from noisy surroundings?

Determine if staff communicate effectively with residents with cognitive impairments, such as referring in a non-contradictory way to what residents are saying, and addressing what residents are trying to express to the agenda behind their behavior.

Probes: §483.15(e)(1)(2)

How have residents' needs been accommodated? Do environmental adaptations enhance residents' independence, self-control, and highest practicable well-being? Is the fit between residents' needs and environment positive?

F248

§483.15(f) Activities

§483.15(f)(1) The facility must provide for an ongoing program of activities designed to meet, in accordance with the comprehensive assessment, the interests and the physical, mental, and psychosocial well-being of each resident.

INTENT: §483.15(f)(1) Activities

The intent of this requirement is that:

- The facility identifies each resident's interests and needs; and
- The facility involves the resident in an ongoing program of activities that is designed to appeal to his or her interests and to enhance the resident's highest practicable level of physical, mental, and psychosocial well-being.

DEFINITIONS

Definitions are provided to clarify key terms used in this guidance.

- "Activities" refer to any endeavor, other than routine ADLs, in which a resident participates that is intended to enhance her/his sense of well-being and to promote or enhance physical, cognitive, and emotional health. These include, but are not limited to, activities that promote self-esteem, pleasure, comfort, education, creativity, success, and independence.

  NOTE: ADL-related activities, such as manicures/pedicures, hair styling, and makeovers, may be considered part of the activities program.

- "One-to-One Programming" refers to programming provided to residents who will not, or cannot, effectively plan their own activity pursuits, or residents needing specialized or extended programs to enhance their overall daily routine and activity pursuit needs.
- "Person Appropriate" refers to the idea that each resident has a personal identity and history that involves more than just their medical illnesses or functional impairments. Activities should be relevant to the specific needs, interests, culture, background, etc. of the individual for whom they are developed.
- "Program of Activities" includes a combination of large and small group, one-to-one, and self-directed activities; and a system that supports the development, implementation, and evaluation of the activities provided to the residents in the facility.[1]

OVERVIEW

In long term care, an ongoing program of activities refers to the provision of activities in accordance with and based upon an individual resident's comprehensive assessment. The Institute of Medicine (IOM)'s 1986 report, "Improving the Quality of Care in Nursing Homes," became the basis for the "Nursing Home Reform" part of OBRA '87 and the current OBRA long term care regulations. The IOM Report identified the need for residents in nursing homes to receive care and/or services to maximize their highest practicable quality of life. However, defining "quality of life" has been difficult, as it is subjective for each person. Thus, it is important for the facility to conduct an individualized assessment of each resident to provide additional opportunities to help enhance a resident's self-esteem and dignity.

Research findings and the observations of positive resident outcomes confirm that activities are an integral component of residents' lives. Residents have indicated that daily life and involvement should be meaningful. Activities are meaningful when they reflect a person's interests and lifestyle, are enjoyable to the person, help the person to feel useful, and provide a sense of belonging.[2]

Residents' Views on Activities

Activities are relevant and valuable to residents' quality of life. In a large-scale study commissioned by CMS, 160 residents in 40 nursing homes were interviewed about what quality of life meant to them. The study found that residents "overwhelmingly assigned priority to dignity, although they labeled this concern in many ways." The researchers determined that the two main components of dignity, in the words of these residents, were "independence" and "positive self-image." Residents listed, under the categories of independence and positive self-image, the elements of "choice of activities" and "activities that amount to something," such as those that produce or teach something; activities using skills from residents' former work; religious activities; and activities that contribute to the nursing home.

The report stated that, "Residents not only discussed particular activities that gave them a sense of purpose but also indicated that a lack of appropriate activities contributes to having no sense of purpose." "Residents rarely mentioned participating in activities as a way to just 'keep busy' or just to socialize. The relevance of the activities to the residents' lives must be considered."

According to the study, residents wanted a variety of activities, including those that are not childish, require thinking (such as word games), are gender-specific, produce something useful, relate to previous work of residents, allow for socializing with visitors and participating in community events, and are physically active. The study found that the above concepts were relevant to both interviewable and non-interviewable residents. Researchers observed that non-interviewable residents appeared "happier" and "less agitated" in homes with many planned activities for them.

Non-traditional Approaches to Activities

Surveyors need to be aware that some facilities may take a non-traditional approach to activities. In neighborhoods/households, all staff may be trained as nurse aides and are responsible to provide activities, and activities may resemble those of a private home.[3] Residents, staff, and families may interact in ways that reflect daily life, instead of in formal activities programs. Residents may be more involved in the ongoing activities in their living area, such as care-planned approaches including chores, preparing foods, meeting with other residents to choose spontaneous activities, and leading an activity. It has been reported that, "some culture changed homes might not have a traditional activities calendar, and instead focus on community life to include activities. Instead of an "activities director," some homes have a Community Life Coordinator, a Community Developer, or other title for the individual directing the activities program.[4]

For more information on activities in homes changing to a resident-directed culture, the following websites are available as resources: www.pioneernetwork.net; www.culturechangenow.com; www.qualitypartnersri.org (click on nursing homes); and www.edenalt.com.

ASSESSMENT

The information gathered through the assessment process should be used to develop the activities component of the comprehensive care plan. The ongoing program of activities should match the skills, abilities, needs, and preferences of each resident with the demands of the activity and the characteristics of the physical, social and cultural environments.[5]

In order to develop individualized care planning goals and approaches, the facility should obtain sufficient, detailed information (even if the Activities RAP is not triggered) to determine what activities the resident prefers and what adaptations, if any, are needed.[6] The facility may use, but need not duplicate, information from other sources, such as the RAI, including the RAPs, assessments by other disciplines, observation, and resident and family interviews. Other sources of relevant information include the resident's lifelong interests, spirituality, life roles, goals, strengths, needs and activity pursuit patterns and preferences.[7] This assessment should be completed by or under the supervision of a qualified professional (see F249 for definition of qualified professional).

NOTE: Some residents may be independently capable of pursuing their own activities without intervention from the facility. This information should be noted in the assessment and identified in the plan of care.

CARE PLANNING

Care planning involves identification of the resident's interests, preferences, and abilities; and any issues, concerns, problems, or needs affecting the resident's involvement/engagement in activities.[8] In addition to the activities component of the comprehensive care plan, information may also be found in a separate activity plan, on a CNA flow sheet, in a progress note, etc.

Activity goals related to the comprehensive care plan should be based on measurable objectives and focused on desired outcomes (e.g., engagement in an activity that matches the resident's ability, maintaining attention to the activity for a specified period of time, expressing satisfaction with the activity verbally or non-verbally), not merely on attendance at a certain number of activities per week.

NOTE: For residents with no discernable response, service provision is still expected and may include one-to-one activities such as talking to the resident, reading to the resident about prior interests, or applying lotion while stroking the resident's hands or feet.

Activities can occur at any time, are not limited to formal activities being provided only by activities staff, and can include activities provided by other facility staff, volunteers, visitors, residents, and family members. All relevant departments should collaborate to develop and implement an individualized activities program for each resident.

Some medications, such as diuretics, or conditions such as pain, incontinence, etc. may affect the resident's participation in activities. Therefore, additional steps may be needed to facilitate the resident's participation in activities, such as:

- If not contraindicated, timing the administration of medications, to the extent possible, to avoid interfering with the resident's ability to participate or to remain at a scheduled activity; or

- If not contraindicated, modifying the administration time of pain medication to allow the medication to take effect prior to an activity the resident enjoys.

The care plan should also identify the discipline(s) that will carry out the approaches. For example:

- Notifying residents of preferred activities;

- Transporting residents who need assistance to and from activities (including indoor, outdoor, and outings);

- Providing needed functional assistance (such as toileting and eating assistance); and

- Providing needed supplies or adaptations, such as obtaining and returning audio books, setting up adaptive equipment, etc.

Concepts the facility should have considered in the development of the activities component of the resident's comprehensive care plan include the following, as applicable to the resident:

- A continuation of life roles, consistent with resident preferences and functional capacity (e.g., to continue work or hobbies such as cooking, table setting, repairing small appliances)[9];

- Encouraging and supporting the development of new interests, hobbies, and skills (e.g., training on using the Internet); and

- Connecting with the community, such as places of worship, veterans' groups, volunteer groups, support groups, wellness groups, athletic or educational connections (via outings or invitations to outside groups to visit the facility).

The facility may need to consider accommodations in schedules, supplies and timing in order to optimize a resident's ability to participate in an activity of choice. Examples of accommodations may include, but are not limited to:

- Altering a therapy or a bath/shower schedule to make it possible for a resident to attend a desired activity that occurs at the same time as the therapy session or bath;

- Assisting residents, as needed, to get to and participate in desired activities (e.g., dressing, toileting, transportation);

- Providing supplies (e.g., books/magazines, music, craft projects, cards, sorting materials) for activities, and assistance when needed, for residents' use (e.g., during weekends, nights, holidays, evenings, or when the activities staff are unavailable); and

- Providing a late breakfast to allow a resident to continue a lifelong pattern of attending religious services before eating.

INTERVENTIONS

The concept of individualized intervention has evolved over the years. Many activity professionals have abandoned generic interventions such as "reality orientation" and large-group activities that include residents with different levels of strengths and needs. In their place, individualized interventions have been developed based upon the assessment of the resident's history, preferences, strengths, and needs. These interventions have changed from the idea of "age-appropriate" activities to promoting "person-appropriate" activities. For example, one person may care for a doll or stroke a stuffed animal, another person may be inclined to reminisce about dolls or stuffed animals they once had, while someone else may enjoy petting a dog but will not be interested in inanimate objects. The surveyor observing these interventions should determine if the facility selected them in response to the resident's history and preferences. Many activities can be adapted in various ways to accommodate the resident's change in functioning due to physical or cognitive limitations.

Some Possible Adaptations that May be Made by the Facility [10, 11]

When evaluating the provision of activities, it is important for the surveyor to identify whether the resident has conditions and/or issues for which staff should have provided adaptations. Examples of adaptations for specific conditions include, but are not limited to the following:

- For the resident with visual impairments: higher levels of lighting without glare; magnifying glasses, light-filtering lenses, telescopic glasses; use of "clock method" to describe where items are located; description of sizes, shapes, colors; large print items including playing cards, newsprint, books; audio books;

- For the resident with hearing impairments: small group activities; placement of resident near speaker/activity leader; use of amplifiers or headphones; decreased background noise; written instructions; use of gestures or sign language to enhance verbal communication; adapted TV (closed captioning, magnified screen, earphones);

- For the resident who has physical limitations, the use of adaptive equipment, proper seating and positioning, placement of supplies and materials[12] (based on clinical assessment and referral as appropriate) to enhance:

    - Visual interaction and to compensate for loss of visual field (hemianopsia);
    - Upper extremity function and range of motion (reach);
    - Hand dexterity (e.g., adapted size of items such as larger handles for cooking and woodworking equipment, built-up paintbrush handles, large needles for crocheting);
    - The ability to manipulate an item based upon the item's weight, such as lighter weight for residents with muscle weakness[13];

- For the resident who has the use of only one hand: holders for kitchen items, magazines/books, playing cards; items (e.g., art work, bingo card, nail file) taped to the table; c-clamp or suction vise to hold wood for sanding;

- For the resident with cognitive impairment: task segmentation and simplification; programs using retained long-term memory, rather than short-term memory; length of activities based on attention span; settings that recreate past experiences or increase/decrease stimulation; smaller groups without interruption; one-to-one activities;

NOTE: The length, duration, and content of specific one-to-one activities are determined by the specific needs of the individual resident, such as several short interventions (rather than a few longer activities) if someone has extremely low tolerance, or if there are behavioral issues.

Examples of one-to-one activities may include any of the following:

- Sensory stimulation or cognitive therapy (e.g., touch/visual/auditory stimulation, reminiscence, or validation therapy) such as special stimulus rooms or equipment; alerting/upbeat music and using alerting aromas or providing fabrics or other materials of varying textures;

- Social engagement (e.g., directed conversation, initiating a resident to resident conversation, pleasure walk or coffee visit);

- Spiritual support, nurturing (e.g., daily devotion, Bible reading, or prayer with or for resident per religious requests/desires);

- Creative, task-oriented activities (e.g., music or pet activities/therapy, letter writing, word puzzles); or

- Support of self-directed activity (e.g., delivering of library books, craft material to rooms, setting up talking book service).

- For the resident with a language barrier: translation tools; translators; or publications and/or audio/video materials in the resident's language;

- For residents who are terminally ill: life review; quality time with chosen relatives, friends, staff, and/or other residents; spiritual support; touch; massage; music; and/or reading to the resident; [8]

NOTE: Some residents may prefer to spend their time alone and introspectively. Their refusal of activities does not necessarily constitute noncompliance.

- For the resident with pain: spiritual support, relaxation programs, music, massage, aromatherapy, pet therapy/pet visits, and/or touch;

- For the resident who prefers to stay in her/his own room or is unable to leave her/his room: in-room visits by staff/other residents/volunteers with similar interests/hobbies; touch and sensory activities such as massage or aromatherapy; access to art/craft materials, cards, games, reading materials; access to technology of interest (computer, DVD, hand held video games, preferred radio programs/stations, audio books); and/or visits from spiritual counselors; [14]

- For the resident with varying sleep patterns, activities are available during awake time. Some facilities use a variety of options when activities staff are not available for a particular resident: nursing staff reads a newspaper with resident; dietary staff makes finger foods available; CNA works puzzle with the resident; maintenance staff take the resident on night rounds; and/or early morning delivery of coffee/juice to residents;

- For the resident who has recently moved-in: welcoming activities and/or orientation activities;

- For the short-stay resident: "a la carte activities" are available, such as books, magazines, cards, word puzzles, newspapers, CDs, movies, and handheld games; interesting/contemporary group activities are offered, such as dominoes, bridge, Pinochle, poker, video games, movies, and travelogues; and/or individual activities designed to match the goals of therapy, such as jigsaw puzzles to enhance fine motor skills;

- For the younger resident: individual and group music offerings that fit the resident's taste and era; magazines, books and movies that fit the resident's taste and era; computer and Internet access; and/or contemporary group activities, such as video games, and the opportunity to play musical instruments, card and board games, and sports; and

    - For residents from diverse ethnic or cultural backgrounds: special events that include meals, decorations, celebrations, or music; visits from spiritual leaders and other individuals of the same ethnic background; printed materials (newspapers, magazines) about the resident's culture; and/or opportunities for the resident and family to share information about their culture with other residents, families, and staff.

Activity Approaches for Residents with Behavioral Symptoms [15, 7]

When the surveyor is evaluating the activities provided to a resident who has behavioral symptoms, they may observe that many behaviors take place at about the same time every day (e.g., before lunch or mid-afternoon). The facility may have identified a resident's pattern of behavior symptoms and may offer activity interventions, whenever possible, prior to the behavior occurring. Once a behavior escalates, activities may be less effective or may even cause further stress to the resident (some behaviors may be appropriate reactions to feelings of discomfort, pain, or embarrassment, such as aggressive behaviors exhibited by some residents with dementia during bathing [16]). Examples of activities-related interventions that a facility may provide to try to minimize distressed behavior may include, but are not limited to the following:

For the resident who is constantly walking:

- Providing a space and environmental cues that encourages physical exercise, decreases exit behavior and reduces extraneous stimulation (such as seating areas spaced along a walking path or garden; a setting in which the resident may manipulate objects; or a room with a calming atmosphere, for example, using music, light, and rocking chairs);

- Providing aroma(s)/aromatherapy that is/are pleasing and calming to the resident; and

- Validating the resident's feelings and words; engaging the resident in conversation about who or what they are seeking; and using one-to-one activities, such as reading to the resident or looking at familiar pictures and photo albums.

For the resident who engages in name-calling, hitting, kicking, yelling, biting, sexual behavior, or compulsive behavior:

- Providing a calm, non-rushed environment, with structured, familiar activities such as folding, sorting, and matching; using one-to-one activities or small group activities that comfort the resident, such as their preferred music, walking quietly with the staff, a family member, or a friend; eating a favorite snack; looking at familiar pictures;

- Engaging in exercise and movement activities; and

- Exchanging self-stimulatory activity for a more socially-appropriate activity that uses the hands, if in a public space.

For the resident who disrupts group activities with behaviors such as talking loudly and being demanding, or the resident who has catastrophic reactions such as uncontrolled crying or anger, or the resident who is sensitive to too much stimulation:

- Offering activities in which the resident can succeed, that are broken into simple steps, that involve small groups or are one-to-one activities such as using the computer, that are short and repetitive, and that are stopped if the resident becomes overwhelmed (reducing excessive noise such as from the television);

- Involving in familiar occupation-related activities. (A resident, if they desire, can do paid or volunteer work and the type of work would be included in the resident's plan of care, such as working outside the facility, sorting supplies, delivering resident mail, passing juice and snacks, refer to F169, Work);

- Involving in physical activities such as walking, exercise or dancing, games or projects requiring strategy, planning, and concentration, such as model building, and creative programs such as music, art, dance or physically resistive activities, such as kneading clay, hammering, scrubbing, sanding, using a punching bag, using stretch bands, or lifting weights; and

- Slow exercises (e.g., slow tapping, clapping or drumming); rocking or swinging motions (including a rocking chair).

For the resident who goes through others' belongings:

- Using normalizing activities such as stacking canned food onto shelves, folding laundry; offering sorting activities (e.g., sorting socks, ties or buttons); involving in organizing tasks (e.g., putting activity supplies away); providing rummage areas in plain sight, such as a dresser; and

- Using non-entry cues, such as "Do not disturb" signs or removable sashes, at the doors of other residents' rooms; providing locks to secure other resident's belongings (if requested).

For the resident who has withdrawn from previous activity interests/customary routines and isolates self in room/bed most of the day:

- Providing activities just before or after meal time and where the meal is being served (out of the room);

- Providing in-room volunteer visits, music or videos of choice;
- Encouraging volunteer-type work that begins in the room and needs to be completed outside of the room, or a small group activity in the resident's room, if the resident agrees; working on failure-free activities, such as simple structured crafts or other activity with a friend; having the resident assist another person;

- Inviting to special events with a trusted peer or family/friend;

- Engaging in activities that give the resident a sense of value (e.g., intergenerational activities that emphasize the resident's oral history knowledge);

- Inviting resident to participate on facility committees;

- Inviting the resident outdoors; and

- Involving in gross motor exercises (e.g., aerobics, light weight training) to increase energy and uplift mood.

For the resident who excessively seeks attention from staff and/or peers: Including in social programs, small group activities, service projects, with opportunities for leadership.

For the resident who lacks awareness of personal safety, such as putting foreign objects in her/his mouth or who is self-destructive and tries to harm self by cutting or hitting self, head banging, or causing other injuries to self:

- Observing closely during activities, taking precautions with materials (e.g., avoiding sharp objects and small items that can be put into the mouth);
- Involving in smaller groups or one-to-one activities that use the hands (e.g., folding towels, putting together PVC tubing);
- Focusing attention on activities that are emotionally soothing, such as listening to music or talking about personal strengths and skills, followed by participation in related activities; and
- Focusing attention on physical activities, such as exercise.

For the resident who has delusional and hallucinatory behavior that is stressful to her/him:

- Focusing the resident on activities that decrease stress and increase awareness of actual surroundings, such as familiar activities and physical activities; offering verbal reassurance, especially in terms of keeping the resident safe; and acknowledging that the resident's experience is real to her/him.

The outcome for the resident, the decrease or elimination of the behavior, either validates the activity intervention or suggests the need for a new approach.

ENDNOTES

[1] Miller, M. E., Peckham, C. W., & Peckham, A. B. (1998). Activities keep me going and going (pp. 217-224). Lebanon, OH: Otterbein Homes.

[2] Alzheimer's Association (n.d.). Activity based Alzheimer care: Building a therapeutic program.
Training presentation made 1998.

[3] Thomas, W.H. (2003). Evolution of Eden. In A. S. Weiner & J. L. Ronch (Eds.), Culture change in long-term care (pp. 146-157). New York: Haworth Press.

[4] Bowman, C. S. (2005). Living Life to the Fullest: A match made in OBRA '87. Milwaukee, WI: Action Pact, Inc.

[5] Glantz, C.G., & Richman, N. (2001). Leisure activities. In Occupational therapy: Practice skills for physical dysfunction. St Louis: Mosby.

[6] Glantz, C.G., & Richman, N. (1996). Evaluation and intervention for leisure activities, ROTE: Role of Occupational Therapy for the Elderly (2nd ed., p. 728). Bethesda, MD.: American Occupational Therapy Association.

[7] Glantz, C.G., & Richman, N. (1998). Creative methods, materials and models for training trainers in alzheimer's education (pp. 156-159). Riverwoods, IL: Glantz/Richman Rehabilitation Associates.

[8] Hellen, C. (1992). Alzheimer's disease: Activity-focused care (pp. 128-130). Boston, MA: Andover.

[9] American Occupatinal Therapy Association. (2002). Occupational therapy practice framework: domain & process. American Journal of Occupational Therapy, 56(6), 616-617. Bethesda, MD: American Occupational Therapy Association.

[10] Henderson, A., Cermak, S., Costner, W., Murray, E., Trombly, C., & Tickle-Gegnen, L. (1991). The issue is: Occupational science is multidimensional. American Journal of Occupational Therapy, 45, 370-372, Bethesda, MD: American Occupational Therapy Association.

[11] Pedretti, L.W. (1996). Occupational performance: A model for practice in physical dysfunction. In L.W. Pedretti (Ed.), Occupational therapy: Practice skills for physical dysfunction (4th ed., pp. 3-11). St. Louis: Mosby-Year Book

[12] Christenson, M.A. (1996). Environmental design, modification, and adaptation, ROTE: Role of occupational therapy for the elderly (2nd ed., pp. 380-408). Bethesda, MD: American Occupational Therapy Association.

[13] Coppard, B.M., Higgins, T., & Harvey, K.D. (2004). Working with elders who have orthopedic conditions. In S. Byers-Connon, H.L. Lohman, and R.L. Padilla (Eds.), Occupational therapy with elders: Strategies for the COTA (2nd ed., p. 293). St. Louis, MO: Elservier Mosby.

[14] Glantz, C.G., & Richman, N. (1992). Activity programming for the resident with mental illness (pp. 53-76). Riverwoods, IL: Glantz/Richman Rehabilitation Associates.

[15] Day, K., & Calkins, M.P. (2002). Design and dementia. In R. B. Bechtel & A. Churchman (Eds.), Handbook of environmental psychology (pp. 374-393). New York: Wiley.

[16] Barrick, A.L., Rader, J., Hoeffer, B., & Sloane, P. (2002). Bathing without a battle: Personal care of individuals with dementia (p. 4). New York: Springer.

INVESTIGATIVE PROTOCOL

ACTIVITIES

Objective

To determine if the facility has provided an ongoing program of activities designed to accommodate the individual resident's interests and help enhance her/his physical, mental and psychosocial well-being, according to her/his comprehensive resident assessment.

Use

Use this procedure for each sampled resident to determine through interview, observation and record review whether the facility is in compliance with the regulation.

Procedures

Briefly review the comprehensive assessment and interdisciplinary care plan to guide observations to be made.

1. Observations

Observe during various shifts in order to determine if staff are consistently implementing those portions of the comprehensive plan of care related to activities. Determine if staff take into account the resident's food preferences and restrictions for activities that involve food, and provide ADL assistance and adaptive equipment as needed during activities programs. For a resident with personal assistive devices such as glasses or hearing aides, determine if these devices are in place, glasses are clean, and assistive devices are functional.

For a resident whose care plan includes group activities, observe if staff inform the resident of the activities program schedule and provide timely transportation, if needed, for the resident to attend in-facility activities and help the resident access transportation to out-of-facility and community activities.

Determine whether the facility provides activities that are compatible with the resident's known interests, needs, abilities and preferences. If the resident is in group activity programs, note if the resident is making attempts to leave, or is expressing displeasure with, or sleeping through, an activity program. If so, determine if staff attempted to identify the reason the resident is attempting to leave, and if they addressed the resident's needs. Determine whether the group activity has been adapted for the resident as needed and whether it is "person appropriate."

NOTE: If you observe an activity that you believe would be age inappropriate for most residents, investigate further to determine the reason the resident and staff selected this activity. The National Alzheimer's Association has changed from endorsing the idea of "age-appropriate" activities to promoting "person-appropriate" activities. In general, surveyors should not expect to see the facility providing dolls or stuffed animals for most residents, but some residents are attached to these items and should be able to continue having them available if they prefer.

Regarding group activities in common areas, determine if the activities are occurring in rooms that have sufficient space, light, ventilation, equipment and supplies. Sufficient space includes enough space for residents to participate in the activity and space for a resident to enter and leave the room without having to move several other residents. Determine if the room is sufficiently free of extraneous noise, such as environmental noises from mechanical equipment and staff interruptions.

For a resident who is involved in individual activities in her/his room, observe if staff have provided needed assistance, equipment and supplies. Observe if the room has sufficient light and space for the resident to complete the activity.

2. Interviews

Resident/Representative Interview. Interview the resident, family or resident representative as appropriate to identify their involvement in care plan development, defining the approaches and goals that reflect the resident's preferences and choices. Determine:

- What assistance, if any, the facility should be providing to facilitate participation in activities of choice and whether or not the assistance is being provided;
- Whether the resident is participating in chosen activities on a regular basis, and if not, why not;
- Whether the resident is notified of activities opportunities and is offered transportation assistance as needed to the activity location within the facility or access to transportation, where available and feasible, to outside activities;
- Whether the facility tried, to the extent possible, to accommodate the resident's choices regarding her/his schedule, so that service provision (for example, bathing and therapy services) does not routinely conflict with desired activities;
- Whether planned activity programs usually occur as scheduled (instead of being cancelled repeatedly); and
- Whether the resident desires activities that the facility does not provide.

If the resident has expressed any concerns, determine if the resident has discussed these with staff and, if so, what was the staff's response.

Activity Staff Interview

Interview activities staff as necessary to determine:

- The resident's program of activities and related goals;
- What assistance/adaptations they provide in group activities according to the resident's care plan;
- How regularly the resident participates; if not participating, what is the reason(s);
- How they assure the resident is informed of, and transported to, group activities of choice;
- How special dietary needs and restrictions are handled during activities involving food;
- What assistance they provide if the resident participates in any individual (non-group) activities; and
- How they assure the resident has sufficient supplies, lighting, and space for individual activities.

CNA Interview

Interview CNAs as necessary to determine what assistance, if needed, the CNA provides to help the resident participate in desired group and individual activities, specifically:

- Their role in ensuring the resident is out of bed, dressed, and ready to participate in chosen group activities, and in providing transportation if needed;
- Their role in providing any needed ADL assistance to the resident while she/he is participating in group activities;
- Their role in helping the resident to participate in individual activities (if the resident's plan includes these), for example, setup of equipment/supplies, positioning assistance, providing enough lighting and space; and
- How activities are provided for the resident at times when activities staff are not available to provide care planned activities.

Social Services Staff Interview

Interview the social services staff member as necessary to determine how they help facilitate resident participation in desired activities; specifically, how the social services staff member:

- Addresses the resident's psychosocial needs that impact on the resident's ability to participate in desired activities;
- Obtains equipment and/or supplies that the resident needs in order to participate in desired activities (for example, obtaining audio books, helping the resident replace inadequate glasses or a hearing aid); and
- Helps the resident access his/her funds in order to participate in desired activities that require money, such as attending concerts, plays, or restaurant dining events.

Nurse Interview

Interview a nurse who supervises CNAs who work with the resident to determine how nursing staff:

- Assist the resident in participating in activities of choice by:
    - Coordinating schedules for ADLs, medications, and therapies, to the extent possible, to maximize the resident's ability to participate;
    - Making nursing staff available to assist with activities in and out of the facility;
- If the resident is refusing to participate in activities, how they try to identify and address the reasons; and
- Coordinate the resident's activities participation when activities staff are not available to provide care planned activities.

3. Record Review

Assessment

Review the RAI, activity documentation/notes, social history, discharge information from a previous setting, and other interdisciplinary documentation that may contain information regarding the resident's activity interests, preferences and needed adaptations.

Compare information obtained by observation of the resident and interviews with staff and the resident/responsible party (as possible), to the information in the resident's record, to help determine if the assessment accurately and comprehensively reflects the resident's status. Determine whether staff have identified:

- Longstanding interests and customary routine, and how the resident's current physical, mental, and psychosocial health status affects her/his choice of activities and her/his ability to participate;

- Specific information about how the resident prefers to participate in activities of interest (for example, if music is an interest, what kinds of music; does the resident play an instrument; does the resident have access to music to which she/he likes to listen; and can the resident participate independently, such as inserting a CD into a player);

- Any significant changes in activity patterns before or after admission;

- The resident's current needs for special adaptations in order to participate in desired activities (e.g., auditory enhancement or equipment to help compensate for physical difficulties such as use of only one hand);

- The resident's needs, if any, for time-limited participation, such as a short attention span or an illness that permits only limited time out of bed;

- The resident's desired daily routine and availability for activities; and

- The resident's choices for group, one-to-one, and self-directed activities.

Comprehensive Care Planning

Review the comprehensive care plan to determine if that portion of the plan related to activities is based upon the goals, interests, and preferences of the resident and reflects the comprehensive assessment. Determine if the resident's care plan:

- Includes participation of the resident (if able) or the resident's representative;

- Considers a continuation of life roles, consistent with resident preferences and functional capacity;

- Encourages and supports the development of new interests, hobbies, and skills;

- Identifies activities in the community, if appropriate;

- Includes needed adaptations that address resident conditions and issues affecting activities participation; and

- Identifies how the facility will provide activities to help the resident reach the goal(s) and who is responsible for implementation (e.g., activity staff, CNAs, dietary staff).

If care plan concerns are noted, interview staff responsible for care planning regarding the rationale for the current plan of care.

Care Plan Revision

Determine if the staff have evaluated the effectiveness of the care plan related to activities and made revisions, if necessary, based upon the following:

- Changes in the resident's abilities, interests, or health;
- A determination that some aspects of the current care plan were unsuccessful (e.g., goals were not being met);
- The resident refuses, resists, or complains about some chosen activities;
- Changes in time of year have made some activities no longer possible (e.g., gardening outside in winter) and other activities have become available; and
- New activity offerings have been added to the facility's available activity choices.

For the resident who refused some or all activities, determine if the facility worked with the resident (or representative, as appropriate) to identify and address underlying reasons and offer alternatives.

DETERMINATION OF COMPLIANCE (Task 6, Appendix P)

Synopsis of Regulation (F248)

This requirement stipulates that the facility's program of activities should accommodate the interests and well-being of each resident. In order to fulfill this requirement, it is necessary for the facility to gain awareness of each resident's activity preferences as well as any current limitations that require adaptation in order to accommodate these preferences.

Criteria for Compliance
The facility is in compliance with this requirement if they:

- Recognized and assessed for preferences, choices, specific conditions, causes and/or problems, needs and behaviors;

- Defined and implemented activities in accordance with resident needs and goals;
- Monitored and evaluated the resident's response; and
- Revised the approaches as appropriate.

If not, cite at F248.

Noncompliance for Tag F248

After completing the Investigative Protocol, analyze the information gained in order to determine whether noncompliance with the regulation exists. Activities (F248) is an outcome-oriented requirement in that compliance is determined separately for each resident sampled. The survey team's review of the facility's activities program is conducted through a review of the individualization of activities to meet each resident's needs and preferences. For each sampled resident for whom activities participation was reviewed, the facility is in compliance if they have provided activities that are individualized to that resident's needs and preferences, and they have provided necessary adaptations to facilitate the resident's participation. Non compliance with F248 may look like, but is not limited to the following:

The facility does not have an activity program and does not offer any activities to the resident;

- A resident with special needs does not receive adaptations needed to participate in individualized activities;
- Planned activities were not conducted or designed to meet the resident's care plan;

Potential Tags for Additional Investigation

During the investigation of the provision of care and services related to activities, the surveyor may have identified concerns with related outcome, process and/or structure requirements. The surveyor is cautioned to investigate these related requirements before determining whether noncompliance may be present. Some examples of requirements that should be considered include the following (not all inclusive):

- 42 CFR 483.10(e), F164, Privacy and Confidentiality
    - Determine if the facility has accommodated the resident's need for privacy for visiting with family, friends, and others, as desired by the resident.
- 42 CFR 483.10(j)(1) and (2), F172, Access and Visitation Rights

    - Determine if the facility has accommodated the resident's family and/or other visitors (as approved by the resident) to be present with the resident as much as desired, even round-the-clock.

- 42 CFR 483.15(b), F242, Self-Determination and Participation

    - Determine if the facility has provided the resident with choices about aspects of her/his life in the facility that are significant to the resident.

- 42 CFR 483.15(e)(1), F246, Accommodation of Needs

    - Determine if the facility has provided reasonable accommodation to the resident's physical environment (room, bathroom, furniture, etc.) to accommodate the resident's individual needs in relation to the pursuit of individual activities, if any.

- 42 CFR 483.15(f)(2), F249, Qualifications of the Activities Director

    - Determine if a qualified activities director is directing the activities program.

- 42 CFR 483.15(g)(1), F250, Social Services

    - Determine if the facility is providing medically-related social services related to assisting with obtaining supplies/equipment for individual activities (if any), and assisting in meeting the resident's psychosocial needs related to activity choices.

- 43 CFR 483.20(b)(1), F272, Comprehensive Assessment

    - Determine if the facility assessed the resident's activity needs, preferences, and interests specifically enough so that an individualized care plan could be developed.

- 43 CFR 483.20(k)(1), F279, Comprehensive Care Plan

    - Determine if the facility developed specific and individualized activities goals and approaches as part of the comprehensive care plan, unless the resident is independent in providing for her/his activities without facility intervention.

- 43 CFR 483.20(k)(2), F280, Care Plan Revision

- Determine whether the facility revised the plan of care as needed with input of the resident (or representative, as appropriate).

- 43 CFR 483.30(a), F353, Sufficient Staff
  - Determine if the facility had qualified staff in sufficient numbers to assure the resident was provided activities based upon the comprehensive assessment and care plan.

- 43 CFR 483.70(g), F464, Dining and Activities Rooms
  - Determine if the facility has provided sufficient space to accommodate the activities and the needs of participating residents and that space is well lighted, ventilated, and adequately furnished.

- 43 CFR 483.75(g), F499, Staff Qualifications
  - Determine if the facility has employed sufficient qualified professional staff to assess residents and to develop and implement the activities approaches of their comprehensive care plans.

V. DEFICIENCY CATEGORIZATION (Part V, Appendix P)

Deficiencies at F248 are most likely to have psychosocial outcomes. The survey team should compare their findings to the various levels of severity on the Psychosocial Outcome Severity Guide at Appendix P, Part V.

F249

§483.15(f)(2) The activities program must be directed by a qualified professional who--

(i) Is a qualified therapeutic recreation specialist or an activities professional who--

(A) Is licensed or registered, if applicable, by the State in which practicing; and

(B) Is eligible for certification as a therapeutic recreation specialist or as an activities professional by a recognized accrediting body on or after October 1, 1990; or

(ii) Has 2 years of experience in a social or recreational program within the last 5 years, 1 of which was full-time in a patient activities program in a health care setting; or

(iii) Is a qualified occupational therapist or occupational therapy assistant; or

(iv) Has completed a training course approved by the State.

INTENT: (F249) §483.15(f)(2) Activities Director

The intent of this regulation is to ensure that the activities program is directed by a qualified professional.

DEFINITIONS

"Recognized accrediting body" refers to those organizations that certify, register, or license therapeutic recreation specialists, activity professionals, or occupational therapists.

ACTIVITIES DIRECTOR RESPONSIBILITIES

An activity director is responsible for directing the development, implementation, supervision and ongoing evaluation of the activities program. This includes the completion and/or directing/delegating the completion of the activities component of the comprehensive assessment; and contributing to and/or directing/delegating the contribution to the comprehensive care plan goals and approaches that are individualized to match the skills, abilities, and interests/preferences of each resident.

Directing the activity program includes scheduling of activities, both individual and groups, implementing and/or delegating the implementation of the programs, monitoring the response and/or reviewing/evaluating the response to the programs to determine if the activities meet the assessed needs of the resident, and making revisions as necessary.

NOTE: Review the qualifications of the activities director if there are concerns with the facility's compliance with the activities requirement at §483.15(f)(1), F248, or if there are concerns with the direction of the activity programs.

A person is a qualified professional under this regulatory tag if they meet any one of the qualifications listed under 483.15(f)(2).

DETERMINATION OF COMPLIANCE (Task 6, Appendix P)

Synopsis of Regulation (F249)

This requirement stipulates that the facility's program of activities be directed by a qualified professional.

Criteria for Compliance

The facility is in compliance with this requirement if they:

- Have employed a qualified professional to provide direction in the development and implementation of activities in accordance with resident needs and goals, and the director:
    - Has completed or delegated the completion of the activities component of the comprehensive assessment;
    - Contributed or directed the contribution to the comprehensive care plan of activity goals and approaches that are individualized to match the skills, abilities, and interests/preferences of each resident;
    - Has monitored and evaluated the resident's response to activities and revised the approaches as appropriate; and
    - Has developed, implemented, supervised and evaluated the activities program.

If not, cite at F249.

Noncompliance for F249

Tag F249 is a tag that is absolute, which means the facility must have a qualified activities professional to direct the provision of activities to the residents. Thus, it is cited if the facility is non-compliant with the regulation, whether or not there have been any negative outcomes to residents.

Noncompliance for F249 may include (but is not limited to) one or more of the following, including:

- Lack of a qualified activity director; or
- Lack of providing direction for the provision of an activity program;

V. DEFICIENCY CATEGORIZATION (Part V, Appendix P)

Once the team has completed its investigation, reviewed the regulatory requirements, and determined that noncompliance exists, the team must determine the severity of each deficiency, based on the resultant effect or potential for harm to the resident. The key elements for severity determination for F249 are as follows:

1. Presence of harm/negative outcome(s) or potential for negative outcomes due to a lack of an activities director or failure of the director to oversee, implement and/or provide activities programming.

    - Lack of the activity director's involvement in coordinating/directing activities; or

    - Lack of a qualified activity director.

2. Degree of harm (actual or potential) related to the noncompliance.

    Identify how the facility practices caused, resulted in, allowed or contributed to the actual or potential for harm:

    - If harm has occurred, determine level of harm; and

    - If harm has not yet occurred, determine the potential for discomfort to occur to the resident.

3. The immediacy of correction required.

    Determine whether the noncompliance requires immediate correction in order to prevent serious injury, harm, impairment, or death to one or more residents.

<u>Severity Level 4 Considerations: Immediate Jeopardy to Resident Health or Safety</u>

Immediate jeopardy is not likely to be issued as it is unlikely that noncompliance with F249 could place a resident or residents into a situation with potential to sustain serious harm, injury or death.

<u>Severity Level 3 Considerations: Actual Harm that is not Immediate Jeopardy</u>

Level 3 indicates noncompliance that results in actual harm, and may include, but is not limited to the resident's inability to maintain and/or reach his/her highest practicable well-being. In order to cite actual harm at this tag, the surveyor must be able to identify a relationship between noncompliance cited at Tag F248 (Activities) and failure of the provision and/or direction of the activity program by the activity director. For Severity Level 3, both of the following must be present:

1. Findings of noncompliance at Severity Level 3 at Tag F248; and

2. There is no activity director; or the facility failed to assure the activity director was responsible for directing the activity program in the assessment, development, implementation and/or revision of an individualized activity program for an individual resident; and/or the activity director failed to assure that the facility's activity program was implemented.

NOTE: If Severity Level 3 (actual harm that is not immediate jeopardy) has been ruled out based upon the evidence, then evaluate as to whether Level 2 (no actual harm with the potential for more than minimal harm) exists.

Severity Level 2 Considerations: No Actual Harm with Potential for more than Minimal Harm that is not Immediate Jeopardy

Level 2 indicates noncompliance that results in a resident outcome of no more than minimal discomfort and/or has the potential to compromise the resident's ability to maintain or reach his or her highest practicable level of well being. The potential exists for greater harm to occur if interventions are not provided. In order to cite Level 2 at Tag F249, the surveyor must be able to identify a relationship between noncompliance cited at Level 2 at Tag F248 (Activities) and failure of the provision and/or direction of activity program by the activity director. For Severity Level 2 at Tag F249, both of the following must be present:

1. Findings of noncompliance at Severity Level 2 at Tag F248; and

2. There is no activity director; or the facility failed to involve the activity director in the assessment, development, implementation and/or revision of an individualized activity program for an individual resident; and/or the activity director failed to assure that the facility's activity program was implemented.

<u>Severity Level 1 Considerations: No Actual Harm with Potential for Minimal Harm</u>
<u>In order to cite Level 1, no actual harm with potential for minimal harm at this tag, the surveyor must be able to identify that:</u>

There is no activity director and/or the activity director is not qualified, however:

- Tag F248 was not cited;
- The activity systems associated with the responsibilities of the activity director are in place;
- There has been a relatively short duration of time without an activity director; and
- The facility is actively seeking a qualified activity director.

§483.15(g) Social Services

F250

§483.15(g)(1) The facility must provide medically-related social services to attain or maintain the highest practicable physical, mental, and psychosocial well-being of each resident.

Intent §483.15(g)

To assure that sufficient and appropriate social service are provided to meet the resident's needs.

Interpretive Guidelines §483.15(g)(1)

Regardless of size, all facilities are required to provide for the medically related social services needs of each resident. This requirement specifies that facilities aggressively identify the need for medically-related social services, and pursue the provision of these services. It is not required that a qualified social worker necessarily provide all of these services. Rather, it is the responsibility of the facility to identify the medically-related social service needs of the resident and assure that the needs are met by the appropriate disciplines.

"Medically-related social services" means services provided by the facility's staff to assist residents in maintaining or improving their ability to manage their everyday physical, mental, and psychosocial needs. These services might include, for example:

- Making arrangements for obtaining needed adaptive equipment, clothing, and personal items;
- Maintaining contact with facility (with resident's permission) to report on changes in health, current goals, discharge planning, and encouragement to participate in care planning;
- Assisting staff to inform residents and those they designate about the resident's health status and health care choices and their ramifications;
- Making referrals and obtaining services from outside entities (e.g., talking books, absentee ballots, community wheelchair transportation);
- Assisting residents with financial and legal matters (e.g., applying for pensions, referrals to lawyers, referrals to funeral homes for preplanning arrangements);

- Discharge planning services (e.g., helping to place a resident on a waiting list for community congregate living, arranging intake for home care services for residents returning home, assisting with transfer arrangements to other facilities);

- Providing or arranging provision of needed counseling services;

- Through the assessment and care planning process, identifying and seeking ways to support residents' individual needs;

- Promoting actions by staff that maintain or enhance each resident's dignity in full recognition of each resident's individuality;

- Assisting residents to determine how they would like to make decisions about their health care, and whether or not they would like anyone else to be involved in those decisions;

- Finding options that most meet the physical and emotional needs of each resident;

- Providing alternatives to drug therapy or restraints by understanding and communicating to staff why residents act as they do, what they are attempting to communicate, and what needs the staff must meet;

- Meeting the needs of residents who are grieving; and

- Finding options which most meet their physical and emotional needs

Factors with a potentially negative effect on physical, mental, and psychosocial well being include an unmet need for:

- Dental /denture care;

- Podiatric care;

- Eye Care;

- Hearing services

- Equipment for mobility or assistive eating devices; and

- Need for home-like environment, control, dignity, privacy

Where needed services are not covered by the Medicaid State plan, nursing facilities are still required to attempt to obtain these services. For example, if a resident requires transportation services that are not covered under a Medicaid state plan, the facility is required to arrange these services. This could be achieved, for example, through obtaining volunteer assistance.

Types of conditions to which the facility should respond with social services by staff or referral include:

- Lack of an effective family/support system;
- Behavioral symptoms;
- If a resident with dementia strikes out at another resident, the facility should evaluate the resident's behavior. For example, a resident may be re-enacting an activity he or she used to perform at the same time everyday. If that resident senses that another is in the way of his re-enactment, the resident may strike out at the resident impeding his or her progress. The facility is responsible for the safety of any potential resident victims while it assesses the circumstances of the residents behavior);
- Presence of a chronic disabling medical or psychological condition (e.g., multiple sclerosis, chronic obstructive pulmonary disease, Alzheimer's disease, schizophrenia);
- Depression
- Chronic or acute pain;
- Difficulty with personal interaction and socialization skills;
- Presence of legal or financial problems
- Abuse of alcohol or other drugs;
- Inability to cope with loss of function;
- Need for emotional support;
- Changes in family relationships, living arrangements, and/or resident's condition or functioning; and
- A physical or chemical restraint.
- For residents with or who develop mental disorders as defined by the "Diagnostic and Statistical Manual for Mental Disorders (DSM-IV)," see §483.45, F406.

Probes: §483.15(g)(1)

For residents selected for a comprehensive or focused review as appropriate:

- How do facility staff implement social services interventions to assist the resident in meeting treatment goals?
- How do staff responsible for social work monitor the resident's progress in improving physical, mental and psychosocial functioning? Has goal attainment been evaluated and the care plan changed accordingly?
- How does the care plan link goals to psychosocial functioning/well-being?
- Have the staff responsible for social work established and maintained relationships with the resident's family or legal representative?
- [NFs] What attempts does the facility make to access services for Medicaid recipients when those services are not covered by a Medicaid State Plan?

Look for evidence that social services interventions successfully address residents' needs and link social supports, physical care, and physical environment with residents' needs and individuality.

For sampled residents, review MDS, section H.

F251

§483.15(g)(2) and (3)

(2) A facility with more than 120 beds must employ a qualified social worker on a full-time basis.

(3) Qualifications of a social worker. A qualified social worker is an individual with-

> **(i) A bachelor's degree in social work or a bachelor's degree in a human services field including but not limited to sociology, special education, rehabilitation counseling, and psychology; and**
>
> **(ii) One year of supervised social work experience in a health care setting working directly with individuals**

Procedures §483.15(g)(2) and (3)

If there are problems with the provision of social services in a facility with over 120 beds, determine if a qualified social worker is employed on a full time basis. See also F250.

F252

§483.15(h) Environment

The facility must provide--

§483.15(h)(1) A safe, clean, comfortable and homelike environment, allowing the resident to use his or her personal belongings to the extent possible;

Interpretive Guidelines §483.15(h)(1)

For "safe" environment, also see Guidelines for §§483.25(h), Accidents, and 483.70(a), Life Safety Code."

For Comfortable Environment, see Guidelines for 483.15(h)(5), Adequate and Comfortable Lighting Levels; 483.15(h)(6), Comfortable and Safe Temperature Levels; and 483.15(h)(7), Comfortable Sound Levels.

A determination of "comfortable and homelike" should include, whenever possible, the resident's or representative of the resident's opinion of the living environment.

The absence of a personalized, homelike environment in a resident's room, is not meaningful unless the survey team determines that the absence of personal belongings is a result of facility practices, rather than the result of resident choice or circumstances (e.g., lack of resident funds, lack of family support system, resident's reason for being in the facility, such as short-term rehabilitation).

A "homelike environment" is one that de-emphasizes the institutional character of the setting, to the extent possible, and allows the resident to use those personal belongings that support a homelike environment. A personalized, homelike environment recognizes the individuality and autonomy of the resident, provides an opportunity for self-expression and encourages links with the past and family members. Use this Tag when the facility fails to allow the resident to personalize his or her individual environment to the extent possible. Use Tag F224, 483.15(c), if the facility fails to have a system in place to prevent the misappropriation of resident's property.

For purposes of this requirement, "environment" refers to any environment in the facility that is frequented by residents, including the residents' rooms, bathrooms, hallways, activity areas, and therapy areas.

If the survey team observes that the rooms of residents with dementia do not appear to be homelike, determine if this decision was made in the context of assessment and care planning; i.e., that this environment assists these residents to maintain their highest practicable functioning levels.

If the team observes non-homelike environments for residents with dementia, determine if each of these residents have the same plan of care and the reason why each of these residents have the same plan of care.

By observing the residents' surroundings, what can the survey team learn about their everyday life and interests? Their life prior to residing in the facility? Observe for family photographs, books and magazines, bedspreads, knickknacks, mementos, and furniture that belong to the residents. For residents who have no relatives or friends, and have few assets, determine the extent to which the facility has assisted these residents to make their rooms homelike, if they so desire.

F253

§483.15(h)(2)

§483.15(h)(2) Housekeeping and maintenance services necessary to maintain a sanitary, orderly, and comfortable interior;

Intent §483.15(h)(2)

The intent of this requirement is to focus on the facility's responsibility to provide effective housekeeping and maintenance services.

Interpretive Guidelines §483.15(h)(2)

"Sanitary" includes, but is not limited to, preventing the spread of disease-causing organisms by keeping resident care equipment clean and properly stored. Resident care equipment includes toothbrushes, dentures, denture cups, glasses and water pitchers, emesis basins, hair brushes and combs, bed pans, urinals, feeding tubes, leg bags and catheter bags, pads and positioning devices.

For kitchen sanitation, see §483.70(h), Other Environmental Conditions.

For facility-wide sanitary practices affecting the quality of care, see §483.65, Infection Control.

"Orderly" is defined as an uncluttered physical environment that is neat and well-kept.

Procedures §483.15(h)(2)

Balance the resident's need for a homelike environment and the requirements of having a "sanitary" environment in a congregate living situation. For example, a resident may prefer a cluttered room, but does this clutter result in unsanitary or unsafe conditions?

Probes: §483.15(h)(2)

Is resident care equipment sanitary?

Is the area orderly?

Is the area uncluttered and in good repair?

Can residents and staff function unimpeded?

F254

§483.15(h)(3)

§483.15(h)(3) Clean bed and bath linens that are in good condition;

Probes: §483.15(h)(3)

Are bed linens clean and in good condition? Are there clean towels and wash cloths in good condition available for the resident?

F255

§483.15(h)(4)

§483.15(h)(4) Private closet space in each resident room, as specified in §483.70(d)(2)(iv) of this part;

Interpretive Guidelines §483.15(h)(4)

§483.70(d)(2)(iv) states: "The facility must provide each resident with individual closet space in his/her bedroom with clothes racks and shelves accessible to the resident."

Probes: §483.15(h)(4)

Are there individual closet spaces with accessible shelves?

Also see F470.

F256

§483.15(h)(5)

§483.15(h)(5) Adequate and comfortable lighting levels in all areas;

Interpretive Guidelines §483.15(h)(5)

"Adequate lighting" is defined as levels of illumination suitable to tasks the resident chooses to perform or the facility staff must perform. For some residents (e.g., those with glaucoma), lower levels of lighting would be more suitable.

"Comfortable" lighting is defined as lighting which minimizes glare and provides maximum resident control, where feasible, over the intensity, location, and direction of illumination so that visually impaired residents can maintain or enhance independent functioning.

Procedures §483.15(h)(5)

Are there adequate and comfortable lighting levels for individual resident and staff work needs?

Consider the illumination available from any source, natural or artificial. For hallways, observe the illumination that is normally present. For resident rooms or for other spaces where residents can control the lighting, turn on the lights and make the rating under these conditions.

F257

§483.15(h)(6)

§483.15(h)(6) Comfortable and safe temperature levels. Facilities initially certified after October 1, 1990 must maintain a temperature range of 71 - 81° F; and

Procedures §483.15(h)(6)

"Comfortable and safe temperature levels" means that the ambient temperature should be in a relatively narrow range that minimizes residents' susceptibility to loss of body heat and risk of hypothermia or susceptibility to respiratory ailments and colds. Although there are no explicit temperatures standards for facilities certified on or before October 1, 1990, these facilities still must maintain safe and comfortable temperature levels.

For facilities certified after October 1, 1990, temperatures may exceed the upper range of 81° F for facilities in geographic areas of the country (primarily at the northernmost latitudes) where that temperature is exceeded only during rare, brief unseasonably hot weather. This interpretation would apply in cases where it does not adversely affect resident health and safety, and would enable facilities in areas of the country with relatively cold climates to avoid the expense of installing air conditioning equipment that would only be needed infrequently. Conversely, the temperatures may fall below 71° F for facilities in areas of the country where that temperature is exceeded only during brief episodes of unseasonably cold weather (minimum temperature must still be maintained at a sufficient level to minimize risk of hypothermia and susceptibility to loss of body heat, respiratory ailments and colds.)

Measure the air temperature above floor level in resident rooms, dining areas, and common areas. If the temperature is out of the 71-81 degree range, then ask staff what actions they take when residents complain of heat or cold, e.g., provide extra fluids during heat waves and extra blankets and sweaters in cold.

F258

§483.15(h)(7)

§483.15(h)(7) For the maintenance of comfortable sound levels.

Interpretive Guidelines §483.15(h)(7)

"Comfortable" sound levels do not interfere with resident's hearing and enhance privacy when privacy is desired, and encourage interaction when social participation is desired. Of particular concern to comfortable sound levels is the resident's control over unwanted noise.

Procedures §483.15(h)(7)

Determine if the sound levels are comfortable to residents. Do residents and staff have to raise their voices to communicate over background sounds? Are sound levels suitable for the activities occurring in that space during observation?

Consider whether residents have difficulty hearing or making themselves heard because of background sounds (e.g., overuse or excessive volume of intercom, shouting, loud TV, cleaning equipment). Consider if it is difficult for residents to concentrate because of distractions or background noises such as traffic, music, equipment, or staff behavior. Consider the comfort of sound levels based on the needs of the residents participating in a particular activity, e.g., the sound levels may have to be turned up for hard of hearing individuals watching TV or listening to the radio. Consider the effect of noise on the comfort of residents with dementia.

During resident reviews, ask residents if during evenings and at nighttime, sounds are at comfortable levels? (If yes) Have you told staff about it and how have they responded?

F271

§483.20(a) Admission Orders

At the time each resident is admitted, the facility must have physician orders for the resident's immediate care.

Intent §483.20(a)

To ensure the resident receives necessary care and services.

Interpretive Guidelines §483.20(a)

"Physician orders for immediate care" are those written orders facility staff need to provide essential care to the resident, consistent with the resident's mental and physical status upon admission. These orders should, at a minimum, include dietary, drugs (if necessary) and routine care to maintain or improve the resident's functional abilities until staff can conduct a comprehensive assessment and develop an interdisciplinary care plan.

F272

§483.20 Resident Assessment

The facility must conduct initially and periodically a comprehensive, accurate, standardized reproducible assessment of each resident's functional capacity.

Intent §483.20

To provide the facility with ongoing assessment information necessary to develop a care plan, to provide the appropriate care and services for each resident, and to modify the care plan and care/services based on the resident's status. The facility is expected to use resident observation and communication as the primary source of information when completing the RAI. In addition to direct observation and communication with the resident, the facility should use a variety of other sources, including communication with licensed and non-licensed staff members on all shifts and may include discussions with the resident's physician, family members, or outside consultants and review of the resident's record.

§483.20(b) Comprehensive Assessments

§483.20(b)(1) Resident Assessment Instrument. A facility must make a comprehensive assessment of a resident's needs, using the RAI specified by the State. The assessment must include at least the following:

(i) Indentification and demographic information
(ii) Customary routine.
(iii) Cognitive patterns.
(iv) Communication.
(v) Vision.
(vi) Mood and behavior patterns.
(vii) Psychological well-being.
(viii) Physical functioning and structural problems.
(ix) Continence.
(x) Disease diagnosis and health conditions.
(xi) Dental and nutritional status.
(xii) Skin Conditions.
(xiii) Activity pursuit.
(xiv) Medications.
(xv) Special treatments and procedures.
(xvi) Discharge potential.
(xvii) Documentation of summary information regarding the additional assessment performed through the resident assessment protocols.
(xviii) Documentation of participation in assessment.

§483.20(b) Intent

To ensure that the RAI is used in conducting comprehensive assessments as part of an ongoing process through which the facility identifies the resident's functional capacity and health status.

§483.20(b) Guidelines

The information required in §483.20(b)(i-xvi) is incorporated into the MDS, which forms the core of each State's approved RAI. Additional assessment information is also gathered using triggered RAPs.

Each facility must use its State-specified RAI (which includes both the MDS and utilization guidelines which include the RAPs) to assess newly admitted residents, conduct an annual reassessment and assess those residents who experience a significant change in status. The facility is responsible for addressing all needs and strengths of residents regardless of whether the issue is included in the MDS or RAPs. The scope of the RAI does not limit the facility's responsibility to assess and address all care needed by the resident. Furthermore:

(i) Identification and demographic information

"Identification and demographic information" corresponds to MDS v 2.0 sections AA, BB and A, and refers to information that uniquely identifies each resident and the facility in which he/she resides, date of entry into the facility and residential history.

(ii) Customary routine

"Customary routine" corresponds to MDS v 2.0 section AC, and refers to information regarding the resident's usual community lifestyle and daily routine in the year prior to the date of entry to the nursing home.

(iii) Cognitive patterns

"Cognitive patterns" (iii) corresponds to MDS v. 2.0 section B. "Cognitive patterns" is defined as the resident's ability to problem solve, decide, remember, and be aware of and respond to safety hazards.

(iv) Communication

"Communication" (iv) corresponds to MDS v. 2.0 section C, and refers to the resident's ability to hear, understand others, make him or herself understood (with assistive devices if they are used).

(v) Vision

"Vision" (v) corresponds to MDS v. 2.0 section D, and I.1.jj, kk, ll and mm, and refers to the resident's visual acuity, limitations and difficulties, and appliances used to enhance vision.

(vi) Mood and behavior patterns

"Mood and behavior patterns" (vi) corresponds to MDS v. 2.0 section E, and refers to the resident's patterns of mood and behavioral symptoms

(vii) Psychosocial well-being

"Psychosocial well-being" (vii) corresponds to MDS v. 2.0 sections E1o and p, and F and refers to the resident's positive or negative feelings about him or herself or his/her social relationships.

(viii) Physical functioning and structural problems

"Physical functioning and structural problems" (viii) corresponds to MDS v. 2.0 section G, and refers to the resident's physical functional status, ability to perform activities of daily living, and the resident's need for staff assistance and assistive devices or equipment to maintain or improve functional abilities.

(ix) Continence

"Continence" (ix) corresponds to MDS v. 2.0, section H, and refers to the resident's patterns of bladder and bowel continence (control), pattern of elimination, and appliances used.

(x) Disease diagnosis and health conditions

"Disease diagnoses and health conditions" (x) corresponds to MDS v. 2.0, sections AB.9 and 10, I.1 and 2, and J.

(xi) Dental and nutritional status

"Dental and nutritional status" (xi) corresponds to MDS v. 2.0, sections K1 and L.

"Dental condition status" refers to the condition of the teeth, gums, and other structures of the oral cavity that may affect a resident's nutritional status, communication abilities, or quality of life. The assessment should include the need for, and use of, dentures or other dental appliances.

"Nutritional status" corresponds to MDS v. 2.0, section K2-6.

Nutritional status refers to weight, height, hematologic and biochemical assessments, clinical observations of nutrition, nutritional intake, resident's eating habits and preferences, dietary restrictions, supplements, and use of appliances.

(xii) Skin conditions

"Skin conditions" (xii) corresponds to MDS v. 2.0 sections M, G1a, G6a, H1a, H1b, and P4c, and refers to the resident's development, or risk of development of a pressure sore.

(xiii) Activity pursuit

"Activity pursuit" (xiii) corresponds to MDS v. 2.0 sections N and AC.

"Activity pursuit" refers to the resident's ability and desire to take part in activities which maintain or improve, physical, mental, and psychosocial well-being. Activity pursuits refer to any activity outside of activities of daily living (ADLs) which a person pursues in order to obtain a sense of well-being. Also, includes activities which provide benefits in self-esteem, pleasure, comfort, health education, creativity, success, and financial or emotional independence. The assessment should consider the resident's normal everyday routines and lifetime preferences.

(xiv) Medications

"Medications" (xiv) corresponds to MDS v. 2.0, section O, and section U, if completed.

"Medications" refers to all prescription and over-the-counter medications taken by the resident, including dosage, frequency of administration, and recognition of significant side effects that would be most likely to occur in the resident. This information need not appear in the assessment. However, it must be in the resident's clinical record and included in the care plan.

(xv) Special treatments and procedures

"Special treatments and procedures" (xv) corresponds to MDS v. 2.0 sections K5, M5, and P1, and section T, if completed.

"Special treatments and procedures" refers to treatments and procedures that are not part of basic services provided. For example, treatment for pressure sores, naso-gastric feedings, specialized rehabilitation services, respiratory care, or devices and restraints.

(xvi) Discharge potential

"Discharge potential" (xvi) corresponds to MDS v. 2.0 section Q.

"Discharge potential" refers to the facility's expectation of discharging the resident from the facility within The next 3 months.

(xvii) Documentation of summary information regarding the additional assessment performed through the resident assessment protocols

"Documentation of summary information (xvii) regarding the additional assessment performed through the resident assessment protocols (RAPs)" corresponds to MDS v. 2.0 section V, and refers to documentation concerning which RAPs have been triggered, documentation of assessment information in support of clinical decision making relevant to the RAP, documentation regarding where, in the clinical record, information related to the RAP can be found, and for each triggered RAP, whether the identified problem was included in the care plan.

(xviii) Documentation of participation in assessment

"Documentation of participation in the assessment" corresponds to MDS v. 2.0 section R, and refers to documentation of who participated in the assessment process. The assessment process must include direct observation and communication with the resident, as well as communication with licensed and nonlicensed direct care staff members on all shifts.

F273

§483.20(b)(2)

§483.20(b)(2) When required, a facility must conduct a comprehensive assessment of a resident as follows:

> **(i) Within 14 calendar days after admission, excluding readmissions in which there is no significant change in the resident's physical or mental condition. (For purposes of this section, "readmission" means a return to the facility following a temporary absence for hospitalization for therapeutic leave.)**

Intent §483.20(b)(2)

To assess residents in a timely manner.

F274

§483.20(b)(2)(ii)

> **(ii) Within 14 days after the facility determines, or should have determined, that there has been a significant change in the resident's physical or mental condition. (For purpose of this section, a "significant change" means a major decline or improvement in the resident's status that will not normally resolve itself without further intervention by staff or by implementing standard disease-related clinical interventions, that has an impact on more than one area of the resident's health status, and requires interdisciplinary review or revision of the care plan, or both.)**

§483.20(b)(2)(ii) Guidelines

The following are the criteria for significant changes:

A significant change reassessment is generally indicated if decline or improvement is consistently noted in 2 or more areas of decline or 2 or more areas of improvement:

Decline:

- Any decline in activities of daily living (ADL) physical functioning where a resident is newly coded as 3, 4 or 8 Extensive Assistance, Total Dependency, activity did not occur (note that even if coding in both columns A and B of an ADL category changes, this is considered 1 ADL change);

- Increase in the number of areas where Behavioral Symptoms are coded as "not easily altered" (e.g., an increase in the use of code 1's for E4B);
- Resident's decision-making changes from 0 or 1, to 2 or 3;
- Resident's incontinence pattern changes from 0 or 1 to 2, 3 or 4, or placement of an indwelling catheter;
- Emergence of sad or anxious mood as a problem that is not easily altered;
- Emergence of an unplanned weight loss problem (5% change in 30 days or 10% change in 180 days);
- Begin to use trunk restraint or a chair that prevents rising for a resident when it was not used before;
- Emergence of a condition/disease in which a resident is judged to be unstable;
- Emergence of a pressure ulcer at Stage II or higher, when no ulcers were previously present at Stage II or higher; or
- Overall deterioration of resident's condition; resident receives more support (e.g., in ADLs or decision making).

Improvement:

- Any improvement in ADL physical functioning where a resident is newly coded as 0, 1, or 2 when previously scored as a 3, 4, or 8;
- Decrease in the number of areas where Behavioral Symptoms or Sad or Anxious Mood are coded as "not easily altered";
- Resident's decision making changes from 2 or 3, to 0 or 1;
- Resident's incontinence pattern changes from 2, 3, or 4 to 0 or 1; or
- Overall improvement of resident's condition; resident receives fewer supports.
- If the resident experiences a significant change in status, the next annual assessment is not due until 366 days after the significant change reassessment has been completed.

F275

§483.20(b)(2)(iii)

(iii) Not less than once every 12 months.

Interpretive Guidelines §483.20(b)(2)(iii):

The annual resident assessment must be completed within 366 days after final completion of the most recent comprehensive resident assessment.

Probes§483.20(b)(2):

- Has each resident in the sample been comprehensively assessed using the State-specified RAI within the regulatory timeframes (i.e., within 14 days after admission, on significant change in status, and at least annually)?
- Has the facility identified, in a timely manner, those residents who have experienced a change?
- Has the facility reassessed residents using the State-specific RAI who had a significant change in status within 14 days after determining the change was significant.
- Has the facility gathered supplemental assessment information based on triggered RAPs prior to establishing the care plan?
- Does information in the RAI correspond with information obtained during observations of and interviews with the resident, facility staff and resident's family?

F276

§483.20(c) Quarterly Review Assessment

A facility must assess a resident using the quarterly review instrument specified by the State and approved by CMS not less frequently than once every 3 months.

Intent §483.20(c):

To assure that the resident's assessment is updated on at least a quarterly basis.

Interpretive Guidelines §483.20(c):

At least each quarter, the facility shall review each resident with respect to those MDS items specified under the State's quarterly review requirement. At a minimum, this would include all items contained in CMS' standard quarterly review form. A Quarterly review assessment must be completed within 92 days of the date at MDS Item R2b of the most recent, clinical assessment (AA8a=1,2,3,4,5 or 10). If the resident has experienced a significant change in status, the next quarterly review is due no later than 3 months after the significant change reassessment.

Probes §483.20(c):

Is the facility assessing and acting, no less than once every 3 months, on the results of resident's functional and cognitive status examinations?

Is the quarterly review of the resident's condition consistent with information in the progress notes, the plan of care and your resident observations and interviews?

F286

§483.20(d) Use

A facility must maintain all resident assessments completed within the previous 15 months in the resident's active record.

Intent §483.20(d):

Facilities are required to maintain 15 months of assessment data in the resident's active clinical record.

Interpretive Guidelines §483.20(d):

The requirement to maintain 15 months of data in the resident's active clinical record applies regardless of form of storage to all MDS forms, RAP Summary forms, Quarterly Assessment forms, Face Sheet Information and Discharge and Reentry Tracking Forms and MDS Correction Request Forms (including signed attestation). MDS assessments must be kept in the resident's active clinical record for 15 months following the final completion date, tracking forms for discharge and reentry must be kept for 15 months following the date of the event, Correction Request Forms must be kept for 15 months following the final completion date of the MDS Correction Request form.

The information must be kept in a centralized location, accessible to all professional staff members (including consultants) who need to review the information in order to provide care to the resident.

After the 15-month period, RAI information may be thinned from the clinical record and stored in the medical records department, provided that it is easily retrievable if requested by clinical staff, the State agency, or CMS.

Whether or not the facility's clinical record system is entirely electronic, a hard copy of all MDS forms, including the signatures of the facility staff attesting to the accuracy and completion of the records, must be maintained in the resident's clinical record.

F287

§483.20(f) Automated Data Processing Requirement

§483.20(f)(1) Encoding Data. Within 7 days after a facility completes a resident's assessment, a facility must encode the following information for each resident in the facility:

(i) Admission assessment.

(ii) Annual assessment updates.

(iii) Significant change in status assessments.

(iv) Quarterly review assessments.

(v) A subset of items upon a resident's transfer, reentry, discharge, and death.

(vi) Background (face-sheet) information, if there is no admission assessment.

§483.20(f)(2) Transmitting data. Within 7 days after a facility completes a resident's assessment, a facility must be capable of transmitting to the State information for each resident contained in the MDS in a format that conforms to standard record layouts and data dictionaries, and that passes standardized edits defined by CMS and the State.

§483.20(f)(3) Monthly transmittal requirements. A facility must electronically transmit, at least monthly, encoded, accurate, complete MDS data to the State for all assessments conducted during the previous month, including the following:

(i) Admission assessment.

(ii) Annual assessment.

(iii) Significant change in status assessment.

(iv) Significant correction of prior full assessment.

(v) Significant correction of prior quarterly assessment.

(vi) Quarterly review.

(vii) A subset of items upon a resident's transfer, reentry, discharge, and death.

(viii) Background (face-sheet) information, for an initial transmission of MDS data on a resident that does not have an admission assessment.

§483.20(f)(4) Data format. The facility must transmit data in the format specified by CMS or, for a State which has an alternate RAI approved by CMS, in the format specified by the State and approved by CMS.

Intent §483.20(f)(1-4):

The intent is to enable a facility to better monitor a resident's decline and progress over time. Computer-aided data analysis facilitates a more efficient, comprehensive and sophisticated review of health data. The primary purpose of maintaining the assessment data is so a facility can monitor resident progress over time. The information should be readily available at all times.

Interpretive Guidelines §483.20(f)(1-4):

"Encoding" means entering MDS information into a computer.

"Transmitting data" refers to electronically sending encoded MDS information, from the facility to the State database, using a modem and communications software.

"Capable of transmitting" means that the facility has encoded and edited according to CMS specifications, the record accurately reflects the resident's overall clinical status as of the assessment reference date, and the record is ready for transmission.

"Passing standard edits" means that the encoded responses to MDS items are consistent and within range, in accordance with CMS specified standards. In general, inconsistent responses are either not plausible or ignore a skip pattern on the MDS. An example of inconsistency would be if one or more MDS items on a list were checked as present, and the "None of the Above" response was also checked for the same list. Out of range responses are invalid responses, such as using a response code of 2 for an MDS item for which the valid responses are zero or 1.

"Monthly Transmittal" means electronically transmitting to the State, an MDS record that passes CMS' standard edits, within 31 days of the final completion date of the record.

"Accurate" means that the encoded MDS data matches the MDS form in the clinical record. Also refer to guidance regarding accuracy at §483.20(g), and the information accurately reflects the resident's status as of the Assessment Reference Date at MDS Item A3a.

"Complete" means that all items required according to the record type, and in accordance with CMS' record specifications and State required edits are in effect at the time the record is completed.

In accordance with the final rule, facilities will be responsible to edit the encoded MDS data to ensure that it meets the standard edit specifications.

We encourage facilities to use software that has a programmed capability to automatically edit MDS records according to CMS' edit specifications.

For §483.20(f)(1)(v), the subset of items required upon a resident's transfer, discharge, and death are contained in the Discharge Tracking form and the items required for reentry are contained in the Reentry Tracking form. Refer to Appendix R for further information about the Discharge Tracking and Reentry Tracking forms.

All nursing homes must computerize MDS information. The facility must edit MDS information using standard CMS-specified edits, revise the information to conform to the edits and to be accurate, and be capable of transmitting that data to the State system within 7 days of:

- Completing a comprehensive assessment (the date at MDS item VB4);
- Completing an assessment that is not comprehensive (the date at MDS item R2b);
- A discharge event (the date at MDS item R4);
- A reentry event (the date at MDS item A4a); or
- Completing a correction request form (the date at MDS item AT6).

Submission must be according to State and Federal time frames. Therefore the facility must:

- Encode the MDS and RAP Summary (where applicable) in machine readable format;
- Edit the MDS and RAP Summary (where applicable) according to edits specified by CMS. Within the 7 day time period specified above for editing, the facility must revise any information on the encoded MDS and RAP Summary (if applicable) that does not pass CMS-specified edits, revise any otherwise inaccurate information, and make the information ready for submission. The MDS Vendor software used at the facility should have an

automated editing process that alerts the user to entries in an MDS record that do not conform with the CMS-specified edits and that prompts the facility to complete revisions within the 7-day editing and revision period. After editing and revision, MDS information and RAP summary information (if applicable) must always accurately reflect the resident's overall clinical status as of the original Assessment Reference date for an assessment or the original event date for a discharge or reentry;

- Print the edited and revised MDS and RAP summary form (where applicable). Discharge or Reentry Tracking form or Correction Request form, and place it in the resident's record. The hard copy of the MDS record must match the record that the facility transmits to the State, and it must accurately reflect the resident's status as of the Assessment Reference date or event date. If a hard copy exists prior to data entry, the facility must correct the hard copy to reflect the changes associated with the editing and revision process.

Electronically submit MDS information to the State MDS database within 31 days of:

- The date the Care Planning Decision process was complete (the date at MDS Item VB4) for comprehensive assessments;
- The date the RN Coordinator certified that the MDS was complete (the date at MDS Item R2b) for assessments that are not comprehensive;
- The date of death or discharge (the date at MDS Item R4) for Discharge Tracking forms;
- The date of reentry (the date at MDS Item A4a) for Reentry Tracking forms; and
- The date of completion of a correction request (the date at MDS Item AT6)

For a discussion of the process that a facility should follow in the event an error is discovered in an MDS record after editing and revision but before it is transmitted to the State, refer to "Correction Policy for MDS Records" in the State Operations Manual, Appendix R, Part IV.

The facility must maintain RAI assessments and Discharge and Reentry Tracking forms, as well as correction information, including Correction Request forms as a part of the resident's clinical record. Whether or not the facility's system is entirely electronic, a hard copy of completed MDS forms, including the signature of the facility staff attesting to the accuracy and completion of the corrected record, must be maintained in the resident's clinical record.

A facility must complete and submit to the State a subset of items when the resident is discharged from the facility (discharge tracking form), or readmitted to the facility (reentry tracking form.

F278

§483.20(g) Accuracy of Assessment

The assessment must accurately reflect the resident's status.

Intent §483.20(g):

To assure that each resident receives an accurate assessment by staff that are qualified to assess relevant care areas and knowledgeable about the resident's status, needs, strengths, and areas of decline.

Interpretive Guidelines §483.20(g):

"The accuracy of the assessment" means that the appropriate, qualified health professional correctly documents the resident's medical, functional, and psychosocial problems and identifies resident strengths to maintain or improve medical status, functional abilities, and psychosocial status. The initial comprehensive assessment provides baseline data for ongoing assessment of resident progress.

§483.20(h) Coordination

A registered nurse must conduct or coordinate each assessment with the appropriate participation of health professionals.

Intent §483.20(h):

The registered nurse will conduct and/or coordinate the assessment, as appropriate. Whether conducted or coordinated by the registered nurse, he or she is responsible for certifying that the assessment has been completed.

Interpretive Guidelines §483.20(h):

According to the Utilization Guidelines for each State's RAI, the physical, mental and psychosocial condition of the resident determines the appropriate level of involvement of physicians, nurses, rehabilitation therapists, activities professionals, medical social workers, dietitians, and other professionals, such as developmental disabilities specialists, in assessing the resident, and in correcting resident assessments. Involvement of other disciplines is dependent upon resident status and needs.

Probes §483.20(g)(h):

Have appropriate health professionals assessed the resident? For example, has the resident's nutritional status been assessed by someone who is knowledgeable in nutrition and capable of correctly assessing a resident?

If the resident's medical status, functional abilities, or psychosocial status declined and the decline was not clinically unavoidable, were the appropriate health professionals involved in assessing the resident?

Based on your total review of the resident, is each portion of the assessment accurate?

Are the appropriate certifications in place, including the RN Coordinator's certification of completion of an assessment or Correction Request form, and the certification of individual assessors of the accuracy and completion of the portion(s) of the assessment, tracking form or face sheet they completed or corrected. On an assessment or correction request, the RN Assessment Coordinator is responsible for certifying overall completion once all individual assessors have completed and signed their portion(s) of the MDS forms. When MDS forms are completed directly on the facility's computer, (e.g., no paper form has been manually completed), the RN Coordinator signs and dates the computer generated hard copy after reviewing it for completeness, including the signatures of all individual assessors. Backdating a completion date is not acceptable.

§483.20(i) Certification

(1) A registered nurse must sign and certify that the assessment is completed.

(2) Each individual who completes a portion of the assessment must sign and certify the accuracy of that portion of the assessment.

Interpretive Guidelines §483.20(i):

Whether the MDS forms are manually completed, or computer generated following data entry, each individual assessor is responsible for certifying the accuracy of responses on the forms relative to the resident's condition and discharge or reentry status. Manually completed forms are signed and dated by each individual assessor the day they complete their portion(s) of the MDS record. When MDS forms are completed directly on the facility's computer (e.g., no paper form has been manually completed), then each individual assessor signs and dates a computer generated hard copy, after they review it for accuracy of the portion(s) they completed. Backdating completion dates is not acceptable.

§483.20(j) Penalty for Falsification

(1) Under Medicare and Medicaid, an individual who willfully and knowingly--

(i) Certifies a material and false statement in a resident assessment is subject to a civil money penalty of not more than $1,000 for each assessment; or

(ii) Causes another individual to certify a material and false statement in a resident assessment is subject to a civil money penalty or not more than $5,000 for each assessment.

(2) Clinical disagreement does not constitute a material and false statement.

Interpretive Guidelines §483.20(j):

MDS information serves as the clinical basis for care planning and delivery. With the introduction of additional uses of MDS information such as for payment rate setting and quality monitoring, MDS information as it is reported impacts a nursing home's payment rate and standing in terms of the quality monitoring process. A pattern within a nursing home of clinical documentation or of MDS assessment or reporting practices that result in higher RUG scores, untriggering RAP(s), or unflagging QI(s), where the information does not accurately reflect the resident's status, may be indicative of payment fraud or avoidance of the quality monitoring process. Such practices may include but are not limited to a pattern or high prevalence of the following:

- Submitting MDS Assessments (including any reason(s) for assessment, routine or non-routine), Discharge or Reentry Tracking forms, where the information does not accurately reflect the resident's status as of the Assessment Reference date, or the Discharge or Reentry date, as applicable;

- Submitting correction(s) to information in the State MDS database where the corrected information does not accurately reflect the resident's status as of the original Assessment Reference date, or the original Discharge or Reentry date, as applicable, or where the record it claims to correct does not appear to have been in error;

- Submitting Significant Correction Assessments where the assessment it claims to correct does not appear to have been in error;

- Submitting Significant Change in Status Assessments where the criteria for significant change in the resident's status do not appear to be met;

- Delaying or withholding MDS Assessments (including any reason(s) for assessment, routine or non-routine), Discharge or Reentry Tracking information, or correction(s) to information in the State MDS database.

When such patterns or practices are noticed, they should be reported by the State Agency to the proper authority.

F279

§483.20(d) (A facility must..) use the results of the assessment to develop, review and revise the resident's comprehensive plan of care.

§483.20(k) Comprehensive Care Plans

(1) The facility must develop a comprehensive care plan for each resident that includes measurable objectives and timetables to meet a resident's medical, nursing, and mental and psychosocial needs that are identified in the comprehensive assessment. The care plan must describe the following:

> **(i) The services that are to be furnished to attain or maintain the resident's highest practicable physical, mental, and psychosocial well-being as required under §483.25; and**
>
> **(ii) Any services that would otherwise be required under §483.25 but are not provided due to the resident's exercise of rights under §483.10, including the right to refuse treatment under §483.10(b)(4).**

Interpretive Guidelines §483.20(k):

An interdisciplinary team, in conjunction with the resident, resident's family, surrogate, or representative, as appropriate, should develop quantifiable objectives for the highest level of functioning the resident may be expected to attain, based on the comprehensive assessment. The interdisciplinary team should show evidence in the RAP summary or clinical record of the following:

- The resident's status in triggered RAP areas;
- The facility's rationale for deciding whether to proceed with care planning; and
- Evidence that the facility considered the development of care planning interventions for all RAPs triggered by the MDS.

The care plan must reflect intermediate steps for each outcome objective if identification of those steps will enhance the resident's ability to meet his/her objectives. Facility staff will use these objectives to monitor resident progress. Facilities may, for some residents, need to prioritize their care plan interventions. This should be noted in the clinical record or on the plan or care.

The requirements reflect the facility's responsibilities to provide necessary care and services to attain or maintain the highest practicable physical, mental and psychosocial well-being, in accordance with the comprehensive assessment and plan of care. However, in some cases, a resident may wish to refuse certain services or treatments that professional staff believe may be indicated to assist the resident in reaching his or her highest practicable level of well-being. Desires of the resident should be documented in the clinical record (see guidelines at §483.10(b)(4) for additional guidance concerning refusal of treatment).

Probes§483.20(k)(1):

Does the care plan address the needs, strengths and preferences identified in the comprehensive resident assessment?

Is the care plan oriented toward preventing avoidable declines in functioning or functional levels? How does the care plan attempt to manage risk factors? Does the care plan build on resident strengths?

Does the care plan reflect standards of current professional practice?

Do treatment objectives have measurable outcomes?

Corroborate information regarding the resident's goals and wishes for treatment in the plan of care by interviewing residents, especially those identified as refusing treatment.

Determine whether the facility has provided adequate information to the resident so that the resident was able to make an informed choice regarding treatment.

If the resident has refused treatment, does the care plan reflect the facility's efforts to find alternative means to address the problem?

For implementation of care plan, see §483.20(k)(3).

F280

§483.10(d)(3) – The resident has the right to -- unless adjudged incompetent or otherwise found to be incapacitated under the laws of the State, participate in planning care and treatment or changes in care and treatment.

Interpretive Guidelines §483.10(d)(3)

"**Participates in planning care and treatment**" means that the resident is afforded the opportunity to select from alternative treatments. This applies both to initial decisions about care and treatment and to decisions about changes in care and treatment. The resident's right to participate in care planning and to refuse treatment are covered in §§483.20(d)(2) and 483.10(b)(4).

A resident whose ability to make decisions about care and treatment is impaired, or a resident who has been formally declared incompetent by a court, should, to the extent practicable, be kept informed and be consulted on personal preferences.

Whenever there appears to be a conflict between a resident's right and the resident's health or safety, determine if the facility attempted to accommodate both the exercise of the resident's rights and the resident's health, including exploration of care alternatives through a thorough care planning process in which the resident may participate.

Procedures §483.10(d)(3)

Look for evidence that the resident was afforded the right to participate in care planning or was consulted about care and treatment changes (e.g., ask residents or their representatives during interviews).

§483.20(k)(2)

§483.20(k)(2) A comprehensive care plan must be--

(i) Developed within 7 days after the completion of the comprehensive assessment;

(ii) Prepared by an interdisciplinary team, that includes the attending physician, a registered nurse with responsibility for the resident, and other appropriate staff in disciplines as determined by the resident's needs, and, to the extent practicable, the participation of the resident, the resident's family or the resident's legal representative; and

(iii) Periodically reviewed and revised by a team of qualified persons after each assessment.

Interpretive Guidelines §483.20(k)(2):

As used in this requirement, "Interdisciplinary" means that professional disciplines, as appropriate, will work together to provide the greatest benefit to the resident. It does not mean that every goal must have an interdisciplinary approach. The mechanics of how the interdisciplinary team meets its responsibilities in developing an interdisciplinary care plan (e.g., a face-to-face meeting, teleconference, written communication) is at the discretion of the facility.

The physician must participate as part of the interdisciplinary team, and may arrange with the facility for alternative methods, other than attendance at care planning conferences, of providing his/her input, such as one-on-one discussions and conference calls.

The resident's right to participate in choosing treatment options, decisions in care planning and the right to refuse treatment are addressed at §483.20(k)(2)(ii) and 483.10(b)(4), respectively, and include the right to accept or refuse treatment. The facility has a responsibility to assist residents to participate, e.g., helping residents, and families, legal surrogates or representatives understand the assessment and care planning process; when feasible, holding care planning meetings at the time of day when a resident is functioning best; planning enough time for information exchange and decision making; encouraging a resident's advocate to attend (e.g. family member, friend) if desired by a resident.

The resident has the right to refuse specific treatments and to select among treatment options before the care plan is instituted. (See §483.20(k)(2)(ii) and 483.10(b)(4).) The facility should encourage residents, legal surrogates and representatives to participate in care planning, including attending care planning conferences if they so desire.

While Federal regulations affirm the resident's right to participate in care planning and to refuse treatment, the regulations do not create the right for a resident, legal surrogate or representative to demand that the facility use specific medical intervention or treatment that the facility deems inappropriate. Statutory requirements hold the facility ultimately accountable for the resident's care and safety, including clinical decisions.

Probes §483.20(k)(2):

1. Was interdisciplinary expertise utilized to develop a plan to improve the resident's functional abilities?

    a. For example, did an occupational therapist design needed adaptive equipment or a speech therapist provide techniques to improve swallowing ability?

    b. Do the dietitian and speech therapist determine, for example, the optimum textures and consistency for the resident's food that provide both a nutritionally adequate diet and effectively use oropharyngeal capabilities of the resident?

    c. Is there evidence of physician involvement in development of the care plan (e.g., presence at care plan meetings, conversations with team members concerning the care plan, conference calls)?

2. In what ways do staff involve residents and families, surrogates, and/or representatives in care planning?

3. Do staff make an effort to schedule care plan meetings at the best time of the day for residents and their families?

4. Ask the ombudsman if he/she has been involved in a care planning meeting as a resident advocate. If yes, ask how the process worked.

5. Do facility staff attempt to make the process understandable to the resident/family?

6. Ask residents whether they have brought questions or concerns about their care to the attention of facility's staff. If so, what happened as a result?

Interpretive Guidelines §483.20(k)(2)(iii):

See §483.75(g)(2)(iii) for "Qualified Person,"

Probes §483.20(k)(2)(iii):

Is the care plan evaluated and revised as the resident's status changes?

F281

§483.20(k)(3)

(3) The services provided or arranged by the facility must--

(i) Meet professional standards of quality and;

Intent §483.20(k)(3)(i):

The intent of this regulation is to assure that services being provided meet professional standards of quality (in accordance with the definition provided below) and are provided by appropriate qualified persons (e.g., licensed, certified).

Interpretive Guidelines §483.20(k)(3)(i):

"Professional standards of quality" means services that are provided according to accepted standards of clinical practice. Standards may apply to care provided by a particular clinical discipline or in a specific clinical situation or setting. Standards regarding quality care practices may be published by a professional organization, licensing board, accreditation body or other regulatory agency. Recommended practices to achieve desired resident outcomes may also be found in clinical literature. Possible reference sources for standards of practice include:

- Current manuals or textbooks on nursing, social work, physical therapy, etc.

- Standards published by professional organizations such as the American Dietetic Association, American Medical Association, American Medical

Directors Association, American Nurses Association, National Association of Activity Professionals, National Association of Social Work, etc.

- Clinical practice guidelines published by the Agency of Health Care Policy and Research.

- Current professional journal articles.

If a negative resident outcome is determined to be related to the facility's failure to meet professional standards, and the team determines a deficiency has occurred, it should be cited under the appropriate quality of care or other relevant requirement.

Probes §483.20(k)(3):

Question only those practices which have a negative outcome or have a potential negative outcome. Ask the facility to produce references upon which the practice is based.

- Do nurses notify physicians, as appropriate, and show evidence of discussions of acute medical problems?

- Are residents with acute conditions who require intensive monitoring and hospital-level treatments that the facility is unable to provide, promptly hospitalized?

- Are there errors in the techniques of medication administration? (Cite actual medication errors at §483.25(m).)

- Is there evidence of assessment and care planning sufficient to meet the needs of newly admitted residents, prior to completion of the first comprehensive assessment and comprehensive care plan?

- Are physicians' orders carried out, unless otherwise indicated by an advanced directive?

F282

§483.20(k)(3)(ii) Be provided by qualified persons in accordance with each resident's written plan of care.

Interpretive Guidelines §483.20(k)(3)(ii):

If you find problems with quality of care, quality of life, or resident rights, are these problems attributable to the qualifications of the facility staff, or lack of, inadequate or incorrect implementation of the care plan?

Probes §483.20(k)(3)(ii):

- Can direct care-giving staff describe the care, services, and expected outcomes of the care they provide; have a general knowledge of the care and services being provided by other therapists; have an understanding of the expected outcomes of this care, and understand the relationship of these expected outcomes to the care they provide?

F283

§483.20(l) Discharge Summary

When the facility anticipates discharge a resident must have a discharge summary that includes:

(1) A recapitulation of the resident's stay;
(2) A final summary of the resident's status to include items in paragraph (b)(2) of this section, at the time of the discharge that is available for release to authorized persons and agencies, with the consent of the resident or legal representative; and

Intent §483.20(l):

To ensure appropriate discharge planning and communication of necessary information to the continuing care provider.

Interpretive Guidelines §483.20(l):

"Anticipates" means that the discharge was not an emergency discharge (e.g., hospitalization for an acute condition) or due to the resident's death.

"Adjust to his or her living environment" means that the post-discharge plan, as appropriate, should describe the resident's and family's preferences for care, how the resident and family will access these services, and how care should be coordinated if continuing treatment involves multiple caregivers. It should identify specific resident needs after discharge such as personal care, sterile dressings, and physical therapy, as well as describe resident/caregiver education needs and ability to meet care needs after discharge.

F284

§483.20(l)(3) A post-discharge plan of care that is developed with the participation of the resident and his or her family, which will assist the resident to adjust to his or her new living environment.

Interpretive Guidelines §483.20(l)(3):

A post-discharge plan of care for an anticipated discharge applies to a resident whom the facility discharges to a private residence, to another NF or SNF, or to another type of residential facility such as a board and care home or an intermediate care facility for individuals with mental retardation. Resident protection concerning transfer and discharge are found at §483.12. A "post-discharge plan of care" means the discharge planning process which includes: assessing continuing care needs and developing a plan designed to ensure the individual's needs will be met after discharge from the facility into the community.

Probes §483.20(l):

- Does the discharge summary have information pertinent to continuing care for the resident?
- Is there evidence of discharge planning in the records of discharged residents who had an anticipated discharge or those residents to be discharged shortly (e.g., in the next 7-14 days)?
- Do discharge plans address necessary post-discharge care?
- Has the facility aided the resident and his/her family in locating and coordinating post-discharge services?
- What types of pre-discharge preparation and education has the facility provided the resident and his/her family?

F285

§483.20(e) Coordination

A facility must coordinate assessments with the pre-admission screening and resident review program under Medicaid in part 483, subpart C to the maximum extent practicable to avoid duplicative testing and effort.

Interpretive Guidelines §483.20(e)

With respect to the responsibilities under the Pre-Admission Screening and Resident Review (PASRR) program, the State is responsible for conducting the screens, preparing the PASRR report, and providing or arranging the specialized services that are needed as a result of conducting the screens. The State is required to provide a copy of the PASRR report to the facility. This report must list the specialized services that the individual requires and that are the responsibility of the State to provide. All other needed services are the responsibility of the facility to provide.

§483.20(m) Preadmission Screening for Mentally Ill Individuals and Individuals With Mental Retardation.

§483.20(m)(1) A nursing facility must not admit, on or after January 1, 1989, any new residents with:

(i) Mental illness as defined in paragraph (m)(2)(i) of this section, unless the State mental health authority has determined, based on an independent physical and mental evaluation performed by a person or entity other than the State mental health authority, prior to admission;

(A) That, because of the physical and mental condition of the individual, the individual requires the level of services provided by a nursing facility; and
(B) If the individual requires such level of services, whether the individual requires specialized services for mental retardation.

(ii) Mental retardation, as defined in paragraph (m)(2)(ii) of this section, unless the State mental retardation or developmental disability authority has determined prior to admission--

(A) That, because of the physical and mental condition of the individual, the individual requires the level of services provided by a nursing facility; and
(B) If the individual requires such level of services, whether the individual requires specialized services for mental retardation.

§483.20(m)(2) Definitions. For purposes of this section:

(i) An individual is considered to have "mental illness" if the individual has a serious mental illness defined at 483.102(b)(1).

(ii) An individual is considered to be "mentally retarded" if the individual is mentally retarded as defined in 483.102(b)(3) or is a person with a related condition as described in 42 CFR 1009.

Intent §483.20(m):

To ensure that individuals with mental illness and mental retardation receive the care and services they need in the most appropriate setting.

"Specialized services" are those services the State is required to provide or arrange for that raise the intensity of services to the level needed by the resident. That is, specialized services are an "add-on" to NF services--they are of a higher intensity and frequency than specialized rehabilitation services, which are provided by the NF.

The statute mandates preadmission screening for all individuals with mental illness (MI) or mental retardation (MR) who apply to NFs, regardless of the applicant's source of payment, except as provided below. (See §1919(b)(3)(F).) Residents readmitted and individuals who initially apply to a nursing facility directly following a discharge from an acute care stay are exempt if:

- They are certified by a physician prior to admission to require a nursing facility stay of less than 30 days; and

- They require care at the nursing facility for the same condition for which they were hospitalized.

The State is responsible for providing specialized services to residents with MI/MR residing in Medicaid-certified facilities. The facility is required to provide all other care and services appropriate to the resident's condition. Therefore, if a facility has residents with MI/MR, do not survey for specialized services, but survey for all other requirements, including resident rights, quality of life, and quality of care.

If the resident's PAS report indicates that he or she needs specialized services but the resident is not receiving them, notify the Medicaid agency. NF services ordinarily are not of the intensity to meet the needs of residents with MI or MR.

Probes §483.20(m):

If sampled residents have MI or MR, did the State Mental Health or Mental Retardation Authority determine:

- Whether the residents needed the services of a NF?

- Whether the residents need specialized services for their MR or MI?

F309

§483.25 Quality of Care

Each resident must receive and the facility must provide the necessary care and services to attain or maintain the highest practicable physical, mental, and psychosocial well-being, in accordance with the comprehensive assessment and plan of care.

Use F309 for quality of care deficiencies not covered by §483.25(a)-(m).

Intent: §483.25

The facility must ensure that the resident obtains optimal improvement or does not deteriorate within the limits of a resident's right to refuse treatment, and within the limits of recognized pathology and the normal aging process.

Definitions: §483.25

- "Highest practicable" is defined as the highest level of functioning and well-being possible, limited only by the individual's presenting functional status and potential for improvement or reduced rate of functional decline. Highest practicable is determined through the comprehensive resident assessment by competently and thoroughly addressing the physical, mental or psychosocial needs of the individual.

- "Skin Ulcer/Wound"

  NOTE: Skin ulcer definitions are included to clarify clinical terms related to skin ulcers. At the time of the assessment and diagnosis, the clinician is expected to document the clinical basis (e.g., underlying condition contributing to the ulceration, ulcer edges and wound bed, location, shape, condition of surrounding tissues) which permit differentiating the ulcer type, especially if the ulcer has characteristics consistent with a pressure ulcer, but is determined not to be one.

  - "Arterial Ulcer" is ulceration that occurs as the result of arterial occlusive disease when non-pressure related disruption or blockage of the arterial blood flow to an area causes tissue necrosis.

    Inadequate blood supply to the extremity may initially present as intermittent claudication. Arterial/Ischemic ulcers may be present in individuals with moderate to severe peripheral vascular disease, generalized arteriosclerosis, inflammatory or autoimmune disorders (such as arteritis), or significant vascular disease elsewhere (e.g., stroke or heart attack). The arterial ulcer is characteristically painful, usually occurs in the distal portion of the lower extremity and may be over the ankle or bony areas of the foot (e.g., top of the foot or toe, outside edge of the foot). The wound bed is frequently dry and pale with minimal or no exudate. The affected foot may exhibit: diminished or absent pedal pulse, coolness to touch, decreased pain when hanging down (dependent) or increased pain when elevated, blanching upon elevation, delayed capillary fill time, hair loss on top of the foot and toes, toenail thickening.

  - "Diabetic neuropathic ulcer" requires that the resident be diagnosed with diabetes mellitus and have peripheral neuropathy. The diabetic ulcer characteristically occurs on the foot, e.g., at mid-foot, at the ball of the foot over the metatarsal heads, or on the top of toes with Charcot deformity.

- "Pressure ulcer". See Guidance at 42 CFR 483.25(c)-F314.

- "Venous insufficiency ulcer" (previously known as "stasis ulcer") is an open lesion of the skin and subcutaneous tissue of the lower leg, usually occurring in the pretibial area of the lower leg or above the medial ankle. Venous ulcers are reported to be the most common vascular ulceration and may be difficult to heal, may occur off and on for several years, and may occur after relatively minor trauma. The ulcer may have a moist, granulating wound bed, may be superficial, and may have minimal to copious serous drainage unless the wound is infected. The resident may experience pain which may be increased when the foot is in a dependent position, such as when a resident is seated with her or his feet on the floor. Recent literature implicates venous hypertension as a causative factor. Earlier, the ulceration was believed to be due to the pooling of blood in the veins.

  Venous hypertension may be caused by one (or a combination of) factor(s) including: loss of (or compromised) valve function in the vein, partial or complete obstruction of the vein (e.g., deep vein thrombosis, obesity, malignancy), and/or failure of the calf muscle to pump the blood (e.g., paralysis, decreased activity). Venous insufficiency may result in edema and induration, dilated superficial veins, cellulitis in the lower third of the leg or dermatitis (typically characterized by change in skin pigmentation). The pigmentation may appear as darkening skin, tan or purple areas in light skinned residents and dark purple, black or dark brown in dark skinned residents.

Interpretive Guidelines §483.25

Use F309 when the survey team determines there are quality of care deficiencies not covered by §§483.25(a)-(m). "Highest practicable" is defined as the highest level of functioning and well-being possible, limited only by the individual's presenting functional status and potential for improvement or reduced rate of functional decline. Highest practicable is determined through the comprehensive resident assessment by competently and thoroughly addressing the physical, mental or psychosocial needs of the individual.

The facility must ensure that the resident obtains optimal improvement or does not deteriorate within the limits of a resident's right to refuse treatment, and within the limits of recognized pathology and the normal aging process.

In any instance in which there has been a lack of improvement or a decline, the survey team must determine if the occurrence was unavoidable or avoidable. A determination of unavoidable decline or failure to reach highest practicable well-being may be made only if all of the following are present:

- An accurate and complete assessment (see §483.20);
- A care plan which is implemented consistently and based on information from the assessment;
- Evaluation of the results of the interventions and revising the interventions as necessary.

Determine if the facility is providing the necessary care and services based on the findings of the RAI. If services and care are being provided, determine if the facility is evaluating the outcome to the resident and changing the interventions if needed. This should be done in accordance with the resident's customary daily routine. Use Tag F309 to cite quality of care deficiencies that are not explicit in the quality of care regulations.

Procedures §483.25

Assess a facility's compliance with these requirements by determining if the services noted in the plan of care, based on a comprehensive and accurate functional assessment of the resident's strengths, weaknesses, risk factors for deterioration and potential for improvement, is continually and aggressively implemented and updated by the facility staff. In looking at assessments, use both the MDS and RAPs information, any other pertinent assessments, and resulting care plans.

If the resident has been in the facility for less than 14 days (before completion of all the RAI is required), determine if the facility is conducting ongoing assessment and care planning, and, if appropriate, care and services are being provided.

If quality of care problems are noted in areas of nurse aide responsibility, review nurse aide competency requirements at §483.75(e).

---

§483.25(a) Activities of Daily Living.

Based on the comprehensive assessment of a resident, the facility must ensure that

Intent §483.25(a)

The intent of this regulation is that the facility must ensure that a resident's abilities in ADLs do not deteriorate unless the deterioration was unavoidable.

F310

§483.25(a)(1) A resident's abilities in activities of daily living do not diminish unless circumstances of the individual's clinical condition demonstrate that diminution was unavoidable. This includes the resident's ability to --

(i) Bathe, dress, and groom;
(ii) Transfer and ambulate;
(iii) Toilet;
(iv) Eat; and
(v) Use speech, language, or other functional communication systems.

Interpretive Guidelines §483.25(a)

The mere presence of a clinical diagnosis, in itself, justify a decline in a resident's ability to perform ADLs. Conditions which may demonstrate unavoidable diminution in ADLs include:

- The natural progression of the resident's disease;

- Deterioration of the resident's physical condition associated with the onset of a physical or mental disability while receiving care to restore or maintain functional abilities; and

- The resident's or his/her surrogate's or representative's refusal of care and treatment to restore or maintain functional abilities after aggressive efforts by the facility to counsel and/or offer alternatives to the resident, surrogate, or representative. Refusal of such care and treatment should be documented in the clinical record. Determine which interventions were identified on the care plan and/or could be in place to minimize or decrease complications. Note also that depression is a potential cause of excess disability and, where appropriate, therapeutic interventions should be initiated.

Appropriate treatment and services includes all care provided to residents by employees, contractors, or volunteers of the facility to maximize the individual's functional abilities. This includes pain relief and control, especially when it is causing a decline or a decrease in the quality of life of the resident.

If the survey team identifies a pattern of deterioration in ADLs, i.e., a number of residents have deteriorated in more than one ADL or a number of residents have deteriorated in only one ADL (one in bathing, one in eating, one in toileting) and it is determined there is deficient practice, cite at F310.

For evaluating a resident's ADLs and determining whether a resident's abilities have declined, improved or stayed the same within the last twelve months, use the following definitions as specified in the State's RAI:

1. **Independent** - No help or staff oversight; or staff help/oversight provided only 1 or 2 times during prior 7 days.

2. **Supervision** - Oversight encouragement or cuing provided 3 or more times during the last 7 days, or supervision plus physical assistance provided only 1 or 2 times during the last 7 days.

3. **Limited Assistance** - Resident highly involved in activity, received physical help in guided maneuvering of limbs, and/or other non-weight bearing assistance 3 or more times; or more help provided only 1 or 2 times over 7-day period.

4. **Extensive Assistance** - While resident performed part of activity, over prior 7-day period, help of following type(s) was provided 3 or more times;

    a. Weight-bearing support; or

    b. Full staff performance during part (but not all) of week.

5. **Total Dependence** - Full staff performance of activity over entire 7-day period.

§483.25(a)(1)(i) Bathing, Dressing, Grooming

Interpretive Guidelines §483.25(a)(1)(i)

This corresponds to MDS section E; version 2.0, section G, when specified for use by the State.

"Bathing" means how resident takes full-body bath, sponge bath, and transfers in/out of tub/shower. Exclude washing of back and hair.

"Dressing" means how resident puts on, fastens, and takes off all items of clothing, including donning/removing prosthesis.

"Grooming" means how resident maintains personal hygiene, including preparatory activities, combing hair, brushing teeth, shaving, applying make-up, washing/drying face, hands and perineum. Exclude baths and showers.

BATHING, DRESSING, GROOMING

Procedures: §483.25(a)(1)(i)

For each sampled resident selected for the comprehensive review or the focused review, as appropriate, determine:

1. Whether the resident's ability to bathe, dress and/or groom has changed since admission, or over the past 12 months;

2. Whether the resident's ability to bathe, dress and groom has improved, declined or stayed the same;

3. Whether any deterioration or lack of improvement was avoidable or unavoidable by:

4. Identifying if resident triggers RAPs for ADL functional/rehabilitation potential.

    a. What risk factors for decline of bathing, dressing, and/or grooming abilities did the facility identify?

    b. What care did the resident receive to address unique needs to maintain his/her bathing, dressing, and/or grooming abilities (e.g., resident needs a button hook to button his shirt; staff teaches the resident how to use it; staff provides resident with dementia with cues that allow him/her to dress him or herself)?

    c. Were individual objectives of the plan of care periodically evaluated, and if the objectives were not met, were alternative approaches developed to encourage maintenance of bathing, dressing, and/or grooming abilities (e.g., resident now unable to button dress, even with encouragement; will ask family if we may use velcro in place of buttons so resident can continue to dress herself)?

Probes: §483.25(a)(1)(i)

If the resident's abilities in bathing, dressing, and grooming have been maintained, what evidence is there that the resident could have improved if appropriate treatment and services were provided:

- Identify relevant sections of the MDS and consider whether assessment triggers the RAPs and the RAPs were followed.

- Are there physical and psychosocial deficits that could affect improvement in functional abilities?

- Was the care plan driven by resident strengths identified in the comprehensive assessment?

- Was the care plan consistently implemented?

- What changes were made in treatment if the resident failed to progress or when initial rehabilitation goals were achieved, but additional progress might have been possible?

TRANSFER AND AMBULATION

§483.25(a)(1)(ii)

Interpretive Guidelines: §483.25(a)(1)(ii)

This corresponds to MDS section E; MDS 2.0 section G when specified for use by the State.

"Transfer" means how resident moves between surfaces - to/from: bed, chair, wheelchair, standing position. (Exclude to/from bath/toilet.)

"Ambulation" means how resident moves between locations in his/her room and adjacent corridor on same floor. If in wheelchair, self-sufficiency once in chair.

Procedures: §483.25(a)(1)(ii)

Determine for each resident selected for a comprehensive review, or a focused review as appropriate, whether the resident's ability to transfer and ambulate has declined, improved or stayed the same and whether any deterioration or decline in function was avoidable or unavoidable.

Probes: §483.25(a)(1)(ii)

If the resident's transferring and ambulating abilities have declined, what evidence is there that the decline was unavoidable:

- What risk factors for decline of transferring or ambulating abilities did the facility identify (e.g., necrotic area of foot ulcer becoming larger, postural hypotension)?

- What care did the resident receive to address risk factors and unique needs to maintain transferring or ambulating abilities (e.g., a transfer board is provided to maintain ability to transfer from bed to wheelchair and staff teaches the resident how to use it)?

- What evidence is there that sufficient staff time and assistance are provided to maintain transferring and ambulating abilities?
- Has resident been involved in activities that enhance mobility skills?
- Were individual objectives of the plan of care periodically evaluated, and if goals were not met, were alternative approaches developed to encourage maintenance of transferring and ambulation abilities (e.g., resident remains unsteady when using a cane, returns to walker, with staff encouraging the walker's consistent use)?
- Identify if resident triggers RAPs for ADL functional/rehabilitation potential, psychosocial well-being, or mood state and the RAPs are followed.

If the resident's abilities in transferring and ambulating have been maintained, is there evidence that the resident could have improved if appropriate treatment and services were provided?

- Are there physical and psychosocial deficits that could affect improvement in functional abilities?
- Was the care plan driven by resident strengths identified in the comprehensive assessment?
- Was the care plan consistently implemented? What changes were made in treatment if the resident failed to progress or when initial rehabilitation goals were achieved, but additional progress seemed possible?

TOILETING

§483.25(a)(1)(ii)

Interpretive Guidelines: §483.25(a)(1)(iii)

This corresponds to MDS sections E; MDS 2.0 sections G and H when specified for use by the State.

"Toilet use" means how the resident uses the toilet room (or commode, bedpan, urinal); transfers on/off the toilet, cleanses self, changes pad, manages ostomy or catheter, adjusts clothes.

Procedures: §483.25(a)(1)(iii)

Determine for each resident selected for a comprehensive review, or focused review as appropriate, whether the resident's ability to use the toilet has improved, declined or stayed the same and whether any deterioration or decline in improvement was avoidable or unavoidable.

Probes: §483.25(a)(1)(iii)

If the resident's toilet use abilities have declined, what evidence is there that the decline was unavoidable.

- What risk factors for the decline of toilet use abilities did the facility identify (e.g., severe arthritis in hands makes use of toilet paper difficult)?
- What care did resident receive to address risk factors and unique needs to maintain toilet use abilities (e.g., assistive devices to maintain ability to use the toilet such as using a removable elevated toilet seat or wall grab bar to facilitate rising from seated position to standing position)?
- Is there sufficient staff time and assistance provided to maintain toilet use abilities (e.g., allowing residents enough time to use the toilet independently or with limited assistance)?
- Were individual objectives of the plan of care periodically evaluated, and if objectives were not met, were alternative approaches developed to encourage maintaining toilet use abilities (e.g., if resident has not increased sitting stability, seek occupational therapy consult to determine the need for therapy to increase sitting balance, ability to transfer safely and manipulate clothing during the toileting process. For residents with dementia, remind periodically to use the toilet)?
- Identify if resident triggers RAPs for urinary incontinence, and ADL functional/rehabilitation potential and the RAPs were used to assess causal factors for decline or potential for decline or lack of improvement.

If the resident's toilet use abilities have been maintained, what evidence is there that the resident could have improved if appropriate treatment and services were provided?

- Are there physical and psychosocial deficits that could affect improvement in functional abilities?
- Was the care plan driven by resident strengths identified in the comprehensive assessment?
- Was the care plan consistently implemented? What changes were made to treatment if the resident failed to progress or when initial rehabilitation goals were achieved, but additional progress seemed possible?
- Identify if resident triggers RAPs for mood state and psychosocial well-being.

EATING

§483.25(a)(1)(iv)

Interpretive Guidelines: §483.25(a)(1)(iv)

This corresponds to MDS sections E, L1 and MI; MDS 2.0, sections G and K when specified for use by the State.

"Eating" means how resident ingests and drinks (regardless of self-feeding skill).

Procedures: §483.25(a)(1)(iv)

Determine for each resident selected for a comprehensive review, or focused review, as appropriate, whether the resident's ability to eat or eating skills has improved, declined, or stayed the same and whether any deterioration or lack of improvement was avoidable or unavoidable.

If the resident's eating abilities have declined, is there any evidence that the decline was unavoidable?

1. What risk factors for decline of eating skills did the facility identify?

    a. A decrease in the ability to chew and swallow food

    b. Deficit in neurological and muscular status necessary for moving food onto a utensil and into the mouth

    c. Oral health status affecting eating ability

    d. Depression or confused mental state

2. What care did the resident receive to address risk factors and unique needs to maintain eating abilities?

    a. Assistive devices to improve resident's grasp or coordination;

    b. Seating arrangements to improve sociability;

    c. Seating in a calm, quiet setting for residents with dementia.

3. Is there sufficient staff time and assistance provided to maintain eating abilities (e.g., allowing residents enough time to eat independently or with limited assistance)?

4. Identify if resident triggers RAPs for ADL functional/rehabilitation potential, feeding tubes, and dehydration/fluid maintenance, and the RAPs were used to assess causal reasons for decline, potential for decline or lack of improvement.

5. Were individual objectives of the plan of care periodically evaluated, and if the objectives were not met, were alternative approaches developed to encourage maintaining eating abilities?

Probes: §483.25(a)(1)(iv)

If the resident's eating abilities have been maintained, what evidence is there that the resident could have improved if appropriate treatment and services were provided:

- Are there physical and psychosocial deficits that could affect improvement in functional abilities?
- Was the care plan driven by resident strengths identified in the comprehensive assessment?
- Was the care plan consistently implemented? What changes are made to treatment if the resident failed to progress or when initial rehabilitation goals were achieved, but additional progress seemed possible?

Interpretive Guidelines: §483.25(a)(1)(v)

This corresponds to MDS, section C; MDS 2.0 sections B and C when specified for use by the State.

"Speech, language or other functional communication systems" is defined as the ability to effectively communicate requests, needs, opinions, and urgent problems; to express emotion, to listen to others and to participate in social conversation whether in speech, writing, gesture or a combination of these (e.g., a communication board or electronic augmentative communication device).

USE OF SPEECH, LANGUAGE, OR OTHER FUNCTIONAL COMMUNCATION SYSTEMS

§483.25(a)(1)(v)

Procedures: §483.25(a)(1)(v)

Determine for each resident selected for a comprehensive review, or focused review, as appropriate, if resident's ability to communicate has declined, improved or stayed the same and whether any deterioration or lack of improvement was avoidable or unavoidable.

Identify if resident triggers RAPs for communication, psychosocial well-being, mood state, and visual function, and if the RAPs were used to assess causal factors for decline, potential for decline or lack of improvement.

Probes: §483.25(a)(1)(v)

If the resident's communication abilities have diminished, is there any evidence that the decline was unavoidable:

- What risk factors for decline of communication abilities did the facility identify and how did they address them (e.g., dysarthria, poor fitting dentures, few visitors, poor relationships with staff, Alzheimer's disease)?
- Has the resident received audiologic and vision evaluation? If not, did the resident refuse such services? (See also §483.10(b)(4).)
- What unique resident needs and risk factors did the facility identify (e.g., does the resident have specific difficulties in transmitting messages, comprehending messages, and/or using a variety of communication skills such as questions and commands; does the resident receive evaluation and training in the use of assistive devices to increase and/or maintain writing skills)?
- What care does the resident receive to improve communication abilities (e.g.,nurse aides communicate in writing with deaf residents or residents with severe hearing problems; practice exercises with residents receiving speech-language pathology services; increase number of resident's communication opportunities; non-verbal means of communication; review of the effect of medications on communication ability)?
- Is there sufficient staff time and assistance provided to maintain communication abilities?
- Were individual objectives of the plan of care periodically evaluated, and if the objectives were not met, were alternative approaches developed to encourage maintenance of communication abilities (e.g., if drill-oriented therapy is frustrating the resident, a less didactic approach should be attempted)?

Probes: §483.25(a)(1)(v)

If the resident's speech, language, and other communication abilities have been maintained, what evidence is there that the resident could have improved if appropriate treatment and services were provided:

- Are there physical and psychosocial deficits that could affect improvement in functional abilities?
- Was the care plan driven by resident strengths identified in the comprehensive assessment?
- Was the care plan consistently implemented?
- What changes were made to treatment if the resident failed to progress or when initial rehabilitation goals were achieved, but additional progress seemed possible?

F311

§483.25(a)(2)

(2) A resident is given the appropriate treatment and services to maintain or improve his or her abilities specified in paragraph (a)(1) of this section; and

Intent §483.25(a)(2)

The intent of this regulation is to stress that the facility is responsible for providing maintenance and restorative programs that will not only maintain, but improve, as indicated by the resident's comprehensive assessment to achieve and maintain the highest practicable outcome.

Procedures §483.25(a)(2)

Use the survey procedures and probes at §483.25(a)(1)(i) through (v) to assist in making this determination

---

F312

§483.25(a)(3)

(3) A resident who is unable to carry out activities of daily living receives the necessary services to maintain good nutrition, grooming, and personal and oral hygiene.

Intent: §483.25(a)(3)

The intent of this regulation is that the resident receives the care and services needed because he/she is unable to do their own ADL care independently.

Interpretive Guidelines: §483.25(a)(3)

This corresponds to MDS section L; MDS 2.0 section K when specified by the State.

"Unable to carry out ADLs" means those residents who need extensive or total assistance with maintenance of nutrition, grooming and personal and oral hygiene, receive this assistance from the facility.

Methods for maintenance of good nutrition may include hand feeding of foods served on dishes; tube feedings provided through naso-gastric, gastrostomy, or other external tubes; or total parenteral nutrition provided through a central intravenous line.

"Grooming" - See §483.25(a)(1)(i) for definition.

"Personal hygiene" - Those activities described in dressing and bathing as defined in §483.25(a)(1)(i).

"Oral hygiene" means maintaining the mouth in a clean and intact condition and treating oral pathology such as ulcers of the mucosa. Services to maintain oral hygiene may include brushing the teeth, cleaning dentures, cleaning the mouth and tongue either by assisting the resident with a mouth wash or by manual cleaning with a gauze sponge; and application of medication as prescribed.

Procedures: §483.25(a)(3)

For residents selected for a comprehensive review, or focused review, as appropriate, who are unable to carry out these ADLs without extensive assistance, determine if poor nutritional status, poor grooming, or lack of effective personal and oral hygiene exist. To what extent are these negative outcomes attributable to the lack of receiving necessary services?

Identify if residents trigger RAPs for nutritional status, ADL functional/rehabilitation potential, behavior problems, and dental care. Consider whether the RAPs were used to assess causal factors for decline, potential for decline, or lack of improvement. Determine if the facility proceeded properly with care planning and delivery of care for these residents.

F313

§483.25(b) Vision and hearing

To ensure that residents receive proper treatment and assistive devices to maintain vision and hearing abilities, the facility must, if necessary, assist the resident --

1. **In making appointments, and**

2. By arranging for transportation to and from the office of a practitioner specializing in the treatment of vision or hearing impairment or the office of a professional specializing in the provision of vision or hearing assistive devices.

Intent: §483.25(b)

The intent of this regulation is to require a facility to assist residents in gaining access to vision and hearing services by making appointments and arranging for transportation, and assistance with the use of any devices needed to maintain vision and hearing.

Interpretive Guidelines: §483.25(b)

This corresponds to MDS, sections C and O; MDS 2.0 sections C, D, and P when specified for use by the State.

Assistive devices to maintain vision include glasses, contact lenses, and magnifying glasses. Assistive devices to maintain hearing include hearing aids.

This requirement does not mean that the facility must provide refractions, glasses, contact lenses, conduct comprehensive audiological evaluations (although screening is a part of the required assessment in §483.20(b)) or provide hearing aids.

The facility's responsibility is to assist residents and their families in locating and utilizing any available resources (e.g., Medicare or Medicaid program payment, local health organizations offering items and services which are available free to the community) for the provision of the services the resident needs. This includes making appointments and arranging transportation to obtain needed services.

Probes: §483.25(b)

- Identify if resident triggers RAPs for visual function, and communication. Consider whether the RAPs were used to assess causal factors for decline, potential for decline or lack of improvement.
- If the resident needs, and/or requests and does not have vision and/or hearing assistive devices, what has the facility done to assist the resident in making appointments and obtaining transportation to obtain these services?
- If the resident has assistive devices but is not using them, why not (e.g., are repairs or batteries needed)?

F314

§483.25(c) Pressure Sores

Based on the comprehensive Assessment of a resident, the facility must ensure that--

(1) A resident who enters the facility without pressure sores does not develop pressure sores unless the individual's clinical condition demonstrates that they were unavoidable; and

(2) A resident having pressure sores receives necessary treatment and services to promote healing, prevent infection and prevent new sores from developing.

Intent: (F314) 42 CFR 483.25(c)

The intent of this requirement is that the resident does not develop pressure ulcers unless clinically unavoidable and that the facility provides care and services to:

- Promote the prevention of pressure ulcer development;
- Promote the healing of pressure ulcers that are present (including prevention of infection to the extent possible); and
- Prevent development of additional pressure ulcers.

NOTE: Although the regulatory language refers to pressure sores, the nomenclature widely accepted presently refers to pressure ulcers, and the guidance provided in this document will refer to pressure ulcers.

DEFINITIONS

Definitions are provided to clarify clinical terms related to pressure ulcers and their evaluation and treatment.

- "Pressure Ulcer"- A pressure ulcer is any lesion caused by unrelieved pressure that results in damage to the underlying tissue(s).[1] Although friction and shear are not primary causes of pressure ulcers, friction and shear are important contributing factors to the development of pressure ulcers.
- "Avoidable/Unavoidable" Pressure Ulcers
    - "Avoidable" means that the resident developed a pressure ulcer and that the facility did not do one or more of the following: evaluate the resident's clinical condition and pressure ulcer risk factors; define and implement interventions that are consistent with resident needs, resident goals, and

recognized standards of practice; monitor and evaluate the impact of the interventions; or revise the interventions as appropriate.

- "Unavoidable" means that the resident developed a pressure ulcer even though the facility had evaluated the resident's clinical condition and pressure ulcer risk factors; defined and implemented interventions that are consistent with resident needs, goals, and recognized standards of practice; monitored and evaluated the impact of the interventions; and revised the approaches as appropriate.

- "Cleansing/Irrigation"
  - "Cleansing" refers to the use of an appropriate device and solution to clean the surface of the wound bed and to remove the looser foreign debris or contaminants in order to decrease microbial growth.[2]
  - "Irrigation" refers to a type of mechanical debridement, which uses an appropriate solution delivered under pressure to the wound bed to vigorously attempt to remove debris from the wound bed.[3]

- "Colonized/Infected" Wound [4, 5]
  - "Colonized" refers to the presence of bacteria on the surface or in the tissue of a wound without the signs and symptoms of an infection.
  - "Infected" refers to the presence of micro-organisms in sufficient quantity to overwhelm the defenses of viable tissues and produce the signs and symptoms of infection.

- "Debridement"- Debridement is the removal of devitalized/necrotic tissue and foreign matter from a wound to improve or facilitate the healing process. [6, 7, 8] Various debridement methods include:
  - "Autolytic debridement" refers to the use of moisture retentive dressings to cover a wound and allow devitalized tissue to self-digest by the action of enzymes present in the wound fluids.
  - "Enzymatic (chemical) debridement" refers to the topical application of substances e.g., enzymes to break down devitalized tissue.
  - "Mechanical debridement" refers to the removal of foreign material and devitalized or contaminated tissue from a wound by physical rather than by chemical or autolytic means.
  - "Sharp or surgical debridement" refers to removal of foreign material or devitalized tissue by a surgical instrument.

  - "Maggot debridement therapy (MDT)" or medicinal maggots refers to a type of sterile intentional biological larval or biosurgical debridement that uses disinfected (sterile) maggots to clean wounds by dissolving the dead and infected tissue and by killing bacteria.[9]

- "Eschar/Slough"

  - "Eschar" is described as thick, leathery, frequently black or brown in color, necrotic (dead) or devitalized tissue that has lost its usual physical properties and biological activity. Eschar may be loose or firmly adhered to the wound.

  - "Slough" is necrotic/avascular tissue in the process of separating from the viable portions of the body and is usually light colored, soft, moist, and stringy (at times).

- "Exudate"

  - "Exudate" is any fluid that has been forced out of the tissues or its capillaries because of inflammation or injury. It may contain serum, cellular debris, bacteria and leukocytes.

  - "Purulent exudate/drainage/discharge" is any product of inflammation that contains pus (e.g., leukocytes, bacteria, and liquefied necrotic debris).

  - "Serous drainage or exudate" is watery, clear, or slightly yellow/tan/pink fluid that has separated from the blood and presents as drainage.

- "Friction/Shearing"

  - "Friction" is the mechanical force exerted on skin that is dragged across any surface.

  - "Shearing" is the interaction of both gravity and friction against the surface of the skin. Friction is always present when shear force is present.[10] Shear occurs when layers of skin rub against each other or when the skin remains stationary and the underlying tissue moves and stretches and angulates or tears the underlying capillaries and blood vessels causing tissue damage.

- "Granulation Tissue"

  - "Granulation tissue" is the pink-red moist tissue that fills an open wound, when it starts to heal. It contains new blood vessels, collagen, fibroblasts, and inflammatory cells.

- "Tunnel/Sinus Tract/Undermining"-Tunnel and sinus tract are often used interchangeably.
  - o "Tunneling" is a passageway of tissue destruction under the skin surface that has an opening at the skin level from the edge of the wound.
  - o A "sinus tract" is a cavity or channel underlying a wound that involves an area larger than the visible surface of the wound.
  - o "Undermining" is the destruction of tissue or ulceration extending under the skin edges (margins) so that the pressure ulcer is larger at its base than at the skin surface. Undermining often develops from shearing forces and is differentiated from tunneling by the larger extent of the wound edge involved in undermining and the absence of a channel or tract extending from the pressure ulcer under the adjacent intact skin.

OVERVIEW

A pressure ulcer can occur wherever pressure has impaired circulation to the tissue. Critical steps in pressure ulcer prevention and healing include: identifying the individual resident at risk for developing pressure ulcers, identifying and evaluating the risk factors and changes in the resident's condition, identifying and evaluating factors that can be removed or modified, implementing individualized interventions to attempt to stabilize, reduce or remove underlying risk factors, monitoring the impact of the interventions, and modifying the interventions as appropriate. It is important to recognize and evaluate each resident's risk factors and to identify and evaluate all areas at risk of constant pressure.

A complete assessment is essential to an effective pressure ulcer prevention and treatment program. A comprehensive individual evaluation helps the facility to:

- Identify the resident at risk of developing pressure ulcers, the level and nature of risk(s); and
- Identify the presence of pressure ulcers.

This information allows the facility to develop and implement a comprehensive care plan that reflects each resident's identified needs.

The care process should include efforts to stabilize, reduce or remove underlying risk factors; to monitor the impact of the interventions; and to modify the interventions as appropriate.

The facility should have a system/procedure to assure: assessments are timely and appropriate; interventions are implemented, monitored, and revised as appropriate; and changes in condition are recognized, evaluated, reported to the practitioner, and addressed. The quality assessment and assurance committee may help the facility evaluate existing strategies to reduce the development and progression of pressure ulcers, monitor the incidence and prevalence of pressure ulcers within the facility, and ensure that facility policies and procedures are consistent with current standards of practice.

Research into appropriate practices for the prevention, management and treatment of pressure ulcers, continues to evolve. As such, there are many recognized clinical resources regarding the prevention and management of pressure ulcers (including wound care, and complications such as infections and pain). Some of these resources include:

- The Clinical Practice Guidelines from the Agency for Healthcare Research and Quality (AHRQ) www.ahrq.gov (Guideline No. 15: Treatment of Pressure Ulcers and Guideline No.3: Pressure Ulcers in Adults: Prediction and Prevention)(AHRQ was previously known as the Agency for Health Care Policy and Research [AHCPR]);
- The National Pressure Ulcer Advisory Panel (NPUAP) www.npuap.org;
- The American Medical Directors Association (AMDA) www.amda.com (Clinical Practice Guidelines: Pressure Ulcers, 1996 and Pressure Ulcer Therapy Companion, 1999);
- The Quality Improvement Organizations, Medicare Quality Improvement Community Initiatives site at www.medqic.org;
- The Wound, Ostomy, and Continence Nurses Society (WOCN) www.wocn.org; and
- The American Geriatrics Society guideline "The Management of Persistent Pain in Older Persons", www.healthinaging.org.

NOTE: References to non-CMS sources or sites on the Internet are provided as a service and do not constitute or imply endorsement of these organizations or their programs by CMS or the U.S. Department of Health and Human Services. CMS is not responsible for the content of pages found at these sites. URL addresses were current as of the date of this publication.

PREVENTION OF PRESSURE ULCERS

The citation at 42 CFR 483.25 (c) requires that a resident who is admitted without a pressure ulcer doesn't develop a pressure ulcer unless clinically unavoidable, and that a resident who has an ulcer receives care and services to promote healing and to prevent additional ulcers.

The first step in prevention is the identification of the resident at risk of developing pressure ulcers. This is followed by implementation of appropriate individualized interventions and monitoring for the effectiveness of the interventions.

ASSESSMENT

An admission evaluation helps identify the resident at risk of developing a pressure ulcer, and the resident with existing pressure ulcer(s) or areas of skin that are at risk for breakdown. Because a resident at risk can develop a pressure ulcer within 2 to 6 hours of the onset of pressure,[11] the at-risk resident needs to be identified and have interventions implemented promptly to attempt to prevent pressure ulcers. The admission evaluation helps define those initial care approaches.

In addition, the admission evaluation may identify pre-existing signs (such as a purple or very dark area that is surrounded by profound redness, edema, or induration)[12] suggesting that deep tissue damage has already occurred and additional deep tissue loss may occur. This deep tissue damage could lead to the appearance of an unavoidable Stage III or IV pressure ulcer or progression of a Stage I pressure ulcer to an ulcer with eschar or exudate within days after admission. Some situations, which may have contributed to this tissue damage, include pressure resulting from immobility during hospitalization or surgical procedures, during prolonged ambulance transport, or while waiting to be discovered or assisted after a debilitating event, such as a fall or a cerebral vascular accident.

Some evidence suggests that because it may be harder to identify erythema in an older adult with darkly pigmented skin, older individuals with darkly pigmented skin may be more at risk for developing pressure ulcers.[13, 14, 15, 16] It may be necessary, therefore, in a darker skinned individual to focus more on other evidence of pressure ulcer development, such as bogginess, induration, coolness, or increased warmth as well as signs of skin discoloration.

Multiple factors, including pressure intensity, pressure duration, and tissue tolerance, significantly affect the potential for the development and healing of pressure ulcers. An individual may also have various intrinsic risks due to aging, for example: decreased subcutaneous tissue and lean muscle mass, decreased skin elasticity, and impaired circulation or innervation.

The comprehensive assessment, which includes the Resident Assessment Instrument (RAI), evaluates the resident's intrinsic risks, the resident's skin condition, other factors (including causal factors) which place the resident at risk for developing pressure ulcers and/or experiencing delayed healing, and the nature of the pressure to which the resident may be subjected. The assessment should identify which risk factors can be removed or modified.

The assessment also helps identify the resident who has multi-system organ failure or an end-of-life condition or who is refusing care and treatment. If the resident is refusing care, an evaluation of the basis for the refusal, and the identification and evaluation of potential alternatives is indicated.

This comprehensive assessment should address those factors that have been identified as having an impact on the development, treatment and/or healing of pressure ulcers, including, at a minimum: risk factors, pressure points, under-nutrition and hydration deficits, and moisture and the impact of moisture on skin. Each of these factors is discussed in additional detail in the following sections.

Risk Factors

Many studies and professional documents identify risk factors that increase a resident's susceptibility to develop or to not heal pressure ulcers.[17, 18, 19] Examples of these risk factors include, but are not limited to:

- Impaired/decreased mobility and decreased functional ability;
- Co-morbid conditions, such as end stage renal disease, thyroid disease or diabetes mellitus;
- Drugs such as steroids that may affect wound healing;
- Impaired diffuse or localized blood flow, for example, generalized atherosclerosis or lower extremity arterial insufficiency;
- Resident refusal of some aspects of care and treatment;
- Cognitive impairment;
- Exposure of skin to urinary and fecal incontinence;
- Under nutrition, malnutrition, and hydration deficits; and
- A healed ulcer. The history of a healed pressure ulcer and its stage [if known] is important, since areas of healed Stage III or IV pressure ulcers are more likely to have recurrent breakdown.

Some residents have many risk factors for developing pressure ulcers, such as diabetic neuropathy, frailty, cognitive impairment, and under nutrition. Not all factors are fully modifiable and some potentially modifiable factors (e.g., under-nutrition) may not be corrected immediately, despite prompt intervention, while other factors such as pressure may be modified promptly. It may be necessary to stabilize, when possible, the underlying causes (e.g., control blood sugars or ensure adequate food and fluid intake).

Although the requirements do not mandate any specific assessment tool, other than the RAI, validated instruments are available to assess risk for developing pressure ulcers. Research has shown that a significant number of pressure ulcers develop within the first four weeks after admission to a long term care facility.[20] Therefore, many clinicians recommend using a standardized pressure ulcer risk assessment tool to assess a resident's pressure ulcer risks upon admission, weekly for the first four weeks after admission for each resident at risk, then quarterly, or whenever there is a change in cognition or functional ability.[21, 22] A resident's risk may increase due to an acute illness or condition change (e.g., upper respiratory infection, pneumonia, or exacerbation of underlying congestive heart failure) and may require additional evaluation.

Regardless of any resident's total risk score, the clinicians responsible for the resident's care should review each risk factor and potential cause(s) individually[23] to: a)Identify those that increase the potential for the resident to develop pressure ulcers; b) Decide whether and to what extent the factor(s) can be modified, stabilized, removed, etc., and c) Determine whether targeted management protocols need to be implemented. In other words, an overall risk score indicating the resident is not at high risk of developing pressure ulcers does not mean that existing risk factors or causes should be considered less important or addressed less vigorously than those factors or causes in the resident whose overall score indicates he or she is at a higher risk of developing a pressure ulcer.

Pressure Points and Tissue Tolerance

Assessment of a resident's skin condition helps define prevention strategies. The skin assessment should include an evaluation of the skin integrity and tissue tolerance (ability of the skin and its supporting structures to endure the effects of pressure without adverse effects) after pressure to that area has been reduced or redistributed.

Tissue closest to the bone may be the first tissue to undergo necrosis. Pressure ulcers are usually located over a bony prominence, such as the sacrum, heel, the greater trochanter, ischial tuberosity, fibular head, scapula, and ankle (malleolus).

An at-risk resident who sits too long on a static surface may be more prone to get ischial ulceration. Slouching in a chair may predispose an at-risk resident to pressure ulcers of the spine, scapula, or elbow (elbow ulceration is often related to arm rests or lap boards). Friction and shearing are also important factors in tissue ischemia, necrosis and pressure ulcer formation.

Pressure ulcers may develop at other sites where pressure has impaired the circulation to the tissue, such as pressure from positioning or use of medical devices. For example, pressure ulcers may develop from pressure on an ear lobe related to positioning of the head; pressure or friction on areas (e.g., nares, urinary meatus, extremities) caused by tubes, casts, orthoses, braces, cervical collars, or other medical devices; pressure on the labia or scrotum related to positioning (e.g., against a pommel type cushion); pressure on the foot related to ill-fitting shoes causing blistering; or pressure on legs, arms and fingers due to contractures or deformity resulting from rheumatoid arthritis, etc.

While pressure ulcers on the sacrum remain the most common location, pressure ulcers on the heel are occurring more frequently,[24] are difficult to assess and heal, and require early identification of skin compromise over the heel.

It is, therefore, important for clinical staff to regularly conduct thorough skin assessments on each resident who is at risk for developing pressure ulcers.

Under-Nutrition and Hydration Deficits

Adequate nutrition and hydration are essential for overall functioning. Nutrition provides vital energy and building blocks for all of the body's structures and processes. Any organ or body system may require additional energy or structural materials for repair or function. The skin is the body's largest organ system. It may affect, and be affected by, other body processes and organs. Skin condition reflects overall body function; skin breakdown may be the most visible evidence of a general catabolic state.

Weight reflects a balance between intake and utilization of energy. Significant unintended weight loss may indicate under-nutrition or worsening health status. Weight stability (in the absence of fluid excess or loss) is a useful indicator of overall caloric balance. Severely impaired organs (heart, lungs, kidneys, liver, etc.) may be unable to use nutrients effectively. A resident with a pressure ulcer who continues to lose weight either needs additional caloric intake or correction (where possible) of conditions that are creating a hypermetabolic state. Continuing weight loss and failure of a pressure ulcer to heal despite reasonable efforts to improve caloric and nutrient intake may indicate the resident is in multi-system failure or an end-stage or end-of-life condition warranting an additional assessment of the resident's overall condition.

Before instituting a nutritional care plan, it helps to summarize resident specific evidence, including: severity of nutritional compromise, rate of weight loss or appetite decline, probable causes, the individual's prognosis and projected clinical course, and the resident's wishes and goals. Because there are no wound-specific nutritional measures, the interdisciplinary team should develop nutritional goals for the whole person. Unless contraindicated, nutritional goals for a resident with nutritional compromise who has a pressure ulcer or is at risk of developing pressure ulcers should include protein intake of approximately 1.2-1.5 gm/kg body weight daily (higher end of the range for those with larger, more extensive, or multiple wounds). A simple multivitamin is appropriate, but unless the resident has a specific vitamin or mineral deficiency, supplementation with additional vitamins or minerals may not be indicated.

NOTE: Although some laboratory tests may help clinicians evaluate nutritional issues in a resident with pressure ulcers, no laboratory test is specific or sensitive enough to warrant serial/repeated testing. Serum albumin, pre-albumin and cholesterol may be useful to help establish overall prognosis; however, they may not correlate well with clinical observation of nutritional status.[25, 26] At his or her discretion, a practitioner may order test(s) that provide useful additional information or help with management of treatable conditions.

Water is essential to maintain adequate body functions. As a major component of blood, water dissolves vitamins, minerals, glucose, amino acids, etc.; transports nutrients into cells; removes waste from the cells; and helps maintain circulating blood volume as well as fluid and electrolyte balance. It is critical that each resident at risk for hydration deficit or imbalance, including the resident with a pressure ulcer or at risk of developing an ulcer, be identified and that hydration needs be addressed.

(The surveyor should refer to the Guidance at 42 CFR 483.25 (i), F325, Nutrition, and 483.25(j), F327 Hydration for investigation of potential non-compliance with the nutrition and hydration requirements. A low albumin level combined with the facility's lack of supplementation, for example, is not sufficient to cite a pressure ulcer deficiency.)

Moisture and Its Impact

Both urine and feces contain substances that may irritate the epidermis and may make the skin more susceptible to breakdown. Some studies have found that fecal incontinence may pose a greater threat to skin integrity,[27] most likely due to bile acids and enzymes in the feces. Irritation or maceration resulting from prolonged exposure to urine and feces may hasten skin breakdown, and moisture may make skin more susceptible to damage from friction and shear during repositioning.

It may be difficult to differentiate dermatitis related to incontinence from partial thickness skin loss (pressure ulcer). This differentiation should be based on the clinical evidence and review of presenting risk factors. A Stage I pressure ulcer usually presents as a localized area of erythema or skin discoloration, while perineal dermatitis may appear as a more diffuse area of erythema or discoloration where the urine or stool has come into contact with the skin. The dermatitis may occur in the area where the incontinence brief or underpad has been used. Also, the dermatitis/rash more typically presents as intense erythema, scaling, itching, papules, weeping and eruptions.[28]

INTERVENTIONS

The comprehensive assessment should provide the basis for defining approaches to address residents at risk of developing or already having a pressure ulcer. A determination that a resident is at high risk to develop a pressure ulcer has significant implications for preventive and treatment strategies, but does not by itself indicate that development of a pressure ulcer was unavoidable. Effective prevention and treatment are based upon consistently providing routine and individualized interventions.

In the context of the resident's choices, clinical condition, and physician input, the resident's plan of care should establish relevant goals and approaches to stabilize or improve co-morbidities, such as attempts to minimize clinically significant blood sugar fluctuations and other interventions aimed at limiting the effects of risk factors associated with pressure ulcers. Alternatively, facility staff and practitioners should document clinically valid reasons why such interventions were not appropriate or feasible. Repeated hospitalizations or emergency room visits within a 6-month period may indicate overall decline or instability.

Resident Choice

In order for a resident to exercise his or her right appropriately to make informed choices about care and treatment or to refuse treatment, the facility and the resident (or the resident's legal representative) must discuss the resident's condition, treatment options, expected outcomes, and consequences of refusing treatment. The facility is expected to address the resident's concerns and offer relevant alternatives, if the resident has refused specific treatments. (See Resident Rights at 42 CFR 483.10(b)(3) and (4), F154 and F155.)

Advance Directive

A resident at the end of life, in terminal stages of an illness or having multiple system failures may have written directions for his or her treatment goals (or a decision has been made by the resident's surrogate or representative, in accordance with state law).

If a resident has a valid Advance Directive, the facility's care must reflect a resident's wishes as expressed in the Directive, in accordance with state law. However, the presence of an Advance Directive does not absolve the facility from giving supportive and other pertinent care that is not prohibited by the Advance Directive. If the facility has implemented individualized approaches for end-of-life care in accordance with the resident's wishes, and has implemented appropriate efforts to try to stabilize the resident's condition (or indicated why the condition cannot or should not be stabilized) and to provide care to prevent or treat the pressure ulcer (including pertinent, routine, lesser aggressive approaches, such as, cleaning, turning, repositioning), then the development, continuation, or progression of a pressure ulcer may be consistent with regulatory requirements.

NOTE: The presence of a "Do Not Resuscitate" (DNR) order is not sufficient to indicate the resident is declining other appropriate treatment and services. It only indicates that the resident should not be resuscitated if respirations and/or cardiac function cease.

Based upon the assessment and the resident's clinical condition, choices and identified needs, basic or routine care should include interventions to: a) Redistribute pressure (such as repositioning, protecting heels, etc); b) Minimize exposure to moisture and keep skin clean, especially of fecal contamination; c) Provide appropriate, pressure-redistributing, support surfaces; d) Provide non-irritating surfaces; and e) Maintain or improve nutrition and hydration status, where feasible. Adverse drug reactions related to the resident's drug regimen may worsen risk factors for development of pressure ulcers or for non-healing pressure ulcers (for example, by causing lethargy or anorexia or creating/increasing confusion) and should be identified and addressed. These interventions should be incorporated into the plan of care and revised as the condition of the resident indicates.

Repositioning

Repositioning is a common, effective intervention for an individual with a pressure ulcer or who is at risk of developing one.[29, 30] Assessment of a resident's skin integrity after pressure has been reduced or redistributed should guide the development and implementation of repositioning plans. Such plans should be addressed in the comprehensive plan of care consistent with the resident's need and goals. Repositioning is critical for a resident who is immobile or dependent upon staff for repositioning. The care plan for a resident at risk of friction or shearing during repositioning may require the use of lifting devices for repositioning. Positioning the resident on an existing pressure ulcer should be avoided since it puts additional pressure on tissue that is already compromised and may impede healing.

Surveyors should consider the following repositioning issues:

- A resident who can change positions independently may need supportive devices to facilitate position changes. The resident also may need instruction about why repositioning is important and how to do it, encouragement to change positions regularly, and monitoring of frequency of repositioning.

- The care plan for a resident who is reclining and is dependent on staff for repositioning should address position changes to maintain the resident's skin integrity. This may include repositioning at least every 2 hours or more frequently depending upon the resident's condition and tolerance of the tissue load (pressure). Depending on the individualized assessment, more frequent repositioning may be warranted for individuals who are at higher risk for pressure ulcer development or who show evidence (e.g., Stage I pressure ulcers) that repositioning at 2-hour intervals is inadequate. With rare exception (e.g., both sacral and ischial pressure ulcers are present) the resident should not be placed directly on the greater trochanter for more than momentary placement. Elevating the head of the bed or the back of a reclining chair to or above a 30 degree angle creates pressure comparable to that exerted while sitting, and requires the same considerations regarding repositioning as those for a dependent resident who is seated.

- Many clinicians recommend a position change "off loading" hourly for dependent residents who are sitting or who are in a bed or a reclining chair with the head of the bed or back of the chair raised 30 degrees or more.[31] Based upon an assessment including evidence of tissue tolerance while sitting (checking for Stage I ulcers as noted above), the resident may not tolerate sitting in a chair in the same position for1 hour at a time and may require a more frequent position change.

- Postural alignment, weight distribution, sitting balance and stability, and pressure redistribution should all be considered when positioning a resident in a chair.[32] A teachable resident should be taught to shift his/her weight approximately every 15 minutes while sitting in a chair.

- Wheelchairs are often used for transporting residents, but they may severely limit repositioning options and increase the risk of pressure ulcer development. Therefore, wheelchairs with sling seats may not be optimal for prolonged sitting during activities or meals, etc. However, available modifications to the seating can provide a more stable surface and provide better pressure reduction.

- There isn't evidence that momentary pressure relief followed by return to the same position (that is a "microshift" of five or 10 degrees or a 10-15 second lift from a seated position) is beneficial. This approach does not allow sufficient capillary refill and tissue perfusion for a resident at risk of developing pressure ulcers. Ongoing monitoring of the resident's skin integrity and tissue tolerance is critical to prevent development or deterioration of pressure ulcers.

Support Surfaces and Pressure Redistribution

Pressure redistribution refers to the function or ability to distribute a load over a surface or contact area. Redistribution results in shifting pressure from one area to another and requires attention to all affected areas. Pressure redistribution has incorporated the concepts of both pressure reduction (reduction of interface pressure, not necessarily below capillary closure pressure) and pressure relief (reduction of interface pressure below capillary closure pressure).

Appropriate support surfaces or devices should be chosen by matching a device's potential therapeutic benefit with the resident's specific situation; for example, multiple ulcers, limited turning surfaces, ability to maintain position. The effectiveness of pressure redistribution devices (e.g., 4-inch convoluted foam pads, gels, air fluidized mattresses, and low loss air mattresses) is based on their potential to address the individual resident's risk, the resident's response to the product, and the characteristics and condition of the product. For example, an overinflated overlay product, or one that "bottoms out" (completely compressing the overlay, when, for example, the caregiver can feel less than one inch between the resident and support material) is unlikely to effectively reduce the pressure risk. These products are more likely to reduce pressure effectively if they are used in accord with the manufacturer's instructions. The effectiveness of each product used needs to be evaluated on an ongoing basis. Surveyors should consider the following pressure redistribution issues:

- Static pressure redistribution devices (e.g., solid foam, convoluted foam, gel mattress) may be indicated when a resident is at risk for pressure ulcer development or delayed healing. A specialized pressure redistribution cushion or surface, for example, might be used to extend the time a resident is sitting in a chair; however, the cushion does not eliminate the necessity for periodic repositioning.

- Dynamic pressure reduction surfaces may be helpful when: 1) The resident cannot assume a variety of positions without bearing weight on a pressure ulcer, 2) The resident completely compresses a static device that has retained its original integrity, or 3) The pressure ulcer is not healing as expected, and it is determined that pressure may be contributing to the delay in healing.

- Because the heels and elbows have relatively little surface area, it is difficult to redistribute pressure on these two surfaces. Therefore, it is important to pay particular attention to reducing the pressure on these areas for the resident at risk in accord with resident's overall goals and condition. Pillows used to support the entire lower leg may effectively raise the heel from contact with the bed, but use of the pillows needs to take into account the resident's other conditions. The use of donut-type cushions is not recommended by the clinicians.

- A resident with severe flexion contractures also may require special attention to effectively reduce pressure on bony prominences or prevent breakdown from skin-to-skin contact.

Some products serve mainly to provide comfort and reduce friction and shearing forces, e.g., sheepskin, heel and elbow protectors. Although these products are not effective at redistributing pressure, they (in addition to pillows, foam wedges, or other measures) may be employed to prevent bony prominences from rubbing together.

MONITORING

At least daily, staff should remain alert to potential changes in the skin condition and should evaluate and document identified changes. For example, a resident's complaint about pain or burning at a site where there has been pressure or a nursing assistant's observation during the resident's bath that there is a change in skin condition should be reported so that the resident may be evaluated further.

After completing a thorough evaluation, the interdisciplinary team should develop a relevant care plan to including prevention and management interventions with measurable goals. Many clinicians recommend evaluating skin condition (e.g., skin color, moisture, temperature, integrity, and turgor) at least weekly, or more often if indicated, such as when the resident is using a medical device that may cause pressure.

The resident should be monitored for condition changes that might increase the risk for breakdown and the defined interventions should be implemented and monitored for effectiveness.

ASSESSMENT AND TREATMENT OF PRESSURE ULCER(S)

It is important that each existing pressure ulcer be identified, whether present on admission or developed after admission, and that factors that influenced its development, the potential for development of additional ulcers or for the deterioration of the pressure ulcer(s) be recognized, assessed and addressed (see discussion under Prevention regarding overall assessment and interventions). Any new pressure ulcer suggests a need to reevaluate the adequacy of the plan for preventing pressure ulcers.

When assessing the ulcer itself, it is important to:

- Differentiate the type of ulcer (pressure-related versus non-pressure-related) because interventions may vary depending on the specific type of ulcer;
- Determine the ulcer's stage;
- Describe and monitor the ulcer's characteristics;
- Monitor the progress toward healing and for potential complications;
- Determine if infection is present;
- Assess, treat and monitor pain, if present; and
- Monitor dressings and treatments.

TYPES OF ULCERS

Three of the more common types of ulcers are pressure, vascular insufficiency/ischemia (venous stasis and arterial ischemic ulcers) and neuropathic. See Guidance to Surveyors at 42 CFR 483.25 (F309) for definition and description of ulcer types other than pressure ulcers.

At the time of the assessment, clinicians (physicians, advance practice nurses, physician assistants, and certified wound care specialists, etc.) should document the clinical basis (for example, type of skin injury/ulcer, location, shape, ulcer edges and wound bed, condition of surrounding tissues) for any determination that an ulcer is not pressure-related, especially if the injury/ulcer has characteristics consistent with a pressure ulcer, but is determined not to be one.

ULCER CHARACTERISTICS

It is important that the facility have a system in place to assure that the protocols for daily monitoring and for periodic documentation of measurements, terminology, frequency of assessment, and documentation are implemented consistently throughout the facility.

When a pressure ulcer is present, daily monitoring, (with accompanying documentation, when a complication or change is identified), should include:

- An evaluation of the ulcer, if no dressing is present;
- An evaluation of the status of the dressing, if present (whether it is intact and whether drainage, if present, is or is not leaking);
- The status of the area surrounding the ulcer (that can be observed without removing the dressing);
- The presence of possible complications, such as signs of increasing area of ulceration or soft tissue infection (for example: increased redness or swelling around the wound or increased drainage from the wound); and
- Whether pain, if present, is being adequately controlled.

The amount of observation possible will depend upon the type of dressing that is used, since some dressings are meant to remain in place for several days, according to manufacturers' guidelines.

With each dressing change or at least weekly (and more often when indicated by wound complications or changes in wound characteristics), an evaluation of the pressure ulcer wound should be documented. At a minimum, documentation should include the date observed and:

- Location and staging;
- Size (perpendicular measurements of the greatest extent of length and width of the ulceration), depth; and the presence, location and extent of any undermining or tunneling/sinus tract;
- Exudate, if present: type (such as purulent/serous), color, odor and approximate amount;
- Pain, if present: nature and frequency (e.g., whether episodic or continuous);
- Wound bed: Color and type of tissue/character including evidence of healing (e.g., granulation tissue), or necrosis (slough or eschar); and
- Description of wound edges and surrounding tissue (e.g., rolled edges, redness, hardness/induration, maceration) as appropriate.

Photographs may be used to support this documentation, if the facility has developed a protocol consistent with accepted standards[33] (e.g., frequency, consistent distance from the wound, type of equipment used, means to assure digital images are accurate and not modified, inclusion of the resident identification/ulcer location/dates/etc. within the photographic image, and parameters for comparison).

STAGES OF PRESSURE ULCERS

The staging system is one method of summarizing certain characteristics of pressure ulcers, including the extent of tissue damage. This is the system used within the RAI.

Stage I pressure ulcers may be difficult to identify because they are not readily visible and they present with greater variability. Advanced technology (not commonly available in nursing homes) has shown that a Stage I pressure ulcer may have minimal to substantial tissue damage in layers beneath the skin's surface, even when there is no visible surface penetration. The Stage I indicators identified below will generally persist or be evident after the pressure on the area has been removed for 30-45 minutes.

The definitions for the stages of pressure ulcers identified below, are from the NPUAP and used with permission.[34]

- **"Stage I"** - An observable, pressure-related alteration of intact skin, whose indicators as compared to an adjacent or opposite area on the body may include changes in one or more of the following parameters:
    - Skin temperature (warmth or coolness);
    - Tissue consistency (firm or boggy);
    - Sensation (pain, itching); and/or
    - A defined area of persistent redness in lightly pigmented skin, whereas in darker skin tones, the ulcer may appear with persistent red, blue, or purple hues.
- **"Stage II"** - Partial thickness skin loss involving epidermis, dermis, or both. The ulcer is superficial and presents clinically as an abrasion, blister, or shallow crater.
- **"Stage III"** - Full thickness skin loss involving damage to, or necrosis of, subcutaneous tissue that may extend down to, but not through, underlying fascia. The ulcer presents clinically as a deep crater with or without undermining of adjacent tissue.
- **"Stage IV"** - Full thickness skin loss with extensive destruction, tissue necrosis, or damage to muscle, bone, or supporting structures (e.g., tendon, joint capsule). Undermining and sinus tracts also may be associated with Stage IV pressure ulcers.

NOTE: If eschar and necrotic tissue are covering and preventing adequate staging of a pressure ulcer, the RAI User's Manual Version 2 instructs the assessor to code the pressure ulcer as a Stage IV. These instructions must be followed for MDS coding purposes until they are revised. Although the AHCPR and NPUAP system for staging pressure ulcers indicates that the presence of eschar precludes accurate staging of the ulcer, the facility must use the RAI directions in order to code the MDS, but not necessarily to render treatment.

THE HEALING PRESSURE ULCER

Ongoing evaluation and research have indicated that pressure ulcers do not heal in a reverse sequence, that is, the body does not replace the types and layers of tissue (e.g., muscle, fat and dermis) that were lost during the pressure ulcer development.

There are different types of clinical documentation to describe the progression of the healing pressure ulcer(s). The regulation at 42 CFR 483.20(b)(1), F272, requires that facilities use the Resident Assessment Instrument (RAI), which includes direction to describe the healing of the pressure ulcer(s)for coding purposes for the MDS: The RAI User's Manual Version 2.0, instructs staff to identify the stages of pressure ulcer(s) by describing depth in reverse order from deepest to lesser stages to describe the healing or improvement of a pressure ulcer (e.g., a Stage IV becomes a Stage III and so forth. This has been referred to as "reverse staging" or "back staging").

Some clinicians utilize validated instruments to describe the healing of a pressure ulcer. Although such instruments are appropriate for making treatment decisions, they may not be utilized for coding the MDS. Until the MDS is revised, the present coding system (reverse staging) must be used for completion of the RAI.

Clinicians may use the National Pressure Ulcer Advisory Panel - Pressure Ulcer Scale for Healing (NPUAP-PUSH) tool. The NPUAP always refers to a healed pressure ulcer as a healed ulcer at the deepest stage of its development (e.g., a healed Stage IV or a healing Stage IV). The NPUAP cautions that the tool does not represent a comprehensive pressure ulcer assessment, and other factors may need to be considered when selecting pressure ulcer treatment options.

Since surveyors may encounter clinician's notes in which the NPUAP-PUSH tool is used as part of the facility's documentation protocol, the following description of the tool is provided. The NPUAP-PUSH tool documents pressure ulcer healing consistent with the healing process, describes a healing pressure ulcer in terms of three ulcer characteristics, and assigns a numeric value to the characteristics: length (cm) x width (cm), exudate amount, and type of tissue (closed with epithelium; new pink, shiny epithelial tissue; clean, pink or beefy red, shiny, moist granulation tissue; slough tissue; or necrotic, eschar tissue).

The 1994 AHCPR Guidelines and current literature[35] indicate that a clean pressure ulcer with adequate blood supply and innervation should show evidence of stabilization or some healing within 2-4 weeks. Evidence accumulating since 1962 indicates that management of wound exudate coupled with a clean, moist wound environment allows a chronic wound (e.g., pressure ulcer) to lay down healthy granulating tissue more efficiently.[36, 37]

If a pressure ulcer fails to show some evidence of progress toward healing within 2-4 weeks, the pressure ulcer (including potential complications) and the resident's overall clinical condition should be reassessed. Re-evaluation of the treatment plan including determining whether to continue or modify the current interventions is also indicated. Results may vary depending on the resident's condition and interventions/treatments used. The complexity of the resident's condition may limit responsiveness to treatment or tolerance for certain treatment modalities. The clinicians, if deciding to retain the current regimen, should document the rationale for continuing the present treatment (for example, why some, or all, of the plan's interventions remain relevant despite little or no apparent healing).

Pressure ulcers may progress or may be associated with complications such as infection of the soft tissues around the wound (cellulitis), infection of the bone (osteomyelitis), infection of a joint (septic arthritis), abscess, spread of bacteria into the bloodstream (bacteremia/septicemia), chronic infection, or development of a sinus tract. Sometimes these complications may occur despite apparent improvement in the pressure ulcer itself. The physician's involvement is integral whenever significant changes in the nature of the wound or overall resident condition are identified.

INFECTIONS RELATED TO PRESSURE ULCERS

Current literature reports that all Stage II, III, and IV pressure ulcers are colonized with bacteria but may not be infected. Identification, diagnosis and treatment of infection, when present, are critical to healing a pressure ulcer.[38] The infection occurs when the bacteria have invaded the tissue surrounding or within the pressure ulcer.

As with any infection, classic signs and symptoms of infection may include purulent exudate, peri-wound warmth, swelling, induration or erythema (erythema may not be readily determined in individuals with dark skin pigmentation), increasing pain or tenderness around the site or delayed wound healing. These classic signs may not be as evident in someone with a granulating, chronic wound or an immuno-compromised or aged resident. Some infections may present primarily with pain or delayed healing without other typical clinical signs of infection.[39] Clinicians have developed some tools, which may facilitate identifying and assessing an infection[40, 41] and documenting progress toward healing.

Wounds may be classified as infected if the signs and symptoms of infection are present and/or a wound culture (obtained in accord with accepted standards, such as sterile tissue aspirate, a "quantitative surface swab" using the Levine technique or semi-quantitative swab) contains 100,000 (10^5) or greater micro-organisms per gram of tissue. A superficial swab may show the presence of bacteria, but is not a reliable method to identify infection.

Findings such as an elevated white blood cell count, bacteremia, sepsis, or fever may signal an infection related to a pressure ulcer area or a co-existing infection from a different source.

PAIN

The assessment and treatment of a resident's pain are integral components of pressure ulcer prevention and management. "The goal of pain management in the pressure ulcer patient is to eliminate the cause of pain, to provide analgesia, or both."[42] Pain that interferes with movement and/or affects mood may contribute to immobility and contribute to the potential for developing a pressure ulcer or for delayed healing or non-healing of an already existing ulcer.

It may be difficult to assess the degree of pain in a resident who is cognitively impaired. Some strategies and tools exist to help determine the presence and characteristics of pain (e.g., nature, intensity and frequency).[43, 44] Recent research suggests that a resident with a Stage IV pressure ulcer can feel as much pain as those with a Stage I or II ulcer.[45] The relationship of pain to the pressure ulcer healing process is not yet clear. Pain is an individual perception and response and an individual's report of pain is a generally valid indicator of pain. One resident may experience pain of varying intensity and frequency (e.g., continually or periodically) or episodically in association with treatments (e.g., debridement, dressing changes) or movement or infection, while another resident may not have or report pain.

DRESSINGS AND TREATMENTS

Research has found that chronic wounds such as pressure ulcers heal differently from acute wounds, primarily because of differing biochemical and cellular characteristics. Current clinical practice indicates that Stage III and Stage IV ulcers should be covered. Determination of the need for a dressing for a Stage I or Stage II ulcer is based upon the individual practitioner's clinical judgment and facility protocols based upon current clinical standards of practice. No particular dressing promotes healing of all pressure ulcers within an ulcer classification.[46]

For those pressure ulcers with significant exudate, management of the exudate is critical for healing. A balance is needed to assure that the wound is moist enough to support healing but not too moist to interfere with healing.[47] Since excess wound exudate generally impairs wound healing, selecting an appropriate absorptive dressing is an important part of managing chronic wound exudate.

Product selection should be based upon the relevance of the specific product to the identified pressure ulcer(s) characteristics, the treatment goals, and the manufacturer's recommendations for use. Current literature does not indicate significant advantages of any single specific product over another, but does confirm that not all products are appropriate for all pressure ulcers. Wound characteristics should be assessed throughout the healing process to assure that the treatments and dressings being used are appropriate to the nature of the wound.

Present literature suggests that pressure ulcer dressing protocols may use clean technique rather than sterile, but that appropriate sterile technique may be needed for those wounds that recently have been surgically debrided or repaired.[48]

Debridement of non-viable tissue is frequently performed to reduce the amount of wound debris or non-viable tissue and to reduce the risk of sepsis. A variety of debridement methods (e.g., mechanical, sharp or surgical, enzymatic, autolytic, MDT) are available. Removal of necrotic tissue should enhance wound healing. Ongoing monitoring (and timely intervention in case of change in the character of the wound) is critical for areas with eschar and those areas that have been debrided.[49] Many clinicians believe that stable, dry, adherent and intact eschar on the foot/heel should not be debrided, unless signs and symptoms of local infection or instability are detected.[50]

Some facilities may use "wet to dry gauze dressings" or irrigation with chemical solutions to remove slough. The use of wet-to-dry dressings or irrigations may be appropriate in limited circumstances, but repeated use may damage healthy granulation tissue in healing ulcers and may lead to excessive bleeding and increased resident pain.

A facility should be able to show that its treatment protocols are based upon current standards of practice and are in accord with the facility's policies and procedures as developed with the medical director's review and approval.

ENDNOTES

(For more information on the references below, visit the CMS Sharing Innovations in Quality website: www.cms.hhs.gov/medicaid/survey-cert/siqhome.asp.

[1] Cuddigan, J., Ayello, E.A., Sussman, C., & Baranoski, S. (Eds.). (2001). Pressure Ulcers in America: Prevalence, Incidence, and Implications for the Future. National Pressure Ulcer Advisory Panel Monograph (pp. 181). Reston, VA: NPUAP.

[2] Gardner, S.E. & Frantz, R.A. (2003). Wound Bioburden. In Baranoski, S. & Ayello, E.A. (Eds.), Wound Care Essentials: Practice Principles. Philadelphia, PA: Lippincott, Williams, & Wilkins.

---

[3] Ayello, E.A. & Cuddigan, J.E. (2004). Debridement: Controlling the Necrotic/Cellular Burden. Advances in Skin and Wound Care, 17(2), 66-75.

[4] Bergstrom N., Bennett, M.A., Carlson, C.E., et al. (1994). Treatment of Pressure Ulcers in Adults (Publication 95-0652). Clinical Practice Guideline, 15, Rockville, MD: U.S. Department of Health and Human Services, Agency for Health Care Policy and Research.

[5] Thompson, P.D. & Smith, D.J. (1994). What is Infection? American Journal of Surgery, 167, 7-11.

[6] Ayello, E.A., Baranoski, S., Kerstein, M.D., & Cuddigan, J. (2003). Wound Debridement. In Baranoski. S. & Ayello, E.A. (Eds.) Wound Care Essentials: Practice Principles. Philadelphia, PA: Lippincott Williams & Wilkins

[7] Bergstrom, N., et al. (1994). Clinical Practice Guideline, 15.

[8] Ayello & Cuddigan. (2004). Advances in Skin and Wound Care, 66-75.

[9] Sherman, R.A. (1998). Maggot Debridement in Modern Medicine. Infections in Medicine, 15(9), 651-656.

[10] Piper, B. (2000). Mechanical Forces: Pressure, Shear, and Friction. In Bryant, R.A. (Ed.) Acute and Chronic Wounds. Nursing Management (2nd ed., pp. 221-264). St.Louis, MO: Mosby.

[11] Kosiak, M. (1961). Etiology of Decubitus Ulcers. Archives of Physical Medicine and Rehabilitation, 42, 19-29.

[12] Frequently Asked Questions: Pressure Ulcer Staging and Assessment, Question 202 (2000, July 28). Retrieved July 1, 2004 from http://www.npuap.org/archive/stagingdefinition.htm.

[13] Lyder, C., Yu C., Emerling, J., Empleo-Frazier, O., Mangat, R., Stevenson, D. & McKay, J. (1999). Evaluating the Predictive Validity of the Braden Scale for Pressure Ulcer Risk in Blacks and Latino/Hispanic Elders. Applied Nursing Research, 12, 60-68.

[14] Lyder, C. (2003). Pressure Ulcer Prevention and Management. Journal of the American Medical Association, 289, 223-226.

[15] Fuhrer M., Garber S., Rintola D., Clearman R., Hart K. (1993). Pressure Ulcers in Community-resident persons with spinal cord injury: Prevalence and Risk Factors. Archives of Physical Medicine Rehabilitation, 74, 1172-1177.

[16] Cuddigan, Ayello, Sussman, & Baranoski S. (Eds.). (2001). NPUAP Monograph, 153.

[17] Ayello, E.A., Braden, B. (May-June 2002). How and Why to do Pressure Ulcer Risk Assessment. Advances in Skin and Wound Care, 15(3), 125-32.

[18] Bergstrom, N. & Braden, B.A. (1992). A Prospective Study of Pressure Sore Risk Among Institutionalized Elderly. Journal of the American Geriatric Society, 40(8), 747-758.

[19] Gosnell S.J. (1973). An Assessment Tool to Identify Pressure Sores. Nursing Research, 22(1), 55-59.

[20] Bergstrom, N., Braden, B., Kemp, M., Champagne, M., Ruby, E. (1998). Predicting Pressure Ulcer Risk: A Multistate Study of the PredictiveValidity of the Braden Scale. Nursing Research, 47(5), 261-269.

[21] Bergstrom N. & Braden, B.A. (1992). Journal of the American Geriatric Society, 747-758.

[22] Braden, B. (2001). Risk Assessment in Pressure Ulcer Prevention. In Krasner, D.L., Rodeheaver, G.T., Sibbeald, R.G. (Eds.) Chronic Wound Care: A Clinical Source Book for Healthcare Professionals (3rd ed., pp. 641-651). Wayne, PA: HMP Communications Pub.

[23] Ayello, E.A., Baranoski, S., Lyder, C.H., Cuddigan, J. (2003). Pressure Ulcers. In Baranoski S. & Ayello, E.A. (Eds.) Wound Care Essentials: Practice Principles (pp. 245). Philadelphia, PA: Lippincott Williams & Wilkins.

[24] Cuddigan, J., Ayello, E.A., Sussman, C., & Baranoski, S. (Eds.). (2001). NPUAP Monograph, 27 & 168.

[25] Ferguson, R., O'Connor, P., Crabtree, B., Batchelor A., Mitchell J., Coppola, D. (1993). Serum Albumin and Pre-albumin as Predictors of Hospitalized Elderly Nursing Home Patients. Journal of the American Geriatric Society, 41, 545-549.

[26] Covinsky, K.E., Covinsky, K.H., Palmer, R.M., & Sehgal, A.R. (2002). Serum Albumin Concentration and Clinical Assessments of Nutritional Status in Hospitalized Older People: Different Sides of Different Coins? Journal of the American Geriatric Society, 50, 631-637.

[27] Maklebust, J. & Sieggreen, M. (2001). Pressure Ulcers: Guidelines for Prevention and Management (3rd ed., pp. 49). Springhouse, PA: Springhouse.

[28] Lyder, C. (1997). Perineal Dermatitis in the Elderly: A Critical Review of the Literature. Journal of Gerontological Nursing, 23(12), 5-10.

[29] Bergstrom N., et al. (1994). Clinical Practice Guideline, 15.

[30] Agency for Health Care Policy and Research (AHCPR). (1992). Pressure Ulcers in Adults: Prediction and Prevention (Publication 92-0050). Clinical Practice Guideline, 3.

[31] Wound Ostomy Continence Nurses Society. (2003). Guidelines for Prevention and Management of Pressure Ulcers (pp. 12). Glenview, IL: Author.

[32] Kloth, L.C. & McCulloch, J.M. (Eds.) (2002). Prevention and Treatment of Pressure Ulcer. Wound Healing: Alternatives in Management (3rd ed., pp. 434-438). Philadelphia: FA Davis Company.

[33] Jones, V., Bale, S., & Harding, K. (2003). Acute and Chronic Wound Healing. In Baranoski, S. & Ayello, E.A. (Eds.), Wound Care Essentials: Practice Principles (pp. 72-73). Philadelphia, PA: Lippincott Williams & Wilkins.

[34] Cuddigan, J., Ayello, E.A., Sussman, C., & Baranoski, S. (Eds.) (2001). NPUAP Monograph,181.

[35] Morrison, M.J. (Ed.). (2001). The Prevention and Treatment of Pressure Ulcers. London: Mosby.

[36] Bullen, E.C., Longaker, M.T., Updike, D.L., Benton, R., Ladin, D., Hou, Z., & Howard, E.W. (1996). Tissue inhibitor of metalloproteinases-1 is decreased and activated gelatinases are increased in chronic wounds. Journal of Investigative Dermatology, 106(2), 335-341.

[37] Ayello, E.A. & Cuddigan, J. (2003). Jump start the healing process. Nursing Made Incredibly Easy! 1(2), 18-26.

[38] Bergstrom N., et al. (1994). Clinical Practice Guideline, 15.

[39] Gardner, S.E., Frantz, R.A., & Doebbeling, B.N. (2001). The Validity of the Clinical Signs and Symptoms Used to Identify Localized Chronic Wound Infection. Wound Repair and Regeneration, 9, 178-186.

[40] Gardner, S.E. & Frantz, R.A. (2001). A Tool to Assess Clinical Signs and Symptoms of Localized Chronic Wound Infection: Development and Reliability. Ostomy/Wound Management, 47(1), 40-47.

[41] Cutting, K.F. & Harding, K.G. (1994). Criteria for Identifying Wound Infection. Journal of Wound Care, 3(4), 198-201.

---

[42] Bergstrom N., et al. (1994). Clinical Practice Guideline, 15.

[43] American Geriatric Society. (2002). American Geriatric Society Guideline: The Management of Persistent Pain in Older Persons. Journal of American Geriatric Society, 50(6), S205-S224.

[44] Gomez, S., Osborn, C., Watkins, T. & Hegstrom, S. (2002). Caregivers team up to manage chronic pain. Provider, 28(4), 51-58.

[45] Dallam, L.E., Barkauskas, C., Ayello, E.A., & Baranoski, S. (2003). Pain Management and Wounds. In Baranoski, S. & Ayello, E.A. (Eds.). Wound Care Essentials: Practice Principles (pp. 223-224). Philadelphia, PA: Lippincott Williams & Wilkins.

[46] Ayello, E.A., Baranoski, S., Lyder, C.H., & Cuddigan, J. (2003). Pressure Ulcers. In Baranoski, S. & Ayello, E.A. Wound Care Essentials: Practice Principles (pp. 257). Philadelphia, PA: Lippincott Williams & Wilkins.

[47] Schultz, G.S., Sibbald, R.G., Falanga, V., Ayello, E.A., Dowsett, C., Harding, K., Romanelli, M., Stacey, M.C., Teot, L., Vanscheidt, W. (2003). Wound Bed Preparation: A systematic Approach to Wound Management. Wound Repair Regeneration, 11,1-28.

[48] Association for Professionals in Infection Control and Epidemiology, Inc. (March/April 2001). Position Statement: Clean vs. Sterile: Management of Chronic Wounds. Retrieved July 6, 2004 from www.apic.org resource center.

[49] Black, J.M. & Black, S.B. (2003). Complex Wounds. In Baranoski, S. & Ayello, E.A. (Eds.). Wound Care Essentials: Practice Principles (pp. 372) Philadelphia, PA: Lippincott Williams & Wilkins.

[50] Bergstrom N., et al. (1994). Clinical Practice Guideline, 15.

INVESTIGATIVE PROTOCOL

PRESSURE ULCER

Objectives

- To determine if the identified pressure ulcer(s) is avoidable or unavoidable; and
- To determine the adequacy of the facility's interventions and efforts to prevent and treat pressure ulcers.

Use

Use this protocol for a sampled resident having--or at risk of developing-- a pressure ulcer.

If the resident has an ulcer, determine if it was identified as non-pressure related, e.g., vascular insufficiency or a neuropathic ulcer. If record review, staff and/or physician interview, and observation (unless the dressing protocol precludes observing the wound) support the conclusion that the ulcer is not pressure related, do not proceed with this protocol unless the resident is at risk for developing, or also has, pressure ulcers. Evaluate care and services regarding non-pressure related ulcers at F309, Quality of Care.

Procedures

Briefly review the assessment, care plan and orders to identify facility interventions and to guide observations to be made. For a newly admitted resident either at risk or with a pressure ulcer, the staff is expected to assess and provide appropriate care from the day of admission. Corroborate observations by interview and record review.

1. Observation

Observe whether staff consistently implements the care plan over time and across various shifts. During observations of the interventions, note and/or follow up on deviations from the care plan as well as potential negative outcomes, including but not limited to the following:

- Erythema or color changes on areas such as the sacrum, buttocks, trochanters, posterior thigh, popliteal area, or heels when moved off an area:
    - If erythema or color change are noted, return approximately ½ - ¾ hours later to determine if the changes or other Stage I characteristics persist;
    - If the changes persist and exhibit tenderness, hardness, or alteration in temperature from surrounding skin, ask staff how they determine repositioning schedules and how they evaluate and address a potential Stage I pressure ulcer;

- Previously unidentified open areas;
- Whether the positioning avoids pressure on an existing pressure ulcer(s);
- Measures taken to prevent or reduce the potential for shearing or friction during transfers, elevation, and repositioning; and
- Whether pressure-redistributing devices for the bed and/or chair, such as gel-type surfaces or overlays are in place, working, and used according to the manufacturer's recommendations.

Observation of Existing Ulcer/Wound Care

If a dressing change is scheduled during the survey, observe the wound care to determine if the record reflects the current status of the ulcer(s) and note:

- Characteristics of the wound and surrounding tissues such as presence of granulation tissue, the Stage, presence of exudates, necrotic tissue such as eschar or slough, or evidence of erythema or swelling around the wound;
- The form or type of debridement, if used;
- Whether treatment and infection control practices reflect current standards of practice; and
- Based on location, steps taken to cleanse and protect the wound from likely contamination by urine or fecal incontinence.

If unable to observe the dressing change due to the dressing protocol, observe the area surrounding the ulcer(s). For ulcers with dressings that are not scheduled to be changed, the surveyor may request that the dressing be removed to observe the wound and surrounding area if other information suggests a possible treatment or assessment problem.

If the resident expresses (or appears to be in) pain related to the ulcer or treatment, determine if the facility:

- Assessed for pain related to the ulcer, addressed and monitored interventions for effectiveness; and/or
- Assessed and took preemptive measures for pain related to dressing changes or other treatments, such as debridement/irrigations, and monitored for effectiveness.

2. Resident/Staff Interviews

Interview the resident, family or responsible party to the degree possible to identify:

- Involvement in care plan, choices, goals, and if interventions reflect preferences;
- Awareness of approaches, such as pressure redistribution devices or equipment, turning/repositioning, weight shifting to prevent or address pressure ulcer(s);
- Presence of pain, if any, and how it is managed;
- If treatment(s) was refused, whether counseling on alternatives, consequences, and/or other interventions was offered; and
- Awareness of current or history of an ulcer(s). For the resident who has or has had a pressure ulcer, identify, as possible, whether acute illness, weight loss or other condition changes occurred prior to developing the ulcer.

Interview staff on various shifts to determine:

- Knowledge of prevention and treatment, including facility-specific guidelines/protocols and specific interventions for the resident;
- If nursing assistants know what, when, and to whom to report changes in skin condition; and
- Who monitors for the implementation of the care plan, changes in the skin, the development of pressure ulcers, and the frequency of review and evaluation of an ulcer.

3. Record Review

Assessment

Review the RAI and other documents such as physician orders, progress notes, nurses' notes, pharmacy or dietary notes regarding the assessment of the resident's overall condition, risk factors and presence of a pressure ulcer(s) to determine if the facility identified the resident at risk and evaluated the factors placing the resident at risk:

- For a resident who was admitted with an ulcer or who developed one within 1 to 2 days, review the admission documentation regarding the wound site and characteristics at the time of admission, the possibility of underlying tissue damage because of immobility or illness prior to admission, skin condition on or within a day of admission, history of impaired nutrition; and history of previous pressure ulcers; and
- For a resident who subsequently developed or has an existing pressure ulcer, review documentation regarding the wound site, characteristics, progress and

complications including reassessment if there were no signs of progression towards healing within 2 to 4 weeks.

In considering the appropriateness of a facility's response to the presence, progression, or deterioration of a pressure ulcer, take into account the resident's condition, complications, time needed to determine the effectiveness of a treatment, and the facility's efforts, where possible, to remove, modify, or stabilize the risk factors and underlying causal factors.

Care Plan

For the resident at risk for developing or who has a pressure ulcer, determine if the facility developed an individualized care plan that addresses prevention, care and treatment of any existing pressure ulcers, including specific interventions, measurable objectives and approximate time frames.

If the facility's care of a specific resident refers to a treatment protocol that contains details of the treatment regimen, the care plan should refer to that protocol. The care plan should clarify any major deviations from, or revisions to, that protocol in a specific resident.

A specific care plan intervention for risk of pressure ulcers is not needed if other components of the care plan address related risks adequately. For example, the risk of skin breakdown posed by fecal/urinary incontinence might be addressed in that part of the care plan that deals with incontinence management.

If the resident refuses or resists staff interventions to reduce risk or treat existing pressure ulcers, determine if the care plan reflects efforts to seek alternatives to address the needs identified in the assessment.

Revision of the Care Plan

Determine if the staff have been monitoring the resident's response to interventions for prevention and/or treatment and have evaluated and revised the care plan based on the resident's response, outcomes, and needs. Review the record and interview staff for information and/or evidence that:

- Continuing the current approaches meets the resident's needs, if the resident has experienced recurring pressure ulcers or lack of progression toward healing and staff did not revise the care plan; and

- The care plan was revised to modify the prevention strategies and to address the presence and treatment of a newly developed pressure ulcer, for the resident who acquired a new ulcer.

4. Interviews with Health Care Practitioners and Professionals

If the interventions defined or care provided appear not to be consistent with recognized standards of practice, interview one or more health care practitioners and professionals as necessary (e.g., physician, charge nurse, director of nursing) who, by virtue of training and knowledge of the resident, should be able to provide information about the causes, treatment and evaluation of the resident's condition or problem. Depending on the issue, ask about:

- How it was determined that chosen interventions were appropriate;
- Risks identified for which there were no interventions;
- Changes in condition that may justify additional or different interventions; or
- How they validated the effectiveness of current interventions.

If the attending physician is unavailable, interview the medical director, as appropriate.

DETERMINATION OF COMPLIANCE (Task 6, Appendix P)

Synopsis of Regulation (F314)

The pressure ulcer requirement has two aspects. The first aspect requires the facility to prevent the development of pressure ulcer(s) in a resident who is admitted without pressure ulcer(s), unless the development is clinically unavoidable. The second aspect requires the facility to provide necessary treatment and services to promote healing, prevent infection and prevent new ulcers from developing. A facility may have non-compliance in either or both aspects of this requirement.

Criteria for Compliance

- Compliance with 42 CFR 483.25(c)(1), F314, Pressure Sore
    - For a resident who developed a pressure ulcer after admission, the facility is in compliance with this requirement, if staff have:
        - Recognized and assessed factors placing the resident at risk for developing a pressure ulcer, including specific conditions, causes and/or problems, needs and behaviors;
        - Defined and implemented interventions for pressure ulcer prevention in accordance with resident needs, goals and recognized standards of practice;
        - Monitored and evaluated the resident's response to preventive efforts; and
        - Revised the approaches as appropriate.

If not, the development of the pressure ulcer is avoidable, cite at F314.

- Compliance with 42 CFR 483.25(c)(2), F314, Pressure Sore
    - For a resident who was admitted with a pressure ulcer, who has a pressure ulcer that is not healing, or who is at risk of developing subsequent pressure ulcers, the facility is in compliance with this requirement if they:
        - Recognized and assessed factors placing the resident at risk of developing a new pressure ulcer or experiencing non-healing or delayed healing of a current pressure ulcer, including specific conditions, causes and/or problems, needs and behaviors;
        - Defined and implemented interventions for pressure ulcer prevention and treatment in accordance with resident needs, goals and recognized standards of practice;
        - Addressed the potential for infection;
        - Monitored and evaluated the resident's response to preventive efforts and treatment interventions; and
        - Revised the approaches as appropriate.

    If not, cite at F314.

Non-compliance for F314

After completing the Investigative Protocol, analyze the data in order to determine whether or not noncompliance with the regulation exists. Non-compliance for F314 may include (but is not limited to) one or more of the following, including failure to:

- Accurately or consistently assess a resident's skin integrity on admission and as indicated thereafter;
- Identify a resident at risk of developing a pressure ulcer(s);
- Identify and address risk factors for developing a pressure ulcer, or explain adequately why they could not or should not do so;
- Implement preventive interventions in accord with the resident's need and current standards of practice;
- Provide clinical justification for the unavoidable development or non-healing/ delayed healing or deterioration of a pressure ulcer;

- Provide appropriate interventions, care and treatment to an existing pressure ulcer to minimize infections and to promote healing;

- Implement interventions for existing wounds;

- Notify the physician of the resident's condition or changes in the resident's wound(s);

- Adequately implement pertinent infection management practices in relation to wound care; and

- Identify or know how to apply relevant policies and procedures for pressure ulcer prevention and treatment.

Potential Tags for Additional Investigation

During the investigation of F314, the surveyor may have determined that concerns may also be present with related outcome, process and/or structure requirements. The surveyor is cautioned to investigate these related requirements before determining whether non-compliance may be present. Some examples of related requirements that should be considered include the following:

- 42 CFR 483.10(b)(11)(i)(B)&(C), F157, Notification of Changes

    - Determine if staff notified the physician of significant changes in the resident's condition or failure of the treatment plan to prevent or heal pressure ulcers; or the resident's representative (if known) of significant changes in the resident's condition in relation to the development of a pressure ulcer or a change in the progression of healing of an existing pressure ulcer.

- 42 CFR 483.20(b)(1), F272, Comprehensive Assessments

    - Determine if the facility comprehensively assessed the resident's skin condition, including existing pressure ulcers, and resident-specific risk factors (including potential causative factors) for the development of a pressure ulcer or non-healing of the ulcer.

- 42 CFR 483.20(k)(1), F279, Comprehensive Care Plans

    - Determine if the facility developed a care plan that was consistent with the resident's specific conditions, risks, needs, behaviors, and preferences and current standards of practice and included measurable objectives and timetables, specific interventions/services to prevent the development of pressure ulcers and/or to treat existing pressures ulcers.

- 42 CFR 483.20(k)(2)(iii), F280, Comprehensive Care Plan Revision
    - Determine if the care plan was periodically reviewed and revised as necessary to prevent the development of pressure ulcers and to promote the healing of existing pressure ulcers.
- 42 CFR 483.20(k)(3)(i), F281, Services Provided Meet Professional Standards
    - Determine if pressure ulcer care was provided in accordance with accepted professional standards.
- 42 CFR 483.25, F309, Quality of Care
    - Determine if staff identified and implemented appropriate measures for the management of pain as indicated as related to pressure ulcers and pressure ulcer treatment.
- 42 CFR 482.30(a), F353, Sufficient Staff
    - Determine if the facility had qualified staff in sufficient numbers to assure the resident was provided necessary care and services, based upon the comprehensive assessment and care plan, to prevent or treat pressure ulcers.
- 42 CFR 483.40(a)(1), F385, Physician Supervision
    - Determine if the physician has assessed and developed a treatment regimen relevant to preventing or healing a pressure ulcer and responded appropriately to the notice of changes in condition.
- 42 CFR 483.75(i)(2), F501, Medical Director
    - Determine whether the medical director assisted the facility in the development and implementation of policies and procedures for pressure ulcer prevention and treatment, and that these are based on current standards of practice; and whether the medical director interacts with the physician supervising the care of the resident if requested by the facility to intervene on behalf of the resident with a pressure ulcer(s).

V. DEFICIENCY CATEGORIZATION (Part V, Appendix P)

Once the team has completed its investigation, analyzed the data, reviewed the regulatory requirement, and identified the deficient practices that demonstrate that the facility failed to provide care and treatment to prevent or treat pressure ulcers and that non-compliance exists, the team must determine the severity of the deficient practice(s) and the resultant harm or potential for harm to the resident. The key elements for severity determination for F314 are as follows:

1. **Presence of harm/negative outcome(s) or potential for negative outcomes because of lack of appropriate treatment and care.** Actual or potential harm/negative outcome for F314 may include but is not limited to:

    - Potential for development of, occurrence or recurrence of (an) avoidable pressure ulcer(s);
    - Complications such as sepsis or pain related to the presence of avoidable pressure ulcer(s); and/or
    - Pressure ulcers that fail to improve as anticipated or develop complications such as sepsis or pain because of the lack of appropriate treatment and care.

2. **Degree of harm (actual or potential) related to the non-compliance**

Identify how the facility practices caused, resulted in, allowed or contributed to the actual or potential for harm:

- If harm has occurred, determine if the harm is at the level of serious injury, impairment, death, compromise or discomfort; and
- If harm has not yet occurred, determine how likely is the potential for serious injury, impairment, death, compromise or discomfort to occur to the resident.

3. **The immediacy of correction required**

Determine whether the non-compliance requires immediate correction in order to prevent serious injury, harm, impairment, or death to one or more residents.

The survey team must evaluate the harm or potential for harm based upon the following levels of severity for tag F314. First, the team must rule out whether Severity Level 4, Immediate Jeopardy to a resident's health or safety exists by evaluating the deficient practice in relation to immediacy, culpability and severity. (Follow the guidance in Appendix Q.)

Severity Level 4 Considerations: Immediate Jeopardy to Resident Health or Safety

Immediate Jeopardy is a situation in which the facility's non-compliance:

- With one or more requirements of participation has caused/resulted in, or is likely to cause, serious injury, harm, impairment or death to a resident; and

- Requires immediate correction as the facility either created the situation or allowed the situation to continue by failing to implement preventative or corrective measures.

Examples of possible avoidable negative outcomes may include:

- Development of avoidable Stage IV pressure ulcer(s): As a result of the facility's non-compliance, permanent tissue damage (whether or not healing occurs) has compromised the resident, increasing the potential for serious complications including osteomyelitits and sepsis.

- Admitted with a Stage IV pressure ulcer(s) that has shown no signs of healing or shows signs of deterioration: As a result of the facility's non-compliance, a Stage IV pressure ulcer has shown signs of deterioration or a failure to progress towards healing with an increased potential for serious complications including osteomyelitis and sepsis.

- Stage III or IV pressure ulcers with associated soft tissue or systemic infection: As a result of the facility's failure to assess or treat a resident with an infectious complication of a pressure ulcer. (See discussion in guidelines and definitions that distinguishes colonization from infection.)

- Extensive failure in multiple areas of pressure ulcer care: As a result of the facility's extensive noncompliance in multiple areas of pressure ulcer care, the resident developed recurrent and/or multiple, avoidable Stage III or Stage IV pressure ulcer(s).

NOTE: If immediate jeopardy has been ruled out based upon the evidence, then evaluate whether actual harm that is not immediate jeopardy exists at Severity Level 3.

Severity Level 3 Considerations: Actual Harm that is not Immediate Jeopardy

Level 3 indicates noncompliance that results in actual harm, and can include but may not be limited to clinical compromise, decline, or the resident's ability to maintain and/or reach his/her highest practicable well-being.

Examples of avoidable negative outcomes may include but are not limited to:

- **The development of avoidable Stage III pressure ulcer(s):** As a result of the facility's non-compliance, Stage III pressure ulcers occurred, which are open wounds in which damage has occurred into the subcutaneous level and may be painful.

- **The development of recurrent or multiple avoidable Stage II pressure ulcer(s):** As a result of the facility's non-compliance, the resident developed multiple and/or recurrent avoidable Stage II ulcers.

- **Failure to implement the comprehensive care plan for a resident who has a pressure ulcer**: As a result of a facility's failure to implement a portion of an existing plan related to pressure ulcer care, such as failure to provide for pressure redistribution, or inappropriate treatment/dressing changes, a wound increased in size or failed to progress towards healing as anticipated, or the resident experienced untreated pain.

NOTE: If Severity Level 3 (actual harm that is not immediate jeopardy) has been ruled out based upon the evidence, then evaluate as to whether Level 2 (no actual harm with the potential for more than minimal harm) exists.

Severity Level 2 Considerations: No Actual Harm with Potential for More Than Minimal Harm that is Not Immediate Jeopardy

Level 2 indicates noncompliance that results in a resident outcome of no more than minimal discomfort and/or has the potential to compromise the resident's ability to maintain or reach his or her highest practicable level of well being. The potential exists for greater harm to occur if interventions are not provided.

Examples of avoidable negative outcomes may include but are not limited to:

- **The development of a single avoidable Stage II pressure ulcer that is receiving appropriate treatment:** As a result of the facility's non-compliance, a resident developed an avoidable Stage II pressure ulcer.
- **The development of an avoidable Stage I pressure ulcer**: As a result of the facility's non-compliance, a resident developed an avoidable Stage I pressure ulcer.

- **Failure to implement an element of the care plan for a resident who has a pressure ulcer however, there has been no evidence of decline or failure to heal.**

- **Failure to recognize or address the potential for developing a pressure ulcer:** As a result of the facility's non-compliance, staff failed to identify the risks, develop a plan of care and/or consistently implement a plan that has been developed to prevent pressure ulcers.

Severity Level 1: No Actual Harm with Potential for Minimal Harm

The failure of the facility to provide appropriate care and services to prevent pressure ulcers or heal existing pressure ulcers is more than minimal harm. Therefore, Severity Level 1 doesn't apply for this regulatory requirement.

F315

§483.25(d) Urinary Incontinence

Based on the resident's comprehensive assessment, the facility must ensure that --

§483.25(d) (1) A resident who enters the facility without an indwelling catheter is not catheterized unless the resident's clinical condition demonstrates that catheterization was necessary; and

§483.25(d) (2) A resident who is incontinent of bladder receives appropriate treatment and services to prevent urinary tract infections and to restore as much normal bladder function as possible.

INTENT: (F315) 42 CFR 483.25 (d) (1) and (2) Urinary Incontinence and Catheters

The intent of this requirement is to ensure that:

- Each resident who is incontinent of urine is identified, assessed and provided appropriate treatment and services to achieve or maintain as much normal urinary function as possible;
- An indwelling catheter is not used unless there is valid medical justification;
- An indwelling catheter for which continuing use is not medically justified is discontinued as soon as clinically warranted;
- Services are provided to restore or improve normal bladder function to the extent possible, after the removal of the catheter; and
- A resident, with or without a catheter, receives the appropriate care and services to prevent infections to the extent possible.

DEFINITIONS

Definitions are provided to clarify clinical terms related to evaluation and treatment of urinary incontinence and catheter use.

- "Bacteremia" is the presence of bacteria in the bloodstream.
- "Bacteriuria" is defined as the presence of bacteria in the urine.
- "Urinary Incontinence" is the involuntary loss or leakage of urine. There are several types of urinary incontinence, and the individual resident may experience more than one type at a time. Some of the more common types include:

- "Functional Incontinence" refers to loss of urine that occurs in residents whose urinary tract function is sufficiently intact that they should be able to maintain continence, but who cannot remain continent because of external factors (e.g., inability to utilize the toilet facilities in time);

- "Mixed Incontinence" is the combination of stress incontinence and urge incontinence;

- "Overflow Incontinence" is associated with leakage of small amounts of urine when the bladder has reached its maximum capacity and has become distended;

- "Stress Incontinence" (outlet incompetence) is associated with impaired urethral closure (malfunction of the urethral sphincter) which allows small amounts of urine leakage when intra-abdominal pressure on the bladder is increased by sneezing, coughing, laughing, lifting, standing from a sitting position, climbing stairs, etc.;

- "Transient Incontinence" refers to temporary episodes of urinary incontinence that are reversible once the cause(s) of the episode(s) is (are) identified and treated; and

- "Urge Incontinence" (overactive bladder) is associated with detrusor muscle overactivity (excessive contraction of the smooth muscle in the wall of the urinary bladder resulting in a sudden, strong urge (also known as urgency) to expel moderate to large amounts of urine before the bladder is full).

- "Urinary Retention" is the inability to completely empty the urinary bladder by micturition.

- "Urinary Tract Infection" (UTI) is a clinically detectable condition associated with invasion by disease causing microorganisms of some part of the urinary tract, including the urethra (urethritis), bladder (cystitis), ureters (ureteritis), and/or kidney (pyelonephritis). An infection of the urethra or bladder is classified as a lower tract UTI and infection involving the ureter or kidney is classified as an upper tract UTI.

- "Urosepsis" refers to the systemic inflammatory response to infection (sepsis) that appears to originate from a urinary tract source. It may present with symptoms such as fever, hypotension, reduced urine output, or acute change in mental status.

OVERVIEW

Urinary incontinence is not normal. Although aging affects the urinary tract and increases the potential for urinary incontinence, urinary incontinence is not a normal part of aging. In the younger person, urinary incontinence may result from a single cause. In the older individual, urinary incontinence generally involves psychological, physiological, pharmacological and/or pathological factors or co-morbid conditions (e.g., later stages of dementia, diabetes, prostatectomy, medical conditions involving dysfunction of the central nervous system, urinary tract infections, etc.). Because urinary incontinence is a symptom of a condition and may be reversible, it is important to understand the causes and to address incontinence to the extent possible. If the underlying condition is not reversible, it is important to treat or manage the incontinence to try to reduce complications.

Many older adults are incontinent of urine prior to admission to a nursing home. Urinary incontinence and related loss of independence are prominent reasons for a nursing home admission. Articles[1] and data currently available, including CMS data (e.g., MDS Active Resident Information Report (Item H1b) at www.cms.hhs.gov/states/mdsreports), indicate that more than 50% of the nursing home population experience some degree of urinary incontinence. Whether the resident is incontinent of urine on admission or develops incontinence after admission, the steps of assessment, monitoring, reviewing, and revising approaches to care (as needed) are essential to managing urinary incontinence and to restoring as much normal bladder function as possible.

Various conditions or situations may aggravate the severity of urinary incontinence in nursing home residents. In addition, urinary incontinence may be associated with changes in skin integrity, skin irritation or breakdown, urinary tract infections, falls and fractures, sleep disturbances, and psychosocial complications including social withdrawal, embarrassment, loss of dignity, feelings of isolation, and interference with participation in activities.

Various factors common to elderly individuals may increase the risk of infection including: underlying diseases (e.g., diabetes mellitus), medications that affect immune responses to infection (e.g., steroids and chemotherapy, history of multiple antibiotic usage), conditions that cause incontinence, and indwelling urinary catheters.

The urinary tract is a common source of bacteremia in nursing home residents. Urinary tract infection (UTI) is one of the most common infections occurring in nursing homes and is often related to an indwelling urinary catheter. Without a valid clinical rationale for an indwelling catheter, its use is not an acceptable approach to manage urinary incontinence. Although UTIs can result from the resident's own flora, they may also be the result of microorganisms transmitted by staff when handling the urinary catheter drainage system and/or providing incontinence care. Hand washing remains one of the most effective infection control tools available.

Resources

It is important for the facility to have in place systems/procedures to assure: assessments are timely and appropriate; interventions are defined, implemented, monitored, and revised as appropriate in accordance with current standards of practice; and changes in condition are recognized, evaluated, reported to the practitioner, and addressed. The medical director and the quality assessment and assurance committee may help the facility evaluate existing strategies for identifying and managing incontinence, catheter use, and UTIs, and ensure that facility policies and procedures are consistent with current standards of practice.

Research into appropriate practices to prevent, manage, and treat urinary incontinence, urinary catheterization, and UTI continues to evolve. Many recognized clinical resources on the prevention and management of urinary incontinence, infection, and urinary catheterization exist. Some of these resources include:

- The American Medical Directors Association (AMDA) at www.amda.com (Clinical Practice Guidelines: Clinical Practice Guidelines, 1996);
- The Quality Improvement Organizations, Medicare Quality Improvement Community Initiatives at www.medqic.org;
- The CMS Sharing Innovations in Quality website at www.cms.hhs.gov/medicaid/survey-cert/siqhome.asp;
- Association for Professionals in Infection Control and Epidemiology (APIC) at www.apic.org;
- Centers for Disease Control at www.cdc.gov;
- The Annals of Long Term Care publications at www.mmhc.com;
- American Foundation for Urologic Disease, Inc. at www.afud.org; and
- The American Geriatrics Society at www.americangeriatrics.org.

NOTE: References to non-CMS sources or sites on the internet are provided as a service and do not constitute or imply endorsement of these organizations or their programs by CMS or the U. S. Department of Health and Human Services. CMS is not responsible for the content of pages found at these sites. URL addresses were current as of the date of this publication.

Resident Choice

In the course of developing and implementing care plan interventions for treatment and services related to achieving the highest practicable level of urinary continence, preventing and treating urinary tract infections, and avoiding the use of indwelling catheters without medical justification, it is important to involve the resident and/or her or his surrogate in care decisions and to consider whether the resident has an advance directive in place.

In order for a resident to exercise his or her right appropriately to make informed choices about care and treatment or to refuse treatment, the facility and the resident (or the resident's legal representative) must discuss the resident's condition, treatment options, expected outcomes, and consequences of refusing treatment. The facility should address the resident's concerns and offer relevant alternatives, if the resident has refused specific treatments. (See Resident Rights 483.10(b) (3) and (4) (F154 and F155).)

Advance Directive. A resident who is at the end of life or in terminal stages of an illness or who has multiple organ system failures may have written directions for his or her treatment goals (or a decision has been made by the resident's surrogate or representative, in accordance with State law).

Although a facility's care must reflect a resident's wishes as expressed in the Directive, in accordance with State law, the presence of an Advance Directive does not absolve the facility from giving supportive and other pertinent care that is not prohibited by the Advance Directive. The presence of a "Do Not Resuscitate" (DNR) order does not indicate that the resident is declining appropriate treatment and services. It only indicates that the resident should not be resuscitated if respirations and/or cardiac function cease.

If the facility has implemented individualized approaches for end-of-life care in accordance with the resident's wishes, and has implemented appropriate efforts to try to stabilize the resident's condition (or indicated why the condition cannot or should not be stabilized), and has provided care based on the assessed needs of the resident, then the development, continuation, or progression of urinary incontinence; the insertion and prolonged use of an indwelling urinary catheter; the development of infection or skin-related complications from urine or an indwelling catheter may be consistent with regulatory requirements.

URINARY INCONTINENCE

42 CFR 483.25 (d) (2) Urinary Incontinence requires that a resident who is incontinent of bladder receives appropriate treatment and services to prevent urinary tract infections and to restore as much normal bladder function as possible.

Urinary incontinence generally involves a number of transitory or chronic progressive factors that affect the bladder and/or the urethral sphincter. Any condition, medication, or factor that affects lower urinary tract function, bladder capacity, urination, or the ability to toilet can predispose residents to urinary incontinence and may contribute to incomplete bladder emptying.

The first steps toward assuring that a resident receives appropriate treatment and services to restore as much bladder function as possible or to treat and manage the incontinence are to identify the resident already experiencing some level of incontinence or at risk of developing urinary incontinence and to complete an accurate, thorough assessment of factors that may predispose the resident to having urinary incontinence. This is followed by implementing appropriate, individualized interventions that address the incontinence, including the resident's capabilities and underlying factors that can be removed, modified, or stabilized, and by monitoring the effectiveness of the interventions and modifying them, as appropriate. The practitioner, may at his or her option, refer residents to various practitioners who specialize in diagnosing and treating conditions that affect urinary function.

Assessment

Factors contributing to urinary incontinence sometimes may be resolved after a careful examination and review of history. In addition, for a resident who is incontinent of urine, determining the type of urinary incontinence can allow staff to provide more individualized programming or interventions to enhance the resident's quality of life and functional status. A resident should be evaluated at admission and whenever there is a change in cognition, physical ability, or urinary tract function. This evaluation is to include identification of individuals with reversible and irreversible (e.g., bladder tumors and spinal cord disease) causes of incontinence. If the resident has urinary incontinence that has already been investigated, documented, and determined to be irreversible or not significantly improvable, additional studies may be of limited value, unless there has been advancement in available treatments.

Documentation of assessment information may be found throughout the medical record, such as in an admission assessment, hospital records, history and physical, and the Resident Assessment Instrument (RAI). The location of RAI assessment information is identified on the Resident Assessment Protocol (RAP) summary form. It is important that staff, when completing the comprehensive assessment, consider the following:

- Prior history of urinary incontinence, including onset, duration and characteristics, precipitants of urinary incontinence, associated symptoms (e.g., dysuria, polyuria, hesitancy) and previous treatment and/or management, including the response to the interventions and the occurrence of persistent or recurrent UTI;

- Voiding patterns (such as frequency, volume, nighttime or daytime, quality of stream) and, for those already experiencing urinary incontinence, voiding patterns over several days;

- Medication review, particularly those that might affect continence, such as medications with anticholinergic properties (may cause urinary retention and possible overflow incontinence), sedative/hypnotics (may cause sedation leading to functional incontinence), diuretics (may cause urgency, frequency, overflow incontinence), narcotics, alpha-adrenergic agonists (may cause urinary retention in men) or antagonists (may cause stress incontinence in women) calcium channel blockers (may cause urinary retention);[2]

- Patterns of fluid intake, such as amounts, time of day, alterations and potential complications, such as decreased or increased urine output;

- Use of urinary tract stimulants or irritants (e.g., frequent caffeine intake);[3]

- Pelvic and rectal examination to identify physical features that may directly affect urinary incontinence, such as prolapsed uterus or bladder, prostate enlargement, significant constipation or fecal impaction, use of a urinary catheter, atrophic vaginitis, distended bladder, or bladder spasms;

- Functional and cognitive capabilities that could enhance urinary continence and limitations that could adversely affect continence, such as impaired cognitive function or dementia, impaired immobility, decreased manual dexterity, the need for task segmentation, decreased upper and lower extremity muscle strength, decreased vision, pain with movement;

- Type and frequency of physical assistance necessary to assist the resident to access the toilet, commode, urinal, etc. and the types of prompting needed to encourage urination;

- Pertinent diagnoses such as congestive heart failure, stroke, diabetes mellitus, obesity, and neurological disorders (e.g., Multiple Sclerosis, Parkinson's Disease or tumors that could affect the urinary tract or its function);

- Identification of and/or potential of developing complications such as skin irritation or breakdown;

- Tests or studies indicated to identify the type(s) of urinary incontinence (e.g., post-void residual(s) for residents who have, or are at risk of, urinary retention, results of any urine culture if the resident has clinically significant systemic or urinary symptoms), or evaluations assessing the resident's readiness for bladder rehabilitation programs; and

- Environmental factors and assistive devices that may restrict or facilitate a resident's ability to access the toilet (e.g., grab bars, raised or low toilet seats, inadequate lighting, distance to toilet or bedside commodes, availability of urinals, use of bed rails or restraints, or fear of falling).

Types of Urinary Incontinence

Identifying the nature of the incontinence is a key aspect of the assessment and helps identify the appropriate program/interventions to address incontinence.

- Urge Incontinence is characterized by abrupt urgency, frequency, and nocturia (part of the overactive bladder diagnosis). It may be age-related or have neurological causes (e.g., stroke, diabetes mellitus, Parkinson's Disease, multiple sclerosis) or other causes such as bladder infection, urethral irritation, etc. The resident can feel the need to void, but is unable to inhibit voiding long enough to reach and sit on the commode. It is the most common cause of urinary incontinence in elderly persons.

- Stress Incontinence is the loss of a small amount of urine with physical activity such as coughing, sneezing, laughing, walking stairs or lifting. Urine leakage results from an increase in intra-abdominal pressure on a bladder that is not over distended and is not the result of detrusor contractions. It is the second most common type of urinary incontinence in older women.

- Mixed Incontinence is the combination of urge incontinence and stress incontinence. Many elderly persons (especially women) will experience symptoms of both urge and stress called mixed incontinence.

- Overflow Incontinence occurs when the bladder is distended from urine retention. Symptoms of overflow incontinence may include: weak stream, hesitancy, or intermittency; dysuria; nocturia; frequency; incomplete voiding; frequent or constant dribbling. Urine retention may result from outlet obstruction (e.g., benign prostatic hypertrophy (BPH), prostate cancer, and urethral stricture), hypotonic bladder (detrusor under activity) or both. Hypotonic bladder may be caused by outlet obstruction, impaired or absent contractility of the bladder (neurogenic bladder) or other causes. Neurogenic bladder may also result from neurological conditions such as diabetes mellitus, spinal cord injury, or pelvic nerve damage from surgery or radiation therapy. In overflow incontinence, post void residual (PVR) volume (the amount of urine remaining in the bladder within 5 to 10 minutes following urination) exceeds 200 milliliters (ml). Normal PVR is usually 50 ml. or less. A PVR of 150 to 200 may suggest a need for retesting to determine if this finding is clinically significant. Overflow incontinence may mimic urge or stress incontinence but is less common than either of those.

- Functional Incontinence refers to incontinence that is secondary to factors other than inherently abnormal urinary tract function. It may be related to physical weakness or poor mobility/dexterity (e.g., due to poor eyesight, arthritis, deconditioning, stroke, contracture), cognitive problems (e.g., confusion, dementia, unwillingness to toilet), various medications (e.g., anti-cholinergics, diuretics) or environmental impediments (e.g., excessive distance of the resident from the toilet facilities, poor lighting, low chairs that are difficult to get out of, physical restraints and toilets that are difficult to access). Refer to 42 CFR 483.15(e) (1) for issues regarding unmet environmental needs (e.g., handicap toilet, lighting, assistive devices).

  NOTE: Treating the physiological causes of incontinence, without attending to functional components that may have an impact on the resident's continence, may fail to solve the incontinence problem.

- Transient Incontinence refers to temporary or occasional incontinence that may be related to a variety of causes, for example: delirium, infection, atrophic urethritis or vaginitis, some pharmaceuticals (such as sedatives/hypnotics, diuretics, anticholinergic agents), increased urine production, restricted mobility or fecal impaction. The incontinence is transient because it is related to a potentially improvable or reversible cause.

Interventions

It is important that the facility follow the care process (accurate assessment, care planning, consistent implementation and monitoring of the care plan with evaluation of the effectiveness of the interventions, and revision, as appropriate). Recording and evaluating specific information (such as frequency and times of incontinence and toileting and response to specific interventions) is important for determining progress, changes, or decline.

A number of factors may contribute to the decline or lack of improvement in urinary continence, for example: underlying medical conditions, an inaccurate assessment of the resident's type of incontinence (or lack of knowledge about the resident's voiding patterns) may contribute to inappropriate interventions or unnecessary use of an indwelling catheter. Facility practices that may promote achieving the highest practicable level of functioning, may prevent or minimize a decline or lack of improvement in degree of continence include providing treatment and services to address factors that are potentially modifiable, such as:

- Managing pain and/or providing adaptive equipment to improve function for residents suffering from arthritis, contractures, neurological impairments, etc;

- Removing or improving environmental impediments that affect the resident's level of continence (e.g., improved lighting, use of a bedside commode or reducing the distance to the toilet);

- Treating underlying conditions that have a potentially negative impact on the degree of continence (e.g., delirium causing urinary incontinence related to acute confusion);

- Possibly adjusting medications affecting continence (e.g., medication cessation, dose reduction, selection of an alternate medication, change in time of administration); and

- Implementing a fluid and/or bowel management program to meet the assessed needs.

Options for managing urinary incontinence in nursing home residents include primarily behavioral programs and medication therapy. Other measures and supportive devices used in the management of urinary incontinence and/or urinary retention may include intermittent catheterization; pelvic organ support devices (pessaries); the use of incontinence products, garments and an external collection system for men and women; and environmental accommodation and/or modification.

Behavioral Programs

Interventions involving the use of behavioral programs are among the least invasive approaches to address urinary incontinence and have no known adverse complications. Behavior programs involve efforts to modify the resident's behavior and/or environment. Critical aspects of a successful behavioral program include education of the caregiver and the resident, availability of the staff and the consistent implementation of the interventions.

NOTE: It is important for the comprehensive assessment to identify the essential skills the resident must possess to be successful with specific interventions being attempted. These skills include the resident's ability to: comprehend and follow through on education and instructions; identify urinary urge sensation; learn to inhibit or control the urge to void until reaching a toilet; contract the pelvic floor muscle (Kegel exercises) to lessen urgency and/or urinary leakage; and/or respond to prompts to void.[4] Voiding records help detect urinary patterns or intervals between incontinence episodes and facilitate planning care to avoid or reduce the frequency of episodes.

Programs that require the resident's cooperation and motivation in order for learning and practice to occur include the following:

- "Bladder Rehabilitation/Bladder Retraining" is a behavioral technique that requires the resident to resist or inhibit the sensation of urgency (the strong desire to urinate), to postpone or delay voiding, and to urinate according to a timetable rather than to the urge to void. Depending upon the resident's successful ability to control the urge to void, the intervals between voiding may be increased progressively. Bladder training generally consists of education, scheduled voiding with systematic delay of voiding, and positive reinforcement. This program is difficult to implement in cognitively impaired residents and may not be successful in frail, elderly, or dependent residents. The resident who may be appropriate for a bladder rehabilitation (retraining) program is usually fairly independent in activities of daily living, has occasional incontinence, is aware of the need to urinate (void), may wear incontinence products for episodic urine leakage, and has a goal to maintain his/her highest level of continence and decrease urine leakage. Successful bladder retraining usually takes at least several weeks. Residents who are assessed with urge or mixed incontinence and are cognitively intact may be candidates for bladder retraining; and

- "Pelvic Floor Muscle Rehabilitation," also called Kegel and pelvic floor muscle exercise, is performed to strengthen the voluntary periuretheral and perivaginal muscles that contribute to the closing force of the urethra and the support of the pelvic organs. These exercises are helpful in dealing with urge and stress incontinence. Pelvic floor muscle exercises (PFME) strengthen the muscular components of urethral supports and are the cornerstone of noninvasive treatment of stress urinary incontinence. PFME requires residents who are able and willing to participate and the implementation of careful instructions and monitoring provided by the facility. Poor resident adherence to the exercises may occur even with close monitoring.

Programs that are dependent on staff involvement and assistance, as opposed to resident function, include the following:

- "Prompted Voiding" is a behavioral technique appropriate for use with dependent or more cognitively impaired residents. Prompted voiding techniques have been shown to reduce urinary incontinence episodes up to 40% for elderly incontinent nursing home residents, regardless of their type of urinary incontinence or cognitive deficit—provided that they at least are able to say their name or reliably point to one of two objects.[5] Prompted voiding has three components: regular monitoring with encouragement to report continence status; prompting to toilet on a scheduled basis; and praise and positive feedback when the resident is continent and attempts to toilet. These methods require training, motivation and continued effort by the resident and caregivers to ensure continued success. Prompted voiding focuses on teaching the resident, who is incontinent, to recognize bladder fullness or the need to void, to ask for help, or to respond when prompted to toilet.

  Residents who are assessed with urge or mixed incontinence and are cognitively impaired may be candidates for prompted voiding. As the resident's cognition changes, the facility should consider other factors, such as mobility, when deciding to conduct a voiding trial to determine feasibility of an ongoing toileting program; and

- "Habit Training/Scheduled Voiding" is a behavioral technique that calls for scheduled toileting at regular intervals on a planned basis to match the resident's voiding habits. Unlike bladder retraining, there is no systematic effort to encourage the resident to delay voiding and resist urges. Habit training includes timed voiding with the interval based on the resident's usual voiding schedule or pattern. Scheduled voiding is timed voiding, usually every three to four hours while awake. Residents who cannot self-toilet may be candidates for habit training or scheduled voiding programs.

Intermittent Catheterization

Sterile insertion and removal of a catheter through the urethra every 3-6 hours for bladder drainage may be appropriate for the management of acute or chronic urinary retention. See additional discussion below in "Catheterization".

Medication Therapy

Medications are often used to treat specific types of incontinence, including stress incontinence and those categories associated with an overactive bladder, which may involve symptoms including urge incontinence, urinary urgency, frequency and nocturia. The current literature identifies classifications and names of medications used for various types of incontinence. When using medications, potentially problematic anticholinergic and other side effects must be recognized. The use of medication therapy to treat urinary incontinence may not be appropriate for some residents because of potential adverse interactions with their other medications or other co-morbid conditions. Therefore, it is important to weigh the risks and benefits before prescribing medications for continence management and to monitor for both effectiveness and side effects. As with all approaches attempting to improve control or management of incontinence, the education and discussion with the resident (or the resident's surrogate) regarding the benefits and risks of pharmacologic therapies is important.

§Pessary

A pessary is an intra-vaginal device used to treat pelvic muscle relaxation or prolapse of pelvic organs. Women whose urine retention or urinary incontinence is exacerbated by bladder or uterine prolapse may benefit from placement of a pessary. Female residents may be admitted to the nursing home with a pessary device. The assessment should note whether the resident has a pessary in place or has had a history of successful pessary use. If a pessary is to be used, it is important to develop a plan of care for ongoing management and for the prevention of and monitoring for complications.

Absorbent Products, Toileting Devices, and External Collection Devices

Absorbent incontinence products include perineal pads or panty liners for slight leakage, undergarments and protective underwear for moderate to heavy leakage, guards and drip collection pouches for men, and products (called adult briefs) for moderate or heavy loss. Absorbent products can be a useful, rational way to manage incontinence; however, every absorbent product has a saturation point. Factors contributing to the selection of the type of product to be used should include the severity of incontinence, gender, fit, and ease of use.

Advantages of using absorbent products to manage urinary incontinence include the ability to contain urine (some may wick the urine away from the skin), provide protection for clothing, and preserve the resident's dignity and comfort.

NOTE: Although many residents have used absorbent products prior to admission to the nursing home and the use of absorbent products may be appropriate, absorbent products should not be used as the primary long term approach to continence management until the resident has been appropriately evaluated and other alternative approaches have been considered.

The potential disadvantages of absorbent products are the impact on the resident's dignity, cost, the association with skin breakdown and irritation, and the amount of time needed to check and change them.[6]

It is important that residents using various toileting devices, absorbent products, external collection devices, etc., be checked (and changed as needed) on a schedule based upon the resident's voiding pattern, accepted standards of practice, and the manufacturer's recommendations.

Skin-Related Complications

Skin problems associated with incontinence and moisture can range from irritation to increased risk of skin breakdown. Moisture may make the skin more susceptible to damage from friction and shear during repositioning.

One form of early skin breakdown is maceration or the softening of tissue by soaking. Macerated skin has a white appearance and a very soft, sometimes "soggy" texture.

The persistent exposure of perineal skin to urine and/or feces can irritate the epidermis and can cause severe dermatitis or skin erosion. Skin erosion is the loss of some or all of the epidermis (comparable to a deep chemical peel) leaving a slightly depressed area of skin.

One key to preventing skin breakdown is to keep the perineal skin clean and dry. Research has shown that a soap and water regimen alone may be less effective in preventing skin breakdown compared with moisture barriers and no-rinse incontinence cleansers.[7] Because frequent washing with soap and water can dry the skin, the use of a perineal rinse may be indicated. Moisturizers help preserve the moisture in the skin by either sealing in existing moisture or adding moisture to the skin. Moisturizers include creams, lotions or pastes. However, moisturizers should be used sparingly—if at all—on already macerated or excessively moist skin.

CATHETERIZATION

42 CFR 483.25 (d) (1) Urinary Incontinence requires that a resident who enters the facility without an indwelling catheter is not catheterized unless the resident's clinical condition demonstrates that catheterization was necessary. Some residents are admitted to the facility with indwelling catheters that were placed elsewhere (e.g., during a recent acute hospitalization). The facility is responsible for the assessment of the resident at risk for urinary catheterization and/or the ongoing assessment for the resident who currently has a catheter. This is followed by implementation of appropriate individualized interventions and monitoring for the effectiveness of the interventions.

Assessment

A resident may be admitted to the facility with or without an indwelling urinary catheter (urethral or suprapubic) and may be continent or incontinent of urine. Regardless of the admission status, a comprehensive assessment should address those factors that predispose the resident to the development of urinary incontinence and the use of an indwelling urinary catheter.

An admission evaluation of the resident's medical history and a physical examination helps identify the resident at risk for requiring the use of an indwelling urinary catheter. This evaluation is to include detection of reversible causes of incontinence and identification of individuals with incontinence caused by conditions that may not be reversible, such as bladder tumors and spinal cord diseases. (See the assessment factors discussed under incontinence.) The assessment of continence/incontinence is based upon an interdisciplinary review. The comprehensive assessment should include underlying factors supporting the medical justification for the initiation and continuing need for catheter use, determination of which factors can be modified or reversed (or rationale for why those factors should not be modified), and the development of a plan for removal. The clinician's decision to use an indwelling catheter in the elderly should be based on valid clinical indicators.

For the resident with an indwelling catheter, the facility's documented assessment and staff knowledge of the resident should include information to support the use of an indwelling catheter. Because of the risk of substantial complications with the use of indwelling urinary catheters, they should be reserved primarily for short-term decompression of acute urinary retention. The assessment should include consideration of the risks and benefits of an indwelling (suprapubic or urethral) catheter; the potential for removal of the catheter; and consideration of complications resulting from the use of an indwelling catheter, such as symptoms of blockage of the catheter with associated bypassing of urine, expulsion of the catheter, pain, discomfort and bleeding.

Intermittent Catheterization

Intermittent catheterization can often manage overflow incontinence effectively. Residents who have new onset incontinence from a transient, hypotonic/atonic bladder (usually seen following indwelling catheterization in the hospital) may benefit from intermittent bladder catheterization until the bladder tone returns (e.g., up to approximately 7 days). A voiding trial and post void residual can help identify when bladder tone has returned.

Indwelling Catheter Use

The facility's documented assessment and staff approach to the resident should be based on evidence to support the use of an indwelling catheter. Appropriate indications for continuing use of an indwelling catheter beyond 14 days may include:[8]

- Urinary retention that cannot be treated or corrected medically or surgically, for which alternative therapy is not feasible, and which is characterized by:
    - Documented post void residual (PVR) volumes in a range over 200 milliliters (ml);
    - Inability to manage the retention/incontinence with intermittent catheterization; and
    - Persistent overflow incontinence, symptomatic infections, and/or renal dysfunction.
- Contamination of Stage III or IV pressure ulcers with urine which has impeded healing, despite appropriate personal care for the incontinence; and

- Terminal illness or severe impairment, which makes positioning or clothing changes uncomfortable, or which is associated with intractable pain.

Catheter-Related Complications

An indwelling catheter may be associated with significant complications, including bacteremia, febrile episodes, bladder stones, fistula formation, erosion of the urethra, epididymitis, chronic renal inflammation and pyelonephritis. In addition, indwelling catheters are prone to blockage. Risk factors for catheter blockage include alkaline urine, poor urine flow, proteinuria, and preexisting bladder stones. In the absence of evidence indicating blockage, catheters need not be changed routinely as long as monitoring is adequate. Based on the resident's individualized assessment, the catheter may need to be changed more or less often than every 30 days.

Some residents with indwelling catheters experience persistent leakage around the catheter. Examples of factors that may contribute to leakage include irritation by a large balloon or by catheter materials, excessive catheter diameter, fecal impaction, and improper catheter positioning. Because leakage around the catheter is frequently caused by bladder spasm, leakage should generally not be treated by using increasingly larger catheter sizes, unless medically justified. Current standards indicate that catheterization should be accomplished with the narrowest, softest tube that will serve the purpose of draining the bladder. Additional care practices related to catheterization include:

- Educating the resident or responsible party on the risks and benefits of catheter use;
- Recognizing and assessing for complications and their causes, and maintaining a record of any catheter-related problems;
- Attempts to remove the catheter as soon as possible when no indications exist for its continuing use;
- Monitoring for excessive post void residual, after removing a catheter that was inserted for obstruction or overflow incontinence;
- Keeping the catheter anchored to prevent excessive tension on the catheter, which can lead to urethral tears or dislodging the catheter; and
- Securing the catheter to facilitate flow of urine.

Research has shown that catheterization is an important, potentially modifiable, risk factor for UTI. By the 30th day of catheterization, bacteriuria is nearly universal.[9] The potential for complications can be reduced by:

- Identifying specific clinical indications for the use of an indwelling catheter;

- Assessing whether other treatments and services would appropriately address those conditions; and

- Assessing whether residents are at risk for other possible complications resulting from the continuing use of the catheter, such as obstruction resulting from catheter encrustation, urethral erosion, bladder spasms, hematuria, and leakage around the catheter.

URINARY TRACT INFECTIONS

Catheter-Related Bacteriuria and UTIs/Urosepsis

Most individuals with indwelling catheters for more than 7 days have bacteriuria. Bacteriuria alone in a catheterized individual should not be treated with antibiotics.

A long term indwelling catheter (>2 to 4 weeks) increases the chances of having a symptomatic UTI and urosepsis. The incidence of bacteremia is 40 times greater in individuals with a long term indwelling catheter than in those without one. For suspected UTIs in a catheterized individual, the literature recommends removing the current catheter and inserting a new one and obtaining a urine sample via the newly inserted catheter.[10]

Clinical Evidence That May Suggest UTI

Clinically, an acute deterioration in stable chronic symptoms may indicate an acute infection. Multiple co-existing findings such as fever with hematuria are more likely to be from a urinary source.

No one lab test alone proves that a UTI is present. For example, a positive urine culture will show bacteriuria but that alone is not enough to diagnose a symptomatic UTI. However, several test results in combination with clinical findings can help to identify UTIs such as the presence of pyuria (more than minimal white cells in the urine) on microscopic urinalysis, or a positive urine dipstick test for leukocyte esterase (indicating significant pyuria) or for nitrites (indicating the presence of Enterobacteriaceae). A negative leukocyte esterase or the absence of pyuria strongly suggests that a UTI is not present. A positive leukocyte esterase test alone does not prove that the individual has a UTI.[11]

In someone with nonspecific symptoms such as a change in function or mental status, bacteriuria alone does not necessarily warrant antibiotic treatment. Additional evidence that could confirm a UTI may include hematuria, fever (which could include a variation from the individual's normal or usual temperature range), or evidence of pyuria (either by microscopic examination or by dipstick test). In the absence of fever, hematuria, pyuria, or local urinary tract symptoms, other potential causes of nonspecific general symptoms, such as fluid and electrolyte imbalance or adverse drug reactions, should be considered instead of, or in addition to, a UTI. Although sepsis, including urosepsis, can cause dizziness or falling, there is not clear evidence linking bacteriuria or a localized UTI to an increased fall risk.[12]

Indications to Treat a UTI

Because many residents have chronic bacteriuria, the research-based literature suggests treating only symptomatic UTIs. Symptomatic UTIs are based on the following criteria:[13]

- Residents without a catheter should have at least three of the following signs and symptoms:
    - Fever (increase in temperature of >2 degrees F (1.1 degrees C) or rectal temperature >99.5 degrees F (37.5 degrees C) or single measurement of temperature >100 degrees F (37.8 degrees C));[14]
    - New or increased burning pain on urination, frequency or urgency;
    - New flank or suprapubic pain or tenderness;
    - Change in character of urine (e.g., new bloody urine, foul smell, or amount of sediment) or as reported by the laboratory (new pyuria or microscopic hematuria); and/or
    - Worsening of mental or functional status (e.g., confusion, decreased appetite, unexplained falls, incontinence of recent onset, lethargy, decreased activity).[15]
- Residents with a catheter should have at least two of the following signs and symptoms:
    - Fever or chills;
    - New flank pain or suprapubic pain or tenderness;
    - Change in character of urine (e.g., new bloody urine, foul smell, or amount of sediment) or as reported by the laboratory (new pyuria or microscopic hematuria); and/or
    - Worsening of mental or functional status. Local findings such as obstruction, leakage, or mucosal trauma (hematuria) may also be present.[16]

Follow-Up of UTIs

The goal of treating a UTI is to alleviate systemic or local symptoms, not to eradicate all bacteria. Therefore, a post-treatment urine culture is not routinely necessary but may be useful in select situations. Continued bacteriuria without residual symptoms does not warrant repeat or continued antibiotic therapy. Recurrent UTIs (2 or more in 6 months) in a noncatheterized individual may warrant additional evaluation (such as a determination of an abnormal post void residual (PVR) urine volume or a referral to a urologist) to rule out structural abnormalities such as enlarged prostate, prolapsed bladder, periurethral abscess, strictures, bladder calculi, polyps and tumors.

Recurrent symptomatic UTIs in a catheterized or noncatheterized individual should lead the facility to check whether perineal hygiene is performed consistently to remove fecal soiling in accordance with accepted practices. Recurrent UTIs in a catheterized individual should lead the facility to look for possible impairment of free urine flow through the catheter, to re-evaluate the techniques being used for perineal hygiene and catheter care, and to reconsider the relative risks and benefits of continuing the use of an indwelling catheter.

Because the major factors (other than an indwelling catheter) that predispose individuals to bacteriuria, including physiological aging changes and chronic comorbid illnesses, cannot be modified readily, the facility should demonstrate that they:

- Employ standard infection control practices in managing catheters and associated drainage system;
- Strive to keep the resident and catheter clean of feces to minimize bacterial migration into the urethra and bladder (e.g., cleaning fecal material away from, rather than towards, the urinary meatus);
- Take measures to maintain free urine flow through any indwelling catheter; and
- Assess for fluid needs and implement a fluid management program (using alternative approaches as needed) based on those assessed needs.

ENDNOTES

[1] Geurrero, P. & Sinert, R. (November 18, 2004). Urinary Incontinence. Retrieved November 29, 2004 from E-Medicine. Website: www.emedicine.com/emerg/topic791.htm.

[2] Delafuente, J.C. & Stewart, R.B. (Eds.). (1995). Therapeutics in the Elderly (2nd ed., pp. 471). Cincinnati, OH: Harvey Whitney Books..

[3] Newman, D.K. (2002). Managing and Treating Urinary Incontinence (pp.106-107). Baltimore, MD: Health Professions Press.

[4] Newman, D.K. (2002). Managing and Treating Urinary Incontinence.

[5] Ouslander, J.G., Schnelle, J.F., Uman, G., Fingold, S., Nigam, J.G., Tuico, E., et al. (1995). Predictors of Successful Prompted Voiding Among Incontinent Nursing Home Residents. Journal of the American Medical Association, 273(17), 1366-1370.

[6] Armstrong, E.P. & Ferguson, T.A. (1998). Urinary Incontinence: Healthcare Resource Consumption in Veteran Affair Medical Centers. Veteran's Health System Journal, October, 37-42.

[7] Byers, P.H., Ryan, P.A., Regan, M.B., Shields, A., & Carta, S.G. (1995). Effects of Incontinence Care Cleansing Regimens on Skin Integrity. Continence Care, 22(4), 187-192.

[8] Niël-Weise BS, van den Broek PJ. Urinary catheter policies for long-term bladder drainage. The Cochrane Database of Systematic Reviews 2005, Issue 1. Art. No.: CD004201. DOI: 10.1002/14651858.CD004201.pub2.

[9] Maki, D.G. & Tambyah, P.A. (2001). Engineering out the Risk of Infection with Urinary Catheters. Emerging Infectious Diseases, 7(2), 342-347.

[10] Grahn, D., Norman, D.C., White, M.L., Cantrell, M. & Thomas, T.T. (1985). Validity of Urinary Catheter Specimen for Diagnosis of Urinary Tract Infection in the Elderly. Archives of Internal Medicine, 145,1858.

[11] Nicolle, L.E. (1999). Urinary Tract Infections in the Elderly. In W.R.Hazzard, J.P. Blass., W.H. Ettinger,, J.B. Halter & J.G. Ouslander (Eds.), Principles of Geriatric Medicine and Gerontology (4th ed., pp.823-833). New York: McGraw-Hill.

[12] Nicolle, L.E. & SHEA Long-term Care Committee. (2001). Urinary tract Infections in Long-Term Care Facilities. Infection Control Hospital Epidemiology, 22, 167-175.

[13] McGreer, A., Campbell, B., Emori, T.G., Hierholzer, W.J., Jackson, M.M., Nicolle, L.E., et al. (1991). Definitions of Infections for Surveillance in Long Term Care Facilities. American Journal of Infection Control, 19(1), 1-7.

[14] AMDA: Common Infections in the Long-term Care Setting. Clinical practice guideline Adapted from Bentley DW, Bradley S, High K, et al. Practice guideline for evaluation of fever and infection in long-term care facilities. Guidelines from the Infectious Diseases Society of America. J Am Med Dir Assoc 2001; 2(5): 246-258.

[15] Ouslander, J.G., Osterweil, D., Morley, J. (1997). Medical Care in the Nursing Home. (2nd ed., pp.303-307). New York: McGraw-Hill.

[16] Nicolle, L.E. (1997). Asymptomatic Bacteriuria in the Elderly. Infectious Disease Clinics of North America, 11, 647-62.

INVESTIGATIVE PROTOCOL

URINARY CONTINENCE AND CATHETERS

Objectives

- To determine whether the initial insertion or continued use of an indwelling catheter is based upon clinical indication for use of a urinary catheter;
- To determine the adequacy of interventions to prevent, improve and/or manage urinary incontinence; and
- To determine whether appropriate treatment and services have been provided to prevent and/or treat UTIs.

Use

Use this protocol for a sampled resident with an indwelling urinary catheter or for a resident with urinary incontinence.

Procedures

Briefly review the assessment, care plan and orders to identify facility interventions and to guide observations to be made. Staff are expected to assess and provide appropriate care from the day of admission, for residents with urinary incontinence or a condition that may contribute to incontinence or the presence of an indwelling urinary catheter (including newly admitted residents). Corroborate observations by interview and record review.

NOTE: Criteria established in this protocol provide general guidelines and best practices which should be considered when making a determination of compliance, and is not an exhaustive list of mandatory elements.

1. Observation

Observe whether staff consistently implemented care plan interventions across various shifts. During observations of the interventions, note and/or follow up on deviations from the care plan or from current standards of practice, as well as potential negative outcomes.

Observe whether staff make appropriate resident accommodations consistent with the assessment, such as placing the call bell within reach and responding to the call bell, in relation to meeting toileting needs; maintaining a clear pathway and ready access to toilet facilities; providing (where indicated) elevated toilet seats, grab bars, adequate lighting, and assistance needed to use devices such as urinals, bedpans and commodes.

Observe whether assistance has been provided to try to prevent incontinence episodes, such as whether prompting, transfer, and/or stand-by assist to ambulate were provided as required for toileting.

For a resident who is on a program to restore continence or is on a prompted void or scheduled toileting program, note:

- The frequency of breakthrough or transient incontinence;
- How staff respond to the incontinence episodes; and
- Whether care is provided in accord with standards of practice (including infection control practices) and with respect for the resident's dignity.

For a resident who has been determined by clinical assessment to be unable to participate in a program to restore continence or in a scheduled toileting program and who requires care due to incontinence of urine, observe:

Whether the resident is on a scheduled check and change program; and

Whether staff check and change in a timely fashion.

For a resident who has experienced an incontinent episode, observe:

The condition of the pads/sheets/clothing (a delay in providing continence care may be indicated by brown rings/circles, saturated linens/clothing, odors, etc.);

The resident's physical condition (such as skin integrity, maceration, erythema, erosion);

The resident's psychosocial outcomes (such as embarrassment or expressions of humiliation, resignation, about being incontinent);

- Whether staff implemented appropriate hygiene measures (e.g., cleansing, rinsing, drying and applying protective moisture barriers or barrier films as indicated) to try to prevent skin breakdown from prolonged exposure of the skin to urine; and

Whether the staff response to incontinence episodes and the provision of care are consistent with standards of practice (including infection control practices) and with respect for the resident's dignity.

For a resident with an indwelling catheter, observe the delivery of care to evaluate:

- Whether staff use appropriate infection control practices regarding hand washing, catheter care, tubing, and the collection bag;

- Whether staff recognize and assess potential evidence of symptomatic UTI or other related changes in urine condition (such as onset of bloody urine, cloudiness, or oliguria, if present);

- How staff manage and assess urinary leakage from the point of catheter insertion to the bag, if present;

- If the resident has catheter-related pain, how staff assess and manage the pain; and

- What interventions (such as anchoring the catheter, avoiding excessive tugging on the catheter during transfer and care delivery) are being used to prevent inadvertent catheter removal or tissue injury from dislodging the catheter.

For a resident experiencing incontinence and who has an indwelling or intermittent catheter, observe whether the resident is provided and encouraged to take enough fluids to meet the resident's hydration needs, as reflected in various measures of hydration status (approximately 30ml/kg/day or as indicated based on the resident's clinical condition). For issues regarding hydration, see Guidance at 42 CFR 483.25(j), F327.

2. Interviews

Interview the resident, family or responsible party to the degree possible to identify:

- Their involvement in care plan development including defining the approaches and goals, and whether interventions reflect preferences and choices;

- Their awareness of the existing continence program and how to use devices or equipment;

- If timely assistance is provided as needed for toileting needs, hydration and personal hygiene and if continence care and/or catheter care is provided according to the care plan;

- If the resident comprehends and applies information and instructions to help improve or maintain continence (where cognition permits);

- Presence of urinary tract-related pain, including causes and management;

- If interventions were refused, whether consequences and/or other alternative approaches were presented and discussed; and

- Awareness of any current UTI, history of UTIs, or perineal skin problems.

If the resident has a skin problem that may be related to incontinence, or staff are not following the resident's care plan and continence/catheter care program, interview the nursing assistants to determine if they:

Are aware of, and understand, the interventions specific to this resident (such as the bladder or bowel restorative/management programs);

Have been trained and know how to handle catheters, tubing and drainage bags and other devices used during the provision of care; and

Know what, when, and to whom to report changes in status regarding bowel and bladder function, hydration status, urine characteristics, and complaints of urinary-related symptoms.

3. Record Review

Assessment and Evaluation. Review the RAI, the history and physical, and other information such as physician orders, progress notes, nurses' notes, pharmacist reports, lab reports and any flow sheets or forms the facility uses to document the resident's voiding history, including the assessment of the resident's overall condition, risk factors and information about the resident's continence status, rationale for using a catheter, environmental factors related to continence programs, and the resident's responses to catheter/continence services. Request staff assistance, if the information is not readily available.

Determine if the facility assessment is consistent with or corroborated by documentation within the record and comprehensively reflects the status of the resident for:

- Patterns of incontinent episodes, daily voiding patterns or prior routines;
- Fluid intake and hydration status;
- Risks or conditions that may affect urinary continence;
- Use of medications that may affect continence and impaired continence that could reflect adverse drug reactions;
- Type of incontinence (stress, urge, overflow, mixed, functional, or transient incontinence) and contributing factors;
- Environmental factors that might facilitate or impede the ability to maintain bladder continence, such as access to the toilet, call bell, type of clothing and/or continence products, ambulation devices (walkers, canes), use of restraints, side rails;
- Type and frequency of physical assistance necessary to facilitate toileting;
- Clinical rationale for use of an indwelling catheter;
- Alternatives to extended use of an indwelling catheter (if possible); and

- Evaluation of factors possibly contributing to chronically recurring or persistent UTIs.

Care Plan. If the care plan refers to a specific facility treatment protocol that contains details of the treatment regimen, the protocol must be available to the direct care staff, so that they may be familiar with it and use it. The care plan should clarify any significant deviations from such a protocol for a specific resident. If care plan interventions that address aspects of continence and skin care related to incontinence are integrated within the overall care plan, the interventions do not need to be repeated in a separate continence care plan.

Review the care plan to determine if the plan is based upon the goals, needs and strengths specific to the resident and reflects the comprehensive assessment. Determine if the plan:

- Identifies quantifiable, measurable objectives with time frames to be able to assess whether the objectives have been met;

- Identifies interventions specific enough to guide the provision of services and treatment (e.g., toilet within an hour prior to each meal and within 30 minutes after meals, or check for episodes of incontinence within 30 minutes after each meal or specific times based upon the assessment of voiding patterns);

- Is based upon resident choices and preferences;

- Promotes maintenance of resident dignity;

- Addresses potential psychosocial complications of incontinence or catheterization such as social withdrawal, embarrassment, humiliation, isolation, resignation;

- Includes a component to inform the resident and representative about the risks and benefits of catheter use, on continence management approaches, medications selected, etc.;

- Addresses measures to promote sufficient fluid intake, including alternatives such as food substitutes that have a high liquid content, if there is reduced fluid intake;

- Defines interventions to prevent skin breakdown from prolonged exposure to urine and stool;

- Identifies and addresses the potential impact on continence of medication and urinary tract stimulants or irritants (e.g., caffeine) in foods and beverages;

- Identifies approaches to minimize risk of infection (personal hygiene measures and catheter/tubing/bag care); and

- Defines environmental approaches and devices needed to promote independence in toileting, to maintain continence, and to maximize independent functioning.

For the resident who is not on a scheduled toileting program or a program to restore normal bladder function to the extent possible, determine if the care plan provides specific approaches for a check and change program.

For the resident who is on a scheduled toileting or restorative program (e.g., retraining, habit training, scheduled voiding, prompted voiding, toileting devices), determine whether the care plan:

- Identifies the type of urinary incontinence and bases the program on the resident's voiding/elimination patterns; and

- Has been developed by considering the resident's medical/health condition, cognitive and functional ability to participate in a relevant continence program, and needed assistance.

For the resident with a catheter, determine whether the care plan:

- Defines the catheter, tubing and bag care, including indications, according to facility protocol, for changing the catheter, tubing or bag;

- Provides for assessment and removal of the indwelling catheter when no longer needed; and

- Establishes interventions to minimize catheter-related injury, pain, encrustation, excessive urethral tension, accidental removal, or obstruction of urine outflow.

Care Plan Revision. Determine if the resident's condition and effectiveness of the care plan interventions have been monitored and care plan revisions were made (or justifications for continuing the existing plan) based upon the following:

- The outcome and/or effects of goals and interventions;

- A decline or lack of improvement in continence status;

- Complications associated with catheter usage;

- Resident failure to comply with a continence program and alternative approaches that were offered to try to maintain or improve continence, including counseling regarding the potential consequences of not following the program;

- Change in condition, ability to make decisions, cognition, medications, behavioral symptoms or visual problems;

- Input by the resident and/or the responsible person; and

- An evaluation of the resident's level of participation in, and response to, the continence program.

4. Interviews with Health Care Practitioners and Professionals

If inconsistencies in care or potential negative outcomes have been identified, or care is not in accord with standards of practice, interview the nurse responsible for coordinating or overseeing the resident's care. Determine:

- How the staff monitor implementation of the care plan, changes in continence, skin condition, and the status of UTIs;

- If the resident resists toileting, how staff have been taught to respond;

- Types of interventions that have been attempted to promote continence (i.e., special clothing, devices, types and frequency of assistance, change in toileting schedule, environmental modifications);

- If the resident is not on a restorative program, how it was determined that the resident could not benefit from interventions such as a scheduled toileting program;

- For the resident on a program of toileting, whether the nursing staff can identify the programming applicable to the resident, and:

    - The type of incontinence;

    - The interventions to address that specific type;

    - How it is determined that the schedule and program is effective (i.e., how continence is maintained or if there has been a decline or improvement in continence, how the program is revised to address the changes); and

    - Whether the resident has any physical or cognitive limitations that influence potential improvement of his/her continence;

- For residents with urinary catheters, whether the nursing staff:

    - Can provide appropriate justification for the use of the catheter;

    - Can identify previous attempts made (and the results of the attempts) to remove a catheter; and

    - Can identify a history of UTIs (if present), and interventions to try to prevent recurrence.

If the interventions defined or care provided do not appear to be consistent with recognized standards of practice, interview one or more health care practitioners and professionals as necessary (e.g., physician, charge nurse, director of nursing) who, by virtue of training and knowledge of the resident, should be able to provide information about the causes, treatment and evaluation of the resident's condition or problem. Depending on the issue, ask about:

- How it was determined that the chosen interventions were appropriate;
- Risks identified for which there were no interventions;
- Changes in condition that may justify additional or different interventions; or how they validated the effectiveness of current interventions; and
- How they monitor the approaches to continence programs (e.g., policies/procedures, staffing requirements, how staff identify problems, assess the toileting pattern of the resident, develop and implement continence-related action plans, how staff monitor and evaluate resident's responses, etc.).

If the attending physician is unavailable, interview the medical director, as appropriate.

DETERMINATION OF COMPLIANCE (Task 6, Appendix P)

Synopsis of regulation (F315)

The urinary incontinence requirement has three aspects. The first aspect requires that a resident who does not have an indwelling urinary catheter does not have one inserted unless the resident's clinical condition demonstrates that it was necessary. The second aspect requires the facility to provide appropriate treatment and services to prevent urinary tract infections; and the third is that the facility attempt to assist the resident to restore as much normal bladder function as possible.

Criteria for Compliance

- Compliance with 42 CFR 483.25(d)(1) and (2), F315, Urinary Incontinence
    - For a resident who was admitted with an indwelling urinary catheter or who had one placed after admission, the facility is in compliance with this requirement, if staff have:
        - Recognized and assessed factors affecting the resident's urinary function and identified the medical justification for the use of an indwelling urinary catheter;

- Defined and implemented pertinent interventions to try to minimize complications from an indwelling urinary catheter, and to remove it if clinically indicated, consistent with resident conditions, goals, and recognized standards of practice;

- Monitored and evaluated the resident's response to interventions; and

- Revised the approaches as appropriate.

If not, the use of an indwelling urinary catheter is not medically justified, and/or the ongoing treatment and services for catheter care were not provided consistent with the resident's needs. Cite F315.

- o For a resident who is incontinent of urine, the facility is in compliance with this requirement if they:

  - Recognized and assessed factors affecting the risk of symptomatic urinary tract infections and impaired urinary function;

  - Defined and implemented interventions to address correctable underlying causes of urinary incontinence and to try to minimize the occurrence of symptomatic urinary tract infections in accordance with resident needs, goals, and recognized standards of practice;

  - Monitored and evaluated the resident's response to preventive efforts and treatment interventions; and

  - Revised the approaches as appropriate.

  If not, the facility is not in compliance with the requirement to assist the resident to maintain or improve the continence status, and/or prevent the decline of the condition of urinary incontinence for the resident. Cite F315.

- o For a resident who has or has had a symptomatic urinary tract infection, the facility is in compliance with this requirement if they have:

  - Recognized and assessed factors affecting the risk of symptomatic urinary tract infections and impaired urinary function;

  - Defined and implemented interventions to try to minimize the occurrence of symptomatic urinary tract infections and to address correctable underlying causes, in accordance with resident needs, goals, and recognized standards of practice;

- Monitored and evaluated the resident's responses to preventive efforts and treatment interventions; and
- Revised the approaches as appropriate.

If not, the development of a symptomatic urinary tract infection, and/or decline of the resident with one, was not consistent with the identified needs of the resident. Cite F315.

Noncompliance for F315

After completing the Investigative Protocol, analyze the data in order to determine whether or not noncompliance with the regulation exists. Noncompliance for F315 may include (but is not limited to) one or more of the following, including failure to:

- Provide care and treatment to prevent incontinence and/or improve urinary continence and restore as much normal bladder function as possible;
- Provide medical justification for the use of a catheter or provide services for a resident with a urinary catheter;
- Assess, prevent (to the extent possible) and treat a symptomatic urinary tract infection (as indicated by the resident's choices, clinical condition and physician treatment plan);
  - Accurately or consistently assess a resident's continence status on admission and as indicated thereafter;
  - Identify and address risk factors for developing urinary incontinence;
  - Implement interventions (such as bladder rehabilitative programs) to try to improve bladder function or prevent urinary incontinence, consistent with the resident's assessed need and current standards of practice;
  - Provide clinical justification for developing urinary incontinence or for the failure of existing urinary incontinence to improve;
  - Identify and manage symptomatic urinary tract infections, or explain adequately why they could or should not do so;
  - Implement approaches to manage an indwelling urinary catheter based upon standards of practice, including infection control procedures;
  - Identify and apply relevant policies and procedures to manage urinary incontinence, urinary catheters and/or urinary tract infections;

- Notify the physician of the resident's condition or changes in the resident's continence status or development of symptoms that may represent a symptomatic UTI (in contrast to asymptomatic bacteriuria).

Potential Tags for Additional Investigation

During the investigation of 42 CFR 483.25(d)(1) and (2), the surveyor may have identified concerns related to outcome, process and/or structure requirements. The surveyor should investigate these requirements before determining whether noncompliance may be present. The following are examples of related outcome, process and/or structure requirements that should be considered:

- 42 CFR 483.10(b)(11), F157, Notification of Changes

  - Determine if staff notified the physician of significant changes in the resident's continence, catheter usage, or the development, treatment and/or change in symptomatic UTIs; or notified the resident or resident's representative (where one exists) of significant changes as noted above.

- 42 CFR 483.15(a), F241, Dignity

  - Determine if staff provide continence care and/or catheter care to the resident in a manner that respects his/her dignity, strives to meet needs in a timely manner, monitors and helps the resident who cannot request assistance, and strives to minimize feelings of embarrassment, humiliation and/or isolation related to impaired continence.

- 42 CFR 483.20(b)(1), F272, Comprehensive Assessments

  - Determine if the facility comprehensively assessed the resident's continence status and resident-specific risk factors (including potential causes), and assessed for the use of continence-related devices, including an indwelling catheter.

- 42 CFR 483.20(k), F279, Comprehensive Care Plans

  - Determine if the facility developed a care plan (1) that was consistent with the resident's specific conditions, risks, needs, behaviors, and preferences and with current standards of practice and (2) that includes measurable objectives, approximate timetables, specific interventions and/or services needed to prevent or address incontinence, provide catheter care; and to prevent UTIs to the extent possible.

- 42 CFR 483.20(k)(2)(iii), F280, Comprehensive Care Plan Revision

  - Determine if the care plan was reviewed and revised periodically, as necessary, related to preventing, managing, or improving incontinence, managing an indwelling urinary catheter, possible discontinuation of an indwelling catheter, and attempted prevention and management of UTIs.

- 42 CFR 483.20(k)(3)(i), F281, Services Provided Meet Professional Standards

    - Determine if services and care were provided for urinary incontinence, catheter care and/or symptomatic UTIs in accordance with accepted professional standards.

- 42 CFR 483.25, F309, Quality of Care

    - Determine if staff identified and implemented appropriate measures to address any pain related to the use of an indwelling urinary catheter or skin complications such as maceration, and to provide the necessary care and services in accordance with the comprehensive assessment plan of care.

- 42 CFR 483.25 (a)(3) F312, Quality of Care

    - Determine if staff identified and implemented appropriate measures to provide good personal hygiene for the resident who cannot perform relevant activities of daily living, and who has been assessed as unable to achieve and/or restore normal bladder function.

- 42 CFR 483.40(a), F385, Physician Supervision

    - Determine if the physician has evaluated and addressed, as indicated, medical issues related to preventing or managing urinary incontinence, catheter usage, and symptomatic UTIs.

- 42 CFR 483.65(b)(3), F444, Infection Control: Hand Washing

    - Determine if staff wash their hands after providing incontinence care, and before and after providing catheter care.

- 42 CFR 483.75(f), F498, Proficiency of Nurse Aides

    - Determine if nurse aides correctly deliver continence and catheter care, including practices to try to minimize skin breakdown, UTIs, catheter-related injuries, and dislodgement.

- 42 CFR 483.30(a), F353, Sufficient Staff

    - Determine if the facility had qualified staff in sufficient numbers to provide necessary care and services on a 24-hour basis, based upon the comprehensive assessment and care plan, to prevent, manage and/or improve urinary incontinence where possible.

- 42 CFR 483.75(i)(2), F501, Medical Director

    - Determine whether the medical director, in collaboration with the facility and based on current standards of practice, has developed policies and procedures for the prevention and management of urinary incontinence, for catheter care, and for the identification and management of symptomatic urinary tract infections; and whether the medical director interacts, if requested by the facility, with the physician supervising the care of the resident related to the management of urinary incontinence, catheter or infection issues.

V. DEFICIENCY CATEGORIZATION (Part V, Appendix P)

Once the team has completed its investigation, analyzed the data, reviewed the regulatory requirements, and determined that non-compliance exists, the team must determine the severity of each deficiency, based on the resultant effect or potential for harm to the resident.

The key elements for severity determination for F315 are as follows:

1. Presence of harm/negative outcome(s) or potential for negative outcomes because of lack of appropriate treatment and care. Actual or potential harm/negative outcome for F315 may include, but is not limited to:

    - Development, recurrence, persistence, or increasing frequency of urinary incontinence, which is not the result of underlying clinical conditions;

    - Complications such as urosepsis or urethral injury related to the presence of an indwelling urinary catheter that is not clinically justified;

    - Significant changes in psychosocial functioning, such as isolation, withdrawal, or embarrassment, related to the presence of un-assessed or unmanaged urinary incontinence and/or a decline in continence, and/or the use of a urinary catheter without a clinically valid medical justification; and

    - Complications such as skin breakdown that are related to the failure to manage urinary incontinence;

2. Degree of harm (actual or potential) related to the noncompliance. Identify how the facility practices caused, resulted in, allowed or contributed to the actual or potential for harm:

    - If harm has occurred, determine if the harm is at the level of serious injury, impairment, death, compromise, or discomfort; and

- If harm has not yet occurred, determine the potential for serious injury, impairment, death, or compromise or discomfort to occur to the resident; and

3. The immediacy of correction required. Determine whether the noncompliance requires immediate correction in order to prevent serious injury, harm, impairment, or death to one or more residents.

The survey team must evaluate the harm or potential for harm based upon the following levels of severity for tag F315. First, the team must rule out whether Severity Level 4, Immediate Jeopardy to a resident's health or safety exists by evaluating the deficient practice in relation to immediacy, culpability, and severity. (Follow the guidance in Appendix Q, Immediate Jeopardy.)

Severity Level 4 Considerations: Immediate Jeopardy to Resident Health or Safety

Immediate Jeopardy is a situation in which the facility's noncompliance with one or more requirements of participation:

- Has allowed/caused/resulted in, or is likely to allow/cause /result in serious injury, harm, impairment, or death to a resident; and

- Requires immediate correction, as the facility either created the situation or allowed the situation to continue by failing to implement preventative or corrective measures.

Examples of possible negative outcomes as a result of the facility's deficient practices may include:

- **Complications resulting from utilization of urinary appliance(s) without medical justification:** As a result of incorrect or unwarranted (i.e., not medically indicated) utilization of a urinary catheter, pessary, etc., the resident experiences injury or trauma (e.g., urethral tear) that requires surgical intervention or repair.

- **Extensive failure in multiple areas of incontinence care and/or catheter management:** As a result of the facility's noncompliance in multiple areas of continence care or catheter management, the resident developed urosepsis with complications leading to prolonged decline or death.

NOTE: If immediate jeopardy has been ruled out based upon the evidence, then evaluate whether actual harm that is not immediate jeopardy exists at Severity Level 3.

Severity Level 3 Considerations: Actual Harm that is not Immediate Jeopardy

Level 3 indicates noncompliance that results in actual harm, and can include but may not be limited to clinical compromise, decline, or the resident's ability to maintain and/or reach his/her highest practicable well-being.

Examples of avoidable negative outcomes may include, but are not limited to:

- **The development of a symptomatic UTI:** As a result of the facility's noncompliance, the resident developed a symptomatic UTI, without long term complications, associated with the use of an indwelling catheter for which there was no medical justification.

- **The failure to identify, assess and mange urinary retention:** As a result of the facility's noncompliance, the resident had persistent overflow incontinence and/or developed recurrent symptomatic UTIs.

- **The failure to provide appropriate catheter care:** As a result of the facility's noncompliance, the catheter was improperly managed, resulting in catheter-related pain, bleeding, urethral tears or urethral erosion.

- **Medically unjustified use of an indwelling catheter with complications:** As a result of the facility's noncompliance, a resident who was admitted with a urinary catheter had the catheter remain for an extended period of time without a valid medical justification for its continued use, or a urinary catheter was inserted after the resident was in the facility and used for an extended time without medical justification, during which the resident experienced significant complications such as recurrent symptomatic UTIs.

- **Decline or failure to improve continence status:** As a result of the facility's failure to assess and/or re-assess the resident's continence status, utilize sufficient staffing to implement continence programs and provide other related services based on the resident's assessed needs, and/or to evaluate the possible adverse effects of medications on continence status, the resident failed to maintain or improve continence status.

- **Complications due to urinary incontinence:** As a result of the facility's failure to provide care and services to a resident who is incontinent of urine, in accordance with resident need and accepted standards of practice, the resident developed skin maceration and/or erosion or declined to attend or participate in social situations (withdrawal) due to embarrassment or humiliation related to unmanaged urinary incontinence.

NOTE: If Severity Level 3 (actual harm that is not immediate jeopardy) has been ruled out based upon the evidence, then evaluate as to whether Level 2 (no actual harm with the potential for more than minimal harm) exists.

Severity Level 2 Considerations: No Actual Harm with potential for more than minimal harm that is Not Immediate Jeopardy

Level 2 indicates noncompliance that results in a resident outcome of no more than minimal discomfort and/or has the potential to compromise the resident's ability to maintain or reach his or her highest practicable level of well being. The potential exists for greater harm to occur if interventions are not provided.

Examples of potentially avoidable negative outcomes may include, but are not limited to:

- **Medically unjustified use of an indwelling catheter:** As a result of the facility's noncompliance, the resident has the potential for experiencing complications, such as symptomatic UTIs, bladder stones, pain, etc.

- **Complications associated with inadequate care and services for an indwelling catheter:** As a result of the facility's noncompliance, the resident has developed potentially preventable non-life-threatening problems related to the catheter, such as leaking of urine due to blockage of urine outflow, with or without skin maceration and/or dermatitis.

- **Potential for decline or complications:** As a result of the facility's failure to consistently implement a scheduled voiding program defined in accordance with the assessed needs, the resident experiences repeated episodes of incontinence but has not demonstrated a decline or developed complications.

Severity Level 1: No actual harm with potential for minimal harm

The failures of the facility to provide appropriate care and services to improve continence, manage indwelling catheters, and minimize negative outcome places residents at risk for more than minimal harm. Therefore, Severity Level 1 does not apply for this regulatory requirement.

---

§483.25(e) Range of motion.

Based on the comprehensive assessment of a resident, the facility must ensure that

(see Tag **F318** for intent, guidelines, procedures, and probes for §483.25(e))

F317

§483.25(e)(1) A resident who enters the facility without a limited range of motion does not experience reduction in range of motion unless the resident's clinical condition demonstrates that a reduction in range of motion is unavoidable; and

SEE INTERPRERTIVE GUIDELINES AT TAG F318

F318

§483.25(e)(2) A resident with a limited range of motion receives appropriate treatment and services to increase range of motion and/or to prevent further decrease in range of motion

Intent §483.25(e)

The intent of this regulation is to ensure that the resident reaches and maintains his or her highest level of range of motion and to prevent avoidable decline of range of motion.

Interpretive Guidelines §483.25(e)

This corresponds to MDS 2.0 sections G and P when specified for use by the State.

"Range of motion (ROM)" is defined as the extent of movement of a joint.

The clinical condition that may demonstrate that a reduction in ROM is unavoidable is: limbs or digits immobilized because of injury or surgical procedures (e.g., surgical adhesions).

Adequate preventive care may include active ROM performed by the resident's passive ROM performed by staff; active-assistive ROM exercise performed by the resident and staff; and application of splints and braces, if necessary.

Examples of clinical conditions that are the primary risk factors for a decreased range of motion are:

- Immobilization (e.g., bedfast);
- Deformities arising out of neurological deficits (e.g., strokes, multiple sclerosis, cerebral palsy, and polio); and
- Pain, spasms, and immobility associated with arthritis or late state Alzheimer's disease.

This clinical condition may demonstrate that a reduction in ROM is unavoidable only if adequate assessment, appropriate care planning, and preventive care was provided, and resulted in limitation in ROM or muscle atrophy.

Procedures §483.25(e)

For each resident selected for a comprehensive review, or focused review, as appropriate, who needs routine preventive care:

- Observe staff providing routine ROM exercises. Are they done according to the care plan?

Probes: §483.25(e)

Is there evidence that there has been a decline in sampled residents' ROM or muscle atrophy that was avoidable?

- Was the resident at risk for decline in ROM? If so, why?
- What care did the facility provide, including routine preventive measures that addressed the resident's unique risk factors (e.g., use muscle strengthening exercises in residents with muscle atrophy)?
  - Was this care provided consistently?

For all sampled residents who have limited ROM, what is the facility doing to prevent further declines in ROM?

- Are passive ROM exercises provided and active ROM exercises supervised per the plan of care?
- Have care plan objectives identified resident's needs and has resident progress been evaluated?
- Is there evidence that care planning is changed as the resident's condition changes?
- Identify if resident triggers RAPs for ADL functional/rehabilitation potential, visual function, and communication. Consider whether the RAPs used to assess causal factors for decline, potential for decline or lack of improvement.

---

§483.25(f) Mental and Psychosocial Functioning

Based on the comprehensive assessment of a resident, the facility must ensure that--

(See **Tag F319** for intent, guidelines, and probes for §483.25(f))

–

F319

§483.25(f)(1) A resident who displays mental or psychosocial adjustment difficulty, receives appropriate treatment and services to correct the assessed problem; and

Intent §483.25(f)

The intent of this regulation is that the resident receives care and services to assist him or her to reach and maintain the highest level of mental and psychosocial functioning.

Interpretive Guidelines §483.25(f)

This corresponds to MDS 2.0 sections B, F, E, and I when specified for use by the State.

"Mental and psychosocial adjustment difficulties" refer to problems residents have in adapting to changes in life's circumstances. The former focuses on internal thought processes; the latter, on the external manifestations of these thought patterns.

Mental and psychosocial adjustment difficulties are characterized primarily by an overwhelming sense of loss of one's capabilities; of family and friends; of the ability to continue to pursue activities and hobbies; and of one's possessions. This sense of loss is perceived as global and uncontrollable and is supported by thinking patterns that focus on helplessness and hopelessness; that all learning and essentially all meaningful living ceases once one enters a nursing home. A resident with a mental adjustment disorder will have a sad or anxious mood, or a behavioral symptom such as aggression.

The "Diagnostic and Statistical Manual of Mental Disorders, Fourth Edition (DSM/IV)," specifies that adjustment disorders develop within 3 months of a stressor (e.g., moving to another room) and are evidenced by significant functional impairment. Bereavement with the death of a loved one is not associated with adjustment disorders developed within 3 months of a stressor.

Other manifestations of mental and psychosocial adjustment difficulties may, over a period of time, include:

- Impaired verbal communication;
- Social isolation (e.g., loss or failure to have relationships);
- Sleep pattern disturbance (e.g., disruptive change in sleep/rest pattern as related to one's biological and emotional needs);
- Spiritual distress (disturbances in one's belief system);
- Inability to control behavior and potential for violence (aggressive behavior directed at self or others); and
- Stereotyped response to any stressor (i.e., the same characteristic response, regardless of the stimulus).

Appropriate treatment and services for psychosocial adjustment difficulties may include providing residents with opportunities for self-governance; systematic orientation programs; arrangements to keep residents in touch with their communities, cultural heritage, former lifestyle, and religious practices; and maintaining contact with friends and family Appropriate treatment for mental adjustment difficulties may include crisis intervention services; individual, group or family psychotherapy, drug therapy and training in monitoring of drug therapy and other rehabilitative services. (See §483.45(a).)

Clinical conditions that may produce apathy, malaise, and decreased energy levels that can be mistaken for depression associated with mental or psychosocial adjustment difficulty are: (This list is not all inclusive.)

- Metabolic diseases (e.g., abnormalities of serum glucose, potassium, calcium, and blood urea nitrogen, hepatic dysfunction);
- Endocrine diseases (e.g., hypothyroidism, hyperthyroidism, diabetes, hypoparathyroidism, hyperparathyroidism, Cushing's disease, Addison's disease);
- Central nervous system diseases (e.g., tumors and other mass lesions, Parkinson's disease, multiple sclerosis, Alzheimer's disease, vascular disease);
- Miscellaneous diseases (e.g., pernicious anemia, pancreatic disease, malignancy, infections, congestive heart failure);
- Over-medication with anti-hypertensive drugs; and
- Presence of restraints.

Probes: §483.25(f)(1)

For sampled residents selected for a comprehensive or focused review, determine, as appropriate, for those residents exhibiting difficulties in mental and psychosocial adjustment:

- Is there a complete accurate assessment of resident's usual and customary routines?
- What evidence is there that the facility makes accommodations for the resident's usual and customary routines?
- What programs/activities has the resident received to improve and maintain maximum mental and psychosocial functioning?

- Has the resident's mental and psychosocial functioning been maintained or improved (e.g., fewer symptoms of distress)? Have treatment plans and objectives been re-evaluated?

- Has the resident received a psychological or psychiatric evaluation to evaluate, diagnose, or treat her/his condition, if necessary?

- Identify if resident triggers RAPs for activities, mood state, psychosocial well-being, and psychotropic drug use. Consider whether the RAPs were used to assess the causal factors for decline, potential for decline or lack of improvement.

- How are mental and psychosocial adjustment difficulties addressed in the care plan?

See §483.45(a), F406 for health rehabilitative services for mental illness and mental retardation.

Psychosocial adjustment difficulty does not display a pattern of decreased social interaction and/or increased withdrawn, angry, or depressive behaviors, unless the resident's clinical condition demonstrates that such a pattern was unavoidable.

F320

§483.25(f)(2)

(2) A resident whose assessment did not reveal a mental or psychosocial adjustment difficulty does not display a pattern of decreased social interaction and/or increased withdrawn, angry, or depressive behaviors, unless the resident's clinical condition demonstrates that such a pattern is unavoidable.

Procedures §483.25(f)(2)

For sampled residents whose assessment did not reveal a mental or psychosocial adjustment difficulty, but who display decreased social interaction or increased withdrawn, angry, or depressed behaviors, determine, as appropriate, was this behavior unavoidable.

Probes: §483.25(f)(2)

- Did the facility attempt to evaluate whether this behavior was attributable to organic causes or other risk factors not associated with adjusting to living in the nursing facility?

- What care did the resident receive to maintain his/her mental or psychosocial functioning?

- Were individual objectives of the plan of care periodically evaluated, and if progress was not made in reducing, maintaining, or increasing behaviors that assist the resident to have his/her needs met, were alternative treatment approaches developed to maintain mental or psychosocial functioning?

- Identify if resident triggers RAPs for behavior problem, cognitive loss/dementia, and psychosocial well-being. Consider whether the RAPs were used to assess causal factors for decline, potential for decline or lack of improvement.

- Did the facility use the RAPs for behavior problems, cognitive loss/dementia, and psychosocial well-being to assess why the behaviors or change in mental or psychosocial functioning was occurring?

---

§483.25(g) Naso-Gastric Tubes

Based on the comprehensive assessment of a resident, the facility must ensure that --

(See Tag F322 for intent, guidelines, and probes for §483.25(g))

F321

§483.25(g)(1) A resident who has been able to eat enough alone or with assistance is not fed by naso-gastric tube unless the resident's clinical condition demonstrates that use of a naso-gastric tube was unavoidable; and

F322

§483.25(g)(2) A resident who is fed by a naso-gastric or gastrostomy tube receives the appropriate treatment and services to prevent aspiration pneumonia, diarrhea, vomiting, dehydration, metabolic abnormalities, and nasal-pharyngeal ulcers and to restore, if possible, normal eating skills.

Intent §483.25(g)

The intent of this regulation is that a naso-gastric tube feeding is utilized only after adequate assessment, and the resident's clinical condition makes this treatment necessary.

Interpretive Guidelines §483.25(g)

This corresponds to MDS 2.0 sections G, K, P when specified for use by the State.

This requirement is also intended to prevent the use of tube feeding when ordered over the objection of the resident. Decisions about the appropriateness of tube feeding for a resident are developed with the resident or his/her family, surrogate or representative as part of determining the care plan.

Complications in tube feeding are not necessarily the result of improper care, but assessment for the potential for complications and care and treatment are provided to prevent complications in tube feeding by the facility.

Clinical conditions demonstrating that nourishment via an naso-gastric tube is unavoidable include:

- The inability to swallow without choking or aspiration, i.e., in cases of Parkinson's disease, pseudobulbar palsy, or esophageal diverticulum;
- Lack of sufficient alertness for oral nutrition (e.g., resident comatose); and
- Malnutrition not attributable to a single cause or causes that can be isolated and reversed. There is documented evidence that the facility has not been able to maintain or improve the resident's nutritional status through oral intake.

Probes: §483.25(g)

For sampled residents who, upon admission to the facility, were not tube fed and now have a feeding tube, was tube feeding unavoidable? To determine if the tube feeding was unavoidable, assess the following:

- Did the facility identify the resident at risk for malnutrition?
- What did the facility do to maintain oral feeding, prior to inserting a feeding tube? Did staff provide enough assistance in eating? Did staff cue resident as needed, assist with the use of assistive devices, or feed the resident, if necessary?
- Is the resident receiving therapy to improve or enhance swallowing skills, as need, is identified in the comprehensive assessment?
- Was an assessment done to determine the cause of decreased oral intake/weight loss or malnutrition?
- If there was a dietitian consultation, were recommendations followed?
- For all sampled residents who are tube fed:
- Is the NG tube properly placed?
- Are staff responsibilities for providing enteral feedings clearly assigned (i.e., who administers the feeding, formula, amount, feeding intervals, flow rate)?

- Do staff monitor feeding complications (e.g., diarrhea, gastric distension, aspiration) and administer corrective actions to allay complications (e.g., changing rate of formula administration)?
- Are there negative consequences of tube use (e.g., agitation, depression, self-extubation, infections, aspiration and restraint use without a medical reason for the restraint)?
- When long term use is anticipated, is G tube placement considered?

Is the potential for complications from feedings minimized by:

- Use of a small bore, flexible naso-gastric tube, unless contraindicated;
- Securely attached the tube to the nose/face;
- Checking for correct tube placement prior to beginning a feeding or administering medications and after episodes of vomiting or suctioning;
- Checking a resident with a newly inserted gastric tube for gastric residual volume every 2-4 hours until the resident has demonstrated an ability to empty his/her stomach;
- Properly elevating the resident's head;
- Providing the type, rate and volume of the feeding as ordered;
- Using universal precautions and clean technique and as per facility/manufacturer's directions when stopping, starting, flushing, and giving medications through the tube;
- Using hang time recommendations by the manufacturer to prevent excessive microbial growth;
- Implement the procedures to ensure cleanliness of supplies, e.g. irrigating syringes changed on a regular bases as per facility policy. It is not necessary to change the irrigating syringe each time it is used;
- Using a pump equipped with a functional alarm (if pump used);
- The facility's criteria for determining that a resident may be able to return to eating by mouth (e.g., a resident whose Parkinson's symptoms have been controlled);
- There are sampled residents meet these criteria;

- If so, the facility has assisted them in returning to normal eating; and
- Identify if resident triggers RAPs for feeding tubes, nutritional status, and dehydration/fluid maintenance. Consider whether the RAPs were used to assess causal factors for decline, potential for decline and lack of improvement.

F323

(Rev. 27; Issued: 08-17-07; Effective/Implementation: 08-17-07)

§483.25(h) Accidents.

The facility must ensure that –

(1) The resident environment remains as free from accident hazards as is possible; and

(2) Each resident receives adequate supervision and assistance devices to prevent accidents.

INTENT: 42 CFR 483.25(H) (1) AND (2) ACCIDENTS AND SUPERVISION

The intent of this requirement is to ensure the facility provides an environment that is free from accident hazards over which the facility has control and provides supervision and assistive devices to each resident to prevent avoidable accidents. This includes:

- *Identifying hazard(s) and risk(s);*
- *Evaluating and analyzing hazard(s) and risk(s);*
- *Implementing interventions to reduce hazard(s) and risk(s); and*
- *Monitoring for effectiveness and modifying interventions when necessary.*

DEFINITIONS

Definitions are provided to clarify terms related to providing supervision and other interventions to prevent accidents.

- *"Accident" refers to any unexpected or unintentional incident, which may result in injury or illness to a resident. This does not include adverse outcomes that are a direct consequence of treatment or care that is provided in accordance with current standards of practice (e.g., drug side effects or reaction).*

- *"Avoidable Accident" means that an accident occurred because the facility failed to:*

  - *Identify environmental hazards and individual resident risk of an accident, including the need for supervision; and/or*
  - *Evaluate/analyze the hazards and risks; and/or*
  - *Implement interventions, including adequate supervision, consistent with a resident's needs, goals, plan of care, and current standards of practice in order to reduce the risk of an accident; and/or*
  - *Monitor the effectiveness of the interventions and modify the interventions as necessary, in accordance with current standards of practice.*

- *"Unavoidable Accident" means that an accident occurred despite facility efforts to:*

  - *Identify environmental hazards and individual resident risk of an accident, including the need for supervision; and*
  - *Evaluate/analyze the hazards and risks; and*
  - *Implement interventions, including adequate supervision, consistent with the resident's needs, goals, plan of care, and current standards of practice in order to reduce the risk of an accident; and*
  - *Monitor the effectiveness of the interventions and modify the interventions as necessary, in accordance with current standards of practice.*

- *"Assistance Device" or "Assistive Device" refers to any item (e.g., fixtures such as handrails, grab bars, and devices/equipment such as transfer lifts, canes, and wheelchairs, etc.) that is used by, or in the care of a resident to promote, supplement, or enhance the resident's function and/or safety.*

  NOTE: *The currently accepted nomenclature refers to "assistive devices." Although the term "assistance devices" is used in the regulation, the Guidance provided in this document will refer to "assistive devices."*

- *"Environment" refers to the resident environment. (See definition for "resident environment.")*

- *"Fall" refers to unintentionally coming to rest on the ground, floor, or other lower level, but not as a result of an overwhelming external force (e.g., resident pushes another resident). An episode where a resident lost his/her balance and would have fallen, if not for staff intervention, is considered a fall. A fall without injury is still a fall. Unless there is evidence suggesting otherwise, when a resident is found on the floor, a fall is considered to have occurred.*[1]

- *"Hazards" refer to elements of the resident environment that have the potential to cause injury or illness.*

    - *"Hazards over which the facility has control" are those hazards in the resident environment where reasonable efforts by the facility could influence the risk for resulting injury or illness.*

    - *"Free of accident hazards as is possible" refers to being free of accident hazards over which the facility has control.*

- *"Resident environment" includes the physical surroundings to which the resident has access (e.g., room, unit, common use areas, and facility grounds, etc.).*

- *"Risk" refers to any external factor or characteristic of an individual resident that influences the likelihood of an accident.*

- *"Supervision/Adequate Supervision" refers to an intervention and means of mitigating the risk of an accident. Facilities are obligated to provide adequate supervision to prevent accidents. Adequate supervision is defined by the type and frequency of supervision, based on the individual resident's assessed needs and identified hazards in the resident environment. Adequate supervision may vary from resident to resident and from time to time for the same resident.*

OVERVIEW

Numerous and varied accident hazards exist in everyday life. Not all accidents are avoidable. The frailty of some residents increases their vulnerability to hazards in the resident environment and can result in life threatening injuries. It is important that all facility staff understand the facility's responsibility, as well as their own, to ensure the safest environment possible for residents.

The facility is responsible for providing care to residents in a manner that helps promote quality of life. This includes respecting residents' rights to privacy, dignity and self determination, and their right to make choices about significant aspects of their life in the facility.

For various reasons, residents are exposed to some potential for harm. Although hazards should not be ignored, there are varying degrees of potential for harm. It is reasonable to accept some risks as a trade off for the potential benefits, such as maintaining dignity, self-determination, and control over one's daily life. The facility's challenge is to balance protecting the resident's right to make choices and the facility's responsibility to comply with all regulations.

The responsibility to respect a resident's choices is balanced by considering the potential impact of these choices on other individuals and on the facility's obligation to protect the residents from harm. The facility has a responsibility to educate a resident, family, and staff regarding significant risks related to a resident's choices. Incorporating a resident's choices into the plan of care can help the facility balance interventions to reduce the risk of an accident, while honoring the resident's autonomy.

Consent by resident or responsible party alone does not relieve the provider of its responsibility to assure the health, safety, and welfare of its residents, including protecting them from avoidable accidents. While Federal regulations affirm the resident's right to participate in care planning and to refuse treatment, the regulations do not create the right for a resident, legal surrogate, or representative to demand the facility use specific medical interventions or treatments that the facility deems inappropriate. The regulations hold the facility ultimately accountable for the resident's care and safety. Verbal consent or signed consent forms do not eliminate a facility's responsibility to protect a resident from an avoidable accident.

An effective way for the facility to avoid accidents is to commit to safety and implement systems that address resident risk and environmental hazards to minimize the likelihood of accidents.[2, 3] *A facility with a commitment to safety:*

- *Acknowledges the high-risk nature of its population and setting;*
- *Develops a reporting system that does not place blame on the staff member for reporting resident risks and environmental hazards;*
- *Involves all staff in helping identify solutions to ensure a safe resident environment;*
- *Directs resources to address safety concerns; and*
- *Demonstrates a commitment to safety at all levels of the organization.*

A SYSTEMS APPROACH

Establishing and utilizing a systematic approach to resident safety helps facilities comply with the regulations at 42 CFR §483.25(h)(1) and (2). Processes in a facility's system approach may include:

- *Identification of hazards, including inadequate supervision, and a resident's risks of potentially avoidable accidents in the resident environment;*
- *Evaluation and analysis of hazards and risks;*

- *Implementation of interventions, including adequate supervision and assistive devices, to reduce individual risks related to hazards in the environment; and*

- *Monitoring for effectiveness and modification of interventions when necessary.*

A key element of a systematic approach is the consistent application of a process to consistently address identified hazards and/or risks. Risks may pertain to individual residents, groups of residents, or the entire facility. Hazards may include, but are not limited to, aspects of the physical plant, equipment, and devices that are defective or are not used properly (per manufacturer's specifications), are disabled/removed, or are not individually adapted or fitted to the resident's needs. An effective system not only identifies environmental hazards and the resident's risk for an avoidable accident, but also the resident's need for supervision.

Identifying and addressing risks, including the potential for accidents, includes consideration of the environment, the resident's risk factors, and the need for supervision, care, and assistive devices. This will allow the facility to communicate information about observed hazards, identify resident-specific information, develop and implement an individualized plan of care to address each resident's needs and goals, and to monitor the results of the planned interventions. The plan of care should strive to balance the resident's wishes with the potential impact on other residents.

A systematic approach allows the facility to adjust its responses depending on the urgency of the situation and the hazards identified. The system includes a means for communicating the observations of hazards and the recording of resident specific information. Risks identified by the facility can pertain to individual residents or groups of residents. The facility-centered approach addresses risks for groups of residents; whereas, the resident-directed approach addresses risks for the individual residents.

Identification of Hazards and Risks

Identification of hazards and risks is the process through which the facility becomes aware of potential hazards in the resident environment and the risk of a resident having an avoidable accident. All staff (e.g., professional, administrative, maintenance, etc.) are to be involved in observing and identifying potential hazards in the environment, while taking into consideration the unique characteristics and abilities of each resident. The facility should make a reasonable effort to identify the hazards and risk factors for each resident. Various sources provide information about hazards and risks in the resident environment. These sources may include, but are not limited to, quality assurance activities, environmental rounds, MDS/RAPs data, medical history and physical exam, and individual observation. This information is to be documented and communicated across all disciplines.

Evaluation and Analysis

Evaluation and analysis is the process of examining data to identify specific hazards and risks and to develop targeted interventions to reduce the potential for accidents.

Interdisciplinary involvement is a critical component of this process. Analysis may include, for example, considering the severity of hazards, the immediacy of risk, and trends such as time of day, location, etc.

Both the facility-centered and resident-directed approaches include evaluating hazard and accident risk data, analyzing potential causes for each hazard and accident risk, and identifying or developing interventions based on the severity of the hazards and immediacy of risk. Evaluations also look at trends such as time of day, location, etc.

Implementation of Interventions

Implementation refers to using specific interventions to try to reduce a resident's risks from hazards in the environment. The process includes: Communicating the interventions to all relevant staff, assigning responsibility, providing training as needed, documenting interventions (e.g., plans of action developed by the Quality Assurance Committee or care plans for the individual resident), and ensuring that the interventions are put into action.

Interventions are based on the results of the evaluation and analysis of information about hazards and risks and are consistent with relevant standards, including evidence-based practice. Development of interim safety measures may be necessary if interventions cannot immediately be implemented fully.

Facility-based interventions may include, but are not limited to, educating staff, repairing the device/equipment, and developing or revising policies and procedures. Resident-directed approaches may include implementing specific interventions as part of the plan of care, supervising staff and residents, etc. Facility records document the implementation of these interventions.

Monitoring and Modification

Monitoring is the process of evaluating the effectiveness of interventions. Modification is the process of adjusting interventions as needed to make them more effective in addressing hazards and risks.

Monitoring and modification processes include:

(1) *Ensuring that interventions are implemented correctly and consistently;*

(2) *Eevaluating the effectiveness of interventions;*

(3) *Modifying or replacing interventions as needed and*

(4) *Evaluating the effectiveness of new interventions.*

An example of facility-specific modification is additional training of staff when equipment has been upgraded. An example of a resident-specific modification is revising the plan of care to reflect the resident's current condition and risk factors that may have changed since the previous assessment.

SUPERVISION

Supervision is an intervention and a means of mitigating accident risk. Facilities are obligated to provide adequate supervision to prevent accidents. Adequacy of supervision is defined by type and frequency, based on the individual resident's assessed needs, and identified hazards in the resident environment. Adequate supervision may vary from resident to resident and from time to time for the same resident. Tools or items such as personal alarms can help to monitor a resident's activities, but do not eliminate the need for adequate supervision.

The resident environment may contain temporary hazards (e.g., construction, painting, housekeeping activities, etc.) that warrant additional supervision or alternative measures such as barriers to prevent access to affected areas of the resident environment.

Adequate supervision to prevent accidents is enhanced when the facility:

- *Accurately assesses a resident and/or the resident environment to determine whether supervision to avoid an accident is necessary; and/or*

- *Determines that supervision of the resident was necessary and provides supervision based on the individual resident's assessed needs and the risks identified in the environment.*

Resident Smoking

Some facilities permit residents to smoke tobacco products. In these facilities, assessment of the resident's capabilities and deficits determines whether or not supervision is required. If the facility identifies that the resident needs supervision for smoking, the facility includes this information in the resident's plan of care, and reviews and revises the plan periodically as needed.

The facility may designate certain areas for resident smoking. The facility must ensure precautions are taken for the resident's individual safety, as well as the safety of others in the facility. Such precautions may include smoking only in designated areas, supervising residents whose assessment and plans of care indicate a need for supervised smoking, and limiting the accessibility of matches and lighters by residents who need supervision when smoking. Smoking by residents when oxygen is in use is prohibited, and any smoking by others near flammable substances is also problematic. Additional measures may include informing all visitors of smoking policies and hazards.

Guidance concerning resident smoking regulations can be found in NFPA 101, the Life Safety Code at 19.7.4, Smoking, including requirements for signage, prohibiting smoking by residents classified as not responsible, and disposal of smoking materials. Refer to the guidance at 42 CFR 483.15(b)(3) [F242] for information about facilities that desire to be smoke-free.

Resident-to-Resident Altercations

NOTE: *An incident involving a resident who willfully inflicts injury upon another resident should be reviewed as abuse under the guidance for 42 CFR §483.13(b) at F223. "Willful" means that the individual intended the action itself that he/she knew or should have known could cause physical harm, pain, or mental anguish. Even though a resident may have a cognitive impairment, he/she could still commit a willful act. However, there are instances when a resident's willful intent cannot be determined. In those cases, a resident-to-resident altercation should be reviewed under this tag, F323.*

It is important that a facility take reasonable precautions, including providing adequate supervision, when the risk of resident-to-resident altercation is identified, or should have been identified. Certain situations or conditions may increase the potential for such altercations, including, but not limited to:

- *A history of aggressive behaviors including striking out, verbal outbursts, or negative interactions with other resident(s); and/or*
- *Behavior that tends to disrupt or annoy others such as constant verbalization (e.g., crying, yelling, calling out for help), making negative remarks, restlessness, repetitive behaviors, taking items that do not belong to them, going into others' rooms, drawers, or closets, and undressing in inappropriate areas. Although these behaviors may not be aggressive in nature, they may precipitate a negative response from others, resulting in verbal, physical, and/or emotional harm.*

The facility is responsible for identifying residents who have a history of disruptive or intrusive interactions, or who exhibit other behaviors that make them more likely to be involved in an altercation. The facility should identify the factors (e.g., illness, environment, etc.) that increase the risks associated with individual residents, including those (e.g., disease, environment) that could trigger an altercation. The care planning team reviews the assessment along with the resident and/or his/her representative, in order to identify interventions to try to prevent altercations.

The interventions listed below include supervision and other actions that could address potential or actual negative interactions:

- *Providing safe supervised areas for unrestricted movement;*
- *Eliminating or reducing underlying causes of distressed behavior such as boredom and pain;*
- *Monitoring environmental influences such as temperatures, lighting, and noise levels;*

- *Evaluating staffing assignments to ensure consistent staff who are more familiar with the resident and who thus may be able to identify changes in a resident's condition and behavior;*

- *Evaluating staffing levels to ensure adequate supervision (if it is adequate, it is meeting the resident's needs); and*

- *Ongoing staff training and supervision, including how to approach a resident who may be agitated, combative, verbally or physically aggressive, or anxious, and how and when to obtain assistance in managing a resident with behavior symptoms.*

RESIDENT RISKS AND ENVIRONMENTAL HAZARDS

This section discusses common, but not all, potential hazards found in the resident environment.

NOTE: *The information included in the following sections is based on current standards of practice or "best practice" models as described in the industry literature.*

The physical plant, devices, and equipment described in this section may not be hazards by themselves. But they can become hazardous when a vulnerable resident interacts with them. Some temporary hazards in the resident environment can affect most residents who have access to them (e.g., construction, painting, and housekeeping activities). Other situations may be hazardous only for certain individuals (e.g., accessible smoking materials).

In order to be considered hazardous, an element of the resident environment must be accessible to a vulnerable resident. Resident vulnerability is based on risk factors including the individual resident's functional status, medical condition, cognitive abilities, mood, and health treatments (e.g., medications). Resident vulnerability to hazards may change over time. Ongoing assessment helps identify when elements in the environment pose hazards to a particular resident.

Certain sharp items, such as scissors, kitchen utensils, knitting needles, or other items, may be appropriate for many residents but hazardous for others with cognitive impairments. Handrails, assistive devices, and any surface that a resident may come in contact with may cause injury, if the surface is not in good condition and free from sharp edges or other hazards.

Improper actions or omissions by staff can create hazards in the physical plant (e.g., building and grounds), environment, and/or with devices and equipment. Examples of such hazards might include fire doors that have been propped open, disabled locks or latches, nonfunctioning alarms, buckled or badly torn carpets, cords on floors, irregular walking surfaces, improper storage and access to toxic chemicals, exposure to unsafe heating unit surfaces, and unsafe water temperatures. Other potential hazards may include furniture that is not appropriate for a resident (e.g., chairs or beds that are too low or unstable as to present a fall hazard) and lighting that is either inadequate or so intense as to create glare. Devices for resident care, such as pumps, ventilators, and assistive devices, may be hazardous when they are defective, disabled, or improperly used (i.e., used in a manner that is not per manufacturer's recommendations or current standards of practice).

Resident Vulnerabilities

Falls and unsafe wandering/elopement are of particular concern. The following section reviews these issues along with some common potential hazards.
Falls - The MDS defines a fall as unintentionally coming to rest on the ground, floor, or other lower level but not as a result of an overwhelming external force (e.g., resident pushes another resident). An episode where a resident lost his/her balance and would have fallen, if not for staff intervention, is considered a fall. A fall without injury is still a fall. Unless there is evidence suggesting otherwise, when a resident is found on the floor, a fall is considered to have occurred.[1]

Some factors that may result in resident falls include (but are not limited to) environmental hazards, underlying medical conditions, medication side effects, and other factors (e.g., lower extremity weakness, balance disorders, poor grip strength, functional and cognitive impairment, visual deficits, etc.).

Older persons have both a high incidence of falls and a high susceptibility to injury.[4] *Falls can have psychological and social consequences, including the loss of self-confidence to try to ambulate. Evaluation of the causal factors leading to a resident fall helps support relevant and consistent interventions to try to prevent future occurrences. Proper actions following a fall include:*

- *Ascertaining if there were injuries, and providing treatment as necessary;*
- *Determining what may have caused or contributed to the fall;*
- *Addressing the factors for the fall; and*
- *Revising the resident's plan of care and/or facility practices, as needed, to reduce the likelihood of another fall.*

NOTE: *A fall by a resident does not necessarily indicate a deficient practice because not every fall can be avoided.*

Unsafe Wandering or Elopement - Wandering is random or repetitive locomotion. This movement may be goal-directed (e.g., the person appears to be searching for something such as an exit) or may be non-goal-directed or aimless. Non-goal-directed wandering requires a response in a manner that addresses both safety issues and an evaluation to identify root causes to the degree possible. Moving about the facility aimlessly may indicate that the resident is frustrated, anxious, bored, hungry, or depressed. Unsafe wandering and elopement can be associated with falls and related injuries.[5]

Unsafe wandering may occur when the resident at risk enters an area that is physically hazardous or that contains potential safety hazards (e.g., chemicals, tools, and equipment, etc.). Entering into another resident's room may lead to an altercation or contact with hazardous items.[5]

While alarms can help to monitor a resident's activities, staff must be vigilant in order to respond to them in a timely manner. Alarms do not replace necessary supervision.

Elopement occurs when a resident leaves the premises or a safe area without authorization (i.e., an order for discharge or leave of absence) and/or any necessary supervision to do so. A resident who leaves a safe area may be at risk of (or has the potential to experience) heat or cold exposure, dehydration and/or other medical complications, drowning, or being struck by a motor vehicle. Facility policies that clearly define the mechanisms and procedures for monitoring and managing residents at risk for elopement can help to minimize the risk of a resident leaving a safe area without authorization and/or appropriate supervision. In addition, the resident at risk should have interventions in their comprehensive plan of care to address the potential for elopement. Furthermore, a facility's disaster and emergency preparedness plan should include a plan to locate a missing resident.[5]

Physical Plant Hazards

Supervision and/or containment of hazards are needed to protect residents from harm caused by environmental hazards. Examples of such hazards can range from common chemical cleaning materials to those caused by adverse water temperatures or improper use of electrical devices.

Chemicals and Toxins - Various materials in the resident environment can pose a potential hazard to residents. Hazardous materials can be found in the form of solids, liquids, gases, mists, dusts, fumes, and vapors. The routes of exposure for toxic materials may include inhalation, absorption, or ingestion.

For a material to pose a safety hazard to a resident, it must be toxic, caustic, or allergenic; accessible and available in a sufficient amount to cause harm. Toxic materials that may be present in the resident environment are unlikely to pose a hazard unless residents have access or are exposed to them. Some materials that would be considered harmless when used as designed could pose a hazard to a resident who accidentally ingests or makes contact with them.

Examples of materials that may pose a hazard to a resident include (but are not limited to):

- *Chemicals used by the facility staff in the course of their duties (e.g., housekeeping chemicals) and chemicals or other materials brought into the resident environment by staff, other residents, or visitors;*

- *Drugs and therapeutic agents;*

- *Plants and other "natural" materials found in the resident environment or in the outdoor environment (e.g., poison ivy).*

One source of information concerning the hazards of a material that a facility may obtain is its Material Safety Data Sheet (MSDS).[6] The Occupational Safety and Health Administration (OSHA) requires employers to have a MSDS available for all hazardous materials that staff use while performing their duties.[7] MSDSs are available on-line for numerous chemicals and non-toxic materials, and should be reviewed carefully to determine if the material is toxic and poses a hazard. Poison control centers are another source of information for potential hazards, including non-chemical hazards such as plants.

NOTE: *Toxicological profiles for a limited number of hazardous materials are accessible on the Agency for Toxic Substances & Disease Registry Web site.[6]*

Water Temperature - Water may reach hazardous temperatures in hand sinks, showers, and tubs. Burns related to hot water/liquids may also be due to spills and/or immersion. Many residents in long-term care facilities have conditions that may put them at increased risk for burns caused by scalding. These conditions include: decreased skin thickness, decreased skin sensitivity, peripheral neuropathy, decreased agility (reduced reaction time), decreased cognition or dementia, decreased mobility, and decreased ability to communicate.[8]

The degree of injury depends on factors including the water temperature, the amount of skin exposed, and the duration of exposure. Some States have regulations regarding allowable maximum water temperature. Table 1 illustrates damage to skin in relation to the temperature of the water and the length of time of exposure.[9]

Table 1. Time and Temperature Relationship to Serious Burns

Water Temperature		*Time Required for a 3rd Degree Burn to Occur*
155°F	*68°C*	*1 sec*
148°F	*64°C*	*2 sec*
140°F	*60°C*	*5 sec*
133°F	*56°C*	*15 sec*
127°F	*52°C*	*1 min*
124°F	*51°C*	*3 min*
120°F	*48°C*	*5 min*
100°F	*37°C*	*Safe Temperatures for Bathing (see Note)*

> ***NOTE:*** *Burns can occur even at water temperatures below those identified in the table, depending on an individual's condition and the length of exposure.*

Based upon the time of the exposure and the temperature of the water, the severity of the harm to the skin is identified by the degree of burn, as follows.[10]

- *First-degree burns involve the top layer of skin (e.g., minor sunburn). These may present as red and painful to touch, and the skin will show mild swelling.*

- *Second-degree burns involve the first two layers of skin. These may present as deep reddening of the skin, pain, blisters, glossy appearance from leaking fluid, and possible loss of some skin.*

- *Third-degree burns penetrate the entire thickness of the skin and permanently destroy tissue. These present as loss of skin layers, often painless (pain may be caused by patches of first- and second-degree burns surrounding third-degree burns), and dry, leathery skin. Skin may appear charred or have patches that appear white, brown, or black.*

Electrical Safety - Any electrical device, whether or not it needs to be plugged into an electric outlet, can become hazardous to the residents through improper use or improper maintenance. Electrical equipment such as electrical cords can become tripping hazards. Halogen lamps or heat lamps can cause burns or fires if not properly installed away from combustibles in the resident environment. The Life Safety Code prohibits the use of portable electrical space heaters in resident areas.

Extension cords should not be used to take the place of adequate wiring in a facility. If extension cords are used, the cords should be properly secured and not be placed overhead, under carpets or rugs, or anywhere that the cord can cause trips, falls, or overheat. Extension cords should be connected to only one device to prevent overloading of the circuit. The cord itself should be of a size and type for the expected electrical load and made of material that will not fray or cut easily. Electrical cords including extension cords should have proper grounding if required and should not have any grounding devices removed or not used if required.

Power strips may not be used as a substitute for adequate electrical outlets in a facility. Power strips may be used for a computer, monitor, and printer. Power strips are not designed to be used with medical devices in patient care areas. Precautions needed if power strips are used include: installing internal ground fault and over-current protection devices; preventing cords from becoming tripping hazards; and using power strips that are adequate for the number and types of devices used. Overload on any circuit can potentially cause overheating and fire. The use of ground fault circuit interruption (GFCIs) may be required in locations near water sources to prevent electrocution of staff or residents.[11]

The proper use of electric blankets and heating pads is essential to avoid thermal injuries. These items should not be tucked in or squeezed. Constriction can cause the internal wires to break. A resident should not go to sleep with an electric blanket or heating pad turned on. Manufacturer's instructions for use should be followed closely. Injuries and deaths have been related to burns and fires related to the use of heating pads. Most deaths are attributable to heating pads that generated fires, but most injuries are burns from prolonged use or inappropriate temperature setting. Prolonged use on one area of the body can cause a severe burn, even when the heating pad is at a low temperature setting.[12]

Lighting - The risk of an accident increases when there is insufficient light or too much light, which often results in glare. Vision among older persons varies widely; therefore, no single level of illumination can ensure safety for all residents. The proper amount of light depends on the resident's visual needs and the task he/she is performing.

An older person typically needs more light to see. However, a resident with cataracts or glaucoma may be overly sensitive to bright light, and excessive lighting could make it more difficult to see clearly and thereby increase his/her fall risk.[13] *Creating transitional zones between light and dark spaces helps to improve sight recovery and enable safer mobility. Providing extra visual cues that clearly define needed items or spaces in areas with limited or variable light can help to enable safe performance of tasks (e.g., turning on a light). Providing supplemental light near beds for patients who are mobile may assist in safe mobility at night.*[14]

NOTE: *Refer to guidance for 42 CFR 483.15(h)(5) [F256] for lighting issues related to Quality of Life.*

Assistive Devices/Equipment Hazards

Assistive devices also can help to prevent accidents. Assistive devices and equipment can help residents move with increased independence, transfer with greater comfort, and feel physically more secure. However, there are risks associated with the use of such devices and equipment, and these risks need to be balanced with the benefits gained from their use. Training of staff, residents, family members and volunteers on the proper use of assistive devices/equipment is crucial to prevent accidents. It is also important to communicate clearly the approaches identified in the care plan to all staff, including temporary staff. It is important to train staff regarding resident assessment, safe transfer techniques, and the proper use of mechanical lifts including device weight limitations.

NOTE: The Safe Medical Devices Act of 1990 (SMDA) requires hospitals, nursing homes, and other user facilities to report deaths, serious illnesses, and injuries associated with the use of medical devices to manufacturers and the Food and Drug Administration.

Assistive Devices for Mobility - Mobility devices include all types of assistive devices, such as, but not limited to, canes, standard and rolling walkers, manual or non-powered wheelchairs, and powered wheelchairs. Three primary factors that may be associated with an increased accident risk related to the use of assistive devices include:

1. *Resident Condition. Lower extremity weakness, gait disturbances, decreased range of motion, and poor balance may affect some residents. These conditions combined with cognitive impairment can increase the accident risks of using mobility devices. Unsafe behavior, such as failure to lock wheelchair brakes and trying to stand or transfer from a wheelchair unsafely, can result in falls and related injuries;*

2. *Personal Fit and Device Condition. Devices can pose a hazard if not fitted and/or maintained properly.*[15] *Personal fit, or how well the assistive device meets the individual needs of the resident, may influence the likelihood of an avoidable accident; and*

3. *Staff Practices. Mobility devices that a resident cannot readily reach may create a hazardous situation. Unsafe transfer technique used by staff may result in an accident. Inadequate supervision by staff of a resident during the initial trial period of assistive device use or after a change in the resident's functional status can increase the risk of falls and/or injury. Additionally, staff needs to ensure assistive devises properly fit the resident and the resident has received proper training in the use of the assistive device.*

Assistive Devices for Transfer - Mechanical assistive devices for transfer include, but are not limited to, portable total body lifts, sit-to-stand devices, and transfer or gait belts. The resident assessment helps to determine the resident's degree of mobility and physical impairment and the proper transfer method; for example, whether one or more caregivers or a mechanical device is needed for a safe transfer. Residents who become frightened during transfer in a mechanical lift may exhibit resistance movements that can result in avoidable accidents. Communicating with the resident and addressing the resident's fear may reduce the risk.

Factors that may influence a resident's risk of accident during transfer include staff availability, resident abilities, and staff training.[16] *The resident's ability to communicate and identify physical limitations or to aid in the transfer will help determine the need for an assistive device, such as a mechanical lift.*

Devices Associated with Entrapment Risks - Devices can be therapeutic and beneficial; however, devices are not necessarily risk free so it is important to weigh the relative risks and benefits of using certain devices. For example, while physical restraints may be used to treat a resident's medical symptom, the devices may create a risk for entrapment. Physical restraints are defined in the SOM at F221 as any manual method, physical or mechanical device, material, or equipment attached or adjacent to the resident's body that the individual cannot remove easily and that restricts freedom of movement or normal access to one's body.

In 1992, the Food and Drug Administration (FDA) issued a Safety Alert entitled "Potential Hazards with Restraint Devices".[17] *Serious injuries, as well as death, have been reported as a result of using physical restraints. Some physical restraints carry a risk of severe injury, strangulation, and asphyxiation. Restrained residents may be injured or die when they try to remove restraints, to ambulate while restrained, or due to an improperly fitted or used device.*

Regardless of the purpose for use, bed rails (also referred to as "side rails," "bed side rails," and "safety rails") and other bed accessories (e.g., transfer bar, bed enclosures), while assisting with transfer and positioning, can increase resident safety risk. Bed rails include rails of various sizes (e.g., full length rails, half rails, quarter rails) that may be positioned in various locations on the bed. In 1995, the FDA issued a Safety Alert entitled "Entrapment Hazards with Hospital Bed Side Rails."[18] Residents most at risk for entrapment are those who are frail or elderly or those who have conditions such as agitation, delirium, confusion, pain, uncontrolled body movement, hypoxia, fecal impaction, acute urinary retention, etc. that may cause them to move about the bed or try to exit from the bed. The timeliness of toileting, appropriateness of positioning, and other care-related activities can contribute to the risk of entrapment.[19]

Entrapment may occur when a resident is caught between the mattress and bed rail or in the bed rail itself. Technical issues, such as the proper sizing of mattresses, fit and integrity of bed rails or other design elements (e.g., wide spaces between bars in the bed rails) can also affect the risk of resident entrapment.[19]

The use of a specialty air-filled mattress or a therapeutic air-filled bed may also present an entrapment risk that is different from rail entrapment with a regular mattress. The high compressibility of an air-filled mattress compared to a regular conventional mattress requires appropriate precautions when used for a resident at risk for entrapment. An air-filled mattress compresses on the side to which a person moves, thus raising the center of the mattress and lowering the side. This may make it easier for a resident to slide off the mattress or against the rail. Mattress compression widens the space between the mattress and rail. When a resident is between the mattress and rail, the mattress can re-expand and press the chest, neck, or head against the rail. While using air therapy to prevent and treat pressure ulcers, facilities should also take precautions to reduce the risk of entrapment. Precautions may include following manufacturer equipment alerts and increasing supervision.[20]

NOTE: *42 CFR 483.13(a), F221, applies to the use of physical restraints. 42 CFR 483.25(h)(2), F323 applies to assistive devices that create hazards (e.g., devices that are defective; not used properly or according to manufacturer's specifications; disabled or removed; not provided or do not meet the resident's needs (poor fit or not adapted); and/or used without adequate supervision when required).*

ENDNOTES

[1] Centers for Medicare & Medicaid Services. (December 2002 revised June 2006). Revised Long-Term Care Facility Resident Assessment Instrument User's Manual. Version 2.0, 3-146.

[2] *Pizzi, L.T., Goldfarb, N.I., Nash, D.B. (2002). Promoting a culture of safety. In: K.G. Shojania, B.W. Duncan, K.M. McDonald , & R.M. Wachter (Eds.), Evidence Report/Technology Assessment, No. 43. Making Health Care Safer: A Critical Analysis of Patient Safety Practices. Rockville, MD: Agency for Healthcare Research and Quality. Retrieved February 9, 2004 from <http://www.ahrq.gov/clinic/ptsafety/chap40.htm>.*

[3] *Singer, S.J., Gaba, D.M., Geppert, J.J., et al. (2003). The culture of safety: Results of an organization-wide survey in 15 California hospitals. Qual Saf Health Care, 12, 112-118.*

[4] *American Geriatrics Society, British Geriatrics Society American Academy of Orthopedic Surgeons Panel on Falls Prevention. (2001). Guideline for the prevention of falls in older persons. J Am Geriatr Soc, 49, 664–672.*

[5] *Boltz, M. (2003). Litigation Issues Related To Wandering and Elopement. The John A. Hartford Foundation Institute for Geriatric Nursing, New York University, The Steinhardt School of Education, Division of Nursing. Retrieved November 30, 2005 from http://www.hartfordign.org/resources/special topics/spectopics.html>*

[6] *Agency for Toxic Substances & Disease Registry web site at http://www.atsdr.cdc.gov/toxpro2.html.*

[7] *US Dept. of Labor, Occupational Safety and Health Standards, 29 CFR 1910.1200 (g)(1) and (2)*

[8] *Katcher, L.K. (1981). Scald Burns from Hot Tap Water. Journal of Am Med Assoc., 246(11), 1219-1222.*

[9] *Moritz, A.R., Henriques F.C. Jr. (1947). Studies of Thermal Injury: II. The Relative Importance of Time and Surface Temperatures in the Causation of Cutaneous Burns. Am J Pathology, 23, 695-720.*

[10] *US Dept. of Health and Human Services. Centers for Disease Control and Prevention. (June 12, 2003). Emergency Preparedness & Response. Burns. Retrieved November 8, 2005 from <http://www.bt.cdc.gov/masstrauma/burns.asp>*

[11] *Electrical Safety Foundation International. Plug into Electrical Safety. Retrieved February 9, 2004 from <http://www.nesf.org/index.html>.*

[12] *US Dept. of Health and Human Services. Food and Drug Administration. (December 12, 1995). Public Health Advisory: Hazards Associated with the Use of Electric Heating Pads.*

[13] *Tideiksaar, R. (1998). Falls in Older Persons: Prevention and Management (2nd Edition). Baltimore, MD: Health Profession Press.*

[14] *Warren, M. (2001), Occupational Therapy Practice Guidelines for Adults with Low Vision, The American Occupational Therapy Association, Inc.*

[15] *Taylor, J.A., Brown, A.K., Meredith, S., Ray, W.A. (2002). The fall reduction program: a comprehensive program for reduction of falls and injuries in long-term care residents. Nashville, TN: Department of Preventive Medicine, Vanderbilt University School of Medicine.*

[16] *US Dept. of Veterans Affairs, Office of Occupational Safety and Health. (January. 2003). Safe Patient Movement and Handling Guide.*

[17] *US Dept. of Health and Human Services. Food and Drug Administration. (July 15, 1992). FDA Safety Alert: Potential Hazards with Restraint Devices.*

[18] *US Dept. of Health and Human Services. Food and Drug Administration. (August 23, 1995). FDA Safety Alert: Entrapment Hazards with Hospital Bed Side Rails.*

[19] *US Dept. of Health and Human Services, Food and Drug Administration, Hospital Bed Safety Workgroup. (April 2003), Clinical Guidance For the Assessment and Implementation of Bed Rails In Hospitals, Long Term Care Facilities, and Home Care Settings. Retrieved November 11, 2005 from http://www.fda.gov/cdrh/beds/.*

[20] *Miles, S. (June 2002). Death between bedrails and air pressured mattresses. J Am Geriatr Soc, 50(6), 1124-5.*

NOTE: References to non-CMS/HHS sources or sites on the Internet included above or later in this document are provided as a service and do not constitute or imply endorsement of these organizations or their programs by CMS or the U.S. Department of Health and Human Services. CMS is not responsible for the content of pages found at these sites. URL addresses were current as of the date of this publication.

INVESTIGATIVE PROTOCOL

ACCIDENTS AND SUPERVISION

Objectives

- *To determine if the facility has identified hazard(s) present in the resident environment and the individual resident's risks for an avoidable accident posed by those hazards;*
- *To determine if a resident accident was avoidable or unavoidable;*
- *To evaluate whether the facility provides an environment that is as free as possible of hazards over which the facility has control, and minimizes the potential for harm; and*
- *To determine if the facility provides adequate supervision and assistive devices to prevent avoidable accidents.*

Use

Use this protocol:

- *For a sampled resident who is at risk for, or who has a history of accidents, falls, or unsafe wandering/elopement, to determine if the facility provided care and services, including assistive devices as necessary, to prevent avoidable accidents and to reduce the resident's risk to the extent possible;*
- *For a sampled resident who is at risk for accidents or who creates a risk to others, to determine if the facility has provided adequate supervision; and*
- *For identified hazards/risks, to determine if there are facility practices in place to identify, evaluate and analyze hazards/risks; implement interventions to reduce or eliminate the hazards/risks, to the extent possible; and monitor the effectiveness of the interventions.*

Procedures

Observe the general environment and sampled resident environment. For a sampled resident, briefly review the assessment and plan of care to determine whether the facility identified resident risks and implemented interventions as necessary to guide observations during the investigation. For a newly admitted resident at risk for avoidable accidents, determine if the staff assessed and provided appropriate care from the day of admission. Corroborate observations through interview and record review.

1. Observation

The survey team should make observations and investigate potential hazards that may be encountered throughout the survey. The existence of hazards may indicate a more serious problem; for example, that the organization lacks an effective system to identify and correct the problem independently. The previous discussion of specific common hazards guides surveyors to look for items indicating a failure or absence of an organization's systems and processes to enable safety.

During observation of the facility, the survey team may see individual residents who are smoking tobacco products. Whether or not these residents are part of the sample, the issue of facility fires is important enough that the survey team should determine if the situation is hazardous, requiring further investigation.

Observe the environment for the presence of potential/actual hazards including, but not limited to, the following:

- *Accessibility of chemicals, toxics or other hazards such as housekeeping chemicals and supplies, medications, sharp utensils/tools, and cigarette lighters/smoking materials;*

- *Environmental conditions such as unstable or slippery floor surfaces, loose hand rails, excessive water temperatures, electrical hazards, insufficient or excessive light (glare), arrangement of living spaces, obstacles in corridors, unsupervised access into or egress out of the facility, low or loose toilet seats, defective or non-functioning beds, or malfunctioning wheelchair brakes;*

- *Staff responses to verbal calls for help and alarms such as door, personal, and equipment alarms, and call bells;*

- *Assistive devices/equipment (e.g., mobility devices, lifts and transfer aids, bed rails, call lights, physical restraints, pumps, belts) that are defective; not used properly or according to manufacturer's specifications; disabled or removed; not provided or do not meet the resident's needs (poor fit or not adapted); and/or used without adequate supervision, in relation to the facility's assessment of the resident; and/or*

- *Staff response to potential/actual hazard(s) (e.g., cleaning up spilled liquids in a resident area, keeping residents away from the hazard).*

For a sampled resident at risk, observe whether staff implement the care plan consistently over time and across various shifts. Observe how staff respond to any identified resident hazards. Observe how staff supervise the resident, such as during transfers and/or meals, and if caregivers have removed or modified observed hazards. During observations of the interventions, follow up on deviations from the plan of care, as well as potential negative outcomes.

For a resident who smokes, the facility's determination regarding the resident's abilities and capabilities would indicate whether supervision is required. If the resident is found to need supervision for smoking, this information is included in the resident's plan of care. Observe sampled resident(s) in the facility's designated smoking area. If the resident's care plan states supervision is required while smoking, confirm that supervision is provided. For others, note any concerns such as difficulty holding or lighting a cigarette or burned areas in clothing that may indicate the need for supervision.

Observe the resident to determine how the resident's risk influences his/her vulnerability to the observed potential hazard(s) and potential for an accident. Evaluate how the resident's risks relate to the observed potential hazards such as:

- *The resident's access to the hazard and the ability to react appropriately; and/or*

- *The adequacy of the supervision provided for the resident who has been assessed to need supervision in relation to the identified potential hazard(s).*

2. Interview

Conduct interviews to determine the relationship between the resident's risk and hazards.

Interview the resident, family, and/or responsible party to the degree possible to identify:

- *If the resident and/or responsible party reported, or helped identify the resident's risks for an accident and significant hazards in the resident's environment;*

- *If the resident and/or responsible party was aware of or identified a potential hazard for other residents;*

- *If the resident and/or responsible party reported a hazard or potential risk to staff; and*

- *How and when staff responded to a hazard once it was identified.*

Interview staff to determine:

- *If they were aware of planned interventions to reduce a resident's risk for an avoidable accident;*

- *If they reported potential resident risks or environmental hazards to the supervisor or others according to facility policy;*

- *If they acted to correct an immediate hazard, such as spilled liquids; and*

- *If they are aware of, and follow facility procedures correctly to remove or reduce hazards.*

3. Record Review

Assessment and Evaluation: Review the RAI and other documents such as progress notes, physician orders, and nurses' and consultants' notes regarding the assessment of the resident's overall condition and risk factors to determine if the facility identified the resident's risk for avoidable accidents, evaluated and analyzed any risks, implemented interventions to try to prevent accidents and reduce the resident's risks, and monitored and modified interventions as necessary.

Determine if the facility assessment is consistent with or corroborated by documentation within the record and reflects the status of the resident for:

- *Behavior such as unsafe wandering, elopement, ingesting nonfood items, altercations with others;*
- *Hearing, visual, and sensory impairments;*
- *Impaired physical functioning, balance, or gait problems;*
- *Diagnoses that could relate to safety awareness and safe practices, such as Alzheimer's and other dementias, arthritis, Parkinson's disease, seizure disorder, osteoporosis, cardiovascular/cerebrovascular diseases, depression/psychosis;*
- *Symptoms/conditions that could affect safety risk, such as vertigo, postural hypotension, or acute illness;*
- *Use of physical restraints and/or other devices that might limit movement;*
- *Medications that could affect function, level of consciousness, gait, balance, visual acuity, or cognitive ability, use such as antidepressants, anticholinergic medications, anti-hypertensives, diuretics, psychotropic medications, or initiation of new medication therapy; and*
- *History of falls.*

Plan of Care: Review the plan of care to determine if the facility developed interventions based on the resident's risks to try to prevent avoidable accidents, and if the plan was modified as needed based on the response, outcomes, and needs of the resident.

If the resident has had an accident, review the record to determine if the accident is:

- *The result of an order not being followed; and/or*
- *A care need not being addressed; and/or*

- *A plan of care not being implemented.*

In addition, determine if the facility (1) investigated the cause of the accident and (2) if indicated, implemented revised interventions to prevent additional avoidable accidents.

Plan of Care Revision: Determine if the facility has monitored a resident's condition and the effectiveness of the plan of care interventions and has made revisions (or has documented justification for continuing the existing plan) based upon the following:

- *The outcome and/or effects of goals and interventions;*

- *Resident failure to comply with the plan of care and interventions;*

- *Input by the resident and/or the responsible person; and*

- *Changes in condition such as the ability to make decisions, cognition, functional impairment, or changes in the medication regimen.*

4. Review of Facility Practices

The presence or absence of effective facility practices to provide a safe resident environment can influence the likelihood of an accident occurring and subsequent harm to a resident(s). Hazards that have been allowed to exist for a long time, or a facility history of similar problems, could indicate inadequate or ineffective facility practices.

If, during the tour, surveyors identify care delivery, hazards or potential hazards, or a history of resident accidents, the survey team should share the findings with the entire team and determine who will lead the investigation of the facility's systems for identifying, evaluating and preventing avoidable accidents or hazards. Review of facility practices may involve a review of policies and procedures, staffing, staff training, and equipment manufacturer's information, as well as interviews with staff and management. If there is a pattern of accidents involving one or more residents, determine how the facility evaluates its responses to the accidents. Determine if the facility ensured that the resident environment remained as free of accident hazards as possible and if each resident received adequate supervision and assistive devices to try to prevent accidents by:

- *Identifying potential hazards and risks (may require various strategies to gather such information);*

- *Evaluating and analyzing the information gathered to identify the underlying causes of the hazard and/or risk;*

- *Implementing interventions that addressed the causes and prioritized actions based on severity of the hazard and immediacy of the risk; and*

- *Monitoring implementation of interventions and determining if modification is needed.*

DETERMINATION OF COMPLIANCE (Task 6, Appendix P)

Synopsis of Regulation

The requirements at 42 CFR 483.25(h)(1) and (2) have three aspects. The first aspect requires that a resident's environment remains as free of accident hazards as possible; the second aspect requires that the facility provide adequate supervision; and the third is that the facility provides assistive devices to prevent accidents.

Criteria for Compliance

The facility's responsibility to accommodate individual needs and preferences and abide by the resident's right to choice and self-determination must be balanced against compliance with F323 to protect the resident. Documentation regarding the resident's choices will assist the survey team in making compliance decisions.

NOTE: *It is important to remember that not all accidents in a facility, regardless of outcome to a resident, are necessarily due to facility noncompliance. A resident can sustain bodily injury as a result of an accident over which the facility had no control (i.e., an unavoidable accident). The survey team needs to review the situation that led to the injury or potential for injury, as well as the facility practices, and resident's rights, preferences, and choices, to determine if the potential or negative outcome was avoidable or unavoidable.*

Compliance with 42 CFR 483.25(h)(1) and (2), F323, Accidents and Supervision

For the resident who has had an accident or was assessed at risk for an avoidable accident, the facility is in compliance with this requirement, if staff have:

- *Identified hazards and risk of an avoidable accident based on the facility's assessment of the resident environment and the resident, including the need for supervision and/or assistive devices;*

- *Evaluated/analyzed the hazards and risks;*

- *Implemented interventions, including adequate supervision and/or assistive devices, to reduce the risks of an accident that were consistent with a resident's needs, goals, plan of care, and current standards of practice;*

- *Provided assistive devices consistent with a resident's needs;*

- *Properly deployed and maintained resident specific equipment (e.g., lifts, canes, wheelchairs, walkers);*

- *Provided a safe environment, such as by monitoring chemicals, wet floors, cords and other equipment;*

- *Operated equipment in accordance with manufacturer's recommendations and resident need;*

- *Provided and maintain a secure environment (e.g., resident room, unit, common use areas, stairs and windows, facility grounds, etc.) to prevent negative outcomes (e.g., prevent falling/tumbling down stairs or jumping from windows or eloping through exit doors) for residents who exhibit unsafe wandering and/or elopement behavior (regardless of whether ambulatory, in wheelchair or using walker); and*

- *Monitored the effectiveness of the interventions and modified the interventions as necessary, in accordance with current standards of practice.*

  If not, cite F323.

Noncompliance for F323

After completing the investigation, determine whether or not compliance with the regulation exists. Noncompliance for F323 may include, but is not limited to, one or more of the following failures to:

- *Provide each resident an environment that is as free as possible from hazards over which the facility has control, such as assuring safe storage of toxic chemicals and medications, and safe use of equipment and electrical appliances;*

- *Provide adequate supervision for a resident who has exhibited unsafe wandering and/or has a risk of and/or a history of elopement;*

- *Identify and correct hazards such as non-functional alarms or call systems, disabled locks, fire doors that have been propped open, irregular walking surfaces, inadequate lighting or unsafe water temperatures;*

- *Supervise and monitor a resident who smokes and whose comprehensive assessment and plan of care indicates a need for supervision;*

- *Provide assistive devices and/or appropriate training for the use of assistive devices, based upon the assessed needs of the resident;*

- *Monitor for defective or disabled equipment, such as pumps, ventilators or other equipment, or the improper use of assistive devices;*

- *Assess, develop interventions, and/or revise the plan of care for a resident who has experienced falls, or who is identified as having risk factors for falling; and*

- *Assess, develop interventions, and/or revise the plan of care for a resident who has exhibited or has a risk for unsafe wandering or elopement.*

Potential Tags for Additional Investigation

During the investigation of 42 CFR 483.25(h)(1) and (2), the surveyor may have identified concerns related to outcome, process, and/or structure requirements. The surveyor should investigate these requirements before determining whether noncompliance may be present. The following are examples of related outcome, process, and/or structure requirements that should be considered:

- *42 CFR 483.13(a), F221, Restraints*
    - *Determine if staff attempted alternative approaches prior to the use of a restraint and if a medical indication for its use is present.*
- *42 CFR 483.13(b), F223, Abuse*
    - *Determine if the resident was free from verbal, sexual, physical, and mental abuse, corporal punishment, and involuntary seclusion.*
- *42 CFR 483.20(b)(1), F272, Comprehensive Assessments*
    - *Determine if the facility comprehensively assessed resident-specific risk factors (including potential causes) and assessed the need for and use of assistive devices.*
- *42 CFR 483.20(k)(1), F279, Comprehensive Care Plans*
    - *Determine if the facility developed a plan of care based on the comprehensive resident assessment consistent with the resident's specific conditions, risks, needs, behaviors, and preferences and with current standards of practice, and that includes measurable objectives and approximate timetables, specific interventions and/or services including necessary supervision and/or any assistive devices needed to prevent accidents to the extent possible.*
- *42 CFR 483.20(k)(2), F280, Comprehensive Care Plan Revision*
    - *Determine if the plan of care was reviewed and revised periodically, as necessary, related to preventing accidents, supervision required, and the use of assistive devices.*
- *42 CFR 483.20(k)(3)(i), F281, Services Provided Meet Professional Standards*

- *Determine if services and care were provided for the use of assistive devices, supervision, and prevention of accidents in accordance with accepted professional standards.*

- *42 CFR 483.30(a), F353, Sufficient Staff*

  - *Determine if the facility had qualified staff in sufficient numbers to provide necessary care and services, including supervision, based upon the comprehensive assessment and care plan, to prevent accidents, as possible.*

- *42 CFR 483.75(o), F520, Quality Assessment and Assurance*

  - *Determine whether the quality assessment and assurance committee has identified issues, and developed and implemented appropriate plans of action to correct identified quality deficiencies in relation to hazards, accident prevention, and supervision of residents.*

V. DEFICIENCY CATEGORIZATION (Part V, Appendix P)

Once the survey team has completed its investigation, analyzed the data, reviewed the regulatory requirements, and determined that noncompliance exists, the team must determine the severity of each deficiency, based on the resultant effect or potential for harm to the resident.

The key elements for severity determination for F323 are as follows:

1. *Presence of harm/negative outcome(s) or potential for negative outcomes because of presence of environmental hazards, lack of adequate supervision to prevent accidents, or failure to provide assistive devices to prevent accidents. Actual or potential harm/negative outcome for F323 may include, but is not limited to:*

   - *Injuries sustained from falls and/or unsafe wandering/elopement;*

   - *Resident-to-resident altercations;*

   - *Thermal burns from spills/immersion of hot water/liquids;*

   - *Falls due to environmental hazards;*

   - *Ingestion of chemical substances; and*

   - *Burns related to smoking materials.*

2. *Degree of harm (actual or potential) related to the noncompliance. Identify how the facility noncompliance caused, resulted in, allowed, or contributed to the actual or potential for harm.*

- *If harm has occurred, determine if the harm is at the level of serious injury, impairment, death, compromise, or discomfort; and*

- *If harm has not yet occurred, determine the potential for serious injury, impairment, death, or compromise or discomfort to occur to the resident.*

3. *The immediacy of correction required. Determine whether the noncompliance requires immediate correction in order to prevent serious injury, harm, impairment, or death to one or more residents.*

The survey team must evaluate the harm or potential for harm based upon the following levels of severity for Tag F323. First, the team must rule out whether Severity Level 4, Immediate Jeopardy to a resident's health or safety, exists by evaluating the deficient practice in relation to immediacy, culpability, and severity. (Follow the guidance in Appendix Q, **Guidelines for Determining Immediate Jeopardy***.)*

Severity Level 4 Considerations: Immediate Jeopardy to Resident Health or Safety

Immediate Jeopardy is a situation in which the facility's noncompliance with one or more requirements of participation:

- *Has allowed, caused, or resulted in (or is likely to allow, cause, or result in) serious injury, harm, impairment, or death to a resident; and*

- *Requires immediate correction, as the facility either created the situation or allowed the situation to continue by failing to implement preventive or corrective measures.*

NOTE: *The death or transfer of a resident, who was harmed or injured as a result of facility noncompliance, does not always remove a finding of Immediate Jeopardy. The facility is required to implement specific actions to correct the noncompliance which allowed or caused the Immediate Jeopardy.*

When considering Severity Level 4, the survey team must have already determined noncompliance in the facility practices to provide a safe resident environment. Examples of negative outcomes that occurred or have the potential to occur as a result of the noncompliance might include the following:

- *Esophageal damage due to ingestion of corrosive substances;*

- *Loss of consciousness related to head injuries;*

- *3rd degree burn, or a 2nd degree burn covering a large surface area;*

- *Fracture or other injury that may require surgical intervention and results in significant decline in mental and/or physical functioning;*

- *Electric shock due to use of unsafe or improperly maintained equipment;*

- *Entrapment of body parts, such as limbs, head, neck, or chest that cause injury or death as a result of defective or improperly latched side rails or spaces within side rails, between split rails, between rails and the mattress, between side rails and the bed frame, or spaces between side rails and the head or foot board of the bed;*

- *Entrapment of body parts, such as limbs, head, neck, or chest that causes or has the potential to cause serious injury, harm, impairment or death as a result of any manual method, physical or mechanical device, material, or equipment;*

- *Fall(s) that resulted in or had the potential to result in serious injury, impairment, harm or death (e.g. fracture or other injury that may require surgical intervention and/or results in significant decline in mental and/or physical functioning), and the facility had no established measure(s) or practice(s), or ineffective measure(s) or practice(s), that would have prevented the fall or limited the resident's injury; or*

- *Unsafe wandering and/or elopement that resulted in or had the potential to result in serious injury, impairment, harm or death (e.g., resident leaves facility or locked unit unnoticed and sustained or had potential to sustain serious injury, impairment, harm or death), and the facility had no established measure(s) or practice(s), or ineffective measure(s) or practice(s), that would have prevented or limited the resident's exposure to hazards.*

NOTE: *If Immediate Jeopardy has been ruled out based upon the evidence, then evaluate whether actual harm that is not immediate jeopardy exists at Severity Level 3.*

Severity Level 3 Considerations: Actual Harm that is Not Immediate Jeopardy

Severity Level 3 indicates noncompliance that results in actual harm and can include but may not be limited to clinical compromise, decline, or the resident's ability to maintain and/or reach his/her highest practicable well-being.

When considering Severity Level 3, the survey team must have already determined noncompliance in the facility practices to provide a safe resident environment. As a result of the noncompliance, a negative outcome occurred. Some examples of compromise include:

- *Short-term disability;*

- *Pain that interfered with normal activities;*

- *2nd degree burn;*

- *Fracture or other injury that may require surgical intervention and does not result in significant decline in mental and/or physical functioning;*

- *Medical evaluation was necessary, and treatment beyond first aid (e.g., sutures) was required;*

- *Fall(s) that resulted in actual harm (e.g., short-term disability; pain that interfered with normal activities; fracture or other injury that may require surgical intervention and does not result in significant decline in mental and/or physical functioning; or medical evaluation was necessary, and treatment beyond first aid (e.g., sutures) was required) and the facility had established measure(s) or practice(s) in place that limited the resident's potential to fall and limited the resident's injury and prevented the harm from rising to a level of immediate jeopardy; or*

- *Unsafe wandering and/or elopement that resulted in actual harm and the facility had established measure(s) or practice(s) in place that limited the resident's exposure to hazards and prevented the harm from rising to a level of immediate jeopardy.*

  NOTE: *Unsafe wandering or elopement that resulted in actual harm and the facility had no established measure(s) or practice(s), or ineffective measure(s) or practice(s) that would have prevented or limited the resident's exposure to hazards should be cited at Level 4, Immediate Jeopardy.*

NOTE: *If Severity Level 3 (actual harm that is not immediate jeopardy) has been ruled out based upon the evidence, evaluate whether Severity Level 2 (no actual harm with the potential for more than minimal harm) exists.*

Severity Level 2 Considerations: No Actual Harm with Potential for More Than Minimal Harm that is Not Immediate Jeopardy

Severity Level 2 indicates noncompliance that results in a resident outcome of no more than minimal discomfort and/or has the potential to compromise the resident's ability to maintain or reach his or her highest practicable level of well being. The potential exists for greater harm to occur if interventions are not provided.

When considering Severity Level 2, the survey team must have already determined noncompliance in the facility practices to provide a safe resident environment. As a result of the noncompliance, a negative outcome occurred, or the potential for a negative outcome exists, such as the following:

- *Bruising, minor skin abrasions, and rashes;*

- *Pain that does not impair normal activities;*

- *1st degree burn;*

- *Medical evaluation or consultation may or may not have been necessary, and treatment such as first aid may have been required;*

- *Fall(s) which resulted in no more than minimal harm (e.g., bruising or minor skin abrasions; pain that does not impair normal activities; or medical evaluation or consultation may or may not have been necessary, and/or treatment such as first aid may have been required) because the facility had additional established measure(s) or practice(s) that limited the resident's potential to fall or limited the injury or potential for injury; or*

- *Unsafe wandering and/or elopement, which resulted in no more than minimal harm because the facility had additional established measure(s) or practice(s) that limited the resident's exposure to hazards. For example, a resident with Alzheimer's disease left the locked unit and was quickly found unharmed on another unit, and the building was considered a safe environment, as there was no way for the resident to leave the building.*

Severity Level 1 Considerations: No Actual Harm with Potential for Minimal Harm

The failure of the facility to provide a safe environment and adequate supervision places residents at risk for more than minimal harm. Therefore, Severity Level 1 does not apply for this regulatory requirement.

---

§483.25(i) Nutrition

Based on a resident's comprehensive assessment, the facility must ensure that a resident--
(See F326 for intent, guidelines, procedures and probes for §483.25(i))

F325

(1) Maintains acceptable parameters of nutritional status, such as body weight and protein levels, unless the resident's clinical condition demonstrates that this is not possible; and

---

F326

§483.25(i)(2) Receives a therapeutic diet when there is a nutritional problem

Intent §483.25(i)

The intent of this regulation is to assure that the resident maintains acceptable parameters of nutritional status, taking into account the resident's clinical condition or other appropriate intervention, when there is a nutritional problem.

Interpretive Guidelines §483.25(i)

This corresponds to MDS 2.0 sections G, I, J, K and L when specified for use by the State.

Parameters of nutritional status which are unacceptable include unplanned weight loss as well as other indices such as peripheral edema, cachexia and laboratory tests indicating malnourishment (e.g., serum albumin levels).

Weight

Since ideal body weight charts have not yet been validated for the institutionalized elderly, weight loss (or gain) is a guide in determining nutritional status. An analysis of weight loss or gain should be examined in light of the individual's former life style as well as the current diagnosis.

Suggested parameters for evaluating significance of unplanned and undesired weight loss are:

Interval	Significant Loss	Severe Loss
1 month	5%	Greater than 5%
3 months	7.5%	Greater than 7.5%
6 months	10%	Greater than 10%

The following formula determines percentage of loss:

% of body weight loss = (usual weight - actual weight) / (usual weight) x 100

In evaluating weight loss, consider the resident's usual weight through adult life; the assessment of potential for weight loss; and care plan for weight management. Also, was the resident on a calorie restricted diet, or if newly admitted and obese, and on a normal diet, are fewer calories provided than prior to admission? Was the resident edematous when initially weighed, and with treatment, no longer has edema? Has the resident refused food?

Suggested laboratory values are:

Albumin >60 yr.: 3.4 - 4.8 g/dl (good for examining marginal protein depletion)

Plasma Transferrin >60 yr.:180-380 g/dl. (Rises with iron deficiency anemia. More persistent indicator of protein status.)

Hemoglobin Males: 14-17 g/dl

	Females: 12-15 g/dl
Hematocrit	Males: 41 - 53
	Females: 36 - 46
Potassium	3.5 - 5.0 mEq/L
Magnesium	1.3 - 2.0 mEg/L

Some laboratories may have different "normals." Determine range for the specific laboratory.

Because some healthy elderly people have abnormal laboratory values, and because abnormal values can be expected in some disease processes, do not expect laboratory values to be within normal ranges for all residents. Consider abnormal values in conjunction with the resident's clinical condition and baseline normal values.

NOTE: There is no requirement that facilities order the tests referenced above.

Clinical Observations

Potential indicators of malnutrition are pale skin, dull eyes, swollen lips, swollen gums, swollen and/or dry tongue with scarlet or magenta hue, poor skin turgor, cachexia, bilateral edema, and muscle wasting.

Risk factors for malnutrition are:

1. Drug therapy that may contribute to nutritional deficiencies such as:

    a. Cardiac glycosides;

    b. Diuretics;

    c. Anti-inflammatory drugs;

    d. Antacids (antacid overuse);

    e. Laxatives (laxative overuse);

    f. Psychotropic drug overuse;

    g. Anticonvulsants;

    h. Antineoplastic drugs;

    i. Phenothiazines;

    j. Oral hypoglycemics;

2. Poor oral health status or hygiene, eyesight, motor coordination, or taste alterations;

3. Depression or dementia;

4. Therapeutic or mechanically altered diet;

5. Lack of access to culturally acceptable foods;

6. Slow eating pace resulting in food becoming unpalatable, or in staff removing the tray before resident has finished eating; and

7. Cancer.

Clinical conditions demonstrating that the maintenance of acceptable nutritional status may not be possible include, but are not limited to:

- Refusal to eat and refusal of other methods of nourishment;
- Advanced disease (i.e., cancer, malabsorption syndrome);
- Increased nutritional/caloric needs associated with pressure sores and wound healing (e.g., fractures, burns);
- Radiation or chemotherapy;
- Kidney disease, alcohol/drug abuse, chronic blood loss, hyperthyroidism;
- Gastrointestinal surgery; and
- Prolonged nausea, vomiting, diarrhea not relieved by treatment given according to accepted standards of practice.

"**Therapeutic diet**" means a diet ordered by a physician as part of treatment for a disease or clinical condition, to eliminate or decrease certain substances in the diet, (e.g., sodium) or to increase certain substances in the diet (e.g., potassium), or to provide food the resident is able to eat (e.g., a mechanically altered diet).

Procedures §483.25(i)

Determine if residents selected for a comprehensive review or focused review as appropriate, have maintained acceptable parameters of nutritional status. Where indicated by the resident's medical status, have clinically appropriate therapeutic diets been prescribed?

Probes: §483.25(i)

For sampled residents whose nutritional status is inadequate, do clinical conditions demonstrate that maintenance of inadequate nutritional status was unavoidable:

- Did the facility identify factors that put the resident at risk for malnutrition?
- Identify if resident triggered RAPs for nutritional status, ADL functional/rehabilitation potential, feeding tubes, psychotropic drug use, and dehydration/fluid balance. Consider whether the RAPs were used to assess the causal factors for decline, potential for decline or lack of improvement.
- What routine preventive measures and care did the resident receive to address unique risk factors for malnutrition (e.g., provision of an adequate diet with supplements or modifications as indicated by nutrient needs)?
- Were staff responsibilities for maintaining nutritional status clear, including monitoring the amount of food the resident is eating at each meal and offering substitutes?
- Was this care provided consistently?
- Were individual goals of the plan of care periodically evaluated and if not met, were alternative approaches considered or attempted?

F327

§483.25(j) Hydration

§483.25(j) Hydration. The facility must provide each resident with sufficient fluid intake to maintain proper hydration and health

Intent §483.25(j)

The intent of this regulation is to assure that the resident receives sufficient amount of fluids based on individual needs to prevent dehydration.

Interpretive Guidelines §483.25(j)

This corresponds to MDS 2.0 sections G, K, I, J and L when specified for use by the State.

"**Sufficient fluid**" means the amount of fluid needed to prevent dehydration (output of fluids far exceeds fluid intake) and maintain health. The amount needed is specific for each resident, and fluctuates as the resident's condition fluctuates (e.g., increase fluids if resident has fever or diarrhea).

Risk factors for the resident becoming dehydrated are:

- Coma/decreased sensorium;
- Fluid loss and increased fluid needs (e.g., diarrhea, fever, uncontrolled diabetes);
- Fluid restriction secondary to renal dialysis;
- Functional impairments that make it difficult to drink, reach fluids, or communicate fluid needs (e.g., aphasia);
- Dementia in which resident forgets to drink or forgets how to drink;
- Refusal of fluids; and
- Did the MDS trigger RAPs on hydration? What action was taken based on the RAP?

Consider whether assessment triggers RAPs and are RAPs used to assess the causal factors for decline, potential for decline or lack of improvement.

A general guideline for determining baseline daily fluids needs is to multiply the resident's body weight in kg times 30cc (2.2 lbs = 1kg), except for residents with renal or cardiac distress. An excess of fluids can be detrimental for these residents.

Procedures §483.25(j)

Identify if resident triggers RAPs for dehydration/fluid maintenance, and cognitive loss.

Probes: §483.25(j)

Do sampled residents show clinical signs of possible insufficient fluid intake (e.g., dry skin and mucous membranes, cracked lips, poor skin turgor, thirst, fever), abnormal laboratory values (e.g., elevated hemoglobin and hematocrit, potassium, chloride, sodium, albumin, transferrin, blood urea nitrogen (BUN), or urine specific gravity)?

Has the facility provided residents with adequate fluid intake to maintain proper hydration and health? If not:

- Did the facility identify any factors that put the resident at risk of dehydration?
- What care did the facility provide to reduce those risk factors and ensure adequate fluid intake (e.g., keep fluids next to the resident at all times and

assisting or cuing the resident to drink)? Is staff aware of need for maintaining adequate fluid intake?

- If adequate fluid intake is difficult to maintain, have alternative treatment approaches been developed, attempt to increase fluid intake by the use of popsicles, gelatin, and other similar non-liquid foods?

F328

§483.25(k) Special Needs

The facility must ensure that residents receive proper treatment and care for the following special services

Intent 483.25(k)

The intent of this provision is that the resident receives the necessary care and treatment including medical and nursing care and services when they need the specialized services as listed below.

Interpretive Guidelines §483.25(k)

This corresponds to MDS 2.0 section P when specified by for use by the State.

The non-availability of program funding does not relieve a facility of its obligation to ensure that its residents receive all needed services listed in §1819(b)(4)(A) of the Act for Medicare and §1919(b)(4)(A) of the Act for Medicaid. For services not covered, a facility is required to assist the resident in securing any available resources to obtain the needed services.

§483.25(k)(1) Injections

Probes: §483.25(k)(1)

For sampled residents receiving one or more of these services within 7 days of the survey:

- Is proper administration technique used (i.e., maintenance of sterility; correct needle size, route)?

- Are there signs of redness, swelling, lesions from previous injections?

- If appropriate, is resident observed for adverse reaction after the injection?

- Are syringes and needles disposed of according to facility policy and accepted Practice (e.g., Centers for Disease Control and Prevention and Occupational Safety and Health Administration guidelines)?
- Do nursing notes indicate, as appropriate, the resident's response to treatment (e.g., side effects/adverse actions; problems at the injection site(s); relief of pain)?

§483.25(k)(2) Parenteral and Enteral Fluids

Probes: §483.25(k)(2)

This corresponds to MDS 2.0 sections K5 and 6 and P1 when specified for use by the State

For residents selected for a comprehensive review, or focused review as appropriate, receiving one or more of these services within 7 days of the survey:

- Are there signs of inflammation or infiltration at the insertion site?
- If the IV site, tubing, or bottle/bag is changed, is sterile technique maintained?
- Is the rate of administration that which is ordered by the Physician
- Has the resident received the amount of fluid during the past 24 hours that he/she should have received according to the physician's orders (allow flexibility up to 150cc unless an exact fluid intake is critical for the resident)?

Procedures §483.25(k)(2)

See §483.25(g) for enteral feedings (includes gastrostomy).

§483.25(k)(3) Colostomy, Ureterostomy, or Ileostomy care

Procedures §483.25(k)(3)

This corresponds to MDS 2.0 sections G, H, and P when specified for use by the State.

Identify if resident triggers RAPs for urinary incontinence, nutritional status, pressure ulcers (skin care).

Probes: §483.25(k)(3)

- If appropriate, is the resident provided with self-care instructions?
- Does the staff member observe and respond to any signs of resident's discomfort about the ostomy or its care?

- Is skin surrounding the ostomy free of excoriation (abrasion, breakdown)?

- If excoriation is present, does the clinical record indicate an onset and a plan of care to treat the excoriation?

§483.25(k)(4) Tracheostomy Care

Procedures §483.25(k)(4) (Includes care of the tracheostomy site)

This corresponds to MDS 2.0 sections M and P when specified for use by the State.

Observations for tracheostomy care are most appropriate for residents with new or relatively new tracheostomies, and may not be appropriate for those with tracheostomies of long standing.

Probes: §483.25(k)(4) (Includes care of the tracheostomy site)

- Is the skin around the tracheostomy clean and dry? Are the dressing and the ties clean and dry, with the cannula secure?

- Does the resident have signs of an obstructed airway or need for suctioning (e.g., secretions draining from mouth or tracheotomy; unable to cough to clear chest; audible crackles or wheezes; dyspneic, restless or agitated)?

- If appropriate for a specific resident, is there a suction machine and catheter immediately available?

- Is there an extra cannula of the correct size at the bedside or other place easily accessible if needed in an emergency?

For sampled residents receiving one or more of these services within 7 days of the survey:

- Is suction machine available for immediate use, clean, working, and available to a source of emergency power?

- Is there an adequate supply of easily accessible suction catheters?

§483.25(k)(5) Standard: Tracheal Suctioning

Probes: §483.25(k)(5)

This corresponds to MDS 2.0 section P when specified for use by the State

§483.25(k)(6) Standard: Respiratory Care

Procedures §483.25(k)(6)

This corresponds to MDS 2.0 section P when specified for use by the State.

Includes use of respirators/ventilators, oxygen, intermittent positive pressure breathing (IPPB) or other inhalation therapy, pulmonary care, humidifiers, and other methods to treat conditions of the respiratory tract.

Identify if resident triggers RAPs for delirium and dehydration/fluid maintenance.

Probes: §483.25(k)(6)

For sampled residents receiving one or more of these services within 7 days of the survey:

- If oxygen is in use, are precautions observed (e.g., proper storage and handling of oxygen cylinders secured)? Secondary "No Smoking" signs are not required in facilities that prohibit smoking and have signs at all major entrances that the facility does not allow smoking.
- If the survey team observes a treatment being administered, is the resident encouraged and instructed on how to assist in the treatment?
- Is the staff following the facility's protocol and/or written procedures for ventilators (e.g., functioning alarms); frequency of staff monitoring; monitoring of resident response (e.g., use of accessory muscles to breathe, cleanliness of mouth, skin irritation), and availability of manual resuscitators?
- If the resident is ventilator dependent, is routine machine maintenance and care done (e.g., water changes/tubing changes, safety checks on alarms, and machine functioning checks)?

§483.25(k)(7) Foot Care

Procedures §483.25(k)(7)

This corresponds with MDS 2.0 sections G and M when specified for use by the State.

Includes treatment of foot disorders by qualified persons, e.g., podiatrist, Doctor of Medicine, Doctor of Osteopathy), including, but not limited, to corns, neuroma, calluses, bunions, heel spurs, nail disorders, preventive care, to avoid foot problems in diabetic residents and residents with circulatory disorders.

Probes: §483.25(k)(7)

For residents selected for a comprehensive review, or focused review, as appropriate:

- Do nails, corns, calluses, and other foot problems appear unattended; do these foot problems interfere with resident mobility?
- Are residents able to see a qualified person when they want?
- What preventive foot care do staff provide diabetic residents?

§483.25(k)(8) Prostheses

Probes: §483.25(k)(8)

MDS 2.0 sections D, G, L, M, and P when specified for use by the State.

Includes artificial limbs, eyes, teeth.

For residents selected for a comprehensive review, or focused review, as appropriate:

- Is resident able to put on the prosthesis by himself/herself or with some assistance?
- Are residents wearing their prostheses?
- Does the prosthesis fit correctly?
- Is skin/mucous membrane in contact with the prosthesis free of abrasions, wounds, irritation?

F329

(Rev. 22, Issued: 12-15-06, Effective/Implementation: 12-18-06)

§483.25(l) Unnecessary Drugs

1. General. Each resident's drug regimen must be free from unnecessary drugs. An unnecessary drug is any drug when used:

(i) In excessive dose (including duplicate therapy); or
(ii) For excessive duration; or
(iii) Without adequate monitoring; or
(iv) Without adequate indications for its use; or
(v) In the presence of adverse consequences which indicate the dose should be reduced or discontinued; or

(vi) Any combinations of the reasons above.

2. Antipsychotic Drugs. Based on a comprehensive assessment of a resident, the facility must ensure that:

(i) Residents who have not used antipsychotic drugs are not given these drugs unless antipsychotic drug therapy is necessary to treat a specific condition as diagnosed and documented in the clinical record; and

(ii) Residents who use antipsychotic drugs receive gradual dose reductions, and behavioral interventions, unless clinically contraindicated, in an effort to discontinue these drugs.

INTENT: §483.25(l) Unnecessary drugs

The intent of this requirement is that each resident's entire drug/medication regimen be managed and monitored to achieve the following goals:

- The medication regimen helps promote or maintain the resident's highest practicable mental, physical, and psychosocial well-being, as identified by the resident and/or representative(s) in collaboration with the attending physician and facility staff;
- Each resident receives only those medications, in doses and for the duration clinically indicated to treat the resident's assessed condition(s);
- Non-pharmacological interventions (such as behavioral interventions) are considered and used when indicated, instead of, or in addition to, medication;
- Clinically significant adverse consequences are minimized; and
- The potential contribution of the medication regimen to an unanticipated decline or newly emerging or worsening symptom is recognized and evaluated, and the regimen is modified when appropriate.

NOTE: This guidance applies to all categories of medications including antipsychotic medications.

Although the regulatory language refers to "drugs," the guidance in this document generally will refer to "medications," except in those situations where the term "drug" has become part of an established pharmaceutical term (e.g., adverse drug event, and adverse drug reaction or consequence).

For purposes of this guidance, references to "the pharmacist" mean the facility's licensed pharmacist, whether employed directly by the facility or through arrangement.

The surveyor's review of medication use is not intended to constitute the practice of medicine. However, surveyors are expected to investigate the basis for decisions and interventions affecting residents.

DEFINITIONS

Definitions are provided to clarify terminology related to medications and to the evaluation and treatment of residents.

- "Adverse consequence" is an unpleasant symptom or event that is due to or associated with a medication, such as impairment or decline in an individual's mental or physical condition or functional or psychosocial status. It may include various types of adverse drug reactions and interactions (e.g., medication-medication, medication-food, and medication-disease).

  NOTE: Adverse drug reaction (ADR) is a form of adverse consequences. It may be either a secondary effect of a medication that is usually undesirable and different from the therapeutic effect of the medication or any response to a medication that is noxious and unintended and occurs in doses for prophylaxis, diagnosis, or treatment. The term "side effect" is often used interchangeably with ADR; however, side effects are but one of five ADR categories, the others being hypersensitivity, idiosyncratic response, toxic reactions, and adverse medication interactions. A side effect is an expected, well-known reaction that occurs with a predictable frequency and may or may not constitute an adverse consequence.

- "Anticholinergic side effect" is an effect of a medication that opposes or inhibits the activity of the parasympathetic (cholinergic) nervous system to the point of causing symptoms such as dry mouth, blurred vision, tachycardia, urinary retention, constipation, confusion, delirium, or hallucinations.

- "Behavioral interventions" are individualized non-pharmacological approaches (including direct care and activities) that are provided as part of a supportive physical and psychosocial environment, and are directed toward preventing, relieving, and/or accommodating a resident's distressed behavior.

- "Clinically significant" refers to effects, results, or consequences that materially affect or are likely to affect an individual's mental, physical, or psychosocial well-being either positively by preventing, stabilizing, or improving a condition or reducing a risk, or negatively by exacerbating, causing, or contributing to a symptom, illness, or decline in status.

- "Distressed behavior" is behavior that reflects individual discomfort or emotional strain. It may present as crying, apathetic or withdrawn behavior, or as verbal or physical actions such as: pacing, cursing, hitting, kicking, pushing, scratching, tearing things, or grabbing others.

- "Dose" is the total amount/strength/concentration of a medication given at one time or over a period of time. The individual dose is the amount/strength/concentration received at each administration. The amount received over a 24-hour period may be referred to as the daily dose.

    - "Excessive dose" means the total amount of any medication (including duplicate therapy) given at one time or over a period of time that is greater than the amount recommended by the manufacturer's label, package insert, current standards of practice for a resident's age and condition, or clinical studies or evidence-based review articles that are published in medical and/or pharmacy journals and that lacks evidence of:

        - A review for the continued necessity of the dose;

        - Attempts at, or consideration of the possibility of, tapering a medication; and

        - A documented clinical rationale for the benefit of, or necessity for, the dose or for the use of multiple medications from the same pharmacological class.

- "Duplicate therapy" refers to multiple medications of the same pharmacological class/category or any medication therapy that substantially duplicates a particular effect of another medication that the individual is taking.

- "Duration" is the total length of time the medication is being received.

    - "Excessive Duration" means the medication is administered beyond the manufacturer's recommended time frames or facility-established stop order policies, beyond the length of time advised by current standards of practice, clinical practice guidelines, clinical studies or evidence-based review articles, and/or without either evidence of additional therapeutic benefit for the resident or clinical evidence that would warrant the continued use of the medication.

- "Extrapyramidal symptoms (EPS)" are neurological side effects that can occur at any time from the first few days of treatment to years later. EPS includes various syndromes such as:

    - Akathisia, which refers to a distressing feeling of internal restlessness that may appear as constant motion, the inability to sit still, fidgeting, pacing, or rocking.

    - Medication-induced Parkinsonism, which refers to a syndrome of Parkinson-like symptoms including tremors, shuffling gait, slowness of movement, expressionless face, drooling, postural unsteadiness and rigidity of muscles in the limbs, neck and trunk.

  - Dystonia, which refers to an acute, painful, spastic contraction of muscle groups (commonly the neck, eyes and trunk) that often occurs soon after initiating treatment and is more common in younger individuals.

- "Gradual Dose Reduction (GDR)" is the stepwise tapering of a dose to determine if symptoms, conditions, or risks can be managed by a lower dose or if the dose or medication can be discontinued.

- "Indications for use" is the identified, documented clinical rationale for administering a medication that is based upon an assessment of the resident's condition and therapeutic goals and is consistent with manufacturer's recommendations and/or clinical practice guidelines, clinical standards of practice, medication references, clinical studies or evidence-based review articles that are published in medical and/or pharmacy journals.

- "Insomnia" is the inability to sleep characterized by difficulty falling asleep, difficulty staying asleep, early waking, or non-restorative sleep, which may result in impaired physical, social, or cognitive function.

- "Medication Interaction" is the impact of another substance (such as another medication, nutritional supplement including herbal products, food, or substances used in diagnostic studies) upon a medication. The interactions may alter absorption, distribution, metabolism, or elimination. These interactions may decrease the effectiveness of the medication or increase the potential for adverse consequences.

- "Medication Regimen Review" (MRR) is a thorough evaluation of the medication regimen by a pharmacist, with the goal of promoting positive outcomes and minimizing adverse consequences associated with medication. The review includes preventing, identifying, reporting, and resolving medication-related problems, medication errors, or other irregularities in collaboration with other members of the interdisciplinary team.[51]

- "Monitoring" is the ongoing collection and analysis of information (such as observations and diagnostic test results) and comparison to baseline data in order to:

  - Ascertain the individual's response to treatment and care, including progress or lack of progress toward a therapeutic goal;

  - Detect any complications or adverse consequences of the condition or of the treatments; and

- Support decisions about modifying, discontinuing, or continuing any interventions.

- "Neuroleptic Malignant Syndrome" (NMS) is a syndrome related to the use of medications, mainly antipsychotics, that typically presents with a sudden onset of diffuse muscle rigidity, high fever, labile blood pressure, tremor, and notable cognitive dysfunction. It is potentially fatal if not treated immediately, including stopping the offending medications.

- "Non-pharmacological interventions" refers to approaches to care that do not involve medications, generally directed towards stabilizing or improving a resident's mental, physical or psychosocial well-being.

- "Psychopharmacological medication" is any medication used for managing behavior, stabilizing mood, or treating psychiatric disorders.

- "Serotonin Syndrome" is a potentially serious clinical condition resulting from overstimulation of serotonin receptors. It is commonly related to the use of multiple serotonin-stimulating medications (e.g., SSRIs, SNRIs, triptans, certain antibiotics). Symptoms may include restlessness, hallucinations, confusion, loss of coordination, fast heart beat, rapid changes in blood pressure, increased body temperature, overactive reflexes, nausea, vomiting and diarrhea.

- "Tardive dyskinesia" refers to abnormal, recurrent, involuntary movements that may be irreversible and typically present as lateral movements of the tongue or jaw, tongue thrusting, chewing, frequent blinking, brow arching, grimacing, and lip smacking, although the trunk or other parts of the body may also be affected.

OVERVIEW

Medications are an integral part of the care provided to residents of nursing facilities. They are administered to try to achieve various outcomes, such as curing an illness, diagnosing a disease or condition, arresting or slowing a disease process, reducing or eliminating symptoms, or preventing a disease or symptom.

A study of 33,301 nursing facility residents found that an average of 6.7 medications were ordered per resident, with 27 percent of residents taking nine or more medications.[52] Analysis of antipsychotic use by 693,000 Medicare nursing home residents revealed that 28.5 percent of the doses received were excessive and 32.2 percent lacked appropriate indications for use.[53]

Proper medication selection and prescribing (including dose, duration, and type of medication(s)) may help stabilize or improve a resident's outcome, quality of life and functional capacity. Any medication or combination of medications—or the use of a medication without adequate indications, in excessive dose, for an excessive duration, or without adequate monitoring—may increase the risk of a broad range of adverse consequences such as medication interactions, depression, confusion, immobility, falls, and related hip fractures.

Intrinsic factors including physiological changes accompanying the aging process, multiple comorbidities, and certain medical conditions may affect the absorption, distribution, metabolism or elimination of medications from the body and may also increase an individual's risk of adverse consequences.

While assuring that only those medications required to treat the resident's assessed condition are being used, reducing the need for and maximizing the effectiveness of medications are important considerations for all residents. Therefore, as part of all medication management (including antipsychotics), it is important for the interdisciplinary team to consider non-pharmacological approaches. Educating facility staff and providers in addition to implementing non-pharmacological approaches to resident conditions prior to, and/or in conjunction with, the use of medications may minimize the need for medications or reduce the dose and duration of those medications.[54]

Examples of non-pharmacological interventions may include:

- Increasing the amount of resident exercise, intake of liquids and dietary fiber in conjunction with an individualized bowel regimen to prevent or reduce constipation and the use of medications (e.g. laxatives and stool softeners);

- Identifying, addressing, and eliminating or reducing underlying causes of distressed behavior such as boredom and pain;

- Using sleep hygiene techniques and individualized sleep routines;

- Accommodating the resident's behavior and needs by supporting and encouraging activities reminiscent of lifelong work or activity patterns, such as providing early morning activity for a farmer used to awakening early;

- Individualizing toileting schedules to prevent incontinence and avoid the use of incontinence medications that may have significant adverse consequences (e.g., anticholinergic effects);

- Developing interventions that are specific to resident's interests, abilities, strengths and needs, such as simplifying or segmenting tasks for a resident who has trouble following complex directions;

- Using massage, hot/warm or cold compresses to address a resident's pain or discomfort; or

- Enhancing the taste and presentation of food, assisting the resident to eat, addressing food preferences, and increasing finger foods and snacks for an individual with dementia, to improve appetite and avoid the unnecessary use of medications intended to stimulate appetite.

The indications for initiating, withdrawing, or withholding medication(s), as well as the use of non-pharmacological approaches, are determined by assessing the resident's underlying condition, current signs and symptoms, and preferences and goals for treatment. This includes, where possible, the identification of the underlying cause(s), since a diagnosis alone may not warrant treatment with medication.

Orders from multiple prescribers can increase the resident's chances of receiving unnecessary medications. Many residents receive orders for medications from several practitioners, for example, attending and on-call physicians, consultants, and nurse practitioner(s). It is important that the facility clearly identify who is responsible for prescribing and identifying the indications for use of medication(s), for providing and administering the medication(s), and for monitoring the resident for the effects and potential adverse consequence of the medication regimen. This is also important when care is delivered or ordered by diverse sources such as consultants, providers, or suppliers (e.g., hospice or dialysis programs).

Staff and practitioner access to current medication references and pertinent clinical protocols helps to promote safe administration and monitoring of medications. One of the existing mechanisms to warn prescribers about risks associated with medications is the Food and Drug Administration (FDA) requirement that manufacturers include within the medication labeling warnings about adverse reactions and potential safety hazards identified both before and after approval of a medication, and what to do if they occur (Visit: www.fda.gov/medwatch/safety.htm). Manufacturers are required to update labels to warn about newly identified safety hazards—regardless of whether causation has been proven and whether the medication is prescribed for a disease or condition that is not included in the "Indications and Usage" section of the labeling (so-called "off-label" or unapproved use). The FDA may require manufacturers to place statements about serious problems in a prominently displayed box (so-called boxed or "black box" warnings), which indicates a need to closely evaluate and monitor the potential benefits and risks of that medication.

The facility's pharmacist is a valuable source of information about medications. Listings or descriptions of most significant risks, recommended doses, medication interactions, cautions, etc. can be found in widely available, standard references, and computer software and systems that provide up-to-date information. It is important to note that some of the medication information found in many of these references is not specific to older adults or institutionalized individuals.

Clinical standards of practice and clinical guidelines established by professional groups are useful to guide clinicians. Some of the recognized clinical resources available for understanding the overall treatment and management of medical problems, symptoms and medication consequences and precautions include the:

- **American Geriatrics Society www.americangeriatrics.org and www.geriatricsatyourfingertips.org;**
- **American Medical Directors Association www.amda.com;**
- **American Psychiatric Association www.psych.org;**
- **American Society of Consultant Pharmacists www.ASCP.com;**
- **Agency for Healthcare Research and Quality (AHRQ) www.ahrq.gov;**
- **American Association for Geriatric Psychiatry www.aagp.org;**
- **Association for Practitioners in Infection Control and Epidemiology www.apic.org;**
- **CMS Sharing Innovations in Quality Web site maintained at: http://siq.air.org;**
- **National Guideline Clearinghouse www.guideline.gov;**
- **Quality Improvement Organizations, Medicare Quality Improvement Community Initiatives www.medqic.org;**
- **U.S. Department of Health and Human Services, Food and Drug Administration Web site www.fda.gov/medwatch/safety.htm;**
- **U.S. Department of Health and Human Services, National Institute of Mental Health Web site, which includes publications and clinical research information www.nimh.nih.gov;**
- **Mace N, Rabins P. The 36-Hour Day: A Family Guide to Caring for Persons with Alzheimer Disease, Related Dementing Illnesses, and Memory Loss in Later Life; and**
- **"Bathing without a battle" www.bathingwithoutabattle.unc.edu.**

NOTE: References to non-CMS sources or sites on the Internet included above or later in this document are provided as a service and do not constitute or imply endorsement of these organizations or their programs by CMS or the U.S. Department of Health and Human Services. CMS is not responsible for the content of pages found at these sites. URL addresses were current as of the date of this publication.

Although these guidelines generally emphasize the older adult resident, adverse consequences can occur in anyone at any age; therefore, these requirements apply to residents of all ages.

MEDICATION MANAGEMENT

Medication management is based in the care process and includes recognition or identification of the problem/need, assessment, diagnosis/cause identification, management/treatment, monitoring, and revising interventions, as warranted. The attending physician plays a key leadership role in medication management by developing, monitoring, and modifying the medication regimen in conjunction with residents and/or representative(s) and other professionals and direct care staff (the interdisciplinary team).
When selecting medications and non-pharmacological interventions, members of the interdisciplinary team participate in the care process to identify, assess, address, advocate for, monitor, and communicate the resident's needs and changes in condition.

This guidance is intended to help the surveyor determine whether the facility's medication management supports and promotes:

- Selection of medications(s) based on assessing relative benefits and risks to the individual resident;

- Evaluation of a resident's signs and symptoms, in order to identify the underlying cause(s), including adverse consequences of medications;

- Selection and use of medications in doses and for the duration appropriate to each resident's clinical conditions, age, and underlying causes of symptoms;

- The use of non-pharmacological interventions, when applicable, to minimize the need for medications, permit use of the lowest possible dose, or allow medications to be discontinued; and

- The monitoring of medications for efficacy and clinically significant adverse consequences.

The resident's clinical record documents and communicates to the entire team the basic elements of the care process. Information about aspects of the care process related to medications may be found in various locations within the record, such as: hospital discharge summaries and transfer notes, progress notes and interdisciplinary notes, history and physical examination, Resident Assessment Instrument (RAI), plan of care, laboratory reports, professional consults, medication orders, Medication Regimen Review (MRR) reports, and Medication Administration Records (MAR).

Resident Choice – A resident and/or representative(s) has the right to be informed about the resident's condition; treatment options, relative risks and benefits of treatment, required monitoring, expected outcomes of the treatment; and has the right to refuse care and treatment. If a resident refuses treatment, the facility staff and physician should inform the resident about the risks related to the refusal, and discuss appropriate alternatives such as offering the medication at another time or in another dosage form, or offer an alternative medication or non-pharmacological approach, if available.

Advance Directives – A resident may have written or verbal directions related to treatment choices (or a decision has been made by the resident's surrogate or representative) in accordance with state law. An advance directive is a means for the resident to communicate his or her wishes, which may include withdrawing or withholding medications. Whether or not a resident has an advanced directive, the facility is responsible for giving treatment, support, and other care that is consistent with the resident's condition and applicable care instructions.

NOTE: Choosing not to be resuscitated (reflected in a "Do Not Resuscitate" (DNR) order) indicates that the resident should not be resuscitated if respirations and/or cardiac function cease. A DNR order by itself does not indicate that the resident has declined other appropriate treatment and services.

Under these regulations, medication management includes consideration of:

I. Indications for use of medication (including initiation or continued use of antipsychotic medication);

II. Monitoring for efficacy and adverse consequences;

III. Dose (including duplicate therapy);

IV. Duration;

V. Tapering of a medication dose/gradual dose reduction for antipsychotic medications; and

VI. Prevention, identification, and response to adverse consequences.

I. Indications for Use of Medication (including Initiation or Continued Use of an Antipsychotic Medication)

An evaluation of the resident helps to identify his/her needs, comorbid conditions, and prognosis to determine factors (including medications and new or worsening medical conditions) that are affecting signs, symptoms, and test results. This evaluation process is important when making initial medication/intervention selections and when deciding whether to modify or discontinue a current medication intervention. Regarding "as needed" (PRN) medications, it is important to evaluate and document the indication(s), specific circumstance(s) for use, and the desired frequency of administration. As part of the evaluation, gathering and analyzing information helps define clinical indications and provide baseline data for subsequent monitoring. The evaluation also clarifies:

- Whether other causes for the symptoms (including behavioral distress that could mimic a psychiatric disorder) have been ruled out;
- Whether the signs, symptoms, or related causes are persistent or clinically significant enough (e.g., causing functional decline) to warrant the initiation or continuation of medication therapy;
- Whether non-pharmacological interventions are considered;
- Whether a particular medication is clinically indicated to manage the symptom or condition; and
- Whether the intended or actual benefit is sufficient to justify the potential risk(s) or adverse consequences associated with the selected medication, dose, and duration.

The content and extent of the evaluation may vary with the situation and may employ various assessment instruments and diagnostic tools. Examples of information to be considered and evaluated may include, but are not limited to, the following:

- An appropriately detailed evaluation of mental, physical, psychosocial, and functional status, including comorbid conditions and pertinent psychiatric symptoms and diagnoses and a description of resident complaints, symptoms, and signs (including the onset, scope, frequency, intensity, precipitating factors, and other important features);
- Each resident's goals and preferences;
- Allergies to medications and foods and potential for medication interactions;
- A history of prior and current medications and non-pharmacological interventions (including therapeutic effectiveness and any adverse consequences);

- Recognition of the need for end-of-life or palliative care; and

- The refusal of care and treatment, including the basis for declining it, and the identification of pertinent alternatives.

  NOTE: The Resident Assessment Protocols (RAPs), an integral part of the comprehensive resident assessment, help identify some possible categories of causes of various symptoms including: behavioral symptoms of distress, delirium, and changes in functional status. Refer to 42 CFR 483.20 and the Minimum Data Set (MDS) and RAPs.

Circumstances that warrant evaluation of the resident and medication(s) may include:

- Admission or re-admission;

- A clinically significant change in condition/status;

- A new, persistent, or recurrent clinically significant symptom or problem;

- A worsening of an existing problem or condition;

- An unexplained decline in function or cognition;

- A new medication order or renewal of orders; and

- An irregularity identified in the pharmacist's monthly medication regimen review.

Specific considerations related to these circumstances may include the following:

- **Admission (or Readmission)** – Some residents may be admitted on medications for an undocumented chronic condition or without a clear indication as to why a medication was begun or should be continued. It is expected that the attending physician, pharmacist, and staff subsequently determine if continuing the medication is justified by evaluating the resident's clinical condition, risks, existing medication regimen, and related factors. If the indications for continuing the medication are unclear, or if the resident's symptoms could represent a clinically significant adverse consequence, additional consideration of the rationale for the medication(s) is warranted.

- **Multiple prescribers** – Regardless of who the prescribers are, the continuation of a medication needs to be evaluated to determine if the medication is still warranted in the context of the resident's other medications and comorbidities. Medications prescribed by a specialist or begun in another care setting, such as the hospital, need to have a clinically pertinent documented rationale.

- **New medication order as an emergency measure** – When a resident is experiencing an acute medical problem or psychiatric emergency (e.g., the resident's behavior poses an immediate risk to the resident or others), medications may be required. In these situations, it is important to identify and address the underlying causes of the problem or symptoms. Once the acute phase has stabilized, the staff and prescriber consider whether medications are still relevant. Subsequently, the medication is reduced or discontinued as soon as possible or the clinical rationale for continuing the medication is documented.

  When psychopharmacological medications are used as an emergency measure, adjunctive approaches, such as behavioral interventions and techniques should be considered and implemented as appropriate. Longer term management options should be discussed with the resident and/or representative(s).

- **Psychiatric disorders or distressed behavior** – As with all symptoms, it is important to seek the underlying cause of distressed behavior, either before or while treating the symptom. Examples of potential causes include:

  - Delirium;
  - Pain;
  - Chronic psychiatric illness such as schizophrenia or schizoaffective disorder;
  - Acute psychotic illness such as brief reactive psychosis;
  - Substance intoxication or withdrawal;
  - Environmental stressors (e.g., excessive heat, noise, overcrowding);
  - Psychological stressors (e.g., disruption of the resident's customary daily routine, grief over nursing home admission or health status, abuse, taunting, intimidation);
  - Neurological illnesses such as Huntington's disease or Tourette's syndrome; or
  - Medical illnesses such as Alzheimer's disease, Lewy body disease, vascular dementia, or frontotemporal dementia.

See Table I below in these guidelines for key issues related to indications for use of antipsychotic agents, monitoring, and adverse consequences.

II. Monitoring for Efficacy and Adverse Consequences

The information gathered during the initial and ongoing evaluations is essential to:

- Incorporate into a comprehensive care plan that reflects appropriate medication related goals and parameters for monitoring the resident's condition, including the likely medication effects and potential for adverse consequences. Examples of this information may include the FDA boxed warnings or adverse consequences that may be rare, but have sudden onset or that may be irreversible. If the facility has established protocols for monitoring specific medications and the protocols are accessible for staff use, the care plan may refer staff to these protocols;

- Optimize the therapeutic benefit of medication therapy and minimize or prevent potential adverse consequences;

- Establish parameters for evaluating the ongoing need for the medication; and

- Verify or differentiate the underlying diagnoses or other underlying causes of signs and symptoms.

The key objectives for monitoring the use of medications are to track progress towards the therapeutic goal(s) and to detect the emergence or presence of any adverse consequences. Effective monitoring relies upon understanding the indications and goals for using the medication, identifying relevant baseline information, identifying the criteria for evaluating the benefit(s) of the medication, and recognizing and evaluating adverse consequences. Monitoring parameters are based on the resident's condition, the pharmacologic properties of the medication being used and its associated risks, individualized therapeutic goals, and the potential for clinically significant adverse consequences.

Adverse consequences related to medications are common enough to warrant serious attention and close monitoring. For example, a study reported that 338 (42%) of 815 adverse drug events were judged preventable, and that common omissions included inadequate monitoring and either lack of response or a delayed response to signs, symptoms, or laboratory evidence of medication toxicity.[55]

Sources of information to facilitate defining the monitoring criteria or parameters may include cautions, warnings, and identified adverse consequences from:

- Manufacturers' package inserts and black-box warnings;

- Facility policies and procedures;

- Pharmacists;

- Clinical practice guidelines or clinical standards of practice;

- Medication references; and

- Clinical studies or evidence-based review articles that are published in medical and/or pharmacy journals.

Monitoring of the resident's response to any medication(s) is essential to evaluate the ongoing benefits as well as risks of various medications. It is important, for example, to monitor the effectiveness of medications used to address behavioral symptoms (e.g., behavioral monitoring) or to treat hypertension (e.g., periodic pulse and blood pressure). Monitoring for adverse consequences involves ongoing vigilance and may periodically involve objective evaluation (e.g., assessing vital signs may be indicated if a medication is known to affect blood pressure, pulse rate and rhythm, or temperature). Using quantitative and qualitative monitoring parameters facilitates consistent and objective collection of information by the facility.

Examples of tools that may be used by facility staff, practitioners, or consultants to determine baseline status as well as to monitor for effectiveness and potential adverse consequences may include, but are not limited to the following:

Common Conditions/ Symptoms	**Examples of Tools**	**Potential Applications**	**Source/Reference**
Diabetes	Blood glucose, Hemoglobin A1C	Diagnose diabetes and determine diabetic control	www.endocrineweb.com/diabetes/diagnosis.html www.diabetes.org/home.jsp www.diabetes.niddk.nih.gov/ www.diabetestoolbox.com/HbA1c.asp
Alzheimer's Disease / Dementia	Mini Mental Status Exam (MMSE)	Determine degree of cognitive impairment	www.emedicine.com/med/topic3358.htm www.fpnotebook.com/NEU75.htm
Functional Decline	Instrumental Activities of Daily Living (IADL)	Assess functional capabilities	www.cdc.gov/nchs/datawh/nchsdefs/iadl.htm www.fpnotebook.com/GER3.htm
	Resident Assessment Instrument (RAI)	Assess aspects of nursing home resident's behavior and function	www.apadiv20.phhp.ufl.edu/fries.htm www.careplans.com/pages/library/RAI_user_guide.pdf
	Functional Alzheimer's Screening Test (FAST)	Assess level of function in individuals with dementia	http://geriatrics.uthscsa.edu/educational/med_students/fastscale_admin.htm

Common Conditions/ Symptoms	Examples of Tools	Potential Applications	Source/Reference
Delirium	Confusion Assessment Method (CAM)	Screen for cognitive impairment and delirium	www.hartfordign.org/publications/trythis/issue13.pdf http://elderlife.med.yale.edu/pdf/The%20Confusion%20Assessment%20Method.pdf
Bipolar Disorder	Mania Rating Scale	Assess severity of mania	www.psychiatryinpractice.com/AssessmentTools/default.aspx?11=3&12=3&13=&13= www.brainexplorer.org/factsheets/Psychiatry%20Rating%20Scales.pdf
Pain	List of pain scales	Assess pain characteristics (e.g., intensity, impact, timing)	www.chcr.brown.edu/pcoc/Physical.htm
Depression	Geriatric Depression Scale	Screen or monitor individuals at risk for depression	www.assessmentpsychology.com/geriatricscales.htm www.hartfordign.org/publications/trythis/issue04.pdf www.merck.com/mrkshared/mmg/tables/33t4.jsp
	Cornell Depression in Dementia Scale	Screen or monitor for depression in individuals with cognitive impairment	www.emoryhealthcare.org/departments/fuqua/CornellScale.pdf
Abnormal Movements	Abnormal Involuntary Movement Scales (AIMS)	Assess presence and severity of involuntary movements that may be due to disease or medications	www.carepaths.com/pages/Instruments_AIMS.asp www.mhsip.org/library/pdfFiles/abnormalinvoluntarymovementscale.pdf

Common Conditions/ Symptoms	Examples of Tools	Potential Applications	Source/Reference
Behavioral Symptoms associated with Dementia	Neuro-psychiatric Inventory-Nursing Home Version (NPI-NH)	Screen or monitor for behavior associated with dementia (e.g., hallucinations, agitation or anxiety)	www.alzheimer-insights.com/insights/vol2no3/vol2no3.htm
	Behavioral Pathology in Alzheimer's Disease Rating Scale (Behave AD)	Provide a global rating of non-cognitive symptoms.	www.alzforum.org/dis/dia/tes/neuropsychological.asp
	Cohen-Mansfield Agitation Inventory (CMAI)	Assess/rate distressed behavior in older individuals	www.researchinstituteonaging.org/assessment.html www.geriatrictimes.com/g010533.html

Monitoring involves several steps, including:

- **Identifying the essential information and how it will be obtained and reported.** It is important to consider who is responsible for obtaining the information, which information should be collected, and how the information will be documented. The information that is collected depends on therapeutic goals, detection of potential or actual adverse consequences, and consideration of risk factors, such as:
    - Medication-medication, medication-food interactions;
    - Clinical condition (for example renal disease);
    - Properties of the medication;
    - Black-box warnings; and
    - History of adverse consequences related to a similar medication.

- **Determining the frequency of monitoring.** The frequency and duration of monitoring needed to identify therapeutic effectiveness and adverse consequences will depend on factors such as clinical standards of practice, facility policies and procedures, manufacturer's specifications, and the resident's clinical condition. Monitoring involves three aspects:

    - Periodic planned evaluation of progress toward the therapeutic goals;
    - Continued vigilance for adverse consequences; and
    - Evaluation of identified adverse consequences.

  For example, when monitoring all psychopharmacological medications and sedative/hypnotics, the facility should review the continued need for them, at least quarterly (i.e., a 3 month period), and document the rationale for continuing the medication, including evidence that the following had been evaluated:

    - The resident's target symptoms and the effect of the medication on the severity, frequency, and other characteristics of the symptoms;
    - Any changes in the resident's function during the previous quarter (e.g., as identified in the Minimum Data Set); and
    - Whether the resident experienced any medication-related adverse consequences during the previous quarter.

  An important aspect of the review would include whether the pharmacological management of the resident's medical and/or psychiatric disorder is consistent with recommendations from relevant clinical practice guidelines, current standards of practice, and/or manufacturer's specifications.

- **Defining the methods for communicating, analyzing, and acting upon relevant information.** The monitoring process needs to identify who is to communicate with the prescriber, what information is to be conveyed, and when to ask the prescriber to evaluate and consider modifying the medication regimen.

  It is important to consider whether a resident's medications are promoting or maintaining a resident's highest practicable level of function. If the therapeutic goals are not being met or the resident is experiencing adverse consequences, it is essential for the prescriber in collaboration with facility staff and pharmacist to consider whether current medications and doses continue to be appropriate or should be reduced, changed, or discontinued.

- **Re-evaluating and updating monitoring approaches.** Modification of monitoring may be necessary when the resident experiences changes, such as:

- o Acute onset of signs or symptoms or worsening of chronic disease;
- o Decline in function or cognition;
- o Addition or discontinuation of medications and/or non-pharmacological interventions;
- o Addition or discontinuation of care and services such as enteral feedings; and
- o Significant changes in diet that may affect medication absorption or effectiveness or increase adverse consequences.

Additional examples of circumstances that may indicate a need to modify the monitoring include: changes in manufacturer's specifications, FDA warnings, pertinent clinical practice guidelines, or other literature about how and what to monitor.

III. Dose (Including Duplicate Therapy)

A prescriber orders medication(s) based on a variety of factors including the resident's diagnoses, signs and symptoms, current condition, age, coexisting medication regimen, review of lab and other test results, input from the interdisciplinary team about the resident, the type of medication(s), and therapeutic goals being considered or used.

Factors influencing the appropriateness of any dose include the resident's clinical response, possible adverse consequences, and other resident and medication-related variables. Often, lab test results such as serum medication concentrations are only a rough guide to dosing. Significant adverse consequences can occur even when the concentration is within the therapeutic range. Serum concentrations alone may not necessarily indicate a need for dose adjustments, but may warrant further evaluation of a dose or the medication regimen.

The route of administration influences a medication's absorption and ultimately the dose received. Examples of factors that can affect the absorption of medications delivered by transdermal patches include skin temperature and moisture, and the integrity of the patch. Similarly, the flow rate of intravenous solutions affects the amount received at a given time.

Duplicate therapy is generally not indicated, unless current clinical standards of practice and documented clinical rationale confirm the benefits of multiple medications from the same class or with similar therapeutic effects. Some examples of potentially problematic duplicate therapy include:

- Use of more than one product containing the same medication can lead to excessive doses of a medication, such as concomitant use of acetaminophen/hydrocodone and acetaminophen, which may increase the risk of acetaminophen toxicity;

- Use of multiple laxatives to improve or maintain bowel movements, which may lead to abdominal pain or diarrhea;
- Concomitant use of multiple benzodiazepines such as lorazepam for anxiety and temazepam for sleep, which may increase fall risk; or
- Use of medications from different therapeutic categories that have similar effects or properties, such as multiple medications with anticholinergic effects (e.g., oxybutynin and diphenhydramine), which may increase the risk of delirium or excessive sedation.

Documentation is necessary to clarify the rationale for and benefits of duplicate therapy and the approach to monitoring for benefits and adverse consequences. This documentation may be found in various areas of the resident's clinical record.

IV. Duration

Many conditions require treatment for extended periods, while others may resolve and no longer require medication therapy. For example:

- Acute conditions such as cough and cold symptoms, upper respiratory condition, nausea and/or vomiting, acute pain, psychiatric or behavioral symptoms;
- Proton pump inhibitors (PPIs)/H2 blockers used for prophylaxis during the acute phase of a medical illness should be tapered and possibly discontinued after the acute phase of the illness has resolved, unless there is a valid clinical indication for prolonged use.

Periodic re-evaluation of the medication regimen is necessary to determine whether prolonged or indefinite use of a medication is indicated. The clinical rationale for continued use of a medication(s) may have been demonstrated in the clinical record, or the staff and prescriber may present pertinent clinical reasons for the duration of use. Common considerations for appropriate duration may include:

- A medication initiated as a result of a time-limited condition (for example, delirium, pain, infection, nausea and vomiting, cold and cough symptoms, or itching) is then discontinued when the condition has resolved, or there is documentation indicating why continued use is still relevant. Failure to review whether the underlying cause has resolved may lead to excessive duration.
- A medication is discontinued when indicated by facility stop order policy or by the prescriber's order, unless there is documentation of the clinical justification for its extended use. A medication administered beyond the stop date established in the prescriber's order or by facility policy, without evidence of clinical

justification for continued use of the medication, may be considered excessive duration.

V. Tapering of a Medication Dose/Gradual Dose Reduction (GDR)

The requirements underlying this guidance emphasize the importance of seeking an appropriate dose and duration for each medication and minimizing the risk of adverse consequences. The purpose of tapering a medication is to find an optimal dose or to determine whether continued use of the medication is benefiting the resident. Tapering may be indicated when the resident's clinical condition has improved or stabilized, the underlying causes of the original target symptoms have resolved, and/or non-pharmacological interventions, including behavioral interventions, have been effective in reducing the symptoms.

There are various opportunities during the care process to evaluate the effects of medications on a resident's function and behavior, and to consider whether the medications should be continued, reduced, discontinued, or otherwise modified. Examples of these opportunities include:

- During the monthly medication regimen review, the pharmacist evaluates resident-related information for dose, duration, continued need, and the emergence of adverse consequences for all medications;

- When evaluating the resident's progress, the practitioner reviews the total plan of care, orders, the resident's response to medication(s), and determines whether to continue, modify, or stop a medication; and

- During the quarterly MDS review, the facility evaluates mood, function, behavior, and other domains that may be affected by medications.

Sometimes, the decision about whether to continue a medication is clear; for example, someone with a history of multiple episodes of depression or recurrent seizures may need an antidepressant or anticonvulsant medication indefinitely. Often, however, the only way to know whether a medication is needed indefinitely and whether the dose remains appropriate is to try reducing the dose and to monitor the resident closely for improvement, stabilization, or decline.

The time frames and duration of attempts to taper any medication depend on factors including the coexisting medication regimen, the underlying causes of symptoms, individual risk factors, and pharmacologic characteristics of the medications. Some medications (e.g., antidepressants, sedative/hypnotics, opioids) require more gradual tapering so as to minimize or prevent withdrawal symptoms or other adverse consequences.

NOTE: If the resident's condition has not responded to treatment or has declined despite treatment, it is important to evaluate both the medication and the dose to determine whether the medication should be discontinued or the dosing should be altered, whether or not the facility has implemented GDR as required, or tapering.

Considerations Specific to Antipsychotics. The regulation addressing the use of antipsychotic medications identifies the process of tapering as a "gradual dose reduction (GDR)" and requires a GDR, unless clinically contraindicated.

Within the first year in which a resident is admitted on an antipsychotic medication or after the facility has initiated an antipsychotic medication, the facility must attempt a GDR in two separate quarters (with at least one month between the attempts), unless clinically contraindicated. After the first year, a GDR must be attempted annually, unless clinically contraindicated.

For any individual who is receiving an antipsychotic medication to treat behavioral symptoms related to dementia, the GDR may be considered clinically contraindicated if:

- The resident's target symptoms returned or worsened after the most recent attempt at a GDR within the facility; and

- The physician has documented the clinical rationale for why any additional attempted dose reduction at that time would be likely to impair the resident's function or increase distressed behavior.

For any individual who is receiving an antipsychotic medication to treat a psychiatric disorder other than behavioral symptoms related to dementia (for example, schizophrenia, bipolar mania, or depression with psychotic features), the GDR may be considered contraindicated, if:

- The continued use is in accordance with relevant current standards of practice and the physician has documented the clinical rationale for why any attempted dose reduction would be likely to impair the resident's function or cause psychiatric instability by exacerbating an underlying psychiatric disorder; or

- The resident's target symptoms returned or worsened after the most recent attempt at a GDR within the facility and the physician has documented the clinical rationale for why any additional attempted dose reduction at that time would be likely to impair the resident's function or cause psychiatric instability by exacerbating an underlying medical or psychiatric disorder.

Attempted Tapering Relative to Continued Indication or Optimal Dose

As noted, attempted tapering is one way to determine whether a specific medication is still indicated, and whether target symptoms and risks can be managed with a lesser dose of a medication. As noted, many medications in various categories can be tapered safely. The following examples of tapering relate to two common categories of concern: sedatives / hypnotics and psychopharmacologic medications (other than antipsychotic and sedatives/hypnotics medications).

Tapering Considerations Specific to Sedatives/Hypnotics.

For as long as a resident remains on a sedative/hypnotic that is used routinely and beyond the manufacturer's recommendations for duration of use, the facility should attempt to taper the medication quarterly unless clinically contraindicated. Clinically contraindicated means:

- The continued use is in accordance with relevant current standards of practice and the physician has documented the clinical rationale for why any attempted dose reduction would be likely to impair the resident's function or cause psychiatric instability by exacerbating an underlying medical or psychiatric disorder; or

- The resident's target symptoms returned or worsened after the most recent attempt at tapering the dose within the facility and the physician has documented the clinical rationale for why any additional attempted dose reduction at that time would be likely to impair the resident's function or cause psychiatric instability by exacerbating an underlying medical or psychiatric disorder.

Considerations Specific to Psychopharmacological Medications (Other Than Antipsychotics and Sedatives/Hypnotics).

During the first year in which a resident is admitted on a psychopharmacological medication (other than an antipsychotic or a sedative/hypnotic), or after the facility has initiated such medication, the facility should attempt to taper the medication during at least two separate quarters (with at least one month between the attempts), unless clinically contraindicated. After the first year, a tapering should be attempted annually, unless clinically contraindicated. The tapering may be considered clinically contraindicated, if:

- The continued use is in accordance with relevant current standards of practice and the physician has documented the clinical rationale for why any attempted dose reduction would be likely to impair the resident's function or cause psychiatric instability by exacerbating an underlying medical or psychiatric disorder; or

- The resident's target symptoms returned or worsened after the most recent attempt at tapering the dose within the facility and the physician has documented the clinical rationale for why any additional attempted dose reduction at that time would be likely to impair the resident's function or cause psychiatric instability by exacerbating an underlying medical or psychiatric disorder.

VI. Adverse Consequences

Any medication or combination of medications (for example interactions between multiple medications with sedative or anticholinergic effects) can cause adverse consequences. Some adverse consequences occur quickly or abruptly, while others are more insidious and develop over time. Adverse consequences may become evident at any time after the medication is initiated, e.g., when there is a change in dose or after another medication has been added.

When reviewing medications used for a resident, it is important to be aware of the medication's recognized safety profile, tolerability, dosing, and potential medication interactions. Although a resident may have an unanticipated reaction to a medication that is not always preventable, many ADRs can be anticipated, minimized, or prevented. Some adverse consequences may be avoided by:

- Following relevant clinical guidelines and manufacturer's specifications for use, dose, administration, duration, and monitoring of the medication;
- Defining appropriate indications for use; and
- Determining that the resident:
    - Has no known allergies to the medication;
    - Is not taking other medications, nutritional supplements including herbal products, or foods that would be incompatible with the prescribed medication; and
    - Has no condition, history, or sensitivities that would preclude use of that medication.

Published studies have sought to identify the frequency, severity, and preventability of adverse consequences. Neuropsychiatric, hemorrhagic, gastrointestinal, renal/electrolyte abnormalities and metabolic/endocrine complications were the most common overall and preventable adverse consequences identified in two nursing home studies. Specifically, a study of 18 community-based nursing homes reported that approximately 50 percent (276/546) of all the adverse consequences—and 72 percent of those characterized as fatal, life-threatening, or serious—were considered preventable.[56] A second study of two academic-based nursing homes reported that inadequate monitoring, failure to act on the monitoring, and errors in ordering, including wrong dose, wrong medication, and medication-medication interactions were the most frequent causes for the preventable adverse consequences.[57]

The risk for adverse consequences increases with both the number of medications being taken regularly and with medications from specific pharmacological classes, such as anticoagulants, diuretics, antipsychotics, anti-infectives, and anticonvulsants.[58,59] See Tables I and II for classes of medications that are associated with frequent or severe adverse consequences. Adverse consequences can range from minimal harm to functional decline, hospitalization, permanent injury, and death.

Delirium (i.e., acute confusional state) is a common medication-related adverse consequence. In many facilities, a majority of the residents have dementia. Individuals who have dementia may be more sensitive to medication effects and may be at greater risk for delirium.[60] Delirium may result from treatable underlying causes including medical conditions and the existing medication regimen. The presence of delirium is associated with higher morbidity and mortality. Some of the classic signs of delirium may be difficult to recognize and may be mistaken for the natural progression of dementia, particularly in the late stages of dementia. Careful observation of the resident (including mental status and level of consciousness), review of the potential causes (e.g., medications, fluid and electrolyte imbalance, infections) of the mental changes and distressed behavior, and appropriate and timely management of delirium are essential.

ENDNOTES

[51] Adapted from American Society of Consultant Pharmacists (ASCP) Guidelines for Assessing the Quality of Drug Regimen Review in Long-Term Care Facilities.

[52] Tobias, DE & Sey, M. (2001). General and psychotherapeutic medication use in 328 nursing facilities: A year 2000 national survey. The Consultant Pharmacist, 15, pp. 34-42.

[53] Briesacher, B.A., Limcangco, M.R., Simoni-Wastila, L., Doshi, J.A., Levens, S.R., Shea, D.G., & Stuart, B. (2005). The quality of antipsychotic drug prescribing in nursing homes. Archives of Internal Medicine, 165, pp. 1280-1285.

[54] Ray, W.A., Taylor, J.A., Meador, K.G., Lichtenstein, M.J., Griffin, M.R., Fought, R., Adams, M.L., & Blazer, D.G. (1993). Reducing antipsychotic drug use in nursing homes. A controlled trial of provider education. Archives of Internal Medicine, 153(6), pp. 713-21.

[55] Gurwitz, J.H., Field, T.S., Judge, J., Rochon, P., Harrold, L.R., Cadoret, C., Lee, M., White, K., LaPrino, J., Erramuspe-Mainard, J., DeFlorio, M., Gavendo, L., Auger, J., & Bates, D.W. (2005). Incidence of adverse drug consequences in two large academic long-term care facilities. American Journal of Medicine, 118, pp. 251-258.

[56] Gurwitz, J.H., Field, T.S., Avorn, J., McCormick, D., Jain, S., Eckler, M., Benser, M., Edmondson, A.C., & Bates, D.W. (2000). Incidence and preventability of adverse drug events in nursing homes. American Journal of Medicine, 109, pp. 87-94.

[57] Gurwitz, J.H., Field, T.S., Avorn, J., McCormick, D., Jain, S., Eckler, M., Benser, M., Edmondson, A.C., & Bates, D.W. (2000). Incidence and preventability of adverse drug events in nursing homes. American Journal of Medicine, 109, pp. 87-94.

[58] Field T.S., Gurwitz J.H., Avorn J., McCormick, D., Shailavi, J., Eckler, M., Benser, M., & Bates, D.W. (2001). Risk factors for adverse drug events among nursing home residents. Archives of Internal Medicine, 161, pp. 1629-34.

[59] Denham, M.J. (1990). Adverse drug reactions. British Medical Bulletin, 46, pp. 53-62.

[60] Rosen's Emergency Medicine: Concepts and Clinical Practice, 5th ed., (2002). Marx, J.A., Hockberger, R.S., Walls, R.M., Adams, J., Barkin, R.M., Danzl, D.F., Gausche-Hill, M., Hamilton, G.C., Ling, L.J., & Newton, E. (Eds.). St Louis: Mosby, Inc., p. 1469.

TABLE I

MEDICATION ISSUES OF PARTICULAR RELEVANCE

This table lists alphabetically, examples of some categories of medications that have the potential to cause clinically significant adverse consequences, that may have limited indications for use, require specific monitoring, and which warrant careful consideration of relative risks and benefit. Inclusion of a medication in this table does not imply that it is contraindicated for every resident. Medications are identified by generic rather than trade names.

NOTE: This table is based on review of a variety of pharmaceutical references. It does not include all categories of medications or all medications within a category, and does not address all issues or considerations related to medication use, such as dosages. Medications other than those listed in this table may present significant issues related to indications, dosage, duration, monitoring, or potential for clinically significant adverse consequences.

Since medication issues continue to evolve and new medications are being approved regularly, it is important to refer to a current authoritative source for detailed medication information such as indications and precautions, dosage, monitoring, or adverse consequences.

The listed doses for psychopharmacological medications are applicable to older individuals. The facility is encouraged to initiate therapy with lower doses and, when necessary, only gradually increase doses. The facility may exceed these doses if it provides evidence to show why higher doses were necessary to maintain or improve the resident's function and quality of life.

Medication	Issues and Concerns
Analgesics	
acetaminophen	**Dosage / Adverse Consequences** • Daily doses greater than 4 grams/day from all sources (alone or as part of combination products) may increase risk of liver toxicity **Monitoring** • For doses greater than the maximum recommended daily dose, documented assessment should reflect periodic monitoring of liver function and indicate that benefits outweigh risks
Non-Steroidal Anti-	**Indications**

Medication	Issues and Concerns
Inflammatory Drugs (NSAIDs) Non-selective NSAIDs, e.g., • aspirin • diclofenac • diflunisal • ibuprofen • indomethacin • ketorolac • meclofenamate • naproxen • piroxicam • salicylates • tolmetin Cyclooxygenase-II (COX-2) inhibitors, e.g., • celecoxib	• NSAID, including COX-2 inhibitors, should be reserved for symptoms and/or inflammatory conditions for which lower risk analgesics (e.g., acetaminophen) have either failed, or are not clinically indicated **Exception:** Use of low dose aspirin (81–325 mg/day) as prophylactic treatment for cardiovascular events such as myocardial infarct or stroke may be appropriate **Interactions** • Aspirin may increase the adverse effects of COX-2 inhibitors on the gastrointestinal (GI) tract • Some NSAIDS (e.g., ibuprofen) may reduce the cardioprotective effect of aspirin **Monitoring** • Monitor closely for bleeding when ASA > 325 mg/day is being used with another NSAID or when NSAIDS are used with other platelet inhibitors or anticoagulants (See See 42 CFR 483.60(c) F428 for Table of Common Medication-Medication Interactions in Long Term Care) **Adverse Consequences** • May cause gastrointestinal (GI) bleeding in anyone with a prior history of, or with increased risk for, GI bleeding. Compared to nonselective NSAIDs, COX-2 inhibitors may reduce—but do not eliminate—risk of gastrointestinal bleeding • May cause bleeding in anyone who is receiving warfarin, heparin, other anticoagulants, or platelets inhibitors (e.g., ticlopidine, clopidogrel, and dipyridamole) • Any NSAID may cause or worsen renal failure, increase blood pressure, or exacerbate heart failure • Prolonged use of indomethacin, piroxicam, tolmetin, and meclofenamate should be avoided because of central nervous system side effects,

Medication	Issues and Concerns
	e.g., headache, dizziness, somnolence, confusion
Opioid analgesics Short-acting, e.g., • codeine • fentanyl • hydrocodone • hydromorphone • meperidine • morphine • oxycodone Long-acting, e.g., • fentanyl, transdermal • methadone • morphine sustained release • oxycodone, sustained release	**Indications** • The initiation of longer-acting opioid analgesics is not recommended unless shorter-acting opioids have been tried unsuccessfully, or titration of shorter-acting doses has established a clear daily dose of opioid analgesic that can be provided by using a long-acting form • Meperidine is not an effective oral analgesic in doses commonly used in older individuals **Adverse Consequences** • May cause constipation, nausea, vomiting, sedation, lethargy, weakness confusion, dysphoria, physical and psychological dependency, hallucinations and unintended respiratory depression, especially in individuals with compromised pulmonary function. These can lead to other adverse consequences such as falls • Meperidine use (oral or injectable) may cause confusion, respiratory depression even with therapeutic analgesic doses • Active metabolite of meperidine (normerperidine) accumulates with repeated use and has been associated with seizures
pentazocine	**Indications** • Limited effectiveness because it is a partial opiate agonist-antagonist; is not recommended for use in older individuals **Adverse Consequences** • This opioid analgesic causes central nervous system side effects (including confusion and hallucinations) more commonly than other opioid analgesics • May cause dizziness, lightheadedness, euphoria, sedation, hypotension, tachycardia, syncope
propoxyphene and	**Indications**

Medication	Issues and Concerns
combination products with aspirin or acetaminophen	• Offers few analgesic advantages over acetaminophen, yet has the adverse effects, including addiction risk, of other opioid medications; is not recommended for use in older individuals **Adverse Consequences** • May cause hypotension and central nervous system effects (e.g., confusion, drowsiness, dizziness) that can lead to other adverse consequences such as falls
Antibiotics	
All antibiotics	**Indications** • Use of antibiotics should be limited to confirmed or suspected bacterial infection **Adverse Consequences** • Any antibiotic may cause diarrhea, nausea, vomiting, anorexia, and hypersensitivity/allergic reactions • Antibiotics are non-selective and may result in the eradication of beneficial microorganisms and the emergence of undesired ones, causing secondary infections such as oral thrush, colitis, and vaginitis
Parenteral vancomycin and aminoglycosides, e.g., • amikacin • gentamycin/ gentamicin • tobramycin	**Monitoring** • Use must be accompanied by monitoring of renal function tests (which should be compared with the baseline) and by serum medication concentrations • Serious adverse consequences may occur insidiously if adequate monitoring does not occur **Exception:** Single dose administration prophylaxis **Adverse Consequences** • May cause or worsen hearing loss and renal failure
nitrofurantoin	**Indications**

<table>
<tr><th>Medication</th><th>Issues and Concerns</th></tr>
<tr><td></td><td><ul><li>It is not the anti-infective/antibiotic of choice for treatment of acute urinary tract infection or prophylaxis in individuals with impaired renal function (CrCl <60 ml/min) because of ineffectiveness and the high risk of serious adverse consequences</li></ul>Adverse Consequences<ul><li>May cause pulmonary fibrosis (e.g., symptoms including dyspnea, cough) and peripheral neuropathy</li></ul></td></tr>
<tr><td>Fluoroquinolones, e.g.,<ul><li>ciprofloxacin</li><li>levofloxacin</li><li>moxifloxacin</li><li>ofloxacin</li></ul></td><td>Indications<ul><li>Use should be avoided in individuals with prolonged QTc intervals or who are receiving antiarrhythmic agents in class Ia (e.g., procainamide), class Ic (e.g., flecainide) or class III (e.g., amiodarone)</li></ul>Adverse Consequences<ul><li>May cause prolonged QTc interval</li><li>May increase risk of hypo- or hyperglycemia in individuals age 65 or older, and in individuals with diabetes mellitus, renal insufficiency (CrCl < 60 ml/min), or those receiving other glucose-altering medications</li><li>May increase risk of acute tendonitis</li></ul></td></tr>
<tr><td>Anticoagulants</td><td></td></tr>
<tr><td>warfarin</td><td>Monitoring<ul><li>Use must be monitored by Prothrombin Time (PT)/International Normalization Ratio (INR), with frequency determined by clinical circumstances, duration of use, and stability of monitoring results</li></ul>Adverse Consequences<ul><li>Multiple medication interactions exist (See 42 CFR 483.60(c) F428 for Table of Common Medication-Medication Interactions in Long Term Care), which may:</li></ul></td></tr>
</table>

Medication	Issues and Concerns
	o Significantly increase PT/INR results to levels associated with life-threatening bleeding, or o Decrease PT/INR results to ineffective levels, or o Increase or decrease the serum concentration of the interacting medication
Anticonvulsants	
All anticonvulsants, e.g., • carbamazepine • gabapentin • lamotrigine • levetiracetam • oxcarbazepine • phenobarbital • phenytoin • primidone • valproic acid	**Indications** • In addition to seizures, may also be used to treat other disorders, such as bipolar disorder, schizoaffective disorder, chronic neuropathic pain, and for prophylaxis of migraine headaches • Need for indefinite continuation should be based on confirmation of the condition (for example, distinguish epilepsy from isolated seizure due to medical cause or distinguish migraine from other causes of headaches) and its potential causes (medications, electrolyte imbalance, hypocalcemia, etc.) **Duration** • If used to manage behavior, stabilize mood, or treat a psychiatric disorder, refer to Section V – Tapering of a Medication Dose/Gradual Dose Reduction (GDR) in the guidance **Monitoring** • Serum medication concentration monitoring is not required or available for all anticonvulsants. Only the following anticonvulsants should be monitored with periodic serum concentrations: phenytoin, phenobarbital, primidone, divalproex sodium (as valproic acid), and carbamazepine • Serum medication concentrations may help identify toxicity, but significant signs and symptoms of toxicity can occur even at normal or low serum concentrations. • When anticonvulsants are used for conditions other than seizure disorders (e.g., as mood

Medication	Issues and Concerns
	stabilizers), the same concerns exist regarding the need for monitoring for effectiveness and side effects; but evaluation of symptoms—not serum concentrations—should be used to adjust doses. High or toxic serum concentrations should, however, be evaluated and considered for dosage adjustments • Symptom control for seizures or behavior can occur with subtherapeutic serum medication concentrations **Adverse Consequences** • May cause liver dysfunction, blood dyscrasias, and serious skin rashes requiring discontinuation of treatment • May cause nausea/vomiting, dizziness, ataxia, somnolence/lethargy, incoordination, blurred or double vision, restlessness, toxic encephalopathy, anorexia, headaches. These effects can increase the risk for falls
Antidepressants	
All antidepressants classes, e.g., Alpha-adrenoceptor antagonist, e.g., • mirtazapine Dopamine-reuptake blocking compounds, e.g., • bupropion Monoamine oxidase inhibitors (MAOIs) Serotonin (5-HT 2) antagonists, e.g., • nefazodone • trazodone Selective serotonin-norepinephrine reuptake inhibitors (SNRIs), e.g., • duloxetine, • venlafaxine	**Indications** • Agents usually classified as "antidepressants" are prescribed for conditions other than depression including anxiety disorders, post-traumatic stress disorder, obsessive compulsive disorder, insomnia, neuropathic pain (e.g., diabetic peripheral neuropathy), migraine headaches, urinary incontinence, and others **Dosage** • Use of two or more antidepressants simultaneously may increase risk of side effects; in such cases, there should be documentation of expected benefits that outweigh the associated risks and monitoring for any increase in side effects **Duration** • Duration should be in accordance with pertinent literature, including clinical practice guidelines

Medication	Issues and Concerns
Selective serotonin reuptake inhibitors (SSRIs), e.g., • citalopram • escitalopram • fluoxetine • fluvoxamine • paroxetine • sertraline Tricyclic (TCA) and related compounds	• Prior to discontinuation, many antidepressants may need a gradual dose reduction or tapering to avoid a withdrawal syndrome (e.g., SSRIs, TCAs) • If used to manage behavior, stabilize mood, or treat a psychiatric disorder, refer to Section V – Tapering of a Medication Dose/Gradual Dose Reduction (GDR) in the guidance **Monitoring** • All residents being treated for depression with any antidepressant should be monitored closely for worsening of depression and/or suicidal behavior or thinking, especially during initiation of therapy and during any change in dosage **Interactions/Adverse Consequences** • May cause dizziness, nausea, diarrhea, anxiety, nervousness, insomnia, somnolence, weight gain, anorexia, or increased appetite. Many of these effects can increase the risk for falls • Bupropion may increase seizure risk and be associated with seizures in susceptible individuals • SSRIs in combination with other medications affecting serotonin (e.g., tramadol, St. John's Wort, linezolid, other SSRI's) may increase the risk for serotonin syndrome and seizures
Monoamine oxidase inhibitors (MAOIs), e.g., • isocarboxazid • phenelzine • tranylcypromine	**Indications/Contraindications** • Should not be administered to anyone with a confirmed or suspected cerebrovascular defect or to anyone with confirmed cardiovascular disease or hypertension • Should not be used in the presence of pheochromocytoma • MAO Inhibitors are rarely utilized due to their potential interactions with tyramine or tryptophan-containing foods, other medications, and their profound effect on blood pressure **Adverse Consequences**

Medication	Issues and Concerns
	• May cause hypertensive crisis if combined with certain foods, cheese, wine **Exception:** Monoamine oxidase inhibitors such as selegiline (MAO-B inhibitors) utilized for Parkinson's Disease, unless used in doses greater than 10 mg per day **Interactions** • Should not be administered together or in rapid succession with other MAO inhibitors, tricyclic antidepressants, bupropion, SSRIs, buspirone, sympathomimetics, meperidine, triptans, and other medications that affect serotonin or norepinephrine
Tricyclic antidepressants (TCAs), e.g., • amitriptyline • amoxapine • doxepin • combination products, e.g., o amitriptyline and chlordiazepoxide o amitripytline and perphenazine	**Indications** • Because of strong anticholinergic and sedating properties, TCAs and combination products are rarely the medication of choice in older individuals **Exception:** Use of TCAs may be appropriate if: o The resident is being treated for neurogenic pain (e.g., trigeminal neuralgia, peripheral neuropathy), based on documented evidence to support the diagnosis; and o The relative benefits outweigh the risks and other, safer agents including non-pharmacological interventions or alternative therapies are not indicated or have been considered, attempted, and failed **Adverse Consequences** • Compared to other categories of antidepressants, TCAs cause significant anticholinergic side effects and sedation (nortriptyline and desipramine are less problematic)
Antidiabetic medications	
Insulin and oral	**Monitoring**

Medication	Issues and Concerns
hypoglycemics, e.g., • acarbose • acetohexamide • chlorpropamide • glimepiride • glipizide • glyburide • metformin • repaglinide • rosiglitazone • tolazamide • tolbutamide Including combination products, e.g., • rosiglitazone/ metformin • glyburide/metformin • glipizide/metformin • pioglitazone/ metformin	• Use of anti-diabetic medications should include monitoring (for example, periodic blood sugars) for effectiveness based on desired goals for that individual and to identify complications of treatment such as hypoglycemia, impaired renal function **NOTE:** Continued or long-term need for sliding scale insulin for non-emergency coverage may indicate inadequate blood sugar control • Residents on rosiglitazone should be monitored for visual deterioration due to new onset and/or worsening of macular edema in diabetic patients **Adverse Consequences** • Metformin has been associated with the development of lactic acidosis (a potentially life threatening metabolic disorder), which is more likely to occur in individuals with: o serum creatinine ≥ 1.5 mg/dL in males or ≥ 1.4 mg/dL in females o abnormal creatinine clearance from any cause, including shock, acute myocardial infarction, or septicemia o age ≥ 80 years unless measurement of creatinine clearance verifies normal renal function o radiologic studies in which intravascular iodinated contrast materials are given o congestive heart failure requiring pharmacological management o acute or chronic metabolic acidosis with or without coma (including diabetic ketoacidosis) • Rosiglitazone and pioglitazone have been associated with edema and weight gain; therefore, their use should be avoided in residents with Stage III or Stage IV heart failure

Medication	Issues and Concerns
	• Sulfonylureas can cause the syndrome of inappropriate antidiuretic hormone (SIADH) and result in hyponatremia
chlorpropamide glyburide	**Indications** • Chlorpropamide and glyburide are not considered hypoglycemic agents of choice in older individuals because of the long half-life and/or duration of action and increased risk of hypoglycemia **Adverse Consequences** • May cause prolonged and serious hypoglycemia (with symptoms including tachycardia, palpitations, irritability, headache, hypothermia, visual disturbances, lethargy, confusion, seizures, and/or coma)
Antifungals	

Imidazoles for systemic use, e.g.,
• fluconazole
• itraconazole
• ketoconazole
	Indications
	
	• Should be used in lowest possible dose for shortest possible duration, especially in anyone receiving other medications known to interact with these medications
	
	Interactions/Adverse Consequences
	
	• Interaction with warfarin can cause markedly elevated PT/INR, increasing bleeding risk
	
	• Multiple potentially significant medication interactions may occur, for example:
	  o These medications when administered concurrently may increase the effect or toxicity of phenytoin, theophylline, sulfonylureas (hypoglycemics)
	  o Other medications such as rifampin and cimetidine may decrease the effect of these antifungals
	
	• May cause hepatotoxicity, headaches, GI distress
	
	Monitoring

Medication	Issues and Concerns
	• Enhanced monitoring may be required to identify and minimize adverse consequences when these antifungals are given with the following: o warfarin (PT/INR) o phenytoin (serum phenytoin levels) o theophylline (serum theophylline levels) o sulfonylureas (fasting blood glucose)
Antimanic medications	
Lithium	**Indications** • Should generally not be given to individuals with significant renal or cardiovascular disease, severe debilitation, dehydration, or sodium depletion **Monitoring** • Toxic levels are very close to therapeutic levels. Serum lithium concentration should be monitored periodically, and dosage adjusted accordingly **Interactions/Adverse Consequences** • May cause potentially dangerous sodium imbalance • Adverse consequences may occur at relatively low serum concentrations (1–1.5 mEq/L) • Serum lithium concentration levels can be affected by many other medications, e.g., thiazide diurectics, ACE inhibitors, NSAIDs
Antiparkinson medications	
All classes, e.g., Catechol-O-Methyl Transferase (COMT) Inhibitors, e.g., • entacapone Dopamine agonists, e.g., • bromocriptine • ropinirole	**Adverse Consequences** • May cause significant confusion, restlessness, delirium, dyskinesia, nausea, dizziness, hallucinations, agitation • Increased risk of postural hypotension and falls, especially when given in conjunction with antihypertensive medications

Medication	Issues and Concerns
• pramipexole MAO inhibitors, e.g., • selegiline Others, e.g., • amantadine Various dopaminergic combinations, e.g., • carbidopa/levodopa • carbidopa/levodopa/ entacapone	
Antipsychotic medications	
All classes, e.g., First generation (conventional) agents, e.g. • chlorpromazine • fluphenazine • haloperidol • loxapine • mesoridazine • molindone • perphenazine • promazine • thioridazine • thiothixene • trifluoperazine • triflupromazine Second generation (atypical) agents, e.g. • aripiprazole • clozapine • olanzapine • quetiapine • risperidone • ziprasidone	**Indications** • An antipsychotic medication should be used only for the following conditions/diagnoses as documented in the record and as meets the definition(s) in the Diagnostic and Statistical Manual of Mental Disorders, Fourth Edition, Training Revision (DSM-IV TR) or subsequent editions): o Schizophrenia o Schizo-affective disorder o Delusional disorder o Mood disorders (e.g. mania, bipolar disorder, depression with psychotic features, and treatment refractory major depression) o Schizophreniform disorder o Psychosis NOS o Atypical psychosis o Brief psychotic disorder o Dementing illnesses with associated behavioral symptoms o Medical illnesses or delirium with manic or psychotic symptoms and/or treatment-related psychosis or mania (e.g.,

Medication	Issues and Concerns
	thyrotoxicosis, neoplasms, high dose steroids) • In addition, the use of an antipsychotic must meet the criteria and applicable, additional requirements listed below: 1. Criteria: o Since diagnoses alone do not warrant the use of antipsychotic medications, the clinical condition must also meet at least one of the following criteria (A or B or C): A. The symptoms are identified as being due to mania or psychosis (such as: auditory, visual, or other hallucinations; delusions (such as paranoia or grandiosity)); OR B. The behavioral symptoms present a danger to the resident or to others; OR C. The symptoms are significant enough that the resident is experiencing one or more of the following: inconsolable or persistent distress (e.g., fear, continuously yelling, screaming, distress associated with end-of-life, or crying); a significant decline in function; and/or substantial difficulty receiving needed care (e.g., not eating resulting in weight loss, fear and not bathing leading to skin breakdown or infection). 2. Additional Requirements: o Acute Psychiatric Situations When an antipsychotic medication is being initiated or used to treat an acute psychiatric emergency (i.e., recent or abrupt onset or exacerbation of symptoms) related to one or more of the aforementioned conditions/diagnoses, that use must meet one of the above criteria and all of the following additional

Medication	Issues and Concerns
	requirements: A. The acute treatment period is limited to seven days or less; and B. A clinician in conjunction with the interdisciplinary team must evaluate and document the situation within 7 days, to identify and address any contributing and underlying causes of the acute psychiatric condition and verify the continuing need for antipsychotic medication; and C. Pertinent non-pharmacological interventions must be attempted, unless contraindicated, and documented following the resolution of the acute psychiatric situation. o Enduring Psychiatric Conditions Antipsychotic medications may be used to treat an enduring (i.e., non-acute, chronic, or prolonged) condition, if the clinical condition/diagnosis meets the criteria in #1 above. In addition, before initiating or increasing an antipsychotic medication for enduring conditions, the target behavior must be clearly and specifically identified and monitored objectively and qualitatively, in order to ensure the behavioral symptoms are: A. Not due to a medical condition or problem (e.g., headache or joint pain, fluid or electrolyte imbalance, pneumonia, hypoxia, unrecognized hearing or visual impairment) that can be expected to improve or resolve as the underlying condition is treated; and B. Persistent or likely to reoccur without continued treatment; and C. Not sufficiently relieved by non-

Medication	Issues and Concerns
	pharmacological interventions; and D. Not due to environmental stressors (e.g., alteration in the resident's customary location or daily routine, unfamiliar care provider, hunger or thirst, excessive noise for that individual, inadequate or inappropriate staff response, physical barriers) that can be addressed to improve the psychotic symptoms or maintain safety; and E. Not due to psychological stressors (e.g., loneliness, taunting, abuse), or anxiety or fear stemming from misunderstanding related to his or her cognitive impairment (e.g., the mistaken belief that this is not where he/she lives or inability to find his or her clothes or glasses) that can be expected to improve or resolve as the situation is addressed • After initiating or increasing the dose of an antipsychotic medication, the behavioral symptoms must be reevaluated periodically to determine the effectiveness of the antipsychotic and the potential for reducing or discontinuing the dose **Exception:** When antipsychotic medications are used for behavioral disturbances related to Tourette's disorder, or for non-psychiatric indications such as movement disorders associated with Huntington's disease, hiccups, nausea and vomiting associated with cancer or cancer chemotherapy, or adjunctive therapy at end of life. **Inadequate Indications** • In many situations, antipsychotic medications are not indicated. They should not be used if the only indication is one or more of the following: 1) wandering; 2) poor self-care; 3) restlessness; 4) impaired memory; 5) mild anxiety; 6) insomnia; 7) unsociability; 8) inattention or indifference to

Medication	Issues and Concerns
	surroundings; 9) fidgeting; 10) nervousness; 11) uncooperativeness; or 12) verbal expressions or behavior that are not due to the conditions listed under "Indications" and do not represent a danger to the resident or others.

Dosage

- Doses for acute indications (for example, delirium) may differ from those used for long-term treatment, but should be the lowest possible to achieve the desired therapeutic effects

Daily Dose Thresholds for Antipsychotic Medications Used to Manage Behavioral Symptoms Related to Dementing Illnesses

Generic Medication	Dosage
First Generation	
chlorpromazine	75 mg
fluphenazine	4 mg
haloperidol	2 mg
loxapine	10 mg
molindone	10 mg
perphenazine	8 mg
pimozide	*
prochloroperazine	*
thioridazine	75 mg
thiothixene	7 mg
trifluoperazine	8 mg
Second Generation	
aripiprazole	10 mg
clozapine	50 mg
olanzapine	7.5 mg
quetiapine	150 mg
risperidone	2 mg
ziprasidone	*

* Not customarily used for the treatment of behavioral symptoms

References:

Katz, I.R. (2004). Optimizing atypical antipsychotic treatment strategies in the elderly. Journal of the American Geriatrics Society, 52, pp. 272-277.

Medication	Issues and Concerns
	Schneider, L.S. (2005). Risk of death with atypical antipsychotic drug treatment for dementia. Meta-analysis of randomized placebo controlled trials. Journal of the American Medical Association, 294, pp. 1934-1943. Saltz, B.L., Woerner, M.G., Robinson, D.G., & Kane, J.M. (2000). Side effects of antipsychotic drugs: Avoiding and minimizing their impact in elderly patients. Postgraduate Medicine, 107, pp. 169-178.
	Duration • If used to manage behavior, stabilize mood, or treat a psychiatric disorder, refer to Section V – Tapering of a Medication Dose/Gradual Dose Reduction (GDR) in the guidance
	Monitoring/Adverse Consequences • The facility assures that residents are being adequately monitored for adverse consequences such as: o anticholinergic effects (see Table II) o increase in total cholesterol and triglycerides o akathisia o parkinsonism o neuroleptic malignant syndrome (NMS) o blood sugar elevation (including diabetes mellitus) o cardiac arrhythmias o orthostatic hypotension o death secondary to heart-related events (e.g., heart failure, sudden death) o cerebrovascular event (e.g., stroke, transient ischemic attack (TIA)) in older individuals with dementia o falls o tardive dyskinesia o lethargy o excessive sedation • When antipsychotics are used without monitoring

Medication	Issues and Concerns
	they may be considered unnecessary medications because of inadequate monitoring.
Anxiolytics	
All Anxiolytics Benzodiazepines, Short-acting, e.g., • alprazolam • estazolam • lorazepam • oxazepam • temazepam Benzodiazepines, Long acting, e.g., • chlordiazepoxide • clonazepam • clorazepate • diazepam • flurazepam • quazepam buspirone Other antidepressants except bupropion	**Indications** • Anxiolytic medications should only be used when: o Use is for one of the following indications as defined in the Diagnostic and Statistical Manual of Mental Disorders, Fourth Edition, Training Revision (DSM-IV TR) or subsequent editions: a. Generalized anxiety disorder b. Panic disorder c. Symptomatic anxiety that occurs in residents with another diagnosed psychiatric disorder d. Sleep disorders (See Sedatives/Hypnotics) e. Acute alcohol or benzodiazepine withdrawal f. Significant anxiety in response to a situational trigger g. Delirium, dementia, and other cognitive disorders with associated behaviors that: – Are quantitatively and objectively documented; – Are persistent; – Are not due to preventable or correctable reasons; and – Constitute clinically significant distress or dysfunction to the resident or represent a danger to the resident or others • Evidence exists that other possible reasons for the

Medication	Issues and Concerns
	individual's distress have been considered; and • Use results in maintenance or improvement in the individual's mental, physical or psychosocial well-being (e.g., as reflected on the MDS or other assessment tools); or • There are clinical situations that warrant the use of these medications such as: – a long-acting benzodiazepine is being used to withdraw a resident from a short-acting benzodiazepine – used for neuromuscular syndromes (e.g., cerebral palsy, tardive dyskinesia, restless leg syndrome or seizure disorders) – symptom relief in end of life situations **Dosage** • Dosage is less than, or equal to, the following listed total daily doses unless higher doses (as evidenced by the resident's response and/or the resident's clinical record) are necessary to maintain or improve the resident's function

Total Daily Dose Thresholds for Anxiolytic Medications

Generic Medication	Dosage
flurazepam	15 mg
chlordiazepoxide	20 mg
clorazepate	15 mg
diazepam	5 mg
clonazepam	1.5 mg
quazepam	7.5 mg
estazolam	0.5 mg
alprazolam	0.75 mg
oxazepam	30 mg
lorazepam	2 mg

Duration

Medication	Issues and Concerns
	• If used to manage behavior, stabilize mood, or treat a psychiatric disorder, refer to Section V – Tapering of a Medication Dose/Gradual Dose Reduction (GDR) in the guidance **Adverse Consequences** • May increase risk of confusion, sedation, and falls
diphenhydramine and hydroxyzine	**Indications** • Not appropriate for use as an anxiolytic
meprobamate	**Indications** • Highly addictive and sedating medication; not indicated for use in older individuals **Dosage/Duration** • Those who have used meprobamate for prolonged periods may be physically and/or psychologically dependent and may need to be withdrawn slowly
Cardiovascular medications (including antihypertensives)	
All antiarrhythmics	**Adverse Consequences** • Cardiac antiarrhythmics can have serious adverse effects in older individuals, including impaired mental function, falls, appetite, behavior, and heart function
amiodarone	**Indications** • Only approved indication for use is to treat documented life-threatening recurrent ventricular arrhythmias that do not respond to other antiarrhythmic agents or when alternative agents are not tolerated • Common off-label use to treat atrial fibrillation; however, literature suggests that in many higher risk individuals, alternative approaches to managing atrial fibrillation (rate control and anticoagulation) are equally effective and less

Medication	Issues and Concerns
	toxic* * Goldschlager, N., Epstein, A.E., Naccarelli, G., Olshansky, B., & Singh, B. (2000). Practical guidelines for clinicians who treat patients with amiodarone. Archives of Internal Medicine, 160, pp. 1741-1748. * Denus, S., Sanoski, C.A., Carlson, J., Opolski, G., & Spinler, S.A. (2005). Rate vs rhythm control in patients with atrial fibrillation: A meta-analysis. Archives of Internal Medicine, 165, pp. 258-262. **Dosage/Monitoring** • It is critical to carefully consider risks and benefits, to use the lowest possible dose for the shortest possible duration, to closely monitor individuals receiving long-term amiodarone, and to seek and identify adverse consequences **Interactions/Adverse Consequences** • May cause potentially fatal toxicities, including pulmonary toxicity (hypersensitivity pneumonitis or interstitial/alveolar pneumonitis) and hepatic injury. May cause hypothyroidism, exacerbate existing arrhythmia, and worsen heart failure. Can also impair mental function and behavior • May cause clinically significant medication interactions; for example, with digoxin and warfarin • Toxicity increases with higher doses and longer duration of use
disopyramide	**Adverse Consequences** • Disopyramide has potent negative inotropic effects (decreased force of heart contraction), which may induce heart failure in older individuals, and is also strongly anticholinergic
All antihypertensives	**Dosage/Monitoring** • Doses of individual antihypertensives may require modification in order to achieve desired effects while minimizing adverse consequences,

Medication	Issues and Concerns
	especially when multiple antihypertensives are prescribed simultaneously • When discontinuing some antihypertensives (e.g., clonidine, beta blockers), gradual tapering may be required to avoid adverse consequences caused by abrupt cessation **Interactions/Adverse Consequences** • May cause dizziness, postural hypotension, fatigue, and an increased risk for falls • Many other medications may interact with antihypertensives to potentiate their effect (e.g., levodopa, nitrates)
Alpha blockers, e.g., • alfuzosin • doxazosin • prazosin • tamsulosin • terazosin	**Adverse Consequences** • Doxazosin, prazosin, and terazosin can cause significant hypotension and syncope during the first few doses. Therefore, these medications should be initiated at bedtime with a slow titration of dose • Prazosin can cause more CNS side effects and generally should be avoided in older individuals
Angiotensin converting enzyme (ACE) inhibitors, e.g., • benazepril • captopril • enalapril • fosinopril • lisinopril • ramipril Angiotensin II receptor blockers, e.g., • candesartan • eprosartan • irbesartan • losartan • olmesartan • valsartan	**Monitoring** • Monitoring of serum potassium is necessary especially in individuals receiving ACE inhibitors with potassium, or potassium sparing diuretics **Adverse Consequences** • May cause angioedema (signs and symptoms of immediate hypersensitivity), chronic persistent nonproductive cough, or may worsen renal failure • Potential for life-threatening elevation of serum potassium concentrations when used in combination with potassium supplements, potassium-sparing diuretics including spironolactone

Medication	Issues and Concerns
Beta adrenergic blockers, e.g., Nonselective, e.g., • propranolol Cardioselective, e.g., • atenolol • esmolol • metoprolol • nadolol • timolol	**Adverse Consequences** • May cause or exacerbate: o Bradycardia, especially in individuals receiving other medications that affect cardiac conduction (e.g., calcium channel blockers); o Dizziness, fatigue; depression, bronchospasm (especially, but not exclusively, propranolol); or o Cardiac decompensation that may require adjusting dose in residents with acute heart failure • May mask tachycardia associated with symptomatic hypoglycemia • May have increased effect or may accumulate in individuals with hepatic impairment
Calcium channel blockers, e.g., • nifedipine • isradipine • amlodipine • nisoldipine • diltiazem • verapamil	**Adverse consequences** • May cause clinically significant constipation • May cause peripheral edema • Some agents may cause generalized aching, headache, muscle pain • Short acting/immediate release nifedipine increases the risk of cardiac complications and should not be used
methyldopa Including combination products such as methyldopa/ hydrochlorothiazide	**Indications** • Alternate treatments for hypertension are preferred **Adverse Consequences** • May cause bradycardia and excessive sedation; may exacerbate depression in older individuals
digoxin	**Indications** • Digoxin is indicated only for the following diagnoses: congestive heart failure, atrial

Medication	Issues and Concerns
	fibrillation, paroxysmal supraventricular tachycardia, or atrial flutter • Should be used with caution in individuals with impaired renal function **Dosage** • Daily doses in older individuals should ordinarily not exceed 0.125 mg/day except when used to control atrial arrhythmia and ventricular rate **Monitoring** • Must be used cautiously in individuals with renal failure or fluid and electrolyte imbalance, with close monitoring for adverse consequences and monitoring, as indicated, of both renal function and serum medication concentration ("digoxin level") • Adverse consequences may occur even with therapeutic serum concentration, especially in older individuals **Interactions/Adverse Consequences** • May interact with many other medications, possibly resulting in digoxin toxicity or elevated serum concentrations of other medications • May cause significant bradycardia, especially when used in individuals taking other medications affecting cardiac conduction • Toxicity may cause fatigue, nausea, vomiting, anorexia, delirium, cardiac arrhythmia
Diuretics, e.g., • bumetanide • ethacrynic acid • furosemide • hydrochlorothiazide • metolazone • spironolactone • torsemide • triamterene	**Adverse Consequences** • May cause fluid and electrolyte imbalance (hypo/hypernatremia, hypo/hyperkalemia, dehydration, etc.), hypotension; may precipitate or exacerbate urinary incontinence, falls

Medication	Issues and Concerns
Nitrates, e.g., • isosorbide mononitrate • isosorbide dinitrate • nitroglycerin	**Adverse Consequences** • May cause headaches, dizziness, lightheadedness, faintness, or symptomatic orthostatic hypotension, especially when initially started or when taken in combination with antihypertensive medications
Cholesterol lowering medications	
HMG-CoA Reductase Inhibitors ("statins"), e.g., • atorvastatin • fluvastatin • lovastatin • pravastatin • rosuvastatin • simvastatin	**Monitoring** • Liver function monitoring should be performed consistent with manufacturer's recommendations, generally accepted as: o Prior to initiation of therapy, at 12 weeks following both initiation of therapy and any increase in dose, and periodically (e.g., semiannually) thereafter **Adverse Consequences** • May impair liver function; liver function tests should be monitored as indicated above • May cause muscle pain, myopathy, and rhabdomyolysis (breakdown of skeletal muscle) that can precipitate kidney failure especially in combination with other cholesterol lowering medications.
cholestyramine	**Interactions** • May reduce the absorption of other medications being taken concurrently. Other medications, including diuretics, beta-blockers, corticosteroids, thyroid hormones, digoxin, valproic acid, NSAIDs, sulfonylureas, and warfarin should be administered one hour before or four hours after cholestyramine administration to avoid this interaction **Adverse Consequences** • May cause constipation, dyspepsia, nausea or vomiting, abdominal pain

Medication	Issues and Concerns
fibrates, e.g., • fenofibrate • clofibrate	**Monitoring** • Fenofibrate and clofibrate require regular monitoring of liver tests as well as evaluating the complete blood count (CBC) prior to and after initiation
niacin	**Monitoring** • Monitor glucose and liver function tests regularly **Adverse Consequences** • Interferes with glucose control and can aggravate diabetes • Can exacerbate active gallbladder disease and gout • Flushing is common
Cognitive Enhancers	
Cholinesterase inhibitors, e.g., • donepezil • galantamine • rivastigmine	**Indications** • As the underlying disorder progresses into advanced stages, the continued use of the medication should be reevaluated **Adverse Consequences** • May affect cardiac conduction, especially in individuals who already have a cardiac conduction disorder or who are taking other medications that affect heart rate • May cause insomnia, dizziness, nausea, vomiting, diarrhea, anorexia, and weight loss • Should be used with caution in individuals with severe asthma or obstructive pulmonary disease
NMDA receptor antagonists, e.g., • memantine	**Indications** • As the underlying disorder progresses into advanced stages, the continued use of the medication should be reevaluated **Adverse Consequences** • May cause restlessness, distress, dizziness,

Medication	Issues and Concerns
	somnolence, hypertension, headache, hallucinations, or increased confusion
Cough, cold, and allergy medications	
All cough, cold, allergy medications	**Indications/Duration** • Should be used only for a limited duration (less than 14 days) unless there is documented evidence of enduring symptoms that cannot otherwise be alleviated and for which a cause cannot be identified and corrected
Antihistamine H-1 blockers, e.g., • chlorpheniramine • cyproheptadine • diphenhydramine • hydroxyzine • meclizine • promethazine	**Indications** • H-1 blocker antihistamines have strong anticholinergic properties and are not considered medications of choice in older individuals • If appropriate and effective, topical instead of oral diphenhydramine should be considered for allergic reactions involving the skin **Dosage/Duration** • Should be used in the smallest possible dosage for the shortest possible duration, especially in individuals who are susceptible to anticholinergic side effects or who are receiving other medications with anticholinergic properties (see Table II) **Adverse Consequences** • May cause excessive sedation, confusion, cognitive impairment, distress, dry mouth, constipation, urinary retention. These may lead to other adverse consequences such as falls
Oral decongestants, e.g., • pseudoephedrine	**Adverse Consequences** • May cause dizziness, nervousness, insomnia, palpitations, urinary retention, elevated blood pressure • Should be used with caution in individuals who have insomnia or hypertension
Gastrointestinal	

Medication	Issues and Concerns
medications	
Phenothiazine-related antiemetics, e.g., • prochlorperazine • promethazine	**Indications** • Use with caution in individuals with Parkinson's disease, narrow-angle glaucoma, BPH, seizure disorder **Adverse Consequences** • May cause sedation, dizziness, drowsiness, postural hypotension, and neuroleptic malignant syndrome • May lower seizure threshold • Promethazine and prochlorperazine may cause anticholinergic effects, such as constipation, dry mouth, blurred vision, urinary retention • May cause extrapyramidal symptoms, including medication-induced parkinsonism, acute dystonic reactions, akathisia, and tardive dyskinesia • May alter cardiac conduction or induce arrhythmias
trimethobenzamide	**Adverse Consequences** • Relatively ineffective antiemetic that can cause significant extrapyramidal side effects in addition to lethargy, sedation, confusion **Exception:** May be indicated in patients with Parkinson's Disease taking apomorphine
metoclopramide	**Indications** • High-risk medication with limited clinical indication and limited demonstrated effectiveness* • Not recommended for first-line treatment of gastroesophageal reflux disease, especially in older individuals • When used for diabetic gastroparesis, or other indications, relative benefits and risks should be assessed and documented

<table>
<tr><th>Medication</th><th>Issues and Concerns</th></tr>
<tr><td></td><td>* Lata, P.F., Pigarelli, D.L. (2003). Chronic metoclopramide therapy for diabetic gastroparesis. Ann Pharmacotherapy, 37(1), pp. 122-126.

Adverse Consequences

• Especially in older individuals, metoclopramide may cause restlessness, drowsiness, insomnia, depression, distress, anorexia, and extrapyramidal symptoms, and may lower the seizure threshold

• May increase seizures in individuals with seizure disorders or exacerbate symptoms in individuals with Parkinson's Disease

Monitoring

• It is essential to closely monitor at-risk individuals for adverse consequences</td></tr>
<tr><td>Proton pump inhibitors (PPI), e.g.,

• esomeprazole
• lansoprazole
• omeprazole
• rabeprazole

H-2 antagonists, e.g.,

• cimetidine
• famotidine
• ranitidine</td><td>Indications

• Indication for use should be based on clinical symptoms and/or endoscopic findings

• When used to treat or prevent NSAID-induced gastritis or esophagitis, documentation should exist that other, less GI-toxic analgesics have been tried or were not indicated

Duration

• If used for greater than 12 weeks, clinical rationale for continued need and/or documentation should support an underlying chronic disease (e.g., GERD) or risk factors (e.g., chronic NSAID use)

Dosage

• Dosing of histamine-H2 antagonists should be based on renal function

Interactions

• Cimetidine has higher incidence of medication interactions and should be avoided in older individuals

Adverse Consequences</td></tr>
</table>

Medication	Issues and Concerns
	• May cause or exacerbate headache, nausea, vomiting, flatulence, dysphagia, abdominal pain, diarrhea, or other gastrointestinal symptoms • H-2 antagonists may cause confusion • PPIs may increase the risk of clostridium difficile colitis
Glucocorticoids	
All glucocorticoids (except topical or inhaled dosage forms), e.g., • dexamethasone • hydrocortisone • methylprednisolone • prednisone	**Duration/Monitoring** • Necessity for continued use should be documented, along with monitoring for and management of adverse consequences **Adverse Consequences** • Intermediate- or longer-term use may cause hyperglycemia, psychosis, edema, insomnia, hypertension, osteoporosis, mood lability, or depression
Hematinics	
Erythropoiesis stimulants, e.g., • darbepoetin • erythropoietin	**Indications** • Assessment of causes and categories of anemia should precede or accompany the use of this medication **Monitoring** • Use must be monitored according to specific manufacturer's instructions including blood pressure, baseline serum iron or ferritin level, and frequent complete blood count (CBCs) to permit tapering or discontinuation when hemoglobin/hematocrit reaches or exceeds target ranges **Adverse Consequences** • May cause or worsen hypertension • Excessive dose or duration can lead to polycythemia, dangerous thrombotic events

Medication	Issues and Concerns
	including myocardial infarction and stroke
Iron	**Indications** • Iron therapy is not indicated in anemia of chronic disease when iron stores and transferrin levels are normal or elevated **Dosage/Duration** • Clinical rationale should be documented for long-term use (greater than two months) or administration more than once daily for greater than a week, because of side effects and the risk of iron accumulation in tissues **Monitoring** • Baseline serum iron or ferritin level and periodic CBC or hematocrit/ hemoglobin **Adverse Consequences** • May cause constipation, dyspepsia • Can accumulate in tissues and cause multiple complications if given chronically despite normal or high iron stores
Laxatives	
All categories including bulk producing laxatives, hyperosmolar agents, saline laxatives, stimulant laxatives, emollient laxatives	**Adverse Consequences** • May cause flatulence, bloating, abdominal pain • Bulk forming laxatives and stool softeners may cause accumulation of stool and possible bowel obstruction, if not used with adequate fluids or in individuals with other causes of impaired bowel motility
Muscle relaxants	
All muscle relaxants, e.g., • baclofen • carisoprodol • chlorzoxazone • cyclobenzaprine • dantrolene	**Indications/Adverse Consequences** • Most are poorly tolerated by older individuals due to anticholinergic side effects (see Table II), sedation, or weakness • Long-term use in individuals with complications

Medication	Issues and Concerns
• metaxalone • methocarbamol • orphenadrine	due to multiple sclerosis, spinal cord injuries, cerebral palsy, and other select conditions may be indicated, although close monitoring is still warranted • Abrupt cessation of some muscle relaxants may cause or predispose individuals to seizures or hallucinations **Exception:** Periodic use (once every three months) for a short duration (not more than seven days) may be appropriate, when other interventions or alternative medications are not effective or not indicated
Orexigenics (appetite stimulants)	
All appetite stimulants, e.g., • megestrol acetate • oxandrolone • dronabinol	**Indications** • Use should be reserved for situations where assessment and management of underlying correctable causes of anorexia and weight loss is not feasible or successful, and after evaluating potential benefits/risks **Monitoring** • Appetite and weight should be monitored at least monthly and agent should be discontinued if there is no improvement. **Adverse Consequences** • Megesterol acetate may cause fluid retention, adrenal suppression, and symptoms of adrenal insufficiency • Oxandrolone may cause virilization of females and feminization of males, excessive sexual stimulation, and fluid retention • Dronabinol may cause tachycardia, orthostatic hypotension, dizziness, dysphoria, and impaired cognition, which may lead to falls
Osteoporosis medications	
Bisphosphonates, e.g.,	**Dosage**

Medication	Issues and Concerns
• alendronate • ibandronate • risedronate	• These medications must be taken according to very specific directions, including time of day, position, and timing relative to other medications and food **Monitoring** • Individuals receiving these medications should be monitored closely for gastrointestinal complications, including esophageal or gastric erosion **Adverse Consequences** • Potential to cause gastrointestinal symptoms including dysphagia, esophagitis, gastritis, or esophageal and gastric ulcers, especially when given to individuals who are also taking oral corticosteroids, aspirin or other nonsteroidal anti-inflammatory drugs (NSAIDs)
Platelet inhibitors	
All platelet inhibitors, e.g., • dipyridamole • dipyridamole extended-release and aspirin (as fixed-dose combination) • aspirin • clopidogrel	**Interactions/Adverse Consequences** • May cause thrombocytopenia and increase risk of bleeding • Common side effects include headache, dizziness, and vomiting • See discussion at NSAIDs regarding aspirin • Concurrent use with warfarin or NSAIDs may increase risk of bleeding
ticlopidine	**Indication** • Use may be appropriate in individuals who have had a previous stroke or have evidence of stroke precursors (i.e., transient ischemic attacks (TIAs)), and who cannot tolerate aspirin or another platelet inhibitor **Adverse Consequences** • Associated with more severe side effects and considerably more toxic than other platelet inhibitors; use should be avoided in older

Medication	Issues and Concerns
	individuals • Most serious side effects involve the hematologic system, including potentially life-threatening neutropenia • May also cause nausea, vomiting, and diarrhea
Respiratory medications	
theophylline	**Interactions** • Potentially significant interactions with many other medications may occur, especially various antibiotics, seizure medications, and cardiac medications **Monitoring/Adverse Consequences** • There should be monitoring for signs and symptoms of toxicity, such as arrhythmia, seizure, GI upset, diarrhea, nausea/vomiting, abdominal pain, nervousness, headache, insomnia, distress, dizziness, muscle cramp, tremor • Periodic monitoring of serum concentrations helps identify or verify toxicity
Inhalant medications classes, e.g., Anticholinergic, e.g., • ipratropium • tiotropium Beta 2 agonists, e.g., • albuterol • formoterol • pirbuterol acetate • salmeterol Corticosteroids, e.g., • beclomethasone • budesonide • flunisolide • fluticasone • triamcinolone acetonide	**Adverse Consequences** • Inhaled anticholinergics can cause xerostomia (dry mouth) • Inhaled beta agonists can cause restlessness, increased heart rate, and anxiety • Inhaled steroids can cause throat irritation and oral candidiasis, especially if the mouth is not rinsed after administration

Medication	Issues and Concerns
Miscellaneous, e.g., • cromolyn • nedocromil sodium	
Sedatives/Hypnotics (sleep medications)	

All hypnotics
 	
Benzodiazepine hypnotics, e.g.,
• estazolam
• flurazepam
• quazepam
• temazepam
• triazolam
 	
Non-benzodiazepine hypnotics, e.g.,
• eszopiclone
• zaleplon
• zolpidem
 	
Melatonin receptor agonists, e.g.,
• ramelteon
 	
Other hypnotics, e.g.,
• chloral hydrate
 	
Miscellaneous agents used for sleep, e.g.,
• sedating antidepressants (e.g., trazodone)
• sedating antihistamines (e.g., hydroxyzine)
	Indications
	
	• Most cases of insomnia are associated with underlying conditions (secondary or co-morbid insomnia) such as psychiatric disorders (e.g., depression), cardiopulmonary disorders (e.g., COPD, CHF), urinary frequency, pain, obstructive sleep apnea, and restless leg syndrome. Insomnia may be further described by the duration of symptoms
	
	• Before initiating medications to treat insomnia, other factors potentially causing insomnia should be evaluated, including, for example:
	    o environment, such as excessive heat, cold, or noise; lighting
	    o inadequate physical activity
	    o facility routines that may not accommodate residents' individual needs (e.g., time for sleep, awakening, toileting, medication treatments)
	    o provision of care in a manner that disrupts sleep
	    o caffeine or medications known to disrupt sleep
	    o pain and discomfort
	    o underlying conditions (secondary or co-morbid insomnia) such as psychiatric disorders (e.g., depression), cardiopulmonary disorders (e.g., COPD, CHF), urinary frequency, pain, obstructive sleep apnea, and restless leg syndrome
	
	• It is expected that interventions (such as sleep

Medication	Issues and Concerns
	hygiene approaches, individualizing the sleep and wake times to accommodate the person's wishes and prior customary routine, and maximizing treatment of any underlying conditions) are implemented to address the causative factor(s) • These guidelines apply to any medication that is being used to treat insomnia. Initiation of medications to induce or maintain sleep should be preceded or accompanied by other interventions to try to improve sleep. All sleep medications should be used in accordance with approved product labeling; for example, timing and frequency of administration relative to anticipated waking time • The use of sedating medications for individuals with diagnosed sleep apnea requires careful assessment, documented clinical rationale, and close monitoring **Exceptions:** • Use of a single dose sedative for dental or medical procedures • During initiation of treatment for depression, pain or other comorbid condition(s), short-term use of a sleep medication may be necessary until symptoms improve or the underlying aggravating factor can be identified and/or effectively treated
	Dosage **Daily Dose Thresholds For Sedative-Hypnotic Medications**

Generic Medication	Oral Dosage
chloral hydrate*	500 mg
diphenhydramine*	25 mg
estazolam	0.5 mg
eszopiclone	1 mg
flurazepam*	15 mg
hydroxyzine*	50 mg
lorazepam	1 mg

<table>
<tr><th>Medication</th><th>Issues and Concerns</th></tr>
<tr><td></td><td>
<table>
<tr><td>oxazepam</td><td>15 mg</td></tr>
<tr><td>quazepam*</td><td>7.5 mg</td></tr>
<tr><td>ramelteon</td><td>8 mg</td></tr>
<tr><td>temazepam</td><td>15 mg</td></tr>
<tr><td>triazolam*</td><td>0.125 mg</td></tr>
<tr><td>zaleplon</td><td>5 mg</td></tr>
<tr><td>zolpidem IR</td><td>5 mg</td></tr>
<tr><td>zolpidem CR</td><td>6.25 mg</td></tr>
</table>
* These medications are not considered medications of choice for the management of insomnia, especially in older individuals.

Reference:

www.ahrq.gov/downloads/pub/evidence/pdf/insomnia/insomnia.pdf
</td></tr>
<tr><td></td><td>
Duration

• If used to induce sleep or treat a sleep disorder, refer to Section V – Tapering of a Medication Dose/Gradual Dose Reduction (GDR) in the guidance
</td></tr>
<tr><td>
Barbiturates, e.g.,

• amobarbital
• butabarbital
• pentobarbital
• secobarbital
• phenobarbital
• amobarbital-secobarbital
• barbiturates with other medications
</td><td>
NOTE: Refers to barbiturates used to induce sleep or treat anxiety disorder

Indications

• Barbiturates should not be initiated in any dose for any individuals to treat anxiety or insomnia; as they are highly addictive and cause numerous adverse effects, especially in older individuals

Exception: These guidelines do not apply to the use of phenobarbital to treat seizure disorders (see Anticonvulsant section)

Interactions/Adverse Consequences

• May increase the metabolism of many medications (e.g., anticonvulants, antipsychotics), which may lead to decreased effectiveness and subsequent worsening of symptoms or decreased control of underlying illness

• May cause hypotension, dizziness, lightheadedness, “hangover” effect, drowsiness, confusion, mental depression, unusual
</td></tr>
</table>

Medication	Issues and Concerns
	excitement, nervousness, headache, insomnia, nightmares, and hallucinations • May increase the risk for falls
Thyroid medications	
All thyroid medications, e.g., • levothyroxine • triiodothryonine	**Interactions** • Many clinically significant medication interactions have been identified; therefore, re-evaluation of medication doses is indicated **Dosage** • Initiation of thyroid supplementation should occur at low doses and be increased gradually to avoid precipitating cardiac failure or adrenal crisis **Monitoring** • Assessment of thyroid function (e.g., TSH, serum T4 or T3) should occur prior to initiation and periodically thereafter, including when new signs and symptoms of hypo- or hyperthyroidism are present
Urinary incontinence medications	
Urinary Incontinence Types and Agents, e.g., Urge incontinence: Anticholinergics, e.g., • darifenacin • oxybutynin • tolterodine • trospium Tricyclic antidepressants, e.g., • desipramine • imipramine Stress incontinence: Alpha adrenergic agonists,	**Indications** • Before or soon after initiating medication(s) to manage urinary incontinence, assessment of underlying causes and identification of the type/category of urinary incontinence needs to be documented • These medications have specific, limited indications based on the cause and type/category of incontinence **Monitoring** • Ongoing assessments of the effects of the medication on the individual's urinary incontinence as well as lower urinary tract symptoms should be done periodically

Medication	Issues and Concerns
e.g., • pseudoephedrine Mixed incontinence, e.g., • estrogen replacement agents • imipramine Overflow incontinence, e.g., • alpha adrenergic antagonists (see antihypertensives) • bethanechol chloride	**Adverse Consequences** • Anticholinergics and TCAs may cause anticholinergic effects (see Table II) • Estrogen Replacement Agents: oral agents may cause systemic side effects and increased risks (e.g., deep venous thrombosis, breast cancer); therefore, topical agents may be preferred • Bethanechol may cause hypotension, increased sweating and salivation, headache, cramps, diarrhea, nausea and vomiting, and worsening of asthma

TABLE II

MEDICATIONS WITH SIGNIFICANT ANTICHOLINERGIC PROPERTIES

Table II lists common medications with significant anticholinergic properties and potential adverse consequences, but is not all-inclusive. Any of the following signs and symptoms may be caused by any of the medications in the lists below, alone or in combination, as well as by other medications not listed here that have anticholinergic properties.

This table is provided because: 1) Medications in many categories have anticholinergic properties; 2) The use of multiple medications with such properties may be particularly problematic because of the cumulative effects; and 3) Anticholinergic side effects are particularly common and problematic, especially in the older individual[61, 62].

Examples of Medications with Anticholinergic Properties

ANTIHISTAMINES (H-1 BLOCKERS)

chlorpheniramine cyproheptadine
diphenhydramine hydroxyzine

ANTIDEPRESSANTS

amoxapine amitriptyline
clomipramine desipramine
doxepin imipramine
nortriptyline protriptyline
paroxetine

CARDIOVASCULAR MEDICATIONS

furosemide digoxin
nifedipine disopyramide

GASTROINTESTINAL MEDICATIONS

Antidiarrheal Medications

diphenoxylate atropine

Antispasmodic Medications

belladonna clidinium
chlordiazepoxide dicyclomine
hyoscyamine propantheline

ANTIPARKINSON MEDICATIONS

amantadine benztropine
biperiden trihexyphenidyl

MUSCLE RELAXANTS

cyclobenzaprine dantrolene
orphenadrine

ANTIVERTIGO MEDICATIONS

meclizine scopolamine

Antiulcer Medications

cimetidine ranitidine

ANTIPSYCHOTIC MEDICATIONS

chlorpromazine clozapine
olanzapine thioridazine

URINARY INCONTINENCE

oxybutynin probantheline
solifenacin tolterodine
trospium

PHENOTHIAZINE ANTIEMETICS

prochlorperazine promethazine

Potential Adverse Consequences of Medications with Anticholinergic Properties

Blood pressure, increased
Clumsiness or unsteadiness
Digestive system changes, e.g.,
- Bloating
- Bowel motility, decreased
- Constipation
- Ileus, paralytic/adynamic
- Nausea or vomiting
- Swallowing difficulty with dry mouth

Delirium
Drowsiness
Headache
Lethargy, fatigue
Muscle weakness, severe
Skin, changes
- Dryness Sweating, decreased
- Flushing Warmth, excessive

Urinary retention or difficulty

Breathing difficulty, changes
Convulsions
Mental status/behavior changes, e.g.,
- Distress, excitement, nervousness
- Attention, impaired
- Cognitive decline
- Confusion/disorientation
- Hallucinations
- Memory loss
- Restlessness or irritability

Dizziness
Fever
Heart rate, increased
Mucous membrane dryness: mouth, nose
Speech, slurring
Vision impairment, changes in acuity
- Blurring Glaucoma, worsening
- Eye pain Light sensitivity

ENDNOTES

[61] Tune, L. Carr, S., Hoag, E. & Cooper, T. (1992). Anticholinergic effects of drugs commonly prescribed for the elderly: Potential means for assessing risk of delirium. American Journal of Psychiatry, 149, pp. 1393-1394.

[62] Tune, L.E. (2000). Serum anticholinergic activity levels and delirium in the elderly. Seminars in Clinical Neuropsychiatry, 5, pp. 149-153.

INVESTIGATIVE PROTOCOL
UNNECESSARY MEDICATIONS - MEDICATION REGIMEN REVIEW

Because they are closely related, the investigations of the requirements for medication regimen review and the review for unnecessary medications have been merged.

Objectives

- To determine whether each resident receives or is provided:
  - Only those medications that are clinically indicated in the dose and for the duration to meet his or her assessed needs;
  - Non-pharmacological approaches when clinically indicated, in an effort to reduce the need for or the dose of a medication; and
  - Gradual dose reduction attempts for antipsychotics (unless clinically contraindicated) and tapering of other medications, when clinically indicated, in an effort to discontinue the use or reduce the dose of the medication.
- To determine if the facility in collaboration with the prescriber:
  - Identifies the parameters for monitoring medication(s) or medication combinations (including antipsychotics) that pose a risk for adverse consequences; and for monitoring the effectiveness of medications (including a comparison with therapeutic goals); and
  - Recognizes and evaluates the onset or worsening of signs or symptoms, or a change in condition to determine whether these potentially may be related to the medication regimen; and follows-up as necessary upon identifying adverse consequences.
- To determine if the pharmacist:
  - Performed the monthly medication regimen review, and identified any existing irregularities regarding indications for use, dose, duration, and the potential for, or the existence of adverse consequences or other irregularities; and
  - Reported any identified irregularities to the attending physician and director of nursing.
- To determine whether the facility and/or practitioner acted on the report of any irregularity.

Use

Use this protocol during every initial and standard survey. In addition, this protocol may be used on revisits or abbreviated survey (complaint investigation) as necessary.

NOTE: This review is not intended to direct medication therapy. However, surveyors are expected to review factors related to the implementation, use, and monitoring of medications.

The surveyor is not expected to prove that an adverse consequence was directly caused by a medication or combination of medications, but rather that there was a failure in the care process related to considering and acting upon such possibilities.

If during the course of this review, the surveyor needs to contact the attending physician regarding questions related to the medication regimen, it is recommended that the facility's staff have the opportunity to provide the necessary information about the resident and the concerns to the physician for his/her review prior to responding to the surveyor's inquiries.

Procedures

Review the medications (prescription, over-the-counter medications, and nutritional supplements such as herbal products) currently ordered and/or discontinued by the prescriber at least back to the most recent signed recapitulation/reorder of all medications. Obtain a copy of the current orders if necessary. Gather information regarding the resident's mental, physical, functional, and psychosocial status and the medication-related therapeutic goals identified in the care plan as the basis for further review.

1. Observation and Record Review

Use the table below to guide observations, record review, and interviews with the resident or representative and relevant staff. Observe whether the medication-related interventions are consistently implemented over time and across various shifts. Note deviations from the care plan as well as potential medication-related adverse consequences. Verify observations by gathering additional information; for example, additional record reviews and/or interviews with the resident or representative, relevant staff, and practitioners.

SYMPTOMS, SIGNS, AND CONDITIONS THAT MAY BE ASSOCIATED WITH MEDICATIONS	REVIEW FOR HOW FACILITY MANAGED MEDICATIONS FOR THE RESIDENT
Determine if the resident has been transferred to	Review the record (including the care

<table>
<tr><th>SYMPTOMS, SIGNS, AND CONDITIONS THAT MAY BE ASSOCIATED WITH MEDICATIONS</th><th>REVIEW FOR HOW FACILITY MANAGED MEDICATIONS FOR THE RESIDENT</th></tr>
<tr><td>acute care since the last survey and/or has recently (e.g., the previous 3 months) experienced a change in condition or currently has signs and symptoms, such as:

• Anorexia and/or unplanned weight loss, or weight gain
• Behavioral changes, unusual behavior patterns (including increased distressed behavior)
• Bleeding or bruising, spontaneous or unexplained
• Bowel dysfunction including diarrhea, constipation and impaction
• Dehydration, fluid/electrolyte imbalance
• Depression, mood disturbance
• Dysphagia, swallowing difficulty
• Falls, dizziness, or evidence of impaired coordination
• Gastrointestinal bleeding
• Headaches, muscle pain, generalized or nonspecific aching or pain
• Mental status changes, (e.g., new or worsening confusion, new cognitive decline, worsening of dementia (including delirium))
• Rash, pruritus
• Respiratory difficulty or changes
• Sedation (excessive), insomnia, or sleep disturbance
• Seizure activity
• Urinary retention or incontinence

If observations or record review indicate symptoms or changes in condition that may be related to medications (refer to Tables I and II, supplemented with current medication references), determine whether the facility considered medications as a potential cause of the change or symptom.</td><td>plan, comprehensive assessment, and other parts of the record as appropriate) to determine whether it reflects the following elements related to medication management for the resident:

• Clinical indications for use of the medication
• Consideration of non-pharmacological interventions
• Dose, including excessive dose and duplicate therapy
• Duration, including excessive duration
• Consideration of potential for tapering/GDR or rationale for clinical contraindication
• Monitoring for and reporting of:
  o Response to medications and progress toward therapeutic goals
  o Emergence of medication-related adverse consequences
• Adverse consequences, if present and potentially medication-related, note if there was:
  o Recognition, evaluation, reporting, and management by the facility
  o Physician action regarding potential medication-related adverse consequences</td></tr>
</table>

2. Interview

Interview the resident and or family/responsible party, to the extent possible, to determine:

- His/her participation in care planning and decision making, including discussions of the goals related to the use of medications;
- Whether approaches other than medications (as indicated) were discussed; and
- His/her evaluation of the results of the medication therapy and other approaches (such as decreasing symptoms of pain, improving functional ability).

If during the review, you identify concerns about the lack of indication for use; the dose or duration of a medication; lack of monitoring; failure to implement the care plan; or condition changes or functional decline that may be related to the medication regimen, interview knowledgeable staff to determine:

- Whether the resident has experienced any changes in the functioning or amount of activity that he/she is able to do;
- The clinical rationale for the use of the medication, dose or duration and how the interdisciplinary team is monitoring the resident's response to the medication;
- What process is in place to assure the care plan interventions for medication use are being implemented;
- Whether they were aware that the signs and symptoms may be adverse consequences related to the medication regimen;
- Whether the staff had contacted the attending physician to discuss the signs and symptoms and the current medication regimen;
- Whether and how the physician responded when informed of suspected adverse medication consequences; and
- Whether the pharmacist performed a medication regimen review and identified related signs and symptoms, or the staff informed the pharmacist of them if they occurred after the last pharmacist visit.

Interview the physician, as appropriate, to determine:

- Whether staff notified him/her of potential medication-related issues and concerns;
- His/her assessment of the significance of medication-related issues and concerns; and
- Rationale for his/her management of the resident's medications and/or medication-related issues or concerns.

3. Medication Regimen Review (MRR)

Review for compliance with the MRR requirements at F428. Determine:

- If the pharmacist had identified and reported to the director of nursing and attending physician any irregularities with the medication regimen such as:
    - The emergence or existence of clinically significant adverse consequences;
    - Excess dose or duration, lack of monitoring, lack of indication for use, lack of GDR (as indicated) or behavioral interventions for residents receiving antipsychotics, medication interactions potentially affecting the medication's effectiveness; and
- Whether the attending physician and the director of nursing acted on any irregularities identified in the report. The responses from the attending physician could include the following:
    - Changed the medication regimen in response to the concern raised in the report (or after additional review of the situation);
    - Provided a clinically pertinent rationale that is relevant to that specific resident's signs and symptoms, prognosis, test results, etc., documenting or indicating why the benefit of the medication(s) or dose(s) outweighed the risks of the adverse consequence;
    - Provided a clinically pertinent rationale for why any gradual dose reduction (for antipsychotic medications) and/or tapering (for other medications) is contraindicated, even for a trial period; or
    - Provided a clinically pertinent rationale for why a particular medication, dose, or duration is appropriate for a resident despite its risks (for example, the resident has had recurrent seizures unless he/she receives anticonvulsant dosing that exceeds the usual recommended serum medication concentration level or therapeutic

range, and the attending physician and facility have been monitoring for and addressing adverse consequences).

- If the pharmacist identified a suspected adverse consequence, and the attending physician did not respond, determine if staff followed up with the attending physician.

  NOTE: If the staff and pharmacist identify a medication that they believe may be causing a serious adverse consequence or a risk of clinically significant adverse consequences for the resident, and the attending physician did not address the risks or harm to the resident, determine what steps staff took; e.g., contacting the medical director to review the situation and address the issue with the attending physician, as necessary. See guidance at 42 CFR 483.75(i) Medical Director (F501) for additional guidance.

If problems are identified with the MRR, interview the pharmacist, as indicated, to determine:

- How he/she conducts the MRR, including the frequency and extent of the medication review and under what circumstances a review might be conducted more often than monthly;
- How the facility communicates with him/her regarding medication-related issues in specific residents; and
- How he/she approaches the MRR process for short stay residents.

DETERMINATION OF COMPLIANCE (Task 6, Appendix P)

Synopsis of Regulation (F329)

The unnecessary medication requirement has six aspects in order to assure that medication therapy is appropriate for the individual resident. The facility must assure that medication therapy (including antipsychotic agents) is based upon:

- An adequate indication for use;
- Use of the appropriate dose;
- Provision of behavioral interventions and gradual dose reduction for individuals receiving antipsychotics (unless clinically contraindicated) in an effort to reduce or discontinue the medication;
- Use for the appropriate duration;

- Adequate monitoring to determine whether therapeutic goals are being met and to detect the emergence or presence of adverse consequences; and

- Reduction of dose or discontinuation of the medication in the presence of adverse consequences, as indicated.

Criteria for Compliance

Compliance with 42 CFR 483.25(l), F329, Unnecessary Medications

For a resident who has been, or is, receiving medication(s), the facility is in compliance if they, in collaboration with the prescriber:

- Assessed the resident to ascertain, to the extent possible, the causes of the condition or symptoms requiring treatment, including recognizing, evaluating, and determining whether the condition or symptoms may have reflected an adverse medication consequence;

- Based on the assessment, determined that medication therapy was indicated and identified the therapeutic goals for the medication;

- Utilized only those medications in appropriate doses for the appropriate duration, which are clinically necessary to treat the resident's assessed condition(s);

- Implemented a gradual dose reduction and behavioral interventions for each resident receiving antipsychotic medications unless clinically contraindicated;

- Monitored the resident for progress towards the therapeutic goal(s) and for the emergence or presence of adverse consequences, as indicated by the resident's condition and the medication(s); and

- Adjusted or discontinued the dose of a medication in response to adverse consequences, unless clinically contraindicated.

If not, cite F329.

Noncompliance for F329

After completing the investigation, determine whether or not compliance with the regulation exists. Noncompliance for F329 may include:

- **Inadequate Indications for Use** – Examples of noncompliance related to a medication being used without adequate indications include, but are not limited to:

- Failure to document a clinical reason or demonstrate a clinically pertinent rationale, verbally or in writing, for using medication(s) for a specific resident.

- Prescribing or administering a medication despite an allergy to that medication, or without clarifying whether a true allergy existed as opposed to other reactions (e.g., idiosyncratic reaction or other side effect).

- Failure to provide a clear clinical rationale for continuing a medication that may be causing an adverse consequence.

- Initiation of an antipsychotic medication to manage distressed behavior without considering a possible underlying medical cause (e.g., UTI, congestive heart failure)or environmental or psychosocial stressor.

- Initiation of a medication presenting clinically significant risks without considering relative risks and benefits or potentially lower risk medications.

- Concomitant use of two or more medications in the same pharmacological class without a clinically pertinent explanation.

• **Inadequate Monitoring** – Examples of noncompliance related to inadequate monitoring include, but are not limited to:

  - Failure to monitor the responses to or effects of a medication and failure to respond when monitoring indicates a lack of progress toward the therapeutic goal (e.g., relief of pain or normalization of thyroid function) or the emergence of an adverse consequence.

  - Failure to monitor a medication consistent with the current standard of practice or manufacturer's guidelines.

  - Failure to carry out the monitoring that was ordered or failure to monitor for potential clinically significant adverse consequences. For example, use of warfarin in conjunction with:

    – Inadequate or absent monitoring of PT/INR during treatment; and/or

    – Failure to recognize and monitor the increased risk of adverse consequences when the resident is receiving other medications that are known to increase the risk of bleeding or to interact with warfarin and increase PT/INR.

Excessive Dose (including duplicate therapy) – Examples of noncompliance related to excessive dose include, but are not limited to:

- Giving a total amount of any medication at one time or over a period of time that exceeds the amount recommended by the manufacturer's recommendations, clinical practice guidelines, evidence-based studies from medical/pharmacy journals, or standards of practice for a resident's age and condition, without a documented clinically pertinent rationale.
- Failure to consider periodically the continued necessity of the dose or the possibility of tapering a medication.
- Failure to provide and/or document a clinical rationale for using multiple medications from the same pharmacological class.

- **Excessive Duration** – Examples of noncompliance related to excessive duration include, but are not limited to:
  - Continuation beyond the manufacturer's recommended time frames, the stop date or duration indicated on the medication order, facility-established stop order policies, or clinical practice guidelines, evidence-based studies from medical/pharmacy journals, or current standards of practice, without documented clinical justification.
  - Continuation of a medication after the desired therapeutic goal has been achieved without evaluating whether the medication can offer any additional benefit, for example:
    - Use of an antibiotic beyond the recommended clinical guidelines or the facility policy without adequate reassessment of the resident and determination of continuing need.
    - Failure to re-evaluate the rationale for continuing antipsychotic medication initiated in an emergency after the acute phase has stabilized.
- **Adverse Consequences** – Examples of noncompliance related to adverse consequences include, but are not limited to:
  - Failure to act upon (i.e., discontinue a medication or reduce the dose or provide clinical justification for why the benefit outweighs the adverse consequences) a report of the risk for or presence of clinically significant adverse consequence(s);
  - Failure to respond to actual or potentially clinically significant adverse consequences related to the use of warfarin when the PT/INR exceeds the

target goal.

- **Antipsychotic Medications without Gradual Dose Reduction and Behavioral Interventions unless Clinically Contraindicated** – Examples of noncompliance related to this requirement include, but are not limited to:
  - o Failure to attempt GDR in the absence of identified and documented clinical contraindications.
  - o Prolonged or indefinite antipsychotic use without attempting gradual dose reductions.
  - o Failure to implement behavioral interventions to enable attempts to reduce or discontinue an antipsychotic medication.

Potential Tags for Additional Investigation

If noncompliance with 483.25(l) has been identified, then concerns with additional requirements may also have been identified. The surveyor is cautioned to investigate these related additional requirements before determining whether noncompliance with the additional requirements may be present. Examples of some of the related requirements that may be considered when noncompliance has been identified include the following:

- 42 CFR 483.10(b)(11), F157, Notification of Changes
  - o Review whether the facility contacted the attending physician regarding a significant change in the resident's condition in relation to a potential adverse consequence of a medication, or if the resident has not responded to medication therapy as anticipated and/or indicated.
- 42 CFR 483.10 (b)(3) and (4), F154, F155, Notice of Rights and Services and (d)(2) Free Choice
  - o Determine whether the resident was advised of her/his medical condition and therapy and was informed about her/his treatment including medications and the right to refuse treatments.
- 42 CFR 483.20(b), F272, Comprehensive Assessments
  - o Review whether the facility's initial and periodic comprehensive assessments include an assessment of the resident's medication regimen.
- 42 CFR 483.20(k)(1) and (2), F279, F280, Comprehensive Care Plans

  - Review whether the resident's comprehensive care plan: a) was based on the assessment of the resident's conditions, risks, needs, and behavior; b) was consistent with the resident's therapeutic goals; (c) considered the need to monitor for effectiveness based on those therapeutic goals and for the emergence or presence of adverse consequences; and (d) was revised as needed to address medication-related issues.

- 42 CFR 483.25(a)(1), F310, Decline in ADL

  - Review whether the facility had identified, evaluated, and responded to a new or rapidly progressive decline in function, development or worsening of movement disorders, increased fatigue and activity intolerance that affected the resident's ADL ability in relation to potential medication adverse consequences.

- 42 CFR 483.25(d), F315, Urinary Incontinence

  - Review whether the facility had identified, evaluated, and responded to a change in urinary function or continence status in relation to potential medication adverse consequences.

- 42 CFR 483.25(f)(1)&(2), F319, F320, Mental and Psychosocial Functioning

  - Review whether the facility had identified, evaluated, and responded to a change in behavior and/or psychosocial changes, including depression or other mood disturbance, distress, restlessness, increasing confusion, or delirium in relation to potential medication adverse consequences.

- 42 CFR 483.25(i)(1), F325, Nutritional Parameters

  - Review if the facility had identified, evaluated, and responded to a change in nutritional parameters, anorexia or unplanned weight loss, dysphagia, and/or swallowing disorders in relation to potential medication adverse consequences.

- 42 CFR 483.25(j), F327, Hydration

  - Review if the facility had identified, evaluated, and responded to a change in hydration or fluid or electrolyte balance (for example, high or low sodium or potassium) in relation to potential medication adverse consequences.

- 42 CFR 483.40(a), F385, Physician Supervision

  - Review if the attending physician supervised the resident's medical treatment, including assessing the resident's condition and medications, identifying the clinical rationale, and monitoring for and addressing adverse consequences.

- 42 CFR 483.40(b), F386, Physician Visits
    - Review if the attending physician or designee reviewed the resident's total program of care and wrote, signed, and dated progress notes covering pertinent aspects of the medication regimen and related issues.
- 42 CFR 483.60(c), F428, Medication Regimen Review
    - Review whether the licensed pharmacist has provided consultation regarding the integrity of medication-related records (e.g., MAR, physician order sheets, telephone orders), and potential or actual medication irregularities.
- 42 CFR 483.75(i), F501, Medical Director
    - Review whether the medical director, when requested by the facility, interacted with the attending physician regarding a failure to respond or an inadequate response to identified or reported potential medication irregularities and adverse consequences; and whether the medical director collaborated with the facility to help develop, implement, and evaluate policies and procedures for the safe and effective use of medications in the care of residents.

IV. DEFICIENCY CATEGORIZATION (Part IV, Appendix P)

Once the team has completed its investigation, analyzed the data, reviewed the regulatory requirement, and identified any deficient practice(s) that demonstrate that noncompliance with the regulation at F329 exists, the team must determine the severity of each deficiency, based on the resultant harm or potential for harm to the resident.

The key elements for severity determination for F329 are as follows:

1. Presence of potential or actual harm/negative outcome(s) due to a failure related to unnecessary medications.

Examples of actual or potential harm/negative outcomes for F329 may include, but are not limited to:

- Potential for life-threatening toxicity from excessive dose or lack of indication for the use of digoxin.
- Complications (such as diarrhea with life threatening fluid loss, nephrotoxicity, hearing loss, or anaphylactic shock) from use of an antibiotic when no clear

indication for use has been established or response to the use has not been monitored.

- Fractures or falls with injury resulting from the continuing use of medications (e.g., hypnotics/sedatives, antipsychotics, antidepressants, antihypertensives) in the presence of predisposing risks or adverse consequences such as persistent dizziness or recurrent falling without intervening or reevaluating the need for and dose of the medication believed to be the cause of the gait instability.

2. **Degree of potential or actual harm/negative outcome(s) due to a failure related to unnecessary medications.**

   Identify how the facility practices caused, resulted in, allowed, or contributed to the actual or potential for harm:

   - If harm has occurred, determine if the harm is at the level of serious injury, impairment, death, compromise, or discomfort; or

   - If harm has not yet occurred, determine how likely is the potential for serious injury, impairment, death, compromise, or discomfort to occur to the resident.

3. **The immediacy of correction required.**

   Determine whether the noncompliance requires immediate correction in order to prevent serious injury, harm, impairment, or death to one or more residents.

The survey team must evaluate the harm or potential for harm based upon the following levels of severity for tag F329. First, the team must rule out whether Severity Level 4, Immediate Jeopardy to a resident's health or safety, exists by evaluating the deficient practice in relation to immediacy, culpability, and severity. (Follow the guidance in Appendix Q.)

> **NOTE:** The death or transfer of a resident who was harmed or injured as a result of facility noncompliance does not remove a finding of immediate jeopardy. The facility is required to implement specific actions to remove the jeopardy and correct the noncompliance which allowed or caused the immediate jeopardy.

Severity Level 4 Considerations: Immediate Jeopardy to Resident Health or Safety

Immediate Jeopardy is a situation in which the facility's noncompliance with one or more requirements of participation:

- Has allowed, caused, or resulted in, or is likely to allow, cause, or result in serious injury, harm, impairment, or death to a resident; and

- Requires immediate correction, as the facility either created the situation or allowed the situation to continue by failing to implement preventative or corrective measures.

Examples may include, but are not limited to:

- Failure to assess or respond appropriately for a resident taking warfarin who had an elevated INR of 9 or greater with or without bleeding, or the elevated INR persisted without assessment/follow-up.

- Failure to monitor PT/INR for a resident on anticoagulant therapy in accordance with current standards of practice and to recognize and/or respond to a life threatening adverse consequence related to anticoagulation.

- Failure to recognize developing serotonin syndrome (e.g., confusion, motor restlessness, tremor) in a resident receiving a SSRI, leading to the addition of medications with additive serotonin effect or medication to suppress the symptoms.

- Failure to recognize and respond to signs and symptoms of neuroleptic malignant syndrome (NMS).

- In the presence of gastrointestinal bleeding, the failure to recognize medication therapies (such as NSAIDs or COX-2 inhibitors, bisphosphonates) as potentially causing or contributing to the gastrointestinal bleed, resulting in the continued administration of the medication, until the resident required hospitalization for severe bleeding.

  NOTE: If immediate jeopardy has been ruled out based upon the evidence, then evaluate whether actual harm that is not immediate jeopardy exists at Severity Level 3.

Severity Level 3 Considerations: Actual Harm that is Not Immediate Jeopardy

Level 3 indicates noncompliance that resulted in actual harm, and may include, but is not limited to, clinical compromise, decline, or the resident's inability to maintain and/or reach his/her highest practicable well-being. Examples may include, but are not limited to:

- Facility failure to take appropriate action (e.g., suspending administration of the anticoagulant) in response to an INR greater than 4 and less than 9 for a resident who is receiving warfarin until spontaneous bruising or frank bleeding occurs, resulting in the need to transfuse or hospitalize the resident.

- Facility failure to evaluate the medication regimen as a potential cause of seizure activity resulting in the addition of anticonvulsants to treat recent-onset seizures that can be adverse consequences of medications.

- Facility failure to implement a GDR that was not contraindicated in a resident receiving prolonged, continuous antipsychotic therapy resulting in functional decline, somnolence, lethargy, tremors, increased falling, or impaired ambulation.

NOTE: If Severity Level 3 (actual harm that is not immediate jeopardy) has been ruled out based upon the evidence, then evaluate as to whether Severity Level 2 (no actual harm with the potential for more than minimal harm) exists.

Severity Level 2 Considerations: No Actual Harm with Potential for More Than Minimal Harm that is Not Immediate Jeopardy

Level 2 indicates noncompliance that resulted in a resident outcome of no more than minimal discomfort and/or has the potential to compromise the resident's ability to maintain or reach his or her highest practicable level of well-being. The potential exists for greater harm to occur if interventions are not provided. Examples may include, but are not limited to:

- Facility failure to take appropriate action (e.g., change or suspend administration of the warfarin dose) for a resident who has an INR greater than 4 and less than 9 without any bleeding.

- Failure to monitor INR for a resident who has been stabilized on warfarin, but who has not had bleeding.

- Facility failure to identify and act upon minor symptoms of allergic response to medications, such as a rash.

- Facility failure to monitor for response to therapy or for the emergence or presence of adverse consequences before the resident has experienced an adverse consequence or decline in function (e.g., monitoring periodically for symptoms of behavioral distress in someone receiving psychopharmacological medication; monitoring thyroid function at least annually in an individual receiving thyroid hormone replacement; and monitoring hydration status and basic metabolic profile for a resident receiving diuretics or ACE inhibitors, who had a change in mental status after the onset of diarrhea).

Severity Level 1: No Actual Harm with Potential for Minimal Harm

The failure of the facility to provide appropriate care and services to manage the resident's medication regimen to avoid unnecessary medications and minimize negative outcome places residents at risk for more than minimal harm. Therefore, Severity Level 1 does not apply for this regulatory requirement.

F332 and F333

§483.25(m) Medication Errors

The facility must ensure that--

[F332] §483.25(m)(1) It is free of medication error rates of 5 percent or greater; and

[F333] §483.25(m)(2) Residents are free of any significant medication errors.

Interpretive Guidelines §483.25(m)

Medication Error -- The observed preparation or administration of drugs or biologicals which is not in accordance with:

1. Physician's orders,
2. Manufacturer's specifications (not recommendations) regarding the preparation and administration of the drug or biological;
3. Accepted professional standards and principles which apply to professionals providing services. Accepted professional standards and principles include the various practice regulations in each State, and current commonly accepted health standards established by national organizations, boards, and councils.

"**Significant medication error**" means one which causes the resident discomfort or jeopardizes his or her health and safety. Criteria for judging significant medication errors as well as examples are provided under significant and non-significant medication errors. Discomfort may be a subjective or relative term used in different ways depending on the individual situation. (Constipation that is unrelieved by an ordered laxative that results in a drug error that is omitted for one day may be slightly uncomfortable or perhaps not uncomfortable at all. When the constipation persists for greater than three days, the constipation may be more significant. Constipation causing obstruction or fecal impaction can jeopardize the resident's health and safety.)

"**Medication error rate**" is determined by calculating the percentage of errors. The numerator in the ratio is the total number of errors that the survey team observes, both significant and nonsignificant. The denominator is called "opportunities for errors" and includes all the doses the survey team observed being administered plus the doses ordered but not administered. The equation for calculating a medication error rate is as follows:

Medication Error Rate = Number of Errors Observed divided by the Opportunities for Errors (doses given plus doses ordered but not given) X 100.

"**Medication error rate**" -- A medication error rate of 5% or greater includes both significant and nonsignificant medication errors. It indicates that the facility may have systemic problems with its drug distribution system and a deficiency should be written.

The error rate must be 5% or greater. Rounding of a lower rate (e.g., 4.6%) to a 5% rate is not permitted.

Significant and Nonsignificant Medication Errors

"**Determining Significance**" -- The relative significance of medication errors is a matter of professional judgment. Follow three general guidelines in determining whether a medication error is significant or not:

"**Resident Condition**" -- The resident's condition is an important factor to take into consideration. For example, a fluid pill erroneously administered to a dehydrated resident may have serious consequences, but if administered to a resident with a normal fluid balance may not. If the resident's condition requires rigid control, a single missed or wrong dose can be highly significant.

"**Drug Category**" -- If the drug is from a category that usually requires the resident to be titrated to a specific blood level, a single medication error could alter that level and precipitate a reoccurrence of symptoms or toxicity. This is especially important with a drug that has a Narrow Therapeutic Index (NTI) (i.e., a drug in which the therapeutic dose is very close to the toxic dose). Examples of drugs with NTI are as follows: Anticonvulsant: phenytoin (Dilantin),carbamazepine (Tegretol), Anticoagulants: warfarin (Coumadin) Antiarrhythmic (digoxin)Lanoxin) Antiasthmatics: theophylline (TheoDur) Antimanic Drigs: lithium salts (Eskalith, Lithobid).

"**Frequency of Error**" -- If an error is occurring with any frequency, there is more reason to classify the error as significant. For example, if a resident's drug was omitted several times, as verified by reconciling the number of tablets delivered with the number administered, classifying that error as significant would be more in order. This conclusion should be considered in concert with the resident's condition and the drug category.

"**Examples of Significant and Non-Significant Medication Errors**" -- Some of these errors are identified as significant. This designation is based on expert opinion without regard to the status of the resident. Most experts concluded that the significance of these errors, in and of themselves, have a high potential for creating problems for the typical long term care facility resident. Those errors identified as nonsignificant have also been designated primarily on the basis of the nature of the drug. Resident status and frequency of error could classify these errors as significant.

Examples of Medication Errors Detected

Omissions Examples (Drug ordered but not administered at least once):

Drug Order	Significance
Haldol 1mg BID	NS
Motrin 400mg TID	NS
Quinidine 200mg TID	S**
Tearisol Drops 2 both eyes TID	NS
Metamucil one packet BID	NS
Multivitamin one daily	NS
Mylanta Susp. one oz., TID AC	NS
Nitrol Oint. one inch	S

* Not Significant

**Significant

Unauthorized Drug Examples (Drugs administered without a physician's order):

Drug Order	Significance
Feosol	NS
Coumadin 4mg	S
Zyloprim 100mg	NS
Tylenol 5 gr	NS
Motrin 400mg	NS

Wrong Dose Examples:

Drug Order	Administered	Significance
Timoptic 0.25% one drop in the left eye TID	Three drops in each eye	NS
Digoxin 0.125mg everyday	0.25mg	S
Amphojel 30ml QID	15ml	NS
Dilantin 125 SUSP 12ml	2ml	S

Wrong Route of Administration Examples:

Drug Order	Administered	Significance
Cortisporin Ear Drops 4 to 5 left ear QID	Left Eye	S

Wrong Dosage Form Examples:

Drug Order	Administered	Significance

Drug Order	Administered	Significance
Colace Liquid 100mg BID	Capsule	NS
Mellaril Tab 10mg	Liquid Concentrate	NS*
Dilantin Kapseals 100 mg three Kapseals p.o. HS	Prompt Phenytoin 100 mg three capsules p.o. HS	S

* If correct dose was given.
** Parke Davis Kapseals have an extended rate of absorption. Prompt phenytoin capsules do not.

Wrong Drug Examples:

Drug Order	Administered	Significance
Tums	Oscal	NS
Vibramycin	Vancomycin	S

Wrong Time Examples:

Drug Order	Administered	Significance
Digoxin 0.25mg daily at 8 a.m.	At 9:30 am	NS
Percocet 2 Tabs 20 min. before painful treatment	2 Tabs given 3 after treatment	S

Medication Errors Due to Failure to Follow Manufacturers Specifications or Accepted Professional Standards

The following situations in drug administration may be considered medication errors:

- Failure to "Shake Well": The failure to "shake" a drug product that is labeled "shake well." This may lead to an under dose or over dose depending on the drug product and the elapsed time since the last "shake." The surveyor should use common sense in determining the adequacy of the shaking of the medication. Some drugs, for example dilantin, are more critical to achieve correct dosage delivery than others.

- Insulin Suspensions: Also included under this category is the failure to "mix" the suspension without creating air bubbles. Some individuals "roll" the insulin suspension to mix it without creating air bubbles. Any motion used is acceptable so long as the suspension is mixed and does not have air bubbles in it prior to the administration.

- Crushing Medications that should not be Crushed: Crushing tablets or capsules that the manufacturer states "do not crush."

Exceptions to the "Do Not Crush" rule:

- If the prescriber orders a drug to be crushed which the manufacturer states should not be crushed, the prescriber or the pharmacist must explain, in the clinical record, why crushing the medication will not adversely affect the resident. Additionally, the pharmacist should inform the facility staff to observe for pertinent adverse effects.

- If the facility can provide literature from the drug manufacturer or from a reviewed health journal to justify why modification of the dosage form will not compromise resident care.

- Adequate Fluids with Medications: The administration of medications without adequate fluid when the manufacturer specifies that adequate fluids be taken with the medication. For example:

    - Bulk laxatives (e.g., Metamucil, Fiberall, Serutan, Konsyl, Citrucel);

    - Nonsteroidal Anti-Inflammatory Drugs (NSAIDs) should be administered with adequate fluid. Adequate fluid is not defined by the manufacturer but is usually four to eight ounces. The surveyor should count fluids consumed during meals or snacks (such as coffee, juice, milk, soft drinks, etc.) as fluids taken with the medication, as long as they have consumed within a reasonable time of taking the medication (e.g., within approximately 30 minutes). If the resident refuses to take adequate fluid, the facility should not be at fault so long as they made a good faith effort to offer fluid, and provided any assistance that may be necessary to drink the fluid. It is important that the surveyor not apply this rule to residents who are fluid restricted; and

    - Potassium supplements (solid or liquid dosage forms) such as: Kaochlor, Klorvess, Kaon, K-Lor, K-Tab, K-Dur, K-Lyte, Slow K, Klotrix, Micro K, or Ten K should be administered with or after meals with a full glass (e.g., approximately 4 - 8 ounces of water or fruit juice). This will minimize the possibility of gastrointestinal irritation and saline cathartic effect. If the resident refuses to take adequate fluid, the facility should not be at fault so long as they made a good faith effort to offer fluid, and provided any assistance that may be necessary to drink the fluid. It is important that the surveyor not apply this rule to residents who are fluid restricted.

- Medications that Must be Taken with Food or Antacids: The administration of medications without food or antacids when the manufacturer specifies that food or antacids be taken with or before the medication is considered a medication error. The most commonly used drugs that should be taken with food or antacids are the Nonsteroidal Anti-Inflammatory Drugs (NSAIDs).

There is evidence that elderly, debilitated persons are at greater risk of gastritis and GI bleeds, including silent GI bleeds. Determine if the time of administration was selected to take into account the need to give the medication with food.

Examples of commonly used NSAIDs are as follows:

Generic Name	**Brand Name**
Diclofenac	Voltaren, Cataflam
Diflunisal	Dolobid
Etodolac	Lodine
Fenoprofen	Nalfon
Ibuprofen	Motrin, Advil
Indomethacin	Indocin
Ketoprofen	Orudis, Oruvail
Mefenamic Acid	Ponstel
Nabumetone	Relafen
Naproxen	Naprosyn, Aleve
Piroxicam	Feldene
Sulindac	Clinoril
Tolmetin	Tolectin

- Medications Administered with Enteral Nutritional Formulas: Administering medications immediately before, immediately after, or during the administration of enteral nutritional formulas (ENFs) without achieving the following minimum objectives:
    - Check the placement of the naso-gastric or gastrostomy tube in accordance with the facility's policy on this subject. **NOTE:** If the placement of the tube is not checked, this is not a medication error; it is a failure to follow accepted professional practice and should be evaluated under Tag F281 requiring the facility to meet professional standards of quality.
    - Flush the enteral feeding tube with at least 30 ml of preferably warm water before and after medications are administered. While it is noted that some facility policies ideally adopt flushing the tube after each individual medication is given, as opposed to after the group of multiple medications is given, unless there are known compatibility problems between medicines being mixed together, a minimum of one

flushing before and after giving the medications is all the surveyor need review. There may be cases where flushing with 30 ml after each single medication is given may overload an individual with fluid, raising the risk of discomfort or stress on body functions. Failure to flush, before and after, would be counted as one medication error and would be included in the calculation for medication errors exceeding 5 percent.

- The administration of enteral nutrition formula and administration of dilantin should be separated to minimize interaction. The surveyor should look for appropriate documentation and monitoring if the two are administered simultaneously. If the facility is not aware that there is a potential for an interaction between the two when given together, and is not monitoring for outcome of seizures or unwanted side effects of dilantin, then the surveyor should consider simultaneous administration a medication error.

- Medications Instilled into the Eye: The administration of eye drops without achieving the following critical objectives:

  - **Eye Contact**: The eye drop, but not the dropper, must make full contact with the conjunctival sac and then be washed over the eye when the resident closes the eyelid; and

  - **Sufficient Contact Time**: The eye drop must contact the eye for a sufficient period of time before the next eye drop is instilled. The time for optimal eye drop absorption is approximately 3 to 5 minutes. (It should be encouraged that when the procedures are possible, systemic effects of eye medications can be reduced by pressing the tear duct for one minute after eye drop administration or by gentle eye closing for approximately three minutes after the administration.)

- Allowing Resident to Swallow Sublingual Tablets: If the resident persists in swallowing a sublingual tablet (e.g., nitroglycerin) despite efforts to train otherwise, the facility should endeavor to seek an alternative dosage form for this drug.

- Medication Administered Via Metered Dose Inhalers (MDI): The use of MDI in other than the following ways (this includes use of MDI by the resident). This is an error if the person administering the drug did not do all the following:

  - Shake the container well;

  - Position the inhaler in front of or in the resident's mouth. Alternatively a spacer may be used;

- For cognitively impaired residents, many clinicians believe that the closed mouth technique is easier for the resident and more likely to be successful. However, the open mouth technique often results in better and deeper penetration of the medication into the lungs, when this method can be used; and

- If more than one puff is required, (whether the same medication or a different medication) wait approximately a minute between puffs.

NOTE: If the person administering the drug follows all the procedures outlined above, and there is a failure to administer the medication because the resident can't cooperate (for example, a resident with dementia may not understand the procedure), this should not be called a medication error. The surveyor should evaluate the facility's responsibility to assess the resident's circumstance, and possibly attempt other dosage forms such as oral dosage forms or nebulizers.

Determining Medication Errors

Timing Errors -- If a drug is ordered before meals (AC) and administered after meals (PC), always count this as a medication error. Likewise, if a drug is ordered PC and is given AC, count as a medication error. Count a wrong time error if the drug is administered 60 minutes earlier or later than its scheduled time of administration, BUT ONLY IF THAT WRONG TIME ERROR CAN CAUSE THE RESIDENT DISCOMFORT OR JEOPARDIZE THE RESIDENT'S HEALTH AND SAFETY. Counting a drug with a long half-life (e.g., digoxin) as a wrong time error when it is 15 minutes late is improper because this drug has a long half-life (beyond 24 hours) and 15 minutes has no significant impact on the resident. The same is true for many other wrong time errors (except AC AND PC errors).

To determine the scheduled time, examine the facility's policy relative to dosing schedules. The facility's policy should dictate when it administers a.m. doses, or when it administers the first dose in a 4-times-a-day dosing schedule.

Prescriber's Orders -- he latest recapitulation of drug orders is sufficient for determining whether a valid order exists provided the prescriber has signed the "recap." The signed "recap," if the facility uses the "recap" system and subsequent orders constitute a legal authorization to administer the drug.

Procedures §483.25(m)

Medication Error Detection Methodology -- Use an observation technique to determine medication errors. The survey team should observe the administration of drugs, on several different drug "passes," when necessary. Record what is observed; and reconcile the record of observation with the prescriber's drug orders to determine whether or not medication errors have occurred.

Do not rely solely on a paper review to determine medication errors. Detection of blank spaces on a medication administration record does not constitute the detection of actual medication errors. Paper review only identifies possible errors in most cases. In some cases paper review can help identify actual errors but research has shown that the procedure is time consuming for the number of actual errors detected.

Observation Technique --The survey team must know without doubt, what drugs, in what strength, and dosage forms, are being administered. This is accomplished prior to drug administration and may be done in a number of ways depending on the drug distribution system used (e.g. unit dose, vial system, punch card).

1. Identify the drug product. There are two principal ways to do this. In most cases, they are used in combination:

    - Identify the product by its size, shape, and color. Many drug products are identifiable by their distinctive size, shape, or color. This technique is problematic because not all drugs have distinctive sizes, shapes, or color.

    - Identify the product by observing the label. When the punch card or the unit dose system is used, the survey team can usually observe the label and adequately identify the drug product. When the vial system is used, observing the label is sometimes more difficult. Ask the nurse to identify the medication being administered.

2. Observe and record the administration of drugs ("pass"). Follow the person administering drugs and observe residents receiving drugs (e.g., actually swallowing oral dosage forms). Be neutral and as unobtrusive as possible during this process.

    - Make every effort to observe residents during several different drug "passes," if possible, so the survey team will have an assessment of the entire facility rather than one staff member on one drug pass.

    - Identifying residents can present a problem. The surveyor should ask appropriate staff to explain the facility policy or system for the identification of residents.

3. Reconcile the surveyor's record of observation with physician's orders. Compare the record of observation with the most current orders for drugs. This comparison involves two distinct activities:

    - For each drug on the surveyor's list: Was it administered according to the prescriber's orders? For example, in the correct strength, by the correct route? Was there a valid order for the drug? Was the drug the correct one?

- For drugs not on the surveyor's list: Are there orders for drugs that should have been administered, but were not? Examine the record for drug orders that were not administered and should have been. Such circumstances may represent omitted doses, one of the most frequent types of errors.

- Ask the person administering drugs, if possible, to describe the system for administering the drugs given. Occasionally, a respiratory therapist may administer inhalers, a designated treatment person may only administer topical treatments, a hospice nurse may administer hospice medications, another person may administer eye drops or as needed drugs, etc. Sometimes people may share medication carts. Under these circumstances, these individuals should be interviewed about the omitted dose, if they were involved, if possible. When persons that were actually responsible for administering the drugs are not available, ask their supervisor for clarification.

The surveyor should now have a complete record of what was observed and what should have occurred according to the prescribers' orders. Determine the number of errors by adding the errors on each resident. Before concluding for certain that an error has occurred, discuss the apparent error with the person who administered the drugs if possible. There may be a logical explanation for an apparent error. For example, the surveyor observed that a resident had received Lasix 20 mg, but the order was for 40 mg. This was an apparent error in dosage. But the nurse showed the surveyor another more recent order which discontinued the 40 mg order and replaced it with a 20 mg order.

4. Reporting Errors -- Describe to the facility each error that the survey team detects (e.g., Mary Jones received digoxin in 0.125 instead of 0.25 mg). The survey team is not required to analyze the errors and come to any conclusions on how the facility can correct them. Do not attempt to categorize errors into various classifications (e.g., wrong dose, wrong resident). Stress that an error occurred and that future errors must be avoided.

5. Observe Many Individuals Administering Medications. Strive to observe as many individuals administering medications as possible. This provides a better picture of accuracy of the facility's entire drug distribution system.

Dose Reconciliation Technique Supplement to the Observation Technique -- When an omission error has been detected through the observation technique, the dose reconciliation technique can sometimes enable the survey team to learn how frequently an error has occurred in the past. Learning about the frequency of an error can assist in judging the significance of the error. (See Significant and Non Significant Medication

Errors above.) The dose reconciliation technique requires a comparison of the number of doses remaining in a supply of drugs with the number of days the drug has been in use and the directions for use. For example, if a drug were in use for 5 days with direction to administer the drug 4 times a day, then 20 doses should have been used. If a count of the supply of that drug shows that only 18 doses were used (i.e., two extra doses exist) and no explanation for the discrepancy exists (e.g., resident refused the dose, or resident was hospitalized), then two omission errors may have occurred.

Use the dose reconciliation technique in facilities that indicate the number of drugs received, and the date and the specific "pass" when that particular drug was started. Unless this information is available, do not use this technique. If this information is not available, there is no Federal authority under which the survey team may require it, except for controlled drugs.

F334

§483.25(n) Influenza and pneumococcal immunizations---

(1) Influenza. The facility must develop policies and procedures that ensure that--

i. Before offering the influenza immunization, each resident or the resident's legal representative receives education regarding the benefits and potential side effects of the immunization;

ii. Each resident is offered an influenza immunization October 1 through March 31 annually, unless the immunization is medically contraindicated or the resident has already been immunized during this time period;

iii. The resident or the resident's legal representative has the opportunity to refuse immunization; and

iv. The resident's medical record includes documentation that indicates, at a minimum, the following:

(A) That the resident or resident's legal representative was provided education regarding the benefits and potential side effects of influenza immunization; and

(B) That the resident either received the influenza immunization or did not receive the influenza immunization due to medical contraindications or refusal.

(2) Pneumococcal disease. The facility must develop policies and procedures that ensure that—

i. **Before offering the pneumococcal immunization, each resident or the resident's legal representative receives education regarding the benefits and potential side effects of the immunization;**

ii. **Each resident is offered an pneumococcal immunization, unless the immunization is medically contraindicate or the resident has already been immunized;**

iii. **The resident or the resident's legal representative has the opportunity to refuse immunization; and**

iv. **The resident's medical record includes documentation that indicates, at a minimum, the following:**

   (A) That the resident or resident's legal representative was provided education regarding the benefits and potential side effects of pneumococcal immunization; and

   (B) That the resident either received the pneumococcal immunization or did not receive the pneumococcal immunization due to medical contraindication or refusal.

v. **Exception. As an alternative, based on an assessment and practitioner recommendation, a second pneumococcal immunization may be given after 5 years following the first pneumococcal immunization, unless medically contraindicated or the resident or the resident's legal representative refuses the second immunization.**

Intent:

The intent of this requirement is to:

- Minimize the risk of residents acquiring, transmitting, or experiencing complications from influenza and pneumococcal pneumonia by assuring that each resident:
    - Is informed about the benefits and risks of immunizations; and
    - Has the opportunity to receive, unless medically contraindicated or refused or already immunized, the influenza and pneumococcal vaccine; and
- Assure documentation in the resident's medical record of the information/education provided regarding the benefits and risks of immunization and the administration or the refusal of or medical contraindications to the vaccine(s).

Definitions

Medical contraindication – A condition or risk that precludes the administration of a treatment or intervention because of the substantial probability that harm to the individual may occur.

Precaution - A condition in a potential recipient that might increase the risk for a serious adverse reaction or that might compromise the vaccine's induction of immunity. However, the risk for this happening is less than expected with a contraindication. For example, as a result of the resident's condition, complications could result, or a person might experience a more severe reaction to the vaccine than would have otherwise been expected; however, the risk for this happening is less than expected with medical contraindications.

Overview

Receipt of vaccinations is essential to the health and well-being of long term care residents. Establishing an immunization program facilitates achievement of this objective. Flu outbreaks place both the residents and the nursing facility staff at risk of infection. Pneumococcal pneumonia, a type of bacterial pneumonia, is a common cause of hospitalization and death in older people. People 65 years or older, are two to three times more likely than the younger population to get pneumococcal infections.

According to the Centers for Disease Control and Prevention (CDC), (see http://www.cdc.gov/mmwr/preview/mmwrhtml/rr54e713a1.htm) "the primary option for reducing the effect of influenza is immuno-prophylaxis with vaccine. Inactivated (i.e., killed virus) influenza vaccine and live, attenuated influenza vaccine are available for use in the United States. Vaccinating persons at high risk for complications and their contacts each year before seasonal increases in influenza virus circulation is the most effective means of reducing the effect of influenza. When vaccine and epidemic strains are well-matched, achieving increased vaccination rates among persons living in closed settings (e.g., nursing homes and other chronic-care facilities) and among staff can reduce the risk for outbreaks by inducing herd immunity. Vaccination of health-care workers and other persons in close contact with persons at increased risk for severe influenza illness can also reduce transmission of influenza and subsequent influenza-related complications. Antiviral drugs used for chemoprophylaxis or treatment of influenza are a key adjunct to vaccine …However, antiviral medications are not a substitute for vaccination."

Because of the clinically complex conditions of most nursing home residents, it is especially important for the facility to have a program in place for the prevention of disease. The Long Term Care regulations at 42 CFR 483.65 (Tag F441) Infection Control, requires that each "facility must establish and maintain an infection control program designed to provide a safe, sanitary, and comfortable environment and to help prevent the development and transmission of disease and infection." The regulation for immunization complements this existing infection control regulation in the areas of prevention of the development and transmission of disease. (For more information on immunizations programs, see http://www.cdc.gov/nip/publications/long-term-care.pdf.)

An effective immunization program involves collaborating with the medical director to develop resident care policies for immunization(s) that reflect current standards of practice and that include:

- Physician approved policies for orders for influenza and pneumococcal polysaccharide vaccines (administration must be based on an assessment of each resident for possible medical contraindications – See Tag F386 for physician orders for vaccinations);
- Identification, of each resident's immunization status, including assessment for potential medical contraindications and record of vaccination;
- The vaccination schedule including mechanisms for recording and monitoring for administration of both influenza and pneumococcal pneumonia vaccines; and
- How pertinent information will be provided to residents. The facility may wish to use educational resources such as those provided by the U. S. Centers for Disease Control (CDC):

  - For trivalent inactivated vaccine (TIV): http://www.cdc.gov/nip/publications/VIS/vis-flu.pdf;
  - For live attenuated vaccine (LAIV) LAIV: http://www.cdc.gov/nip/publications/VIS/vis-flulive.pdf; and
  - For pneumococcal polysaccharide vaccine; http://www.cdc.gov/nip/publications/vis/vis-ppv.pdf.

For information on the influenza vaccines, the following site contains information on the background, types of vaccines, medical contraindications and other information: http://www.cdc.gov/mmwr/preview/mmwrhtml/rr54e713a1.htm.

PROVISION OF IMMUNIZATIONS

In order for a resident to exercise his or her right to make informed choices, it is important for the facility to provide the resident with education regarding the benefits and potential side effects of immunizations. Facilities are required by 42 CFR 483.25(n)(1)(iv) and 42 CFR 483.25(n)(2)(iv) to document the provision of this education and the administration or refusal of the immunization or the medical contraindication of the immunization. There may be clinical indications or other reasons that a resident may not have received immunizations. Examples may include, but are not limited to the following:

- A decision may have been made to delay vaccination for a resident because a precaution is present. According to the CDC, "under normal circumstances, vaccinations should be deferred when a precaution is present. However, a vaccination might be indicated in the presence of a precaution because the benefit of protection from the vaccine outweighs the risk for an adverse reaction. The presence of a moderate or severe acute illness with or without a fever is a precaution to administration of all vaccines;"

- A resident may be in the end stages of a terminal illness and receiving care that is limited to comfort or palliative measures only. Vaccination decisions for residents in the end stages of a terminal illness should be made jointly by the physician and resident;

- A resident may have medical contraindications for live attenuated influenza vaccine (LAIV) that, according to the Centers for Disease Control and Prevention (www.cdc.gov/flu/professionals/vaccination/shouldnotlaiv.htm) include, but are not limited to:

    - Persons who are 50 years of age or older, have asthma, reactive airway disease, or other chronic disorders of the pulmonary or cardiovascular systems;

    - Persons with underlying medical conditions, including such metabolic diseases such as diabetes, renal dysfunction, and hemoglobinopathies;

    - Persons with known or suspected immunodeficiency diseases or who are receiving immuno-suppressive therapies; and

    - Persons with a history of hypersensitivity, including anaphylaxis, to any of the components of LAIV or to eggs;

- A resident may have already received the influenza vaccine for this season; and the pneumococcal immunization status is current; and

- The resident refused the immunization.

  NOTE: Inactivated influenza vaccine contains noninfectious killed viruses and cannot cause influenza. Since there is a delay in developing antibodies after vaccination, the resident may develop influenza if there was exposure prior to receiving the vaccine. Coincidental respiratory disease unrelated to influenza vaccination can occur at any time after vaccination.

Following vaccination with inactivated vaccine a person may experience local reaction and/or systemic reactions. Local reactions typically include soreness at the vaccination site and body aches. Systemic reactions include fever, malaise and myalgia and persons who have had no previous exposure to the influenza virus antigens in the vaccine are most often affected.

Other reactions as identified by the CDC, which may occur immediately, presumably allergic reactions (e.g., hives, angioedema, allergic asthma, and systemic anaphylaxis) rarely are due to the influenza component of the vaccination, but probably result from hypersensitivity to other vaccine components; the majority of reactions probably are caused by residual egg protein. Persons who have had hives or swelling of the lips or tongue, or who have experienced acute respiratory distress or collapse after eating eggs should consult a physician for appropriate evaluation to help determine if vaccine should be administered. Persons who have documented immunoglobulin E (IgE)-mediated hypersensitivity to eggs, including those who have had occupational asthma or other allergic responses to egg protein, might also be at increased risk for allergic reactions to influenza vaccine, and consultation with a physician should be considered.

The following resource contains information on side effects of influenza vaccines:

http://www.cdc.gov/mmwr/preview/mmwrhtml/rr54e713a1.htm

The resident's record should show vaccination administration to the resident unless the record contains documentation as to why vaccine was not administered, including but not limited to:

- Precautions necessitating delay in administering the vaccination;
- Medical contraindications to the use of the vaccines;
- The eligible resident refused the vaccine; or
- The resident has already been immunized.

NOTE: The influenza vaccine is given seasonally. Although the vaccines usually are representative of the influenza viruses likely to circulate during the flu season, occasionally the vaccine may not be as closely representative. The CDC indicates that administering the vaccine during October or November is generally most effective. However, residents admitted late in the influenza season, February or March, should be offered the influenza vaccine as late season outbreaks do occur. If a resident was admitted outside the influenza season (which is October 1 through March 31), the facility is not expected to offer the influenza vaccine to the resident, but they may, at their discretion.

There should be documentation in the medical record if there is reason to believe that the pneumococcal vaccine was given previously but the date cannot be verified and this had an impact upon the decision regarding administration of the vaccine.

According to the CDC, "Pneumococcal polysaccharide vaccine generally is considered safe based on clinical experience since 1977, when the pneumococcal polysaccharide vaccine was licensed in the United States. Approximately half of persons who receive pneumococcal vaccine develop mild, local side effects (e.g., pain at the injection site, erythema, and swelling). These reactions usually persist for less than 48 hours. Moderate systemic reactions (e.g., fever and myalgia) and more severe local reactions (e.g., local induration) are rare. Intradermal administration may cause severe local reactions and is inappropriate. Severe systemic adverse effects (e.g., anaphylactic reactions) rarely have been reported after administration of pneumococcal vaccine. For more information for the pneumococcal vaccine, see http://www.cdc.gov/mmwr/preview/mmwrhtml/00047135.htm

The pneumococcal vaccine does not prevent or lessen the impact of other types of pneumonia, such as aspiration, fungal, or viral.

INVESTIGATIVE PROTOCOL

Immunizations for Influenza and Pneumococcal Pneumonia

Objectives:

- To determine if the facility's immunization program has been implemented and assures that residents are offered vaccines, and that residents or legal representatives receive related education;
- To determine if education regarding the benefits and potential side effects of immunization(s) was provided to the resident or legal representative each time a vaccine was offered; and
- To determine if each resident received the influenza and/or pneumococcal immunization(s) unless medically contraindicated, refused, or already immunized, or because of circumstances outside of the facility's control, such as vaccine production delays.

Sampling:

For surveys during influenza season (October 1-March 31), follow the Procedure below for all residents who are selected for Comprehensive Reviews in Task 5C – Resident Review. If this number is below 5 residents, select additional residents from the Phase 1 Focused Review sample residents to meet the minimum number of 5 residents.

For surveys conducted outside influenza season, select 5 residents from the list the facility provided (see Task 2 – Entrance Conference) of all current residents who were in the facility during the previous influenza season. Give precedence in selection to those residents whom the survey team has selected as Phase 1 sample residents.

Procedure

For all residents selected for this review, determine the following:

For the provision of Pneumococcal Pneumonia Vaccine, review all selected residents for:

- The provision of education related to the vaccine; and
- Either documentation of the administration of the vaccine; or
- If not provided, documentation as to why the vaccine was not provided, such as medical contraindications, refusal, or vaccine was already given prior to admission.

For the provision of Influenza Vaccine:

- For surveys occurring outside of influenza season, review selected residents for the provision of influenza education and immunization during the previous influenza season.
- For surveys occurring during influenza season, review all selected residents for the provision of influenza education and immunization during the current influenza season.

Review residents for:

- o The provision of education for the vaccine; and
- o The administration of the vaccine, or if the vaccine was not provided, the reason why the vaccine was not provided, such as medical contraindications, refusal, unavailability of the vaccine, or vaccine was already given prior to admission.

NOTE: (For surveys occurring during influenza season) - Unavailability of the influenza vaccine can be a valid reason why a facility has not implemented the influenza vaccine program, especially during the early weeks of the influenza season. It is also likely that a facility surveyed during October may not have administered the vaccine, yet. In these instances, ask the facility to demonstrate that:

- The vaccine has been ordered and the facility received either the vaccine or a confirmation of the order indicating that the vaccine has been shipped or that the product is not available but will be shipped when the supply is available;

- Plans are developed on how and when the vaccines are to be administered;
- Residents have been screened to determine how many and which residents are eligible and wish to receive the vaccine; and
- Education regarding immunizations has been implemented.

For surveys occurring during influenza season, review the facility's immunization program if:

- There has been no shortage or lack of availability of the vaccines and residents have not refused the vaccine, but the residents have not yet been vaccinated;
- The resident(s), have not been evaluated for vaccination status, or
- The resident(s) has not received information/education about the benefits and potential risks of the immunizations.

For all facilities, determine if the facility developed influenza and pneumococcal vaccine policies and procedures including, but not limited to the following:

- The type of information/education provided to the resident prior to administration of the immunization(s);
- How the influenza vaccine program is implemented during the influenza season (October through March), including physician orders and standing orders (if standing orders are used);
- How the pneumococcal vaccine will be provided (i.e., throughout the calendar year);
- How residents and families are educated about the benefits and risks of the vaccines;
- Processes to address issues that are out of the facility's control such as non-availability of vaccines due to production delay or distribution problems, or the presence of a precaution in a resident that may warrant a delay in vaccine;
- The identification and tracking/monitoring of a resident's vaccination status (including medical contraindications or delayed administrations); and
- The location of documentation of education and administration of the vaccines.

If there are significant discrepancies between the facility's policies and procedures and the follow through for the vaccine program, ask the person responsible for implementing the procedures to explain the discrepancies.

Determination of Compliance (Task 6, Appendix P)

Synopsis of Regulation (F334)

The influenza and pneumococcal vaccination requirement has five aspects:

1. The resident is provided education regarding the benefits and potential side effects of the vaccinations;

2. The facility must offer each resident influenza and pneumococcal immunizations unless the immunization is medically contraindicated, or the resident's immunization status is current;

3. The resident, or the resident's legal representative, has the right to refuse the vaccinations;

4. Each eligible resident is administered the influenza and pneumococcal vaccine (unless refused or contraindicated or the resident has already been immunized); and

5. The facility must document that education was provided and that the resident either received the vaccine(s) or, if not received, that the vaccines(s) was (were) refused or medically contraindicated or the resident had already been immunized.

Criteria for Compliance

- Compliance with 42 CFR 483.25 (n), F334, Influenza and Pneumococcal Immunizations

    - The facility is in compliance with this requirement:

        - If each resident receives education regarding the benefits and potential side effects of the vaccine(s);

        - If each resident has been evaluated for eligibility to receive the vaccine(s);

        - If each resident is offered, unless medically contraindicated or already vaccinated, an influenza vaccine October 1 through March 31 annually, and a pneumococcal vaccine;

- If the resident has the opportunity to refuse; and
- If the record includes documentation that indicates, at a minimum:
  - The resident was provided education regarding the benefits and potential side effects; and
  - That the resident received the immunizations, refused the vaccination(s), or did not receive the vaccine(s) because of already being immunized, or as a result of a medical contraindication (including the nature of the resident's medical contraindications), unavailability, or a precaution that delayed the administration and a later date for administration has been planned.

If the facility is not in compliance with each of these aspects of the requirement, cite F334.

Non-compliance for F334

After completing the investigative protocol, determine whether noncompliance with the regulation exists. Noncompliance for F334 may include, but is not limited to, one or more of the following:

- An eligible resident did not receive either the influenza and/or the pneumococcal vaccines without a valid reason;
- The facility did not evaluate to identify potential medical contraindications to the vaccines;
- The facility administered either of the vaccines to a resident who had refused them;
- The facility administered the influenza vaccine to a resident with medical contraindications, without physician involvement and/or approval;
- The facility administered the vaccine(s) to a resident who had an identified precaution, such as moderate or severe acute illness with or without fever, without physician involvement and/or approval;
- The facility administered the live attenuated influenza vaccine without physician approval to a resident who has a medical contraindication for live attenuated influenza vaccine;

- The facility failed to provide the pertinent information regarding the immunizations to the resident;
- The facility failed to document that the resident or resident's legal representative was provided education regarding the benefits and potential side effects of the influenza and, as applicable, the pneumococcal immunization; and
- The facility failed to document that the resident either received the vaccine(s) or did not receive the vaccine(s) due to medical contraindications or refusal.

Potential Tags for Additional Investigation

During the investigation of F334, the surveyor may have identified concerns with additional requirements related to outcome, process, and/or structure requirements. The surveyor is cautioned to investigate these related requirements before determining whether non-compliance may be present. Examples of some of the related requirements that may be considered when non-compliance F334 has been identified include the following:

- 42 CFR 483.20(b), F272, Comprehensive Assessments
    - Review whether the resident's comprehensive assessment documented whether the influenza and/or pneumococcal vaccines were administered in the facility, including the reason(s) why a vaccine may not have been received in the facility.
- 42 CFR 483.65, F441, Infection Control Program
    - Review whether the facility's program for infection control includes the prevention of the development and transmission of disease and infections including influenza and pneumococcal pneumonia.
- 42 CFR 483.75(i)(2), F501, Medical Director
    - Determine whether the medical director has collaborated with the facility to develop policies and procedures based on current standards of practice for an immunization program, including the assessment of the resident, identification of medical contraindications/precautions and emergency medical interventions in the case of allergic reactions to the vaccines.

IV. DEFICIENCY CATEGORIZATION (Part IV, Appendix P)

Once the team has completed its investigation, analyzed the data, reviewed the regulatory requirement, and identified any deficient practice(s) that demonstrate that non-compliance with the regulation at F334 exists, the team must determine the severity of the deficient practice(s) and the resultant harm or potential for harm to the resident. The key elements for severity determination for F334 are as follows:

1. **Presence of harm/negative outcome(s) or potential for negative outcomes because of lack of appropriate treatment and care.**

   Non-compliance related to an actual or potential harm/negative outcome for F334 may include, but is not limited to:

   - A resident who is not eligible to receive the vaccines is administered the vaccine and has a reaction;
   - A resident who is eligible for the vaccine refuses the immunization, however, the resident is administered the vaccine; or
   - The facility fails to implement the immunization program and the residents experience an outbreak of influenza.

2. **Degree of harm (actual or potential) related to the non-compliance.**

   Identify how the facility practices caused, resulted in, allowed, or contributed to the actual or potential for harm:

   - If harm has occurred, determine if the harm is at the level of serious injury, impairment, death, compromise, or discomfort; or
   - If harm has not yet occurred, determine how likely is the potential for serious injury, impairment, death, or compromise or discomfort to occur to the resident.

3. **The immediacy of correction required.**

Determine whether the non-compliance requires immediate correction in order to prevent serious injury, harm, impairment, or death to one or more residents.

The survey team must evaluate the harm or potential for harm based upon the following levels of severity for Tag F334. First, the team must rule out whether Severity Level 4, Immediate Jeopardy to a resident's health or safety, exists by evaluating the deficient practice in relation to immediacy, culpability, and severity. (Follow the guidance in Appendix Q.)

> **NOTE:** The death or transfer of a resident who was harmed or injured as a result of facility non-compliance does not remove a finding of immediate jeopardy. The facility is required to implement specific actions to correct the non-compliance which allowed or caused the immediate jeopardy.

Severity Level 4 Considerations: Immediate Jeopardy to Resident Health or Safety

Immediate Jeopardy is a situation in which the facility's non-compliance with one or more requirements of participation:

- Has allowed/caused/resulted in, or is likely to cause/allow/result in serious injury, harm, impairment, or death to a resident; and
- Requires immediate correction as the facility either created the situation or allowed the situation to continue by failing to implement preventative or corrective measures.

Examples of the facility's non-compliance that may cause or contribute to negative outcomes at severity level 4 include:

- A resident who is not eligible to receive the vaccine due to medical contraindications is administered the vaccine and experiences a life threatening reaction, such as anaphylactic shock; or
- Residents who were eligible to receive vaccines did not receive them as a result of the facility's failure to have any program for vaccinating residents.

NOTE: If immediate jeopardy has been ruled out based upon the evidence, then evaluate whether actual harm that is not immediate jeopardy exists at severity level 3.

Severity Level 3 Considerations: Actual Harm that is not Immediate Jeopardy

Level 3 indicates non-compliance that results in actual harm, and can include, but may not be limited to clinical compromise, decline, or the resident's ability to maintain and/or reach his/her highest practicable well-being. Examples of negative outcomes may include, but are not limited to:

- A resident who was not eligible to receive the vaccine due to medical contraindications receives the vaccine and experiences a reaction that is not life threatening, but requires treatment; or
- Because of an unwarranted delay (e.g., several weeks after it is available to the facility) in administering the influenza vaccine despite its availability, an eligible resident who has agreed to receive the influenza vaccine develops influenza.

  NOTE: If severity level 3 (actual harm that is not immediate jeopardy) has been ruled out based upon the evidence, then evaluate as to whether level 2 (no actual harm with the potential for more than minimal harm) exists.

Severity Level 2 Considerations: No Actual Harm with Potential for more than Minimal Harm that is not Immediate Jeopardy

Level 2 indicates non-compliance that results in a resident outcome of no more than minimal discomfort and/or has the potential to compromise the resident's ability to maintain or reach his or her highest practicable level of well being. The potential exists for greater harm to occur if interventions are not provided. Examples of outcomes may include, but are not limited to:

- An eligible resident did not receive the vaccine, but did not develop symptoms of influenza;
- An eligible resident received two doses of the pneumococcal vaccine, due to a failure to document the receipt of the first dose, but did not experience any untoward reactions; or
- The staff did not assess for medical contraindications prior to providing the vaccines, but there were no reactions to the vaccine.

Severity Level 1: No Actual Harm with Potential for Minimal Harm

The facility failed to document that information/education was provided to the resident prior to administering the immunizations.

F353

§483.30 Nursing Services

The facility must have sufficient nursing staff to provide nursing and related services to attain or maintain the highest practicable physical, mental, and psychosocial well-being of each resident, as determined by resident assessments and individual plans of care.

Intent §483.30

To assure that sufficient qualified nursing staff are available on a daily basis to meet residents' needs for nursing care in a manner and in an environment which promotes each resident's physical, mental and psychosocial well-being, thus enhancing their quality of life.

Procedures §483.30

§483.30(a) and (b) are to be reviewed during the standard survey whenever quality of care problems have been discovered (see Appendix P, Survey Protocol, Task 4, for further information and Task 5C for the investigative protocol to complete this review).

In addition, fully review requirements of nursing services during an extended survey or when a waiver of RN and/or licensed nurse (RN/LPN) staffing has been requested or granted. Except as licensed nursing personnel are specifically required by the regulation (e.g., an RN for 8 consecutive hours a day, 7 days a week), the determination of sufficient staff will be made based on the staff's ability to provide needed care to residents that enable them to reach their highest practicable physical, mental and psychosocial well-being. The ability to meet the requirements of §§483.13, 483.15(a), 483.20, 483.25 and 483.65 determines sufficiency of nurse staffing.

§483.30(a) Sufficient Staff

§483.30(a)(1) The facility must provide services by sufficient numbers of each of the following types of personnel on a 24-hour basis to provide nursing care to all residents in accordance with resident care plans:

(i) Except when waived under paragraph (c) of this section, licensed nurses; and
(ii) other nursing personnel.

§483.30(a)(2) Except when waived under paragraph (c) of this section, the facility must designate a licensed nurse to serve as a charge nurse on each tour of duty.

For Interpretive Guidelines and Probes on §483.30(a) see Tag F354

F354

§483.30(b) Registered Nurse

§483.30(b)(1) Except when waived under paragraph (c) or (d) of this section, the facility must use the services of a registered nurse for at least 8 consecutive hours a day, 7 days a week.

§483.30(b)(2) Except when waived under paragraph (c) or (d) of this section, the facility must designate a registered nurse to serve as the director of nursing on a full time basis.

§483.30(b)(3) The director of nursing may serve as a charge nurse only when the facility has an average daily occupancy of 60 or fewer residents.

Interpretive Guidelines §483.30(a) and (b)

At a minimum, "**staff**" is defined as licensed nurses (RNs and/or LPNs/LVNs), and nurse aides. Nurse aides must meet the training and competency requirements described in §483.75(e).

"**Full-time**" is defined as working 35 or more hours a week.

Except for licensed staff noted above, the determining factor in sufficiency of staff (including both numbers of staff and their qualifications) will be the ability of the facility to provide needed care for residents. A deficiency concerning staffing should ordinarily provide examples of care deficits caused by insufficient quantity and quality of staff. If, however, inadequate staff (either the number or category) presents a clear threat to residents reaching their highest practicable level of well-being, cite this as a deficiency. Provide specific documentation of the threat.

The facility is required to designate an RN to serve as DON on a full time basis. This requirement can be met when RNs share the position. If RNs share the DON position, the total hours per week must equal 40. Facility staff must understand the shared responsibilities. The facility can only be waived from this requirement if it has a waiver under subsection (c) or (d).

Probes: §483.30(a) and (b)

Determine nurse staffing sufficiency for each unit:

- Is there adequate staff to meet direct care needs, assessments, planning, evaluation, supervision?
- Do work loads for direct care staff appear reasonable?
- Do residents, family, and ombudsmen report insufficient staff to meet resident needs?
- Are staff responsive to residents' needs for assistance, and call bells answered promptly?
- Do residents call out repeatedly for assistance?
- Are residents, who are unable to call for help, checked frequently (e.g., each half hour) for safety, comfort, positioning, and to offer fluids and provision of care?
- Are identified care problems associated with a specific unit or tour of duty?
- Is there a licensed nurse that serves as a charge nurse (e.g., supervises the provision of resident care) on each tour of duty (if facility does not have a waiver of this requirement)?
- What does the charge nurse do to correct problems in nurse staff performance?

- Does the facility have the services of an RN available 8 consecutive hours a day, 7 days a week (if this requirement has not been waived)?
- How does the facility assure that each resident receives nursing care in accordance with his/her plan of care on weekends, nights, and holidays?
- How does the sufficiency (numbers and categories) of nursing staff contribute to identified quality of care, resident rights, quality of life, or facility practices problems?

F355 – Nursing Waivers

§483.30(c) Nursing facilities

Waiver of requirement to provide licensed nurses on a 24-hour basis.

To the extent that a facility is unable to meet the requirements of paragraphs (a)(2) and (b)(1) of this section, a State may waive such requirements with respect to the facility if--

(1) The facility demonstrates to the satisfaction of the State that the facility has been unable, despite diligent efforts (including offering wages at the community prevailing rate for nursing facilities), to recruit appropriate personnel;

(2) The State determines that a waiver of the requirement will not endanger the health or safety of individuals staying in the facility;

(3) The State finds that, for any periods in which licensed nursing services are not available, a registered nurse or a physician is obligated to respond immediately to telephone calls from the facility;

(4) A waiver granted under the conditions listed in paragraph (c) of this section is subject to annual State review;

(5) In granting or renewing a waiver, a facility may be required by the State to use other qualified, licensed personnel;

(6) The State agency granting a waiver of such requirements provides notice of the waiver to the State long term care ombudsman (established under section 307 (a)(12) of the Older Americans Act of 1965) and the protection and advocacy system in the State for the mentally ill and mentally retarded; and

(7) The nursing facility that is granted such a waiver by a State notifies residents of the facility (or, where appropriate, the guardians or legal representatives of such residents) and members of their immediate families of the waiver.

Intent §483.30(c)

To give the facility flexibility, in limited circumstances, when the facility cannot meet nurse staffing requirements.

Interpretive Guidelines §483.30(c)

The facility may request a waiver of the RN requirement, and/or the 24-hour licensed nurse requirement. If the facility is Medicaid-certified only, the State has the authority to grant the waiver. If the facility is dually-participating, CMS has the delegated authority to grant the waiver. (See guidelines for §483.30(d).)

A survey of Nursing Services must be conducted if a waiver has been granted or requested.

Probes: §483.30(c)

Before granting a continuation of this waiver, or during the annual review, at a minimum, determine:

- Is a continuing effort being made to obtain licensed nurses?
- How does the facility ensure that residents' needs are being met?
- Are all nursing policies and procedures followed on each shift during times when licensed services are waived?
- Is there a qualified person to assess, evaluate, plan and implement resident care?
- Is care being carried out according to professional practice standards on each shift?
- Can the survey team ensure the State that the absence of licensed nurses will NOT endanger the health or safety of residents?
- Are there trends in the facility, which might be indicators of decreased quality of care as a result of insufficient staffing to meet resident needs (e.g., increases in incident reports, the infection rate, hospitalizations)?
- Are there increases in loss of function, pressure sores, tube feedings, catheters, weight loss, mental status?

- Is there evidence that preventive measures (e.g., turning, ambulating are taken to avoid poor quality of care outcomes and avoidable sudden changes in health status?

- Is there evidence that sudden changes in resident health status and emergency needs are being properly identified and managed by appropriate facility staff and in a timely manner?

- If the facility has a waiver of the requirement to provide licensed nurses on a 24-hour basis, have they notified the ombudsman, residents, surrogates or legal representatives, and members of their immediate families of the waiver, and are there services residents need that are not provided because licensed nurses are not available?

- Is there an increase in hospitalizations because licensed personnel are not available to provide appropriate services?

- Does the facility meet all applicable requirements to continue to receive a waiver?

- Does the staff indicate that an RN or physician is available to respond immediately to telephone calls when licensed nurses are not available?

§483.30(d) SNFs

Waiver of the requirement to provide services of a registered nurse for more than 40 hours a week.

§483.30(d)(1) The Secretary may waive the requirement that a SNF provide the services of a registered nurse for more than 40 hours a week, including a director of nursing specified in paragraph (b) of this section, if the Secretary finds that --

(i) The facility is located in a rural area and the supply of skilled nursing facility services in the area is not sufficient to meet the needs of individuals residing in the area;

(ii) The facility has one full-time registered nurse who is regularly on duty at the facility 40 hours a week; and
(iii) The facility either--

(A) Has only patients whose physicians have indicated (through physicians' orders or admission notes) that they do not require the services of a registered nurse or a physician for a 48-hours period or;

(B) Has made arrangements for a registered nurse or a physician to spend time at the facility, as determined necessary by the physician, to provide

necessary skilled nursing services on days when the regular full-time registered nurse is not on duty;

(iv) The Secretary provides notice of the waiver to the State long term care ombudsman (established under section 307(a)(12) of the Older Americans Act of 1965) and the protection and advocacy system in the State for the mentally ill and mentally retarded; and

(v) The facility that is granted such a waiver notifies residents of the facility (or, where appropriate, the guardians or legal representatives of such residents) and members of their immediate families of the waiver.

(2) A waiver of the registered nurse requirement under paragraph (d)(1) of this section is subject to annual renewal by the Secretary.

Interpretive Guidelines §483.30(d)

CMS is delegated the waiver authority for SNFs, including dually-participating facilities (SNF/NFs). The Medicare waiver authority is far more limited than is the States' authority under Medicaid since a State may waive any element of the nurse staffing requirement, whereas the Secretary may waive only the RN requirement. The requirements that a registered nurse provide services for 8 hours a day, 7 days a week (more than 40 hours a week), and that there be an RN designated as director of nursing on a full-time basis, may be waived by the Secretary in the following circumstances:

- The facility is located in a rural area with an inadequate supply of SNF services to meet area needs. Rural is defined as "all areas not delineated as `urban` by the Bureau of Census, based on the most recent census;

- The facility has one full-time registered nurse regularly working 40 hours a week. This may be the same individual, or part-time individuals. This nurse may or may not be the DON, and may perform some DON and some clinical duties if the facility so desires; **and either**;

- The facility has only residents whose physicians have noted, in writing, do not need RN or physician care for a 48 hour period. This does not relieve the facility from responsibility for providing for emergency availability of a physician, when necessary, nor does it relieve the facility from being responsible for meeting all needs of the residents during those 48 hours;

OR

- A physician or RN will spend the necessary time at the facility to provide care residents need during the days that an RN is not on duty. This requirement refers to clinical care of the residents that need skilled nursing services.

- If a waiver of this requirement has been granted, conduct a survey of nursing services during each certification survey. Dually-participating facilities must meet the waiver provisions of the SNF.

Probes: §483.30(d)

If the SNF has a waiver of the more than 40 hours a week RN requirement:

- Is there an RN on duty 40 hours a week?
- If more than one RN provides the 40 hour per week coverage, how is information exchanged that maintains continuity of resident care?
- Does each clinical record have documentation by the physician that the resident does not need services of a physician or an RN for a 48 hour period each week.
- Are there any emergency or routine services that should be, but are not, provided to residents during the days that a registered nurse is not on duty?
- If specific skilled care is necessary for a resident during the time that an RN is not on duty, does an RN or physician provide that service on an "as needed" basis?
- Did the facility notify residents (or their legal guardians) and their immediate families about the waiver and the ombudsman?

See also probes at §483.30(c).

If the SNF requests continuation of the waiver to provide the services of a registered nurse for more than 40 hours a week, the survey team is to provide the Secretary with information needed to grant this continuation.

- Does the SNF meet all requirements necessary for continuation of the waiver?

Procedures §483.30(a)-(d)

If the facility has an approved nurse staffing waiver, it is **not** considered a deficiency. The facility does not need to submit a POC.

The following procedure should be used to document that a facility has a waiver of nurse staffing requirements.

When a facility does not meet the nurse staffing requirements, cite the appropriate tag. If the facility does have a waiver, reference the tag number based on the type of facility. The type of facility (SNF, NF, or SNF/NF) determines what type of waiver is granted:

- For SNFs and SNF/NFs which may be waived from the requirement to provide more than 40 hours of registered nurse services a week, and for NFs which have been granted a waiver from the 56 hour registered nurse requirement, cite F354;
    - For NFs that have a waiver of the 24-hour licensed nursing requirement, cite F353, or
    - Both facility types could be waived for the requirement to designate a registered nurse as the director of nursing on a full-time basis. Cite F355.

When the Form CMS-2567 is entered into OSCAR, code the waived tag as a "W." Enter the tag number, leave the correction date blank, and enter a "W" in the CP field. This will indicate that this is not a deficiency--that the requirement has been waived.

F356

§483.30(e) Nurse Staffing Information--

(1) Data requirements. The facility must post the following information on a daily basis:

(i) Facility name.

(ii) The current date.

(iii) The total number and the actual hours worked by the following categories of licensed and unlicensed nursing staff directly responsible for resident care per shift:

(A) Registered nurses.

(B) Licensed practical nurses or licensed vocational nurses (as defined under State law).

(C) Certified nurse aides.

(iv) Resident census.

(2) Posting requirements.

(i) The facility must post the nurse staffing data specified in paragraph (e)(1) of this section on a daily basis at the beginning of each shift.

(ii) Data must be posted as follows:

(A) Clear and readable format.

(B) In a prominent place readily accessible to residents and visitors.

- **Public access to posted nurse staffing data. The facility must, upon oral or written request, make nurse staffing data available to the public for review at a cost not to exceed the community standard.**

- **Facility data retention requirements. The facility must maintain the posted daily nurse staffing data for a minimum of 18 months, or as required by State law, whichever is greater.**

F360

§483.35 Dietary Services

The facility must provide each resident with a nourishing, palatable, well-balanced diet that meets the daily nutritional and special dietary needs of each resident.

F361

§483.35(a) Staffing

The facility must employ a qualified dietitian either full-time, part-time, or on a consultant basis.

§483.35(a)(1) If a qualified dietitian is not employed full-time, the facility must designate a person to serve as the director of food service who receives frequently scheduled consultation from a qualified dietitian.

§483.35(a)(2) A qualified dietitian is one who is qualified based upon either registration by the Commission on Dietetic Registration of the American Dietetic Association, or on the basis of education, training, or experience in identification of dietary needs, planning, and implementation of dietary programs.

Intent: §483.35(a)

The intent of this regulation is to ensure that a qualified dietitian is utilized in planning, managing and implementing dietary service activities in order to assure that the residents receive adequate nutrition.

A director of food services has no required minimum qualifications, but must be able to function collaboratively with a qualified dietitian in meeting the nutritional needs of the residents.

Interpretive Guidelines: §483.35(a)

A dietitian qualified on the basis of education, training, or experience in identification of dietary needs, planning and implementation of dietary programs has experience or training which includes:

- Assessing special nutritional needs of geriatric and physically impaired persons;
- Developing therapeutic diets;
- Developing "regular diets" to meet the specialized needs of geriatric and physically impaired persons;
- Developing and implementing continuing education programs for dietary services and nursing personnel;
- Participating in interdisciplinary care planning;
- Budgeting and purchasing food and supplies; and
- Supervising institutional food preparation, service and storage.

Procedures: §483.35(a)

If resident reviews determine that residents have nutritional problems, determine if these nutritional problems relate to inadequate or inappropriate diet nutrition/assessment and monitoring. Determine if these are related to dietitian qualifications.

Probes: §483.35(a)

If the survey team finds problems in resident nutritional status:

- Do practices of the dietitian or food services director contribute to the identified problems in residents' nutritional status? If yes, what are they?
- What are the educational, training, and experience qualifications of the facility's dietitian?

F362

§483.35 (b) Standard Sufficient Staff

The facility must employ sufficient support personnel competent to carry out the functions of the dietary service

Interpretive Guidelines: §483.35(b)

"**Sufficient support personnel**" is defined as enough staff to prepare and serve palatable, attractive, nutritionally adequate meals at proper temperatures and appropriate times and support proper sanitary techniques being utilized.

Procedures: §483.35(b)

For residents who have been triggered for a dining review, do they report that meals are palatable, attractive, served at the proper temperatures and at appropriate times?

Probes: §483.35(b)

Sufficient staff preparation:

- Is food prepared in scheduled timeframes in accordance with established professional practices?

Observe food service:

- Does food leave kitchen in scheduled timeframes? Is food served to residents in scheduled timeframes?

F363

§483.35(c) Menus and Nutritional Adequacy

Menus must:

(1) Meet the nutritional needs of residents in accordance with the recommended dietary allowances of the Food and Nutrition Board of the National Research Council, National Academy of Sciences;

Intent: §483.35(c)(1)(2)(3)

The intent of this regulation is to assure that the meals served meet the nutritional needs of the resident in accordance with the recommended dietary allowances (RDAs) of the Food and Nutrition Board of the National Research Council, of the National Academy of

Sciences. This regulation also assures that there is a prepared menu by which nutritionally adequate meals have been planned for the resident and followed.

Procedures: §483.35(c)(1)

For sampled residents who have a comprehensive review or a focused review, as appropriate, observe if meals served are consistent with the planned menu and care plan in the amounts, types and consistency of foods served.

If the survey team observes deviation from the planned menu, review appropriate documentation from diet card, record review, and interviews with food service manager or dietitian to support reason(s) for deviation from the written menu.

Probes: §483.35(c)(1)

Are residents receiving food in the amount, type, consistency and frequency to maintain normal body weight and acceptable nutritional values?

If food intake appears inadequate based on meal observations, or resident's nutritional status is poor based on resident review, determine if menus have been adjusted to meet the caloric and nutrient-intake needs of each resident.

If a food group is missing from the resident's daily diet, does the facility have an alternative means of satisfying the resident's nutrient needs? If so, does the facility perform a follow-up?

Menu adequately provides the daily basic food groups:

- Does the menu meet basic nutritional needs by providing daily food in the groups of the food pyramid system and based on individual nutritional assessment taking into account current nutritional recommendations?

NOTE: A standard meal planning guide is used primarily for menu planning and food purchasing. It is not intended to meet the nutritional needs of all residents. This guide must be adjusted to consider individual differences. Some residents will need more due to age, size, gender, physical activity, and state of health. There are many meal planning guides from reputable sources, i.e., American Diabetes Association, American Dietetic Association, American Medical Association, or U.S. Department of Agriculture, that are available and appropriate for use when adjusted to meet each resident's needs.

§483.35(c)(2) and (3) Menus and Nutritional Adequacy

§483.35(c)(2) Be prepared in advance; and

Probes: §483.35(c)(2)

Menu prepared in advance:
Are there preplanned menus for both regular and therapeutic diets?

§483.35(c)(3) Be followed.

Probes: §483.35(c)(3)

Menu followed:

- Is food served as planned? If not, why? There may be legitimate and extenuating circumstances why food may not be available on the day of the survey and must be considered before a concern is noted.

F364

§483.35(d) Food

Each resident receives and the facility provides:

(1) Food prepared by methods that conserve nutritive value, flavor, and appearance;

(2) Food that is palatable, attractive, and at the proper temperature;
Intent: §483.35(d)(1)(2)

The intent of this regulation is to assure that the nutritive value of food is not compromised and destroyed because of prolonged food storage, light, and air exposure; prolonged cooking of foods in a large volume of water and prolong holding on steam table, and the addition of baking soda. Food should be palatable, attractive, and at the proper temperature as determined by the type of food to ensure resident's satisfaction. Refer to §483.15(e) and/or §483.15(a).

Interpretive Guidelines: §483.35(d)(1)

"**Food-palatability**" refers to the taste and/or flavor of the food.

"**Food attractiveness**" refers to the appearance of the food when **served** to residents.

Procedures: §483.35(d)(1)

Evidence for palatability and attractiveness of food, from day to day and meal to meal, may be strengthened through sources such as: additional observation, resident and staff interviews, and review of resident council minutes. Review nutritional adequacy in §483.25(i)(1).

Probes: §483.35(d)(1)(2)

Does food have a distinctly appetizing aroma and appearance, which is varied in color and texture?

Is food generally well seasoned (use of spices, herbs, etc.) and acceptable to residents?

Conserves nutritive value:

- Is food prepared in a way to preserve vitamins? Method of storage and preparation should cause minimum loss of nutrients.

Food temperature:

- Is food served at preferable temperature (hot foods are served hot and cold foods are served cold) as discerned by the resident and customary practice? Not to be confused with the proper holding temperature.

F365

§483.35(d)(3) Food prepared in a form designed to meet individual needs; and

---

F366

§483.35(d)(4) Substitutes offered of similar nutritive value to residents who refuse food served

Therapeutic diets must be prescribed by the attending physician.

Procedures §483.35(d)(3)(4)

Observe trays to assure that food is appropriate to resident according to assessment and care plan. Ask the resident how well the food meets their taste needs. Ask if the resident is offered or is given the opportunity to receive substitutes when refusing food on the original menu.

Probes: §483.35(d)(3)(4)

Is food cut, chopped, or ground for individual resident's needs?

Are residents who refuse food offered substitutes of similar nutritive value?

Interpretive Guidelines §483.35(d)(4)

A food substitute should be consistent with the usual and ordinary food items provided by the facility. For example, if a facility never serves smoked salmon, they would not be required to serve this as a food substitute; or the facility may, instead of grapefruit juice, substitute another citrus juice or vitamin C rich juice that the resident likes.

F367

§483.35(e) Therapeutic Diets

Therapeutic diets must be prescribed by the attending physician.

Intent §483.35(e)

The intent of this regulation is to assure that the resident receives and consumes foods in the appropriate form and/or the appropriate nutritive content as prescribed by a physician and/or assessed by the interdisciplinary team to support the treatment and plan of care.

Interpretive Guidelines: §483.35(e)

"**Therapeutic Diet**" is defined as a diet ordered by a physician as part of treatment for a disease or clinical condition, or to eliminate or decrease specific nutrients in the diet, (e.g., sodium) or to increase specific nutrients in the diet (e.g., potassium), or to provide food the resident is able to eat (e.g., a mechanically altered diet).

"**Mechanically altered diet**" is one in which the texture of a diet is altered. When the texture is modified, the type of texture modification must be specific and part of the physicians' order.

Procedures: §483.35(e)

If the resident has inadequate nutrition or nutritional deficits that manifests into and/or are a product of weight loss or other medical problems, determine if there is a therapeutic diet that is medically prescribed.

Probes: §483.35(e)

Is the therapeutic diet that the resident receives prescribed by the physician?

Also, see §483.25(i), Nutritional Status.

F368

§483.35(f) Frequency of Meals

(1) Each resident receives and the facility provides at least three meals daily, at regular times comparable to normal mealtimes in the community.

(2) There must be no more than 14 hours between a substantial evening meal and breakfast the following day, except as provided in (4) below.

(3) The facility must offer snacks at bedtime daily.

(4) When a nourishing snack is provided at bedtime, up to 16 hours may elapse between a substantial evening meal and breakfast the following day if a resident group agrees to this meal span, and a nourishing snack is served.

Intent: §483.35(f)(1-4)

The intent of this regulation is to assure that the resident receives his/her meals at times most accepted by the community and that there are not extensive time lapses between meals. This assures that the resident receives adequate and frequent meals.

Interpretive Guidelines: §483.35(f)(1-4)

A "**substantial evening meal**" is defined as an offering of three or more menu items at one time, one of which includes a high-quality protein such as meat, fish, eggs, or cheese. The meal should represent no less than 20 percent of the day's total nutritional requirements.

"**Nourishing snack**" is defined as a verbal offering of items, single or in combination, from the basic food groups. Adequacy of the "nourishing snack" will be determined both by resident interviews and by evaluation of the overall nutritional status of residents in the facility, (e.g., Is the offered snack usually satisfying?)

Procedures: §483.35(f)(1-4)

Observe meal times and schedules and determine if there is a lapse in time between meals. Ask for resident input on meal service schedules, to verify if there are extensive lapses in time between meals

F369

§483.35(g) Assistive Devices

The facility must provide special eating equipment and utensils for residents who need them.

Intent: §483.35(g)

The intent of this regulation is to provide residents with assistive devices to maintain or improve their ability to eat independently. For example, improving poor grasp by enlarging silverware handles with foam padding, aiding residents with impaired coordination or tremor by installing plate guards, or providing postural supports for head, trunk, and arms.

Procedures: §483.35(g)

Review sampled residents comprehensive assessment for eating ability. Determine if recommendations were made for adaptive utensils and if they were, determine if these utensils are available and utilized by resident. If recommended but not used, determine if this is by resident's choice. If utensils are not being utilized, determine when these were recommended and how their use is being monitored by the facility and if the staff is developing alternative recommendations

§483.35(h) Paid Feeding Assistants- F373

(Rev. 26; Issued: 08-17-07; Effective/Implementation Dates: 08-17-07)

§483.35(h) - Paid Feeding Assistants

(1) State-approved training course. A facility may use a paid feeding assistant, as defined in §488.301 of this chapter, if—

(i) The feeding assistant has successfully completed a State-approved training course that meets the requirements of §483.160 before feeding residents; and

(ii) The use of feeding assistants is consistent with State law.

(2) Supervision.

(i) A feeding assistant must work under the supervision of a registered nurse (RN) or licensed practical nurse (LPN).

(ii) In an emergency, a feeding assistant must call a supervisory nurse for help on the resident call system.

(3) Resident selection criteria.

(i) A facility must ensure that a feeding assistant feeds only residents who have no complicated feeding problems.

(ii) Complicated feeding problems include, but are not limited to, difficulty swallowing, recurrent lung aspirations, and tube or parenteral/IV feedings.

(iii) The facility must base resident selection on the charge nurse's assessment and the resident's latest assessment and plan of care.

NOTE: *One of the specific features of the regulatory requirement for this tag is that paid feeding assistants must complete a training program with the following minimum content as specified at §483.160:*

a. Minimum training course contents. A State-approved training course for paid feeding assistants must include, at a minimum, 8 hours of training in the following:

(1) Feeding techniques;

(2) Assistance with feeding and hydration;

(3) Communication and interpersonal skills;

(4) Appropriate responses to resident behavior;

(5) Safety and emergency procedures, including the Heimlich maneuver;

(6) Infection control;

(7) Resident rights; and

(8) Recognizing changes in residents that are inconsistent with their normal behavior and the importance of reporting those changes to the supervisory nurse.

b. *Maintenance of records. A facility must maintain a record of all individuals, used by the facility as feeding assistants, who have successfully completed the training course for paid feeding assistants.*

Intent: §483.35(h)

The intent of this regulation is to ensure that employees who are used as paid feeding assistants are:

- *Properly trained (in accordance with the requirements at §483.160, including maintenance of records);*
- *Adequately supervised;*
- *Assisting only those residents without complicated feeding problems and who have been selected as eligible to receive these services from a paid feeding assistant; and*
- *Providing assistance in accordance with the resident's needs, based on individualized assessment and care planning.*

Definitions

"Paid feeding assistant" is defined in the regulation at 42 CFR 488.301 as "an individual who meets the requirements specified at 42 CFR 483.35(h)(1)(i) of this chapter and who is paid to feed residents by a facility, or who is used under an arrangement with another agency or organization."

> ***NOTE:*** *The regulation uses the term, "paid feeding assistant." While we are not using any other term, facilities and States may use whatever term they prefer, such as dining assistant, meal assistant, resident assistant, nutritional aide, etc. in order to convey more respect for the resident. Facilities may identify this position with other titles; however, the facility must be able to identify those employees who meet the requirements under the paid feeding assistant regulation. These requirements do not apply to family and/or volunteers who may be providing the resident with assistance.*

"Resident call system," for the purposes of this requirement includes not only the standard hard-wired call system, but other means in an emergency situation by which a paid feeding assistant can achieve timely notification of a supervisory nurse (when not present in the room).

OVERVIEW

The intent behind the use of paid feeding assistants by nursing homes is to provide nutrition and hydration support to residents who may be at risk for unplanned weight loss and dehydration. These are residents with no complicated problems associated with eating or drinking, who cannot or do not eat independently due to physical or cognitive disabilities, or those who simply need cueing or encouragement to eat. The use of paid feeding assistants is intended to supplement certified nurse aides, not substitute for nurse aides or licensed nursing staff. Use of paid feeding assistants is an option for nursing homes if their state approves the use of paid feeding assistants and establishes a mechanism to approve training programs for paid feeding assistants.

Interpretive Guidelines §483.35(h)

> ***NOTE:*** *The regulation at §483.30(a)(2) requires that "Except when waived under paragraph (c) of this section, the facility must designate a licensed nurse to service as a charge nurse on each tour of duty." In the paid feeding assistant regulation, the term charge nurse is used to identify who is responsible for assessing the eligibility of a resident to be assisted by a paid feeding assistant. The regulation also states that a paid feeding assistant must work under the supervision of an RN or LPN, and they must call the supervisory nurse in case of an emergency. Therefore, a facility that has received a waiver and does not have either an RN or LPN available in the building cannot use paid feeding assistants during those times.*

Charge Nurse Assessment of Resident Eligibility for Feeding Assistance

The facility must base resident selection on the charge nurse's (RN, or LPN if allowed by State law) current assessment of the resident's condition and the resident's latest comprehensive assessment and plan of care. Charge nurses may wish to consult with interdisciplinary team members, such as speech-language pathologists or other professionals, when making their decisions.

Paid feeding assistants are permitted to assist only those residents who have no complicated eating or drinking problems. This includes residents who are dependent in eating and/or those who have some degree of dependence, such as needing cueing or partial assistance, as long as they do not have complicated eating or drinking problems.

Paid feeding assistants are not permitted to assist residents who have complicated eating problems, such as (but not limited to) difficulty swallowing, recurrent lung aspirations, or who receive nutrition through parenteral or enteral means. Nurses or nurse aides must continue to assist residents to eat or drink who require the assistance of staff with more specialized training.

Facilities may use paid feeding assistants to assist eligible residents to eat and drink at meal times, snack times, or during activities or social events as needed, whenever the facility can provide the necessary supervision.

Supervision (by RN/LPN) of Paid Feeding Assistants

A paid feeding assistant must work under the supervision of an RN or LPN. While we are not prescribing the exact means by which facility RNs and LPNs assert their supervisory responsibilities, we expect that facilities will do so in a way that avoids negative outcomes for their residents. If a facility chooses to use paid feeding assistants, it is the facility's responsibility to ensure that adequate supervisory nursing staff are available to supervise these assistants.

The supervisory nurse should monitor the provision of the assistance provided by paid feeding assistants to evaluate on an ongoing basis:

- *Their use of appropriate feeding techniques;*
- *Whether they are assisting assigned residents according to their identified eating and drinking needs;*
- *Whether they are providing assistance in recognition of the rights and dignity of the resident; and*
- *Whether they are adhering to safety and infection control practices.*

Adequate supervision by a supervising nurse does not necessarily mean constant visual contact or being physically present during the meal/snack time, especially if a feeding assistant is assisting a resident to eat in his or her room. However, whatever the location, the feeding assistant must be aware of and know how to access the supervisory nurse immediately in the event that an emergency should occur. Should an emergency arise, a paid feeding assistant must immediately call a supervisory nurse for help on the resident call system.

The charge nurse and the supervisory nurse may or may not be the same individuals

Resident Call System

The regulatory language at this Tag states that, "in an emergency, a feeding assistant must call a supervisory nurse for help on the resident call system." Residents may be receiving assistance in eating or drinking in various locations throughout the facility, such as dining areas, activity rooms, or areas such as patios or porches in which a resident call system is not readily available. The resident call system requirement at §483.70(f), F463, only specifies that the call system be available in the residents rooms and bathrooms. Regardless of where a resident is being assisted to eat or drink, in the case of an emergency, the facility needs to have a means for a paid feeding assistant to obtain timely help of a supervisory nurse. Therefore, for the purposes of this requirement, a "resident call system" includes not only the standard hard-wired or wireless call system, but other means in an emergency situation by which a paid feeding assistant can achieve timely notification of a supervisory nurse.

Use of Existing Staff as Paid Feeding Assistants

Facilities may use their existing staff to assist eligible residents to eat and drink. These employees must have successfully completed a State-approved training course for paid feeding assistants, which has a minimum of 8 hours of training as required in §483.160. Staff may include, for example, administrative, clerical, housekeeping, dietary staff, or activity specialists. Employees used as paid feeding assistants, regardless of their position, are subject to the same training and supervisory requirements as any other paid feeding assistant.

Maintenance of Training Records

The facility must maintain a record of all employees used by the facility as paid feeding assistants. The record should include verification that they have successfully completed a State-approved training course for paid feeding assistants.

INVESTIGATIVE PROTOCOL

Use of Paid Feeding Assistants

Objectives

The objectives of this protocol are to determine, for a facility that uses paid feeding assistants:

- *If individuals used as paid feeding assistants successfully completed a State-approved training course;*
- *If sampled residents who were selected to receive assistance from paid feeding assistants were assessed by the charge nurse and determined to be eligible to receive these services based on the latest assessment and plan of care; and*
- *If the paid feeding assistants are supervised by an RN or LPN.*

Use

This protocol is used when a surveyor identifies concerns through observation; interview with residents, family, or staff; or record review, that the facility may not be following the requirements regarding paid feeding assistants, including proper training and supervision of feeding assistants, and proper selection of residents for feeding assistance.

Procedures

Briefly review the comprehensive assessment and interdisciplinary care plan to guide observations to be made. The team coordinator assigns one surveyor to obtain the facility's records of all employees, used by the facility as paid feeding assistants, for review for completion of the training course for paid feeding assistants.

Observations

If the concern was discovered through resident or family interview, observe the resident while they are being assisted to eat and drink by a paid feeding assistant. Determine if the assistant is using proper feeding technique and is providing the type of assistance specified in the resident's care plan. Note the resident's condition and observe for the presence of complicated feeding problems.

If the concern was discovered through observations that were already made, only conduct additional observations if necessary to complete the investigation.

<u>Interviews</u>

Resident and Family Interviews

If a resident is selected for this protocol through surveyor observation that they are having difficulties in eating or drinking and they are being assisted by a paid feeding assistant, interview the resident if the resident is interviewable. Ask questions to gain information about why the resident is receiving these services and the resident's experience with receiving assistance to eat and drink. If concerns are identified, inquire if they have reported these problems to a nurse. If the resident is not interviewable, ask these questions of a family member.

If the concern was discovered through resident or family interviews already conducted as part of Task 5D, focus any additional interview on questions specific to the investigation.

Paid Feeding Assistant Interviews

Interview the paid feeding assistant who was assisting the selected resident. Determine whether there are concerns with the paid feeding assistant's training, supervision, or the selection of the resident such as:

- *What training did you successfully complete in providing feeding assistance?*
- *What information did you receive about this resident's needs for assistance (type of assistance needed, any precautions)?*
- *In what manner and by whom are you supervised while assisting residents?*
- *What issues/problems do you report (such as coughing, choking, changes in the resident's usual responses, or level of alertness) and to whom do you report?*
- *What would you do if an emergency occurred while you were assisting a resident to eat or drink? Who would you contact and how would you contact them if you are not near the resident call system?*

Charge Nurse Interview

Interview the charge nurse who is responsible for assessing this resident as eligible to receive assistance by a paid feeding assistant. Ask:

- *How they determined that this resident has no complicated feeding problems and is eligible to be assisted by a paid feeding assistant;*
- *How they determine that each eligible resident remains free of emergent complicated feeding problems;*
- *Who supervises paid feeding assistants and how is the supervision accomplished;*
- *Describe the processes in place to handle emergencies when a supervisor is not present in the area where paid feeding assistants are assisting residents.*

Supervisory Nurse Interview

Interview the nurse who is supervising the resident during the meal or other times when the paid feeding assistant is assisting the resident to eat or drink. Ask how they supervise paid feeding assistants.

Review of Assessment of Eligibility to Receive Assistance from a Paid Feeding Assistant

Determine whether the charge nurse based her/his assessment of the resident's ongoing eligibility to be assisted by a paid feeding assistant on identification of the current condition of the resident and any additional or new risk factors or condition changes that may impact on the resident's ability to eat or drink. This information may be contained in the RAI or in other supporting documents such as progress notes, etc. The assessment of eligibility to receive assistance from a paid feeding assistant is ongoing and should be in place from the day of admission.

Requirements for Training of Paid Feeding Assistants

Determine how the facility identifies that paid feeding assistants have successfully completed a State-approved training course that meets the requirements at 42 CFR 483.160 before they are allowed to assist eligible residents with eating and drinking.

If the facility uses temporary (agency) staff as paid feeding assistants, request documentation that these staff have met the minimum training requirements specified by the State.

DETERMINATION OF COMPLIANCE (TASK 6, APPENDIX P)

The information below should be used by the survey team for their deficiency determination at Task 6 in Appendix P. The survey team must evaluate the evidence documented during the survey to determine if a deficiency exists due to a failure to meet a requirement, and if there are any negative resident outcomes or potential for negative outcomes due to the failure.

Synopsis of Regulation (42 CFR 483.35)

The paid feeding assistant requirement has five aspects:

- *Staff who are used as paid feeding assistants must have completed a State-approved training course;*
- *The facility must base resident selection to be fed by a paid feeding assistant on the charge nurse's assessment and resident's latest assessment and care plan;*
- *Paid feeding assistants must work under the supervision of an RN or LPN, and, in an emergency, must call a supervisory nurse for help on the resident call system;*
- *Paid feeding assistants assist only residents who have no complicated health problems related to eating or drinking that make them ineligible for these services; and*
- *The facility must maintain a record of all individuals used by the facility as paid feeding assistants, and must maintain documentation of successful completion of a State-approved training course by these individuals.*

Criteria for Compliance

Compliance with 42 CFR 483.35(h), F373, Paid Feeding Assistants

The facility is in compliance with this requirement if all the following are met:

- *The facility only employs paid feeding assistants who have successfully completed a State-approved training course before providing assistance;*
- *The facility selected qualified residents based on the charge nurse's ongoing assessment and the latest assessment and plan of care;*
- *The facility provides supervision by an RN or LPN;*
- *The facility provides in cases of emergency a working call system (and other means for areas without a call system) for the paid feeding assistant to summon help in an emergency;*

- *The facility ensures that the paid feeding assistant only assists residents who have no complicated health problems related to eating or drinking that make them ineligible for these services; and*

- *The facility maintains a record of all individuals used by the facility as paid feeding assistants, and maintains documentation of each paid feeding assistant's successful completion of a State-approved training course.*

  If not, cite F373.

Non-compliance for F373

After completing the investigative protocol, determine whether or not noncompliance with the regulation exists. Noncompliance for F373 may include, but is not limited to, one or more of the following:

- *An employee of the facility (permanent or temporary) who has not successfully completed the State-approved training course is assisting a resident to eat/drink;*

- *The facility allowed an employee who has completed a course that is not State-approved to assist a resident to eat or drink;*

- *A paid feeding assistant was observed assisting a resident in a location without a call system available or other means of emergency notification;*

- *A resident who was assessed by the charge nurse as ineligible for services due to complicated eating/drinking problems, or a resident who has not been assessed for eligibility, is being assisted by a paid feeding assistant;*

- *A paid feeding assistant was not being supervised by a RN or LPN;*

- *RN or LPN staff members assigned to supervise paid feeding assistants were observed to be unavailable (e.g., not in reach of contact);*

- *The clinical record of a resident being assisted by a paid feeding assistant did not show evidence that the resident was eligible to receive assistance from a paid feeding assistant;*

- *The facility did not maintain records of paid feeding assistants working in the facility; or*

- *The facility did not maintain documentation of a paid feeding assistant's successful completion of a State-approved paid feeding training course.*

Potential Tags for Additional Investigation

During the investigation of F373, the surveyor may have identified concerns with additional requirements related to outcome, process, and/or structure requirements. The surveyor is cautioned to investigate these related requirements before determining whether non-compliance may be present at these other tags. Examples of some of the related requirements that may be considered when non-compliance has been identified include the following (but are not limited to):

- *42 CFR 483.15(a), F241, Dignity*

o *Determine if staff are attentive and responsive to the resident's requests, and if they provide assistance to eat in a manner that respects the resident's dignity, meets needs in a timely manner, and minimizes potential feelings of embarrassment, humiliation, and/or isolation related to inability to assist themselves with food or fluid intake.*

- *42 CFR 483.20(b), F272, Comprehensive Assessments*
    - *Review whether the facility initially and periodically conducted a comprehensive, accurate assessment of the resident's ability to eat and drink with or without assistance and/or identified a condition that makes the resident ineligible for this service.*
- *42 CFR 483.20(k)(1), F279, Comprehensive Care Plans*
    - *Review whether the facility developed a comprehensive care plan that was based on the assessment of the resident's conditions, needs, and behaviors, and was consistent with the resident's goals in order to provide assistance with nutrition and hydration as necessary.*
- *42 CFR 483.20(k)(2)(iii), F280, Comprehensive Care Plan Revision*

o *Determine if the care plan was reviewed and revised periodically, as necessary, related to eligibility to eat and drink with assistance of a paid feeding assistant.*

- *42 CFR 483.25(i)(1), F325, Nutritional Parameters*
    - *Review if the facility had identified, evaluated, and responded to a change in nutritional parameters, anorexia, or unplanned weight loss, dysphagia, and/or swallowing disorders in relation to the resident's ability to eat.*
- *42 CFR 483.25(i)(2), F327, Hydration*
    - *Review if the facility had identified, evaluated, and responded to a change in the resident's ability to swallow liquids.*
- *42 CFR 483.25 (a)(3) F312, ADL Assistance for Dependent Residents*

- *Determine if staff identified and implemented appropriate measures to provide food and fluids for the resident who cannot perform relevant activities of daily living.*

- *42 CFR 483.30(a), F353, Sufficient Staff*

    - *Determine if the facility has qualified staff in sufficient numbers to provide assistance to eat or drink to those residents who require such assistance. For residents who are not eligible to receive assistance from paid feeding assistants, determine if there are sufficient CNAs to provide this assistance to these residents in a timely fashion.*

- *42 CFR 483.75(i)(2), F501, Medical Director*

- *Determine whether the medical director collaborates with the facility to help develop, implement, and evaluate resident care policies and procedures based on current standards of practice, e.g., the use of paid feeding assistants, their supervision, and the criteria for determining which residents are eligible to receive assistance to eat or drink from paid feeding assistants.*

IV. DEFICIENCY CATEGORIZATION (Part IV, Appendix P)

Once the team has completed its investigation, analyzed the data, reviewed the regulatory requirement, and identified any deficient practice(s) that demonstrate that non-compliance with the regulation at F373 exists, the team must determine the severity of the deficient practice(s) and the resultant harm or potential for harm to the resident. The key elements for severity determination for F373 are as follows:

1. ***Presence of harm/negative outcome(s) or potential for negative outcomes because of lack of appropriate use of paid feeding assistants.***

   Non-compliance related to an actual or potential harm/negative outcome for F373 may include, but is not limited to:

   - *A resident who is not eligible to receive these services is assisted by a paid feeding assistant; or*

   - *A resident who is eligible to receive these services is assisted by a paid feeding assistant and develops coughing and/or choking episodes related to the paid feeding assistant using poor techniques indicating lack of appropriate supervision*

2. ***Degree of harm (actual or potential) related to the non-compliance:***

   Identify how the facility practices caused, resulted in, allowed, or contributed to the actual or potential for harm:

- *If harm has occurred, determine if the harm is at the level of serious injury, impairment, death, compromise, or discomfort; or*

- *If harm has not yet occurred, determine how likely is the potential for serious injury, impairment, death, or compromise or discomfort to occur to the resident.*

3. ***The immediacy of correction required:***

   Determine whether the non-compliance requires immediate correction in order to prevent serious injury, harm, impairment, or death to one or more residents.

The survey team must evaluate the harm or potential for harm based upon the following levels of severity for tag F373. First, the team must rule out whether Severity Level 4, Immediate Jeopardy to a resident's health or safety exists by evaluating the deficient practice in relation to immediacy, culpability, and severity. (Follow the guidance in Appendix Q, Guidelines for Determining Immediate Jeopardy.)

> ***NOTE:*** *The death or transfer of a resident who was harmed or injured as a result of facility non-compliance does not remove a finding of immediate jeopardy. The facility is required to implement specific actions to correct the non-compliance which allowed or caused the immediate jeopardy.*

Severity Level 4 Considerations: Immediate Jeopardy to Resident Health or Safety

Immediate Jeopardy is a situation in which the facility's non-compliance with one or more requirements of participation:

- *Has allowed/caused/resulted in, or is likely to cause/allow/result in serious injury, harm, impairment, or death to a resident; and*

- *Requires immediate correction as the facility either created the situation or allowed the situation to continue by failing to implement preventative or corrective measures.*

Examples of the facility's non-compliance that may cause or contribute to negative outcomes at severity level 4 include, but are not limited to:

- *An eligible resident in an activity room who is being improperly assisted to eat by a paid feeding assistant, experiences choking, there was no call system readily available, and/or the supervising nurse was not available to assist, and the resident expired;*

- *A resident who is not eligible to receive these services due to complicated feeding problems is assisted by a paid feeding assistant, whether or not the resident has experienced negative outcomes.*

NOTE: *If immediate jeopardy has been ruled out based upon the evidence, then evaluate whether actual harm that is not immediate jeopardy exists at severity level 3.*

Severity Level 3 Considerations: Actual Harm that is not Immediate Jeopardy

Level 3 indicates non-compliance that results in actual harm, and can include but may not be limited to clinical compromise, decline, or the failure to maintain and/or reach the resident's highest practicable well-being.

Examples of the facility's non-compliance that may cause or contribute to negative outcomes at severity level 3 include, but are not limited to:

- *An eligible resident who was assessed to have the potential to improving their eating ability was assisted to eat by a paid feeding assistant. The assistant provided too much food, too quickly and the resident was pocketing the food in her cheeks. The resident experienced choking and coughing and subsequently vomited. As a result, the resident became fearful, refused solid foods, and would only consume liquid dietary supplements.*

  NOTE: *If severity level 3 (actual harm that is not immediate jeopardy) has been ruled out based upon the evidence, then evaluate as to whether level 2 (no actual harm with the potential for more than minimal harm) exists.*

Severity Level 2 Considerations: No Actual Harm with potential for more than minimal harm that is Not Immediate Jeopardy

Level 2 indicates non-compliance that results in a resident outcome of no more than minimal discomfort and/or has the potential to compromise the resident's ability to maintain or reach his or her highest practicable level of well being. The potential exists for greater harm to occur if interventions are not provided.

Examples of the facility's non-compliance that may cause or contribute to negative outcomes at severity level 2 include, but are not limited to:

- *Paid feeding assistants are assisting eligible residents to eat in an area with no call system, and the supervising nurses are not nearby, but there have been no resident outcomes; and*

- *Eligible residents are being assisted to eat by employees who have not successfully completed a State-approved paid feeding assistant training course and who otherwise by State law would not be allowed to feed residents (such as RNs, LPNs or CNAs), and there were no resident negative outcomes.*

Severity Level 1: No actual harm with potential for minimal harm

Level 1 is a deficiency that has the potential for causing no more than a minor negative impact on the resident(s).

Examples of the facility's non-compliance that may cause or contribute to negative outcomes at severity level 1 include, but are not limited to:

Facility did not maintain a record of employees who had completed a State approved paid feeding assistant training program and were used by the facility as paid feeding assistants.

---

§483.35(i) Sanitary Conditions

The facility must--

F370

§483.35(i)(1) Procure food from sources approved or considered satisfactory by Federal, State or local authorities;

F371

§483.35(i)(2) Store, prepare, distribute, and serve food under sanitary conditions; and

Intent: §483.35(i)(2)

The intent of this regulation is to prevent the spread of food borne illness and reduce those practices which result in food contamination and compromised food safety in nursing homes. Since foodborne illness is often fatal to nursing home residents, it can and must be avoided.

Interpretive Guidelines: §483.35(i)(2)

"**Sanitary conditions**" is defined as storing, preparing, distributing, and serving food properly to prevent food borne illness. Potentially hazardous foods must be subject to continuous time/temperature controls in order to prevent either the rapid and progressive growth of infectious or toxigenic micro-organisms such as Salmonella or the slower growth of Clostridium Botulinum. In addition, foods of plant origin become potentially hazardous when the skin, husk, peel, or rind is breached, thereby possibly contaminating the fruit or vegetable with disease causing micro-organisms. Potentially hazardous food tends to focus on animal products, including but not limited to milk, eggs and poultry.

Improper holding temperature is a common contributing factor of foodborne illness. The facility must follow proper procedures in cooking, cooling, and storing food according to time, temperatures, and sanitary guidelines. Improper handling of food can cause salmonella and E-Coli contamination. The 1993 FDA Food Code advises the following precautions:

> **NOTE:** The 1993 FDA Food Code is not regulation and cannot be enforced as such. The food temperatures cited that are recommended in the 1993 FDA Food Code are target temperatures and give a margin of safety in temperature ranges and to avoid known harmful temperatures.

Refrigerator storage of food to prevent food borne illness includes storing raw meat away from vegetables and other foods. Raw meat should be separated from cooked foods and other foods when refrigerated on its own tray on a bottom shelf so meat juices do not drip on other foods. Foods of both plant and animal origin must be cooked, maintained and stored at appropriate temperatures.

- Foods of both plant and animal origin must be cooked, and maintained, and stored at appropriate temperatures. These temperatures are better utilized as food hold temperatures rather than the food temperatures as residents receive the food.

- Hot foods which are potentially hazardous should leave the kitchen (or steam table) above 140° F, and cold foods at or below 41° F and freezer temperatures should be at 0° F or below. Refrigerator temperatures should be maintained at 41° F or below. The 1993 FDA Food Code can be used as an authoritative guide to clarify regulatory requirements on how to prepare and serve food to prevent foodborne illness. As the public becomes more informed and educated on how to prevent foodborne illness, this code will become the standard of practice the same as the 1976 Food Service Sanitation Manual did prior to 1993.

Procedures: §483.35(i)(2)

Observe storage, cooling, and cooking of food. Record the time and date of all observations. If a problem is noted, conduct additional observations to verify findings.

Observe that employees are effectively cleaning their hands prior to preparing, serving and distributing food. Observe that food is covered to maintain temperature and protect from other contaminants when transporting meals to residents.

Refrigerated storage:

- Check all refrigerators and freezers for temperatures. Use the facility's or the surveyor's own properly sanitized thermometer to evaluate the internal temperatures of potentially hazardous foods with a focus on the quantity of leftovers and the container sizes in which bulk leftovers are stored.

Food preparation:

- Use a sanitized thermometer to evaluate food temperatures.

In addition, how do kitchen staff process leftovers?

- Are they heated to the appropriate temperatures?
- How is frozen food thawed?
- How is potentially hazardous food handled during multi-step food preparation (e.g., chicken salad, egg salad)?
- Is hand contact with food minimized?

Food service:

- Using a properly sanitized thermometer, check the temperatures of hot and cold food prior to serving.
- How long is milk held without refrigeration prior to distribution?

Food distribution:

- Is the food protected from contamination as it is transported to the dining rooms and residents' rooms?

Pest free:

- Is the area pest free? (See §483.70(h)(4).) Look for signs of pests such as mice, roaches, rates, flies.

Preventing Contamination:

- Are handwashing facilities convenient and properly equipped for dietary services staff Use? (Staff uses good hygienic practices and staff with communicable disease or infected skin lesions do not have contact with food if that contact will transmit the disease.)

Hazard Free

- Are toxic items (such as insecticides, detergent, polishes) properly stored, labeled, and used separate from the food?

Probes: §483.35(i)(2)

Observe food storage rooms and food storage in the kitchen.

- Are containers of food stored off the floor and on clean surfaces in a manner that protects it from contamination?

- Are other areas under storage shelves monitored for cleanliness to reduce attraction of pest.

- Are potentially hazardous foods stored at 41° F or below and frozen foods kept at 0° F or below?

- Do staff handle and cook potentially hazardous foods properly?

- Are potentially hazardous foods kept at an internal temperature of 41° F or below in cold food storage unit, or at an internal temperature of 140° F or above in a hot food storage unit during display and service?

- Is food transported in a way that protects against contamination (i.e., covered containers, wrapped, or packaged)?

- Is there any sign of rodent or insect infestation.

Dishwashing:

- The current 1993 Food Code, DHHS, FDA, PHS recommends the following water temperature and manual washing instructions:

Machine:

1. Hot Water:

   a. 140° F Wash (or according to the manufacturer's specifications or instructions).

   b. 180° F Rinse (180°, 160° or greater at the rack and dish/utensils surfaces.

2. Low Temperature:

    a. 120° F +25 ppm (parts per million) Hypochlorite (household bleach) on dish Surface.

Manual:

1. 3 Compartment Sink (wash, rinse and sanitize): Sanitizing solution used according to manufacturer's instructions.

    a. 75 degrees F - 50 ppm Hypochlorite (household bleach) or equivalent, or 12.5 ppm of Iodine.

    b. Hot Water Immersion at 170□ F for at least 30 seconds.

Are food preparation equipment, dishes, and utensils effectively sanitized and cleaned to destroy potential disease carrying organisms and stored in a protected manner?

F372

§483.35(i)(3) Dispose of Garbage and Refuse Properly

Interpretive Guidelines: §483.35(i)(3)

The intent of this regulation is to assure that garbage and refuse be properly disposed.

Procedures: §483.35(i)(3)

Garbage/refuse:
Observe garbage and refuse container construction, and outside storage receptacles.

Probes: §483.35(i)(3)

Are garbage and refuse containers in good condition (no leaks) and is waste properly contained in dumpsters or compactors with lids or otherwise covered?

Are areas such as loading docks, hallways, and elevators used for both garbage disposal and clean food transport kept clean, free of debris and free of foul odors and waste fat?

Is the garbage storage area maintained in a saunter condition to prevent the harborage and feeding of pests?

Are garbage receptacles covered when being removed from the kitchen area to the dumpster?

F385

§483.40 Physician Services

A physician must personally approve in writing a recommendation that an individual be admitted to a facility. Each resident must remain under the care of a physician.

§483.40(a) Physician Supervision

The facility must ensure that--

(1) The medical care of each resident is supervised by a physician; and

(2) Another physician supervises the medical care of residents when their attending physician is unavailable.

Intent §483.40

The intent of this regulation is to ensure the medical supervision of the care of nursing home residents by a personal physician.

Interpretive Guidelines §483.40

A physician's "personal approval" of an admission recommendation must be in written form. The physician's admission orders for the resident's immediate care as required in §483.20(a) will be accepted as "personal approval" of the admission.

"**Supervising the medical care of residents**" means participating in the resident's assessment and care planning, monitoring changes in resident's medical status, and providing consultation or treatment when called by the facility. It also includes, but is not limited to, prescribing new therapy, ordering a resident's transfer to the hospital, conducting required routine visits or delegating and supervising follow-up visits to nurse practitioners or physician assistants. Each resident should be allowed to designate a personal physician. (See §483.10(d)(1).) The facility's responsibility in this situation is to simply assist the resident, when necessary, in his or her efforts to obtain those services. For example, the facility could put the resident in touch with the county medical society for the purpose of obtaining referrals to practicing physicians in the area.

Facilities should share MDS and other assessment data with the physician.

Procedures §483.40

If there is a deficiency in §483.10, Resident Rights; §483.13, Resident Behavior and Facility Practices; §483.15, Quality of Life; or §483.25, Quality of Care, fully review all of the tags under this requirement.

Probes: §483.40(a)

- How was the supervising physician involved in the resident's assessment and care planning?
- If staff reported a significant change in medical status to the supervising physician, did the physician respond?
- If the supervising physician was unavailable and could not respond, did the facility have a physician on call? Did this physician respond?
- Are residents sent to hospital emergency rooms routinely because the facility does not always have a physician on call?

F386

§483.40(b) Physician Visits

The physician must--

(1) Review the resident's total program of care, including medications and treatments, at each visit required by paragraph (c) of this section;

(2) Write, sign, and date progress notes at each visit; and

(3) Sign and date all orders with the exception of influenza and pneumococcal polysaccharide vaccines, which may be administered per physician-approved facility policy after an assessment for contraindications.

Intent §483.40(b)

The intent of this regulation is to have the physician take an active role in supervising the care of residents. This should not be a superficial visit, but should include an evaluation of the resident's condition and a review of and decision about the continued appropriateness of the resident's current medical regime.

Interpretive Guidelines §483.40(b)

Total program of care includes all care the facility provides residents to maintain or improve their highest practicable mental and physical functional status, as defined by the comprehensive assessment and plan of care. Care includes medical services and medication management, physical, occupational, and speech/language therapy, nursing care, nutritional interventions, social work and activity services that maintain or improve psychosocial functioning.

The physician records residents' progress and problems in maintaining or improving their mental and physical functional status. The physician need not review the total plan of care at each visit, but must review the total plan of care at visits required by §483.40(c). There is no requirement for physician renewal of orders.

In cases where facilities have created the option for a resident's record to be maintained by computer, rather than hard copy, electronic signatures are acceptable. See Guidelines for §483.75(l)(1) for information on facility safeguards concerning electronic signatures.

Physician orders may be transmitted by facsimile machine if the following conditions are met:

- The physician should have signed and retained the original copy of the order from which the facsimile was transmitted and be able to provide it upon request. Alternatively, the original may be sent to the facility at a later time and substituted for the facsimile.

- The facility should photocopy the faxed order since some facsimiles fade over time. The facsimile copy can be discarded after facility photocopies it.

- A facility using such a system should establish adequate safeguards to assure that it is not subject to abuse.

It is not necessary for a physician to re-sign the facsimile order when he/she visits the facility.

When rubber stamp signatures are authorized by the facility's management, the individual whose signature the stamp represents shall place in the administrative offices of the facility a signed statement to the effect that he/she is the only one who has the stamp and uses it. A list of computer codes and written signatures must be readily available and maintained under adequate safeguards.

Probes: §483.40(b)

- Do services ordered by a physician show a pattern of care to maintain or improve the resident's level of independent functioning? For example, how do physician orders reflect the resident's nutritional status and needs?

- Does documentation reflect continuity of care in maintaining or improving a resident's mental and physical functional status? For example, do the attending physician's rehabilitation service orders show a pattern of consistent restorative programming?

F387

§483.40(c) Frequency of Physician Visits

(1) The residents must be seen by a physician at least once every 30 days for the first 90 days after admission, and at least once every 60 thereafter.

(2) A physician visit is considered timely if it occurs not later than 10 days after the date the visit was required.

F388

§483.40(c)(3) Expect as provided in paragraphs (c)(4) and (f) of this section, all required physician visits must be made by the physician personally.

§483.40(c) (4) At the option of the physician, required visits in SNFs, after the initial visit, may alternate between personal visits by the physician and visits by a physician assistant, nurse practitioner or clinical nurse specialist in accordance with paragraph (e) of this section.

Interpretive Guidelines §483.40(c)

"**Must be seen**" means that the physician must make actual face-to-face contact with the resident. There is no requirement for this type of contact at the time of admission, since the decision to admit an individual to a nursing facility (whether from a hospital or from the individual's own residence) generally involves physician contact during the period immediately preceding the admission.

After the initial physician visit in SNFs, where States allow their use, a qualified nurse practitioner (NP), clinical nurse specialist or physician assistant (PA) may make every other required visit. (See §483.40(e) Physician delegation of tasks in SNFs.)

In a NF, the physician visit requirement, in accordance with the State law, may be satisfied by NP, clinical nurse specialist or PA. (See §483.40(f).)

The timing of physician visits is based on the admission date of the resident. Visits will be made within the first 30 days, and then at 30 day intervals up until 90 days after the admission date. Visits will then be at 60 day intervals. Permitting up to 10 days slippage of a due date will not affect the next due date. However, do not specifically look at the timetables for physician visits unless there is indication of inadequate medical care. The regulation states that the physician (or his/her delegate) must visit the resident **at least** every 30 or 60 days. There is no provision for physicians to use discretion in visiting at intervals longer than those specified at §483.40(c).

Policy that allows an NP, clinical nurse specialist, or PA to make every other required visit, and that allows a 10 day slippage in the time of the visit, does not relieve the physician of the obligation to visit a resident when the resident's medical condition makes that visit necessary.

It is expected that visits will occur at the facility rather than the doctor's office unless office equipment is needed or a resident specifically requests an office visit. If the facility has established policy that residents leave the grounds for medical care, the resident does not object, and this policy does not infringe on his/her rights, there is no prohibition to this practice. The facility should inform the resident of this practice, in accordance with §483.10(b).

Probes: §483.40(c)

- How does the scheduling and frequency of physician visits relate to any identified quality of care problems?
- When a PA, clinical nurse specialist, or NP performs a delegate physician visit, and determines that the resident's condition warrants direct contact between the physician and the resident, does the physician follow-up promptly with a personal visit?

F389

§483.40(d) Availability of Physicians for Emergency Care

The facility must provide or arrange for the provision of physician services 24 hours a day, in case of emergency.

Interpretive Guidelines §483.40(d)

If a resident's own physician is unavailable, the facility should attempt to contact that physician's designated referral physician before assuming the responsibility of assigning a physician. Arranging for physician services may include assuring resident transportation to a hospital emergency room/ward or other medical facility if the facility is unable to provide emergency medical care at the facility.

Probes: §483.40(d)

- Does the facility have a physician on call for medical emergencies? Does this physician respond?
- For what reasons are residents sent to hospital emergency rooms?
- Did medical management of the emergency affect the resident's maintaining or improving their functional abilities?
- If the resident refused the physician's visit, what has the facility done to explain to the resident the results and alternatives that may be available?

F390

§483.40(e) Physician Delegation of Tasks in SNFs

(1) Except as specified in paragraph (e)(2) of this section, a physician may delegate tasks to a physician assistant, nurse practitioner, or clinical nurse specialist who--

(i) Meets the applicable definition in §491.2 of this chapter or, in the case of a clinical nurse specialist, is licensed as such by the State;

(ii) Is acting within the scope of practice as defined by State law; and

(iii) Is under the supervision of the physician.

(2) A physician may not delegate a task when the regulations specify that the physician must perform it personally, or when the delegation is prohibited under State law or by the facility's own policies.

Interpretive Guidelines §483.40(e)

"**Nurse practitioner**" is a registered professional nurse now licensed to practice in the State and who meets the State's requirements governing the qualification of nurse practitioners.

"**Clinical nurse specialist**" is a registered professional nurse currently in practice in the State and who meets the State's requirements governing the qualifications of clinical nurse specialists.

"**Physician assistant**" is a person who meets the applicable State requirements governing the qualifications for assistants to physician.

When **personal** performance of a particular task by a physician is specified in the regulations, performance of that task cannot be delegated to anyone else. The tasks of examining the resident, reviewing the resident's total program of care, writing progress notes, and signing orders may be delegated according to State law. The extent to which physician services are delegated to physician extenders in SNFs will continue to be determined by the provisions of §483.40(e), while the extent to which these services are performed by physician extenders in NFs will be determined by the individual States under §483.40(f).

Probes: §483.40(e)

- Do the facility's attending physicians delegate to NPs, clinical nurse specialists, or PAs?

- Do NP/clinical nurse specialist/PA progress notes and orders follow the scope of practice allowed by State law?

- What evidence is there of physician supervision of NPs or PAs? For example, do physicians countersign NP/PA orders, if required by State law?

§483.40(f) Performance of Physician Tasks in NFs

At the option of State, any required physician task in a NF (including tasks which the regulations specify must be performed personally by the physician) may also be satisfied when performed by a nurse practitioner, clinical nurse specialist, or physician assistant who is not an employee of the facility but who is working in collaboration with a physician.

Interpretive Guidelines §483.40(f)

If delegation of physician tasks is permitted in your State and the physician extender does not meet the qualifications listed here, cite F388.

Procedures §483.40(f)

If a nurse practitioner, clinical nurse specialist, or physician assistant is performing required physician tasks in a NF, is this allowed by the State? Is this person an employee of the facility? (Facility employees are prohibited from serving in this capacity.)

Probes: §483.40(f)

Is this person working in collaboration with the physician?

F406

§483.45(a) Provision of Services

If specialized rehabilitative services such as, but not limited to physical therapy, speech-language pathology, occupational therapy, and mental health rehabilitative services for mental illness and mental retardation, are required in the resident's comprehensive plan of care, the facility must--

(1) Provide the required services; or

(2) Obtain the required services from an outside resource (in accordance with §483.75(h) of this part) from a provider of specialized rehabilitative services.

Intent: §483.45(a)(1)(2)

The intent of this regulation is to assure that residents receive necessary specialized rehabilitative services as determined by the comprehensive assessment and care plan, to prevent avoidable physical and mental deterioration and to assist them in obtaining or maintaining their highest practicable level of functional and psycho-social well-being.

"**Specialized rehabilitative services**" are differentiated from restorative services which are provided by nursing staff. Specialized rehabilitative services are provided by or coordinated by qualified personnel.

Specialized rehabilitative services are considered a facility service and are, thus, included within the scope of facility services. They must be provided by or coordinated by qualified personnel. They must be provided to residents who need them even when the services are not specifically enumerated in the State plan. No fee can be charged a Medicaid recipient for specialized rehabilitative services because they are covered facility services.

A facility is not obligated to provide specialized rehabilitative services if it does not have residents who require these services. If a resident develops a need for these services after admission, the facility must either provide the services, or, where appropriate, obtain the services from an outside resource.

For a resident with MI or MR to have his or her specialized needs met, the individual must receive all services necessary to assist the individual in maintaining or achieving as much independence and self-determination as possible. They are:

"**Specialized services for MI or MR**" refers to those services to be **provided by the State** which can only be delivered by personnel or programs other than those of the NF (e.g., outside the NF setting), because the overall level of NF services is not as intense as necessary to meet the individual's needs.

The Preadmission Screening and Annual Resident Review (PASARR) report indicates specialized services required by the resident. The State is required to list those services in the report, as well as provide or arrange for the provision of the services. If the State determines that the resident does not require specialized services, the facility is responsible to provide all services necessary to meet the resident's mental health or mental retardation needs.

"**Mental health rehabilitative services for MI and MR**" refers to those services of lesser frequency or intensity to be implemented by all levels of nursing facility staff who come into contact with the resident who is mentally ill or who has mental retardation. These services are necessary regardless of whether or not they are required to be subject to the PASARR process and whether or not they require additional services to be provided or arranged for by the State as specialized services.

The facility should provide interventions which complement, reinforce and are consistent with any specialized services (as defined by the resident's PASARR) the individual is receiving or is required to receive by the State. The individual's plan of care should specify how the facility will integrate relevant activities throughout all hours of the individual's day at the NF to achieve this consistency and enhancement of PASARR goals. The surveyor should see competent interaction by staff at all times, in both formal and informal settings in accordance with the individual's needs.

Mental health rehabilitative services for MI and MR may include, but are not limited to:

- Consistent implementation during the resident's daily routine and across settings, of systematic plans which are designed to change inappropriate behaviors;
- Drug therapy and monitoring of the effectiveness and side effects of medications which have been prescribed to change inappropriate behavior or to alter manifestations of psychiatric illness;
- Provision of a structured environment for those individuals who are determined to need such structure (e.g., structured socialization activities to diminish tendencies toward isolation and withdrawal);
- Development, maintenance and consistent implementation across settings of those programs designed to teach individuals the daily living skills they need to be more independent and self-determining including, but not limited to, grooming, personal hygiene, mobility, nutrition, vocational skills, health, drug therapy,

mental health education, money management, and maintenance of the living environment;

- Crisis intervention service;
- Individual, group, and family psychotherapy;
- Development of appropriate personal support networks; and
- Formal behavior modification programs.

Procedures: §483.45(a)(1)(2)

For sampled residents, whose comprehensive assessment indicates physical, psychosocial, and/or communications rehabilitation potential (See MDS 2.0, sections G, C, F, E), observe for unmet needs for rehabilitative services. Determine the extent of follow through with comprehensive care plan using probes outlined below. Verify from the chart that resident is receiving frequency and type of therapy as outlined in the care plan.

Probes: §483.45(a)(1)(2)

1. For physical therapy

    a. What did the facility do to improve the resident's muscle strength? The resident's balance?

    b. What did the facility do to determine if as assistive device would enable the resident to reach or maintain his/her highest practicable level of physical function?

    c. If the resident has an assistive device, is he/she encouraged to use it on a regular basis?

    d. What did the facility do to increase the amount of physical activity the resident could do (for example, the number of repetitions of an exercise, the distance walked)?

    e. What did the facility do to prevent or minimize contractures, which could lead to decreased mobility and increased risk of pressure ulcer occurrence?

2. For occupational therapy

    a. What did the facility do to decrease the amount of assistance needed to perform a task?

    b. What did the facility do to decrease behavioral symptoms?

    c. What did the facility do to improve gross and fine motor coordination?

    d. What did the facility do to improve sensory awareness, visual-spatial awareness, and body integration?

    e. What did the facility do to improve memory, problem solving, attention span, and the ability to recognize safety hazards?

3. For speech-language pathology.

    a. What did the facility do to improve auditory comprehension such as understanding common, functional words, concepts of time and place, and conversation?

    b. What did the facility do to improve speech production?

    c. What did the facility do to improve the expressive behavior such as the ability to name common, functional items?

    d. What did the facility do to improve the functional abilities of residents with moderate to severe hearing loss who have received and audiologic evaluation? For example, did the facility instruct the resident how to effectively and independently use environmental controls to compensate for hearing loss such as eye contact, preferential seating, use of the better ear?

    e. For the resident who cannot speak, did the facility assess for a communication board or an alternate means of communication?

4. For health rehabilitative services for MI and MR

    a. What did the facility do to decrease incidents of inappropriate behaviors, for individuals with MR, or behavioral symptoms for persons with MI? To increase appropriate behavior?

    b. What did the facility do to identify and treat the underlying factors behind tendencies toward isolation and withdrawal?

c. What did the facility do to develop and maintain necessary daily living skills?

d. How has the facility modified the training strategies it uses with its residents to account for the special learning needs of its residents with MI or MR?

e. Questions to ask individuals with MI or MR:

(1) Who do you talk to when you have a problem or need something?

(2) What do you do when you feel happy? Feel sad? Can't sleep at night?

(3) In what activities are you involved, and how often?

F407

§483.45(b) Qualifications

Specialized rehabilitative services must be provided under the written order of a physician by qualified personnel.

Intent: §485.45(b)

The intent of this regulation is to assure that the rehabilitative services are medically necessary as prescribed by a physician and provided by qualified personnel to maximize potential outcomes.

Specialized rehabilitative services are provided for individual's under a physician's order by a qualified professional. Once the assessment for specialized rehabilitative services is completed, a care plan must be developed, followed, and monitored by a licensed professional. Once a resident has met his or her care plan goals, a licensed professional can either discontinue treatment or initiate a maintenance program which either nursing or restorative sides will follow to maintain functional and physical status.

Interpretive Guidelines: §483.45(b)

"**Qualified personnel**" means that professional staff are licensed, certified or registered to provide specialized therapy/rehabilitative services in accordance with applicable State laws.

Health rehabilitative services for MI and MR must be implemented consistently by all staff unless the nature of the services is such that they are designated or required to be implemented only by licensed or credentialed personnel.

Procedures: §483.45(b)

Determine if there are any problems in quality of care related to maintaining or improving functional abilities. Determine if these problems are attributable in part to the qualifications of specialized rehabilitative services staff.

Determine from the care plan and record that rehabilitative services are provided under the written order of a physician and by qualified personnel. If a problem in a resident's rehabilitative care is identified that is related to the qualifications of the care providers, it may be necessary to validate the care providers qualification.

Probes: §483.45(b)

If the facility does not employ professional staff who have experience working directly with or designing training or treatment programs to meet the needs of individuals with MI or MR, how has the facility arranged for the necessary direct or staff training services to be provided?

F411

§483.55 Dental Services

The facility must assist residents in obtaining routine and 24-hour emergency dental care.

§483.55(a) Skilled Nursing Facilities

A facility--

(1) Must provide or obtain from an outside resource, in accordance with §483.75(h) of this part, routine and emergency dental services to meet the needs of each resident;

(2) May charge a Medicare resident an additional amount for routine and emergency dental services;

(3) Must if necessary assist the resident--

(i) In making appointments; and

(ii) By arranging for transportation to and from the dentist's office; and

(4) Promptly refer residents with lost or damaged dentures to a dentist.

Intent: §483.55

The intent of this regulation is to ensure that the facility be responsible for assisting the resident in obtaining needed dental services, including routine dental services.

Interpretive Guidelines: §483.55

This requirement makes the facility directly responsible for the dental care needs of its residents. The facility must ensure that a dentist is available for residents, i.e., employ a staff dentist or have a contract (arrangement) with a dentist to provide services.

For Medicare and private pay residents, facilities are responsible for having the services available, but they may impose an additional charge for the services.

For all residents of the facility, if they are unable to pay for needed dental services, the facility should attempt to find and alternative funding sources or alternative service delivery systems so that the resident is able to maintain his/her highest practicable level of well-being. (See §483.15(g).)

The facility is responsible for selecting a dentist who provides dental services in accordance with professional standards of quality and timeliness under §483.75(h)(2).

"**Routine dental services**" means an annual inspection of the oral cavity for signs of disease, diagnosis of dental disease, dental radiographs as needed, dental cleaning, fillings (new and repairs), minor dental plate adjustments, smoothing of broken teeth, and limited prosthodontic procedures, e.g., taking impressions for dentures and fitting dentures.
"**Emergency dental services**" includes services needed to treat an episode of acute pain in teeth, gums, or palate; broken, or otherwise damaged teeth, or any other problem of the oral cavity by a dentist that required immediate attention.

"**Prompt referral**" means, within reason, as soon as the dentures are lost or damaged. Referral does not mean that the resident must see the dentist at that time, but does mean that an appointment (referral) is made, or that the facility is aggressively working at replacing the dentures.

Probes: §483.55

Do residents selected for comprehensive or focused reviews, as appropriate, with dentures use them?

Are residents missing teeth and may be in need of dentures?

Do sampled residents have problems eating and maintaining nutritional status because of poor oral health or oral hygiene?

Are resident's dentures intact? Proper fit?

F412

§483.55(b) Nursing Facilities

The facility--

(1) Must provide or obtain from an outside resource, in accordance with §483.75(h) of this part, the following dental services to meet the needs of each resident:

(i) Routine dental services (to the extent covered under the State plan); and

(ii) Emergency dental services;

(2) Must, if necessary, assist the resident--

(i) In making appointments; and

(ii) By arranging for transportation to and from the dentist's office; and

(3) Must promptly refer residents with lost or damaged dentures to a dentist.

Interpretive Guidelines: §483.55(b)(1)(i)

For Medicaid residents, the facility must provide the resident, without charge, all emergency dental services, as well as those routine dental services that are covered under the State plan.

F425

(Rev. 22, Issued: 12-15-06, Effective/Implementation: 12-18-06)

§483.60 Pharmacy Services

The facility must provide routine and emergency drugs and biologicals to its residents, or obtain them under an agreement described in §483.75(h) of this part. The facility may permit unlicensed personnel to administer drugs if State law permits, but only under the general supervision of a licensed nurse.

(a) Procedures. A facility must provide pharmaceutical services (including procedures that assure the accurate acquiring, receiving, dispensing, and administering of all drugs and biologicals) to meet the needs of each resident.

(b) Service Consultation. The facility must employ or obtain the services of a licensed pharmacist who--

(1) Provides consultation on all aspects of the provision of pharmacy services in the facility;

INTENT (F425) 42 CFR 483.60, 483.60(a) & (b)(1)

The intent of this requirement is that:

- In order to meet the needs of each resident, the facility accurately and safely provides or obtains pharmaceutical services, including the provision of routine and emergency medications and biologicals, and the services of a licensed pharmacist;
- The licensed pharmacist collaborates with facility leadership and staff to coordinate pharmaceutical services within the facility, and to guide development and evaluation of the implementation of pharmaceutical services procedures;
- The licensed pharmacist helps the facility identify, evaluate, and address/resolve pharmaceutical concerns and issues that affect resident care, medical care or quality of life such as the:
  - Provision of consultative services by a licensed pharmacist between the pharmacist's visits, as necessary; and
  - Coordination of the pharmaceutical services if multiple pharmaceutical service providers are utilized (e.g., pharmacy, infusion, hospice, prescription drug plans [PDP]); and
- The facility utilizes only persons authorized under state requirements to administer medications.

NOTE: Although the regulatory language refers to "drugs," the guidance in this document generally will refer to "medications," except in those situations where the term "drug" has become part of an established pharmaceutical term (e.g., adverse drug event, adverse drug reaction or consequence).

For purposes of this guidance, references to "the pharmacist" mean the licensed pharmacist, whether employed directly by the facility or through arrangement.

DEFINITIONS

Definitions are provided to clarify terminology related to pharmaceutical services and the management of each resident's medication regimen for effectiveness and safety.

- "Acquiring medication" is the process by which a facility requests and obtains a medication.
- "Administering medication" is the process of giving medication(s) to a resident.
- "Biologicals" are products isolated from a variety of natural sources—human, animal, or microorganism—or produced by biotechnology methods and other cutting-edge technologies. They may include a wide range of products such as vaccine, blood and blood components, allergenics, somatic cells, gene therapy, tissues, and recombinant therapeutic proteins.
- "Current standards of practice" refers to approaches to care, procedures, techniques, treatments, etc., that are based on research and/or expert consensus and that are contained in current manuals, textbooks, or publications, or that are accepted, adopted or promulgated by recognized professional organizations or national accrediting bodies.
- "Dispensing" is a process that includes the interpretation of a prescription; selection, measurement, and packaging or repackaging of the product (as necessary); and labeling of the medication or device pursuant to a prescription/order.
- "Disposition" is the process of returning, releasing and/or destroying discontinued or expired medications.
- "Pharmaceutical Services" refers to:
    - The process (including documentation, as applicable) of receiving and interpreting prescriber's orders; acquiring, receiving, storing, controlling, reconciling, compounding (e.g., intravenous antibiotics), dispensing, packaging, labeling, distributing, administering, monitoring responses to, using and/or disposing of all medications, biologicals, chemicals (e.g., povidone iodine, hydrogen peroxide);
    - The provision of medication-related information to health care professionals and residents;

  - The process of identifying, evaluating and addressing medication-related issues including the prevention and reporting of medication errors; and
  - The provision, monitoring and/or the use of medication-related devices.

- "Pharmacy assistant or technician" refers to the ancillary personnel who work under the supervision and delegation of the pharmacist, consistent with state requirements.

- "Receiving medication"—for the purpose of this guidance—is the process of accepting a medication from the facility's pharmacy or an outside source (e.g., vending pharmacy delivery agent, Veterans Administration, family member).

OVERVIEW

The provision of pharmaceutical services is an integral part of the care provided to nursing home residents. The management of complex medication regimens is challenging and requires diverse pharmaceutical services to minimize medication-related adverse consequences or events. The overall goal of the pharmaceutical services system within a facility is to ensure the safe and effective use of medications.

Preventable medication-related adverse consequences and events are a serious concern in nursing homes. Gurwitz and colleagues evaluated the incidence and preventability of adverse drug events in 18 nursing homes in Massachusetts noting that 51% of the adverse drug events were judged to be preventable including 171 (72%) of the 238 fatal, life threatening or serious events and 105 (34%) of the 308 significant events. If these findings are extrapolated to all US nursing homes, approximately 350,000 adverse drug events may occur annually among this patient population, including 20,000 fatal or life threatening events.[63,64]

Factors that increase the risk of adverse consequences associated with medication use in the nursing home setting include complex medication regimens, numbers and types of medication used, physiological changes accompanying the aging process, as well as multiple comorbidities.

The consultative services of a pharmacist can promote safe and effective medication use. A pharmacist evaluates and coordinates all aspects of pharmaceutical services provided to all residents within a facility by all providers (e.g., pharmacy, prescription drug plan, prescribers). A pharmacist can also help in the development of medication-related documentation procedures, such as identification of abbreviations approved for use in the facility and can help guide the selection and use of medications in accordance with the authorized prescriber's orders, applicable state and federal requirements, manufacturers' specifications, characteristics of the resident population, and individual resident conditions.

Providing pharmaceutical consultation is an ongoing, interactive process with prospective, concurrent, and retrospective components. To accomplish some of these consultative responsibilities, pharmacists can use various methods and resources, such as technology, additional personnel (e.g., dispensing pharmacists, pharmacy technicians), and related policies and procedures.

Numerous recognized resources address different aspects of pharmaceutical services and medication utilization, such as:

- The American Society of Consultant Pharmacists (ASCP) www.ascp.com;
- The American Society of Health System Pharmacists (ASHP) www.ashp.com;
- The American Medical Directors Association (AMDA) www.amda.com;
- The National Coordinating Council for Medication Error Reporting and Prevention (NCCMERP) www.nccmerp.org;
- US Department of Health and Human Services (DHHS), Food and Drug Administration (FDA) www.fda.gov/cder; and
- The DHHS, CMS Sharing Innovations in Quality website at: http://siq.air.org.

NOTE: References to non-CMS sources or sites on the Internet are provided as a service and do not constitute or imply endorsement of these organizations or their programs by CMS or the U.S. Department of Health and Human Services. CMS is not responsible for the content of pages found at these sites. URL addresses were current as of the date of this publication.

PROVISION OF ROUTINE AND/OR EMERGENCY MEDICATIONS

The regulation at 42 CFR 483.60 (F425) requires that the facility provide or obtain routine and emergency medications and biologicals in order to meet the needs of each resident. Facility procedures and applicable state laws may allow the facility to maintain a limited supply of medications in the facility for use during emergency or after-hours situations. Whether prescribed on a routine, emergency, or as needed basis, medications should be administered in a timely manner. Delayed acquisition of a medication may impede timely administration and adversely affect a resident's condition. Factors that may help determine timeliness and guide acquisition procedures include:

- Availability of medications to enable continuity of care for an anticipated admission or transfer of a resident from acute care or other institutional settings;

- Condition of the resident including the severity or instability of his/her condition, a significant change in condition, discomfort, risk factors, current signs and symptoms, and the potential impact of any delay in acquiring the medications;

- Category of medication, such as antibiotics or analgesics;

- Availability of medications in emergency supply, if applicable; and

- Ordered start time for a medication.

SERVICES OF A LICENSED PHARMACIST

The facility is responsible for employing or contracting for the services of a pharmacist to provide consultation on all aspects of pharmaceutical services. The facility may provide for this service through any of several methods (in accordance with state requirements) such as direct employment or contractual agreement with a pharmacist. Whatever the arrangement or method employed, the facility and the pharmacist identify how they will collaborate for effective consultation regarding pharmaceutical services. The pharmacist reviews and evaluates the pharmaceutical services by helping the facility identify, evaluate, and address medication issues that may affect resident care, medical care, and quality of life.

The pharmacist is responsible for helping the facility obtain and maintain timely and appropriate pharmaceutical services that support residents' healthcare needs, that are consistent with current standards of practice, and that meet state and federal requirements. This includes, but is not limited to, collaborating with the facility and medical director to:

- Develop, implement, evaluate, and revise (as necessary) the procedures for the provision of all aspects of pharmaceutical services;

- Coordinate pharmaceutical services if and when multiple pharmaceutical service providers are utilized (e.g., pharmacy, infusion, hospice, prescription drug plans [PDP])

- Develop intravenous (IV) therapy procedures if used within the facility (consistent with state requirements) may include determining competency of staff, facility-based IV admixture procedures that address sterile compounding, dosage calculations, IV pump use, and flushing procedures;

- Determine (in accordance with or as permitted by state law) the contents of the emergency supply of medications and monitor the use, replacement, and disposition of the supply;

- Develop mechanisms for communicating, addressing, and resolving issues related to pharmaceutical services;

- Strive to assure that medications are requested, received, and administered in a timely manner as ordered by the authorized prescriber (in accordance with state requirements), including physicians, advanced practice nurses, pharmacists, and physician assistants;

- Provide feedback about performance and practices related to medication administration and medication errors;

- Participate on the interdisciplinary team to address and resolve medication-related needs or problems;

- Establish procedures for:
    - conducting the monthly medication regimen review (MRR) for each resident in the facility,
    - addressing the expected time frames for conducting the review and reporting the findings,
    - addressing the irregularities,
    - documenting and reporting the results of the review (See F428 for provision of the review.); and

- Establish procedures that address medication regimen reviews for residents who are anticipated to stay less than 30 days or when the resident experiences an acute change of condition as identified by facility staff.

  NOTE: Facility procedures should address how and when the need for a consultation will be communicated, how the medication review will be handled if the pharmacist is off-site, how the results or report of their findings will be communicated to the physician, expectations for the physician's response and follow up, and how and where this information will be documented.

In addition, the pharmacist may collaborate with the facility and medical director on other aspects of pharmaceutical services including, but not limited to:

- Developing procedures and guidance regarding when to contact a prescriber about a medication issue and/or adverse effects, including what information to gather before contacting the prescriber;

- Developing the process for receiving, transcribing, and recapitulating medication orders;

- Recommending the type(s) of medication delivery system(s) to standardize packaging, such as bottles, bubble packs, tear strips, in an effort to minimize medication errors;

- Developing and implementing procedures regarding automated medication delivery devices or cabinets, if automated devices or cabinets are used, including: the types or categories of medications, amounts stored, location of supply, personnel authorized to access the supply, record keeping, monitoring for expiration dates, method to ensure accurate removal of medications and the steps for replacing the supply when dosages are used, and monitoring the availability of medications within the system;

- Interacting with the quality assessment and assurance committee to develop procedures and evaluate pharmaceutical services including delivery and storage systems within the various locations of the facility in order to prevent, to the degree possible, loss or tampering with the medication supplies, and to define and monitor corrective actions for problems related to pharmaceutical services and medications, including medication errors;

- Recommending current resources to help staff identify medications and information on contraindications, side effects and/or adverse effects, dosage levels, and other pertinent information; and

- Identifying facility educational and informational needs about medications and providing information from sources such as nationally recognized organizations to the facility staff, practitioners, residents, and families.

  NOTE: This does not imply that the pharmacist must personally present educational programs.

PHARMACEUTICAL SERVICES PROCEDURES

The pharmacist, in collaboration with the facility and medical director helps develop and evaluate the implementation of pharmaceutical services procedures that address the needs of the residents, are consistent with state and federal requirements, and reflect current standards of practice. These procedures address, but are not limited to, acquiring; receiving; dispensing; administering; disposing; labeling and storage of medications; and personnel authorized to access or administer medications.

Acquisition of Medications

Examples of procedures addressing acquisition of medications include:

- Availability of an emergency supply of medications, if allowed by state law, including the types or categories of medications; amounts, dosages/strengths to be provided; location of the supply; personnel authorized to access the supply; record keeping; monitoring for expiration dates; and the steps for replacing the supply when medications are used;

- When, how to, and who may contact the pharmacy regarding acquisition of medications and the steps to follow for contacting the pharmacy for an original routine medication order, emergency medication order, and refills;

- The availability of medications when needed, that is, the medication is either in the facility (in the emergency supply) or obtained from a pharmacy that can be reached 24 hours a day, seven days a week;

- The receipt, labeling, storage, and administration of medications dispensed by the physician, if allowed by state requirements;

- Verification or clarification of an order to facilitate accurate acquisition of a medication when necessary (e.g., clarification when the resident has allergies to, or there are contraindications to the medication being ordered);

- Procedure when delivery of a medication will be delayed or the medication is not or will not be available; and

- Transportation of medications from the dispensing pharmacy or vendor to the facility consistent with manufacturer's specifications, state and federal requirements, and standards of professional practice to prevent contamination, degradation, and diversion of medications.

Receiving Medication(s)

Examples of procedures addressing receipt of medications include:

- How the receipt of medications from dispensing pharmacies (and family members or others, where permitted by state requirements) will occur and how it will be reconciled with the prescriber's order and the requisition for the medication;

- How staff will be identified and authorized in accordance with applicable laws and requirements to receive the medications and how access to the medications will be controlled until the medications are delivered to the secured storage area; and

- Which staff will be responsible for assuring that medications are incorporated into the resident's specific allocation/storage area.

Dispensing Medication(s)

Examples of procedures to assure compatible and safe medication delivery, to minimize medication administration errors, and to address the facility's expectations of the in-house pharmacy and/or outside dispensing pharmacies include:

- Delivery and receipt;
- Labeling; and
- The types of medication packaging (e.g., unit dose, multi-dose vial, blister cards).

Administering Medications

Examples of procedures addressing administration of medications include:

- Providing continuity of staff to ensure that medications are administered without unnecessary interruptions;
- Reporting medication administration errors, including how and to whom to report;
- Authorizing personnel, consistent with state requirements, to administer the medications, including medications needing intravenous administration (see Authorized Personnel and Staff Qualifications section within this document);
- Assuring that the correct medication is administered in the correct dose, in accordance with manufacturer's specifications and with standards of practice, to the correct person via the correct route in the correct dosage form and at the correct time;
- Defining the schedules for administering medications to:
    - Maximize the effectiveness (optimal therapeutic effect) of the medication (for example, antibiotics, antihypertensives, insulins, pain medications);
    - Avoid potential significant medication interactions such as medication-food or medication-medication interactions; and
    - Recognize resident choices and activities, to the degree possible, consistent with the medical plan of care;
- Defining general guidelines for specific monitoring related to medications, when ordered or indicated, including specific item(s) to monitor (e.g., blood pressure, pulse, blood sugar, weight), frequency (e.g., weekly, daily), timing (e.g., before or after administering the medication), and parameters for notifying the prescriber;

- Defining pertinent techniques and precautions for administering medications through alternate routes such as eye, ear, buccal, injection, intravenous, atomizer/aerosol/ inhalation therapy, or enteral tubes;

- Documenting the administration of medications, including:

  - The administration of routine medication(s), and if not administered, an explanation of why not;

  - The administration of "as-needed" medications including the justification and response;

  - The route, if other than oral (intended route may be preprinted on MAR); and

  - Location of administration sites such as transdermal patches and injections;

- Providing accessible current information about medications (e.g., medication information references) and medication-related devices and equipment (e.g., user's manual);

- Clarifying any order that is incomplete, illegible, or presents any other concerns, prior to administering the medication; and

- Reconciling medication orders including telephone orders, monthly or other periodic recapitulations, medication orders to the pharmacy, and medication administration record (MAR), including who may transcribe prescriber's orders and enter the orders onto the MAR.

Disposition of Medications

Examples of procedures addressing the disposition of medications include:

- Timely identification and removal (from current medication supply) of medications for disposition;

- Identification of storage method for medications awaiting final disposition;

- Control and accountability of medications awaiting final disposition consistent with standards of practice;

- Documentation of actual disposition of medications to include: resident name, medication name, strength, prescription number (as applicable), quantity, date of disposition, and involved facility staff, consultant(s) or other applicable individuals; and

- Method of disposition consistent with applicable state and federal requirements, local ordinances, and standards of practice.

Labeling and Storage of Medications, including Controlled Substances

Examples of procedures addressing accurate labeling of the medications (including appropriate accessory and cautionary instructions) include:

- Labeling medications prepared by facility staff, such as IV solutions prepared in the facility;

- Requirements for labeling medications not labeled by a pharmacy, such as bulk supplies/bottles of over-the counter (OTC) medications (as permitted);

- Modifying labels due to changes in the medication orders or directions, in accordance with state and federal requirements; and

- Labeling multi-dose vials to assure product integrity, considering the manufacturer's specifications (e.g., modified expiration dates upon opening the multi-dose vial).

Examples of procedures addressing the safe storage of medications include:

- Location, security (locking), and authorized access to the medication rooms, carts and other storage areas;

- Temperatures and other environmental considerations of medication storage area(s) such as the medication room(s) and refrigerators; and

- Location, access, and security for discontinued medications awaiting disposal.

Examples of procedures addressing controlled medications include:

- Location, access, and security for controlled medications, including the separately locked permanently affixed compartment for those Schedule II medications or preparations with Schedule II medications needing refrigeration;

- A system of records of receipt and disposition of all controlled medications that accounts for all controlled medications; and

- Periodic reconciliation of controlled medications including the frequency, method, by whom, and pertinent documentation.

Authorized Personnel

The facility may permit unlicensed personnel to administer medications if state law permits, but only under the general supervision of a licensed nurse.

The facility assures that all persons administering medications are authorized according to state and federal requirements, oriented to the facility's procedures, and have access to current information regarding medications being used within the facility, including side effects of medications, contraindications, doses, etc.

Examples of procedures addressing authorized personnel include:

- How the facility assures ongoing competency of all staff (including temporary, agency, or on-call staff) authorized to administer medications and biologicals;
- Training regarding the operation, limitations, monitoring, and precautions associated with medication administration devices or other equipment, if used, such as:
    - IV pumps or other IV delivery systems including calculating dosage, infusion rates, and compatibility of medications to be added to the IV;
    - Blood glucose meters, including calibration and cleaning between individual residents; and
    - Using, maintaining, cleaning, and disposing of the various types of devices for administration including nebulizers, inhalers, syringes, medication cups, spoons, and pill crushers;
- Identifying pharmacy personnel in addition to the pharmacist (e.g., pharmacy technicians, pharmacist assistants) who are authorized under state and federal requirements to access medications and biologicals.

INVESTIGATIVE PROTOCOL

For investigating compliance with the requirements at 42 CFR 483.60 and 483.60(a) & (b), see State Operations Manual, Appendix P, II.B., The Traditional Standard Survey, Task 5, Sub-Task 5E Investigative Protocol: Medication Pass and Pharmacy Services.

DETERMINATION OF COMPLIANCE (Task 6, Appendix P)

Synopsis of Regulation (F425)

The Pharmaceutical Services, Procedures and Consultation requirement has four aspects. First, the facility must provide routine and/or emergency medications and biologicals or obtain them under an agreement described in 42 CFR 483.75(h). Second, the facility must have procedures for pharmaceutical services to meet the resident's needs. The procedures must assure accurate acquisition, receipt, dispensing, and administration of all medications and biologicals. Third, the facility must have a licensed pharmacist who provides consultation and oversees all aspects of the pharmaceutical services. Fourth, the facility must follow applicable laws and regulations about who may administer medications.

Criteria for Compliance

Compliance with 42 CFR 483.60, F425, Pharmaceutical Services

The facility is in compliance with this requirement, if they provide or arrange for:

- Each resident to receive medications and/or biologicals as ordered by the prescriber;
- The development and implementation of procedures for the pharmaceutical services;
- The services of a pharmacist who provides consultation regarding all aspects of pharmaceutical services; and
- Personnel to administer medications, consistent with applicable state law and regulations.

If not, cite F425.

Noncompliance for F425

After completing the Investigative Protocol, analyze the data and review the regulatory requirement in order to determine whether or not compliance with F425 exists. As the requirements for F425 include both process and structural components, a determination of noncompliance with F425 does not require a finding of harm to the resident. If the survey team identifies noncompliance at other tags which may be related to the roles and responsibilities of the pharmacist or the provision of pharmaceutical services, the team must also decide whether there is noncompliance with this requirement. Noncompliance for F425 may include (but is not limited to) the facility failure to:

- Utilize the services of a pharmacist;
- Ensure that only appropriate personnel administer medications;
- Provide medications and/or biologicals to meet the needs of the resident; and

- Develop or implement procedures for any of the following: acquiring, receiving, dispensing or accurately administering medications.

Potential Tags for Additional Investigation

If noncompliance with 42 CFR 483.60 and 483.60(a) & (b) has been identified, then concerns with additional requirements may also have been identified. The surveyor is cautioned to investigate these related additional requirements before determining whether noncompliance with the additional requirements may be present. Examples of some of the related requirements that should be considered when noncompliance has been identified include the following:

- 42 CFR 483.30(a), F353, Sufficient Staff
    - Determine if the facility had qualified staff in sufficient numbers to provide medications on a 24-hour basis to meet the needs of the residents, based upon the comprehensive assessment and care plan.
- 42 CFR 483.75(i)(2), F501, Medical Director
    - Determine whether the medical director, in collaboration with the facility and the pharmacist, and based on current standards of practice, helped the facility develop procedures for the safe and accurate provision of medications to meet the needs of the residents.
- 42 CFR 483.75 (o), F520, Quality Assessment and Assurance
    - Determine whether the quality assessment and assurance committee, if concerns regarding pharmaceutical services have been identified, has identified those concerns, responded to the concerns and, as appropriate, has developed, implemented, and monitored appropriate plans of action to correct identified quality deficiencies.
- 42 CFR 483.75(l)(1), F514, Clinical Records
    - Determine whether the facility has maintained clinical records, including medication administration, in accordance with accepted professional standards and practices that are complete, accurately documented, and readily accessible.

IV. DEFICIENCY CATEGORIZATION (Part IV, Appendix P)

Once the survey team has completed its investigation, reviewed the regulatory requirements, and determined that noncompliance exists, the team must determine the severity of each deficiency, based on the resultant harm or potential for harm to the resident.

The key elements for severity determination for F425 are as follows:

1. **Presence of potential or actual harm/negative outcome(s) due to a facility failure related to pharmaceutical services.**

   Identify actual or potential harm/negative outcomes for F425 which may include, but are not limited to:

   - The facility's failure to involve a pharmacist in developing, implementing, and evaluating pharmaceutical procedures including procedures for accurately acquiring, receiving, storing, controlling, dispensing, and administering routine and emergency medications and biologicals resulted in the lack of specific procedures or in procedures that were not consistent with current standards of practice, for example:
     - Absent or inadequate IV infusion procedures led to a resident developing congestive heart failure as a result of an IV infusing too quickly.
   - The facility's failure to provide medications needed by a resident in a timely manner resulted in continued pain or worsening symptoms.
   - The use of unauthorized personnel to administer medications created the potential for harm.

2. **Degree of potential or actual harm/negative outcome(s) due to a facility failure related to pharmaceutical services.**

   Identify how the facility's practices caused, resulted in, allowed, or contributed to the actual or potential for harm:

   - If harm has occurred, determine if the harm is at the level of serious injury, impairment, death, compromise, or discomfort.
   - If harm has not yet occurred, determine how likely is the potential for serious injury, impairment, death, compromise, or discomfort to occur to the resident.

3. **The immediacy of correction required.**

   Determine whether the noncompliance requires immediate correction in order to prevent serious injury, harm, impairment, or death to one or more residents.

The survey team must evaluate the harm or potential for harm based upon the following levels of severity for tag F425. First, the team must rule out whether Severity Level 4,

Immediate Jeopardy to a resident's health or safety, exists by evaluating the deficient practice in relation to immediacy, culpability, and severity. (Follow the guidance in Appendix Q, Guidelines for Determining Immediate Jeopardy.)

NOTE: The death or transfer of a resident who was harmed or injured as a result of facility noncompliance does not remove a finding of immediate jeopardy. The facility is required to implement specific actions to remove the jeopardy and correct the noncompliance which allowed or caused the immediate jeopardy.

Severity Level 4 Considerations: Immediate Jeopardy to Resident Health or Safety

Immediate Jeopardy is a situation in which the facility's noncompliance with one or more requirements of participation:

- Has caused/resulted in, or is likely to cause, serious injury, harm, impairment, or death to a resident; and
- Requires immediate correction as the facility either created the situation or allowed the situation to continue by failing to implement preventative or corrective measures.

Examples may include, but are not limited to:

- Severity Level 4 (Immediate Jeopardy) deficiency at another tag (e.g., F309, F329, F332, F333, F428) and the noncompliance is related to a failure of the facility to provide or obtain the service of a pharmacist or to collaborate with the pharmacist to establish and implement procedures for using medications, resulting in the potential for significant adverse consequences.
- The facility, in collaboration with the pharmacist, failed to establish effective procedures to meet the needs of the residents, such as:
    - Assuring that pain medications were available to meet the needs of the resident. For example, failure to assure availability of pain medication for a recently admitted resident resulting in the resident complaining of excruciating pain (e.g., a pain score of 9 on a 10-point scale).
    - Assuring that devices used to administer medications (such as IV pumps) were working properly, leading to an adverse consequence at the immediate jeopardy level.
    - Identifying medication errors, for example, medications were being dispensed without a valid prescriber's order, resulting in a resident incorrectly receiving three medications over two consecutive months.

NOTE: If immediate jeopardy has been ruled out based upon the evidence, then evaluate whether actual harm that is not immediate jeopardy exists at Severity Level 3.

Severity Level 3 Considerations: Actual Harm that is Not Immediate Jeopardy

Level 3 indicates noncompliance that results in actual harm, and may include, but is not limited to, clinical compromise, decline, or the resident's inability to maintain and/or reach his/her highest practicable well-being. Examples may include, but are not limited to:

- Severity Level 3 deficiency at another tag (e.g., F309, F329, F332, F333, F428) and the noncompliance is related to a failure of the facility to provide or obtain the services of a pharmacist or to collaborate with the pharmacist to develop and implement procedures for monitoring medication therapy, resulting in a failure to monitor treatment and the resident experiencing actual harm.

- The facility in collaboration with the pharmacist failed to assure that procedures were developed and implemented, such as:

  - An effective procedure/mechanism to assure that all medication orders were processed consistently and accurately through the stages of ordering, receiving, and administering medications (including transfer orders, admission orders, telephone orders, order renewals, and the MAR). For example, a transcription error led to an incorrect dose of a medication being administered and the resident experiencing spontaneous bruising and epistaxis requiring medical intervention.

  - Provisions to assure that staff were trained or competent to use new medication-related devices (e.g., intravenous pump). This resulted in a resident receiving an excessive dose of medication requiring subsequent hospitalization or receiving a sub-therapeutic dose of medication with consequential exacerbation of a condition (e.g., infection), continuation of treatment beyond the expected time frame, and subsequent functional decline.

NOTE: If Severity Level 3 (actual harm that is not immediate jeopardy) has been ruled out based upon the evidence, then evaluate as to whether Severity Level 2 (no actual harm with the potential for more than minimal harm) exists.

Severity Level 2 Considerations: No Actual Harm with Potential for More Than Minimal Harm that is Not Immediate Jeopardy

Level 2 indicates noncompliance that results in a resident outcome of no more than minimal discomfort and/or has the potential to compromise the resident's ability to maintain or reach his or her highest practicable level of well-being. The potential exists for greater harm to occur if interventions are not provided. Examples may include, but are not limited to:

- A Severity Level 2 deficiency at another tag (e.g., F309, F329, F332, F333, F428) and the noncompliance is related to a failure of the facility to implement established medication administration procedures. For example, as a result of failure of licensed staff to supervise medication administration by authorized unlicensed personnel, errors occurred in providing timely oral antibiotic therapy.

- The facility failed to obtain or provide the services of a pharmacist or to collaborate with the pharmacist to assure that effective policies and procedures were established and implemented including, for example:

    - As a result of not reordering medications often enough to maintain an adequate supply, a resident did not receive medication for heartburn for seven days and had difficulty sleeping due to nocturnal heartburn. The level of discomfort did not interfere with the resident's participating in activities or performing activities of daily living.

    - As a result of failure to identify medications that should not be crushed for administration, a resident received a medication that was crushed, contrary to the manufacturer's specifications (e.g., an enteric coated aspirin). While the resident did not experience any harm, the potential for harm was present.

NOTE: If Severity Level 2 (no actual harm with potential for more than minimal harm that is not immediate jeopardy) has been ruled out based upon the evidence, then evaluate as to whether Severity Level 1 (no actual harm with the potential for minimal harm) exists.

Severity Level 1 Considerations: No Actual Harm with Potential for Minimal Harm

In order to cite no actual harm with potential for minimal harm at this tag, the surveyor must verify that no resident harm or potential for more than minimal harm identified at other requirements was related to lack of pharmaceutical services, absence of or failure to implement pharmaceutical procedures, or absence of oversight by the pharmacist.

Examples of noncompliance for Severity Level 1 may include:

- The facility and the pharmacist failed to collaborate to:

    - Implement pharmaceutical procedures, but there were no negative resident outcomes or potential for more than minimal negative outcomes as a result of that deficient practice.

- There is no pharmacist; and
  - There were no negative resident outcomes or potential for more than minimal negative outcomes related to pharmaceutical services; and
  - Pharmaceutical procedures were in place; and
  - The facility was actively seeking a new pharmacist.

  NOTE: If there is no pharmacist and there were negative outcomes, or procedures were not in place or if the facility was not looking for a replacement, cite at a Severity Level 2 or higher severity.

- There was a short term failure to provide medications that posed minimal risk to the resident, such as a routine order for a daily multivitamin.

F428

(Rev. 22, Issued: 12-15-06, Effective/Implementation: 12-18-06)

§483.60(c) Drug Regimen Review

(1) The drug regimen of each resident must be reviewed at least once a month by a licensed pharmacist.

(2) The pharmacist must report any irregularities to the attending physician, and the director of nursing, and these reports must be acted upon.

INTENT (F428) 42 CFR 483.60(c)(1)(2) Medication Regimen Review

The intent of this requirement is that the facility maintains the resident's highest practicable level of functioning and prevents or minimizes adverse consequences related to medication therapy to the extent possible, by providing:

- A licensed pharmacist's review of each resident's regimen of medications at least monthly; or
  - A more frequent review of the regimen depending upon the resident's condition and the risks or adverse consequences related to current medication(s);
- The identification and reporting of irregularities to the attending physician and the director of nursing; and

- Action taken in response to the irregularities identified.

NOTE: Although the regulatory language refers to "drugs," the guidance in this document generally will refer to "medications," except in those situations where the term "drug" has become part of an established pharmaceutical term (e.g., adverse drug event, and adverse drug reaction or consequence).

For purposes of this guidance, references to "the pharmacist" mean the licensed pharmacist, whether employed directly by the facility or through arrangement.

DEFINITIONS

Definitions are provided to clarify terminology related to pharmaceutical services and the management of each resident's medication regimen for effectiveness and safety.

- "Adverse consequence" refers to an unpleasant symptom or event that is due to or associated with a medication, such as impairment or decline in an individual's mental or physical condition or functional or psychosocial status. It may include various types of adverse drug reactions and interactions (e.g., medication-medication, medication-food, and medication-disease).

  NOTE: Adverse drug reaction (ADR) is a form of adverse consequence. It may be either a secondary effect of a medication that is usually undesirable and different from the therapeutic and helpful effects of the medication or any response to a medication that is noxious and unintended and occurs in doses used for prophylaxis, diagnosis, or therapy. The term "side effect" is often used interchangeably with ADR; however, side effects are but one of five ADR categories. The others are hypersensitivity, idiosyncratic response, toxic reactions, and adverse medication interactions. A side effect is an expected, well-known reaction that occurs with a predictable frequency and may or may not rise to the level of being an adverse consequence.

- **"Clinically significant" means effects, results, or consequences that materially affect or are likely to affect an individual's mental, physical, or psychosocial well-being either positively by preventing, stabilizing, or improving a condition or reducing a risk, or negatively by exacerbating, causing, or contributing to a symptom, illness, or decline in status.**

- **"Dose" is the total amount/strength/concentration of a medication given at one time or over a period of time. The individual dose is the amount/strength/concentration received at each administration. The amount received over a 24-hour period may be referred to as the daily dose.**

- "Excessive dose" (including duplicate therapy) means the total amount of any medication given at one time or over a period of time that is greater than the amount recommended by the manufacturer's label, package insert, or current standards of practice for a resident's age and condition; without evidence of a review for the continued necessity of the dose or of attempts at, or consideration of the possibility of, tapering a medication; and there is no documented clinical rationale for the benefit of, or necessity for the dose or for the use of multiple medications from the same class.

- **"Duration" is the total length of time the medication is being received.**

  - "Excessive Duration" means the medication is administered beyond the manufacturer's recommended time frames or facility-established stop order policies, beyond the length of time advised by current standards of practice, and/or without either evidence of additional therapeutic benefit for the resident or clear clinical factors that would warrant the continued use of the medication.

- **"Irregularity" refers to any event that is inconsistent with usual, proper, accepted, or right approaches to providing pharmaceutical services (see definition in F425), or that impedes or interferes with achieving the intended outcomes of those services.**

- **"Medication Interaction" is the impact of another substance (such as another medication, herbal product, food or substances used in diagnostic studies) upon a medication. The interactions may alter absorption, distribution, metabolism, or elimination. These interactions may decrease the effectiveness of the medication or increase the potential for adverse consequences.**

- **"Medication Regimen Review" (MRR) is a thorough evaluation of the medication regimen of a resident, with the goal of promoting positive outcomes and minimizing adverse consequences associated with medication. The review includes preventing, identifying, reporting, and resolving medication-related problems, medication errors, or other irregularities, and collaborating with other members of the interdisciplinary team.**[65]

- "Monitoring" is the ongoing collection and analysis of information (such as observations and diagnostic test results) and comparison to baseline data in order to:

  - **Ascertain the individual's response to treatment and care, including progress or lack of progress toward a therapeutic goal;**

- **Detect any complications or adverse consequences of the condition or of the treatments; and**
- **Support decisions about modifying, discontinuing, or continuing any interventions.**

- "Pharmacy Assistant or Technician" refers to ancillary personnel who work under the supervision and delegation of the pharmacist as consistent with state requirements.

OVERVIEW

Many nursing home residents require multiple medications to address their conditions, leading to complex medication regimens. Medications are used for their therapeutic benefits in diagnosing, managing, and treating acute and/or chronic conditions, for maintaining and/or improving a resident's functional status, and for improving or sustaining the resident's quality of life. The nursing home population may be quite diverse and may include geriatric residents as well as individuals of any age with special needs, such as those who are immunocompromised or who have end stage renal disease or spinal cord or closed head injuries. Regardless, this population has been identified as being at high risk for adverse consequences related to medications. Some adverse consequences may mimic symptoms of chronic conditions, the aging process, or a newly emerging condition.

Transitions in care such as a move from home or hospital to the nursing home, or vice versa, increases the risk of medication-related issues. Medications may be added, discontinued, omitted, or changed. It is important, therefore, to review the medications. Currently, safeguards to help identify medication issues include:

- The physician providing and reviewing the orders and total program of care on admission and the prescriber reviewing at each visit;

- The nurse reviewing medications when transmitting the orders to the pharmacy and/or prior to administering medications;

- The interdisciplinary team reviewing the medications as part of the comprehensive assessment for the Resident Assessment Instrument (RAI) and/or care plan;

- The pharmacist reviewing the prescriptions prior to dispensing; and

- The pharmacist performing the medication regimen review at least monthly.

During the MRR, the pharmacist applies his/her understanding of medications and related cautions, actions and interactions as well as current medication advisories and information. The pharmacist provides consultation to the facility and the attending physician(s) regarding the medication regimen and is an important member of the interdisciplinary team. Regulations prohibit the pharmacist from delegating the medication regimen reviews to ancillary staff.

Some resources are available to facilitate evaluating medication concerns related to the performance of the MRR, such as:

- American Society of Consultant Pharmacists (ASCP) www.ascp.com;
- American Medical Directors Association (AMDA) www.amda.com;
- National Coordinating Council for Medication Error Reporting and Prevention (NCCMERP) www.nccmerp.org;
- American Geriatrics Society (AGS) www.americangeriatrics.org;
- U.S. Department of Health and Human Services, Food and Drug Administration (FDA) http://www.fda.gov/medwatch/safety.htm; and
- DHHS, CMS Sharing Innovations in Quality website at: http://siq.air.org.

NOTE: References to non-CMS sources or sites on the Internet are provided as a service and do not constitute or imply endorsement of these organizations or their programs by CMS or the U.S. Department of Health and Human Services. CMS is not responsible for the content of pages found at these sites. URL addresses were current as of the date of this publication.

This guidance is not intended to imply that all adverse consequences related to medications are preventable, but rather to specify that a system exists to assure that medication usage is evaluated on an ongoing basis, that risks and problems are identified and acted upon, and that medication-related problems are considered when the resident has a change in condition. This guidance will discuss the following aspects of the facility's MRR component of the pharmaceutical services systems:

- A pharmacist's review of the resident's medication regimen to identify and report irregularities; and
- Acting upon identified irregularities in order to minimize or prevent adverse consequences, to the extent possible.

NOTE: The surveyor's review of medication use is not intended to constitute the practice of medicine. However, surveyors are expected to investigate the basis for decisions and interventions affecting residents.

MEDICATION REGIMEN REVIEW (MRR)

The MRR is an important component of the overall management and monitoring of a resident's medication regimen. The pharmacist must review each resident's medication regimen at least once a month in order to identify irregularities; and to identify clinically significant risks and/or adverse consequences resulting from or associated with medications. It may be necessary for the pharmacist to conduct the MRR more frequently, for example weekly, depending on the resident's condition and the risks for adverse consequences related to current medications.

Generally, MRRs are conducted in the facility because important information about indications for use, potential medication irregularities or adverse consequences (such as symptoms of tardive dyskinesia, dizziness, anorexia, or falls) may be attainable only by talking to the staff, reviewing the medical record, and observing and speaking with the resident. However, electronic health and medication records and other available technology may permit the pharmacist to conduct some components of the review outside the facility.

Important aspects of the MRR include identification of irregularities, including medication-related errors and adverse consequences, location and notification of MRR findings, and response to identified irregularities. This guidance discusses these aspects and also provides some examples of clinically significant medication interactions.

Identification of Irregularities

An objective of the MRR is to try to minimize or prevent adverse consequences by identifying irregularities including, for example: syndromes potentially related to medication therapy, emerging or existing adverse medication consequences, as well as the potential for adverse drug reactions and medication errors. The resident's record may contain information regarding possible and/or actual medication irregularities. Possible sources to obtain this information include: the medication administration records (MAR); prescribers' orders; progress, nursing and consultants' notes; the Resident Assessment Instrument (RAI); laboratory and diagnostic test results, and other sources of information about behavior monitoring and/or changes in condition. The pharmacist may also obtain information from the Quality Measures/Quality Indicator reports, the attending physician, facility staff, and (as appropriate) from interviewing, assessing, and/or observing the resident.

The pharmacist's review considers factors such as:

- Whether the physician and staff have documented objective findings, diagnoses and/or symptom(s) to support indications for use;
- Whether the physician and staff have identified and acted upon, or should be notified about, the resident's allergies and/or potential side effects and significant

medication interactions (such as medication-medication, medication-food, medication-disease, medication-herbal interactions);

- Whether the medication dose, frequency, route of administration, and duration are consistent with the resident's condition, manufacturer's recommendations, and applicable standards of practice;

- Whether the physician and staff have documented progress towards, or maintenance of, the goal(s) for the medication therapy;

- Whether the physician and staff have obtained and acted upon laboratory results, diagnostic studies, or other measurements (such as bowel function, intake and output) as applicable;

- Whether medication errors exist or circumstances exist that make them likely to occur; and

- Whether the physician and staff have noted and acted upon possible medication-related causes of recent or persistent changes in the resident's condition such as worsening of an existing problem or the emergence of new signs or symptoms. The following are examples of changes potentially related to medication use that could occur at any age, however, some of the changes are more common in the geriatric population and may be unrelated to medications:

    - Anorexia and/or unplanned weight loss, or weight gain;

    - Behavioral changes, unusual behavior patterns (including increased distressed behavior);

    - Bowel function changes including constipation, ileus, impaction;

    - Confusion, cognitive decline, worsening of dementia (including delirium) of recent onset;

    - Dehydration, fluid/electrolyte imbalance;

    - Depression, mood disturbance;

    - Dysphagia, swallowing difficulty;

    - Excessive sedation, insomnia, or sleep disturbance;

    - Falls, dizziness, or evidence of impaired coordination;

    - Gastrointestinal bleeding;

- Headaches, muscle pain, generalized aching or pain;
- Rash, pruritus;
- Seizure activity;
- Spontaneous or unexplained bleeding, bruising;
- Unexplained decline in functional status (e.g., ADLs, vision); and
- Urinary retention or incontinence.

Upon conducting the MRR, the pharmacist may identify and report concerns in one or more of the following categories:[66] (See F329 for additional discussion of irregularities relating to dose, duration, indications for use, monitoring, and adverse consequences.)

- The use of a medication without identifiable evidence of adequate indications for use;
- The use of a medication to treat a clinical condition without identifiable evidence that safer alternatives or more clinically appropriate medications have been considered;
- The use of an appropriate medication that is not helping attain the intended treatment goals because of timing of administration, dosing intervals, sufficiency of dose, techniques of administration, or other reasons;
- The use of a medication in an excessive dose (including duplicate therapy) or for excessive duration, thereby placing the resident at greater risk for adverse consequences or causing existing adverse consequences;
- The presence of an adverse consequence associated with the resident's current medication regimen;
- The use of a medication without evidence of adequate monitoring; i.e., either inadequate monitoring of the response to a medication or an inadequate response to the findings;
- Presence of medication errors or the risk for such errors;
- Presence of a clinical condition that might warrant initiation of medication therapy; and

NOTE: The presence of a diagnosis or symptom does not necessarily warrant medication, but often depends on the consideration of many factors simultaneously.

- A medication interaction associated with the current medication regimen.

The following table provides examples of some problematic medication interactions in the long-term care population. These examples represent common interactions but are not meant to be all inclusive.

NOTE: Concomitant use of these medication combinations is not necessarily inappropriate and these examples are not intended to imply that the medications cannot be used simultaneously. Often, several medications with documented interactions can be given together safely. However, concomitant use of such medications warrants careful consideration of potential alternatives, possible need to modify doses, and diligent monitoring.

Common Medication-Medication Interactions in Long Term Care[67]

Medication 1	Medication 2	Impact
warfarin	NSAIDs such as ibuprofen, naproxen, COX-2 inhibitors	Potential for serious gastrointestinal bleeding
warfarin	sulfonamides such as trimethoprim/ sulfamethoxazole	Increased effects of warfarin, with potential for bleeding
warfarin	macrolides such as clarithromycin, erythromycin	Increased effects of warfarin, with potential for bleeding
warfarin	fluoroquinolones such as ciprofloxacin, levofloxacin, ofloxacin	Increased effects of warfarin, with potential for bleeding
warfarin	phenytoin	Increased effects of warfarin and/or phenytoin
ACE Inhibitors such as benazepril, captopril, enalapril, and lisinopril	potassium supplements	Elevated serum potassium levels
ACE Inhibitors such as benazepril, captopril, enalapril, and lisinopril	spironolactone	Elevated serum potassium levels
digoxin	amiodarone	digoxin toxicity
digoxin	verapamil	digoxin toxicity
theophylline	fluoroquinolones such as ciprofloxacin, levofloxacin, ofloxacin	theophylline toxicity

Location and Notification of Medication Regimen Review Findings

The pharmacist is expected to document either that no irregularity was identified or the nature of any identified irregularities. The pharmacist is responsible for reporting any identified irregularities to the attending physician and director of nursing. The timeliness of notification of irregularities depends on factors including the potential for or presence of serious adverse consequences; for example, immediate notification is indicated in cases of bleeding in a resident who is receiving anticoagulants or in cases of possible allergic reactions to antibiotic therapy. If no irregularities were identified during the review, the pharmacist includes a signed and dated statement to that effect. The facility and the pharmacist may collaborate to identify the most effective means for assuring appropriate notification. This notification may be done electronically.

The pharmacist does not need to document a continuing irregularity in the report each month if the pharmacist has deemed the irregularity to be clinically insignificant or evidence of a valid clinical reason for rejecting the pharmacist's recommendation was provided. In this situation, the pharmacist need only reconsider annually whether to report the irregularity again or make a new recommendation.

The pharmacist's findings are considered part of each resident's clinical record. If documentation of the findings is not in the active record, it is maintained within the facility and is readily available for review. The interdisciplinary team is encouraged to review the reports and to get the pharmacist's input on resident problems and issues. Establishing a consistent location for the pharmacist's findings and recommendations can facilitate communication with the attending physician, the director of nursing, the remainder of the interdisciplinary team, the medical director, the resident and his or her legal representative (in accord with 42 CFR 483.10(b)(2),(d)(2)), ombudsman (with permission of the resident in accord with 42 CFR 483.10(j)(3)), and surveyors.

Response to Irregularities Identified in the MRR

Throughout this guidance, a response from a physician regarding a medication problem implies appropriate communication, review, and resident management, but does not imply that the physician must necessarily order tests or treatments recommended or requested by the staff, unless the physician determines that those are medically valid and indicated.

For those issues that require physician intervention, the physician either accepts and acts upon the report and potential recommendations or rejects all or some of the report and provides a brief explanation of why the recommendation is rejected, such as in a dated progress note. It is not acceptable for a physician to document only that he/she disagrees with the report, without providing some basis for disagreeing.

If there is the potential for serious harm and the attending physician does not concur with or take action on the report, the facility and the pharmacist should contact the facility's medical director for guidance and possible intervention to resolve the issue. The facility should have a procedure to resolve the situation when the attending physician is also the medical director. For those recommendations that do not require a physician intervention, such as one to monitor vital signs or weights, the director of nursing or designated licensed nurse addresses and documents action(s) taken.

INVESTIGATIVE PROTOCOL

Refer to the Investigative Protocol at F329 for evaluation of medication regimen review.

DETERMINATION OF COMPLIANCE (Task 6, Appendix P)

Synopsis of regulation (F428)

This requirement has four aspects relating to the safety of the resident's medication regimen, including:

- A review by the pharmacist of each resident's medication regimen at least once a month or more frequently depending upon the resident's condition and the risks or adverse consequences related to current medication(s);
- The identification of any irregularities;
- Reporting irregularities to the attending physician and the director of nursing; and
- Action in response to irregularities reported.

Criteria for compliance

Compliance with 42 CFR 483.60(c)(1) and (2), F428, Medication Regimen Review

The facility is in compliance with this requirement if:

- The pharmacist has performed a medication regimen review on each resident at least once a month or more frequently depending upon the resident's condition and/or risks or adverse consequence associated with the medication regimen;
- The pharmacist has identified any existing irregularities;
- The pharmacist has reported any identified irregularities to the director of nursing and attending physician; and
- The report of any irregularities has been acted upon.

If not, cite F428.

Noncompliance for F428

After completing the Investigative Protocol, analyze the data in order to determine whether or not compliance with F428 exists. A determination of noncompliance with F428 does not require a finding of harm to the resident. Noncompliance may include (but is not limited to) one or more of the following:

- The pharmacist failed to conduct an MRR at least monthly (or more frequently, as indicated).
- The pharmacist failed to identify or report the absence of or inadequate indications for use of a medication, or a medication or medication combination with significant potential for adverse consequences or medication interactions.

- The pharmacist failed to identify or report medications in a resident's regimen that could (as of the review date) be causing or associated with new, worsening, or progressive signs and symptoms.
- The pharmacist failed to identify and report the absence of any explanation as to why or how the benefit of a medication(s) with potential for clinically significant adverse consequences outweighs the risk.
- The pharmacist failed to identify and report the lack of evidence or documentation regarding progress toward treatment goals.
- The facility failed to act upon a report of clinically significant risks or existing adverse consequences or other irregularities.

Potential Tags for Additional Investigation

If noncompliance with 483.60(c)(1) and (2) has been identified, then concerns with additional requirements may also have been identified. The surveyor is cautioned to investigate these related additional requirements before determining whether noncompliance with the additional requirements may be present. Examples of some of the related requirements that should be considered when noncompliance has been identified include the following:

- 42 CFR 483.10(b)(11), F157, Notification of Changes
    - Review whether the facility contacted the attending physician regarding a significant change in the resident's condition in relation to a potential adverse consequence of a medication, or a need to alter treatment significantly (i.e., a need to discontinue an existing form of treatment due to adverse consequences, or to commence a different form of treatment).
- 42 CFR 483.25(l), F329, Unnecessary Medications
    - Review whether the resident is receiving any medications without an indication for use, in excessive dose or duration, with inadequate monitoring, or in the presence of any adverse consequences that indicate that the dose should be reduced or discontinued.
- 42 CFR 483.40(a), F385, Physician Supervision
    - Review whether the attending physician supervised the resident's medical treatment, including assessing the resident's condition, identifying the need for and continuing use of medication to address the resident's needs, and identifying and addressing adverse consequences related to

medications.

- 42 CFR 483.40(b), F385, Physician Visits

    - Review whether the attending physician or another designated practitioner reviewed the resident's total program of care including the beneficial and adverse effects of medications and treatment, and provided a relevant progress note at each visit.

- 42 CFR 483.60(a)(b)(1), F425, Pharmacy Services

    - Review whether the licensed pharmacist has provided consultation regarding all aspects of pharmaceutical services.

- 42 CFR 483.75(i), F501, Medical Director

    - Review whether the medical director, when requested by the facility, interacted with the attending physician regarding an inadequate response to identified or reported potential medication irregularities and adverse consequences.

IV. DEFICIENCY CATEGORIZATION (Part IV, Appendix P)

Once the survey team has completed its investigation, analyzed the data, reviewed the regulatory requirements, and determined that noncompliance exists, the team must determine the severity of each deficiency, based on the resultant harm or potential for harm to the resident. The survey team must identify whether noncompliance cited at other tags (e.g., F329, F332/333) was the direct result of or related to inadequate or absent MRR or response to notification regarding irregularities.

The key elements for severity determination for F428 are as follows:

1. Presence of potential or actual harm/negative outcome(s) due to a facility failure related to the MRR.

Identify actual or potential harm/negative outcomes which for F428 may include, but are not limited to:

- The resident experienced a clinically significant adverse consequence associated with a medication.

- Irregularities within the medication regimen or inaccuracy of medication-related documents created the potential for adverse consequences such as overdose, respiratory depression, rash, or anorexia.

2. **Degree of potential or actual harm/negative outcome(s) due to a facility failure related to the MRR.**

   Identify to what degree the facility practices caused, resulted in, allowed, or contributed to the actual or potential harm:

- If harm has occurred, determine if the harm is at the level of serious injury, impairment, death, compromise, or discomfort; or
- If harm has not yet occurred, determine the potential for serious injury, impairment, death, compromise, or discomfort to occur to the resident.

3. **The immediacy of correction required.**

   Determine whether the noncompliance requires immediate correction in order to prevent serious injury, harm, impairment, or death to one or more residents.

The survey team must evaluate the harm or potential for harm based upon the following levels of severity for tag F428. First, the team must rule out whether Severity Level 4, Immediate Jeopardy, to a resident's health or safety, exists by evaluating the deficient practice in relation to immediacy, culpability, and severity. (Follow the guidance in Appendix Q, Guidelines for Determining Immediate Jeopardy.)

NOTE: The death or transfer of a resident who was harmed or injured as a result of facility noncompliance does not remove a finding of immediate jeopardy. The facility is required to implement specific actions to remove the jeopardy and correct the noncompliance which allowed or caused the immediate jeopardy.

Severity Level 4 Considerations: Immediate Jeopardy to Resident Health or Safety

Immediate Jeopardy is a situation in which the facility's noncompliance with one or more requirements of participation:

- Has allowed, caused, or resulted in, or is likely to allow, cause, or result in serious injury, harm, impairment, or death to a resident; and
- Requires immediate correction, as the facility either created the situation or allowed the situation to continue by failing to implement preventative or corrective measures.

Examples may include, but are not limited to:

- Despite identifying irregularities with the potential for serious harm or death, the pharmacist did not report the irregularities to the attending physician or no action was taken on the irregularities reported.

- Findings of noncompliance at Severity Level 4 at Tag(s) F309, F329, F332, or F333 that show evidence of process failures for conducting the MRR.

- Repeated or cumulative failures in multiple areas of the medication regimen review process (e.g., failure to identify, report, or act upon) that resulted in the resident(s) experiencing actual or potential harm.

NOTE: If immediate jeopardy has been ruled out based upon the evidence, then evaluate whether actual harm that is not immediate jeopardy exists at Severity Level 3.

Severity Level 3 Considerations: Actual Harm that is Not Immediate Jeopardy

Level 3 indicates noncompliance that resulted in actual harm, and may include, but is not limited to, clinical compromise, decline, or the resident's inability to maintain and/or reach his/her highest practicable well-being. Examples may include, but are not limited to:

- The pharmacist's MRR failed to identify the indication for continued use for opioid analgesics that had been prescribed for a resident's acute pain which had resolved. As a result of prolonged duration of use, the resident became more lethargic, withdrawn, and anorectic.

- The pharmacist's MRR identified that the staff were crushing medications that should not be crushed, based on inappropriate standing orders to crush all medications. As a result of facility failure to act upon the notification, the resident experienced clinically significant adverse consequences such as hypoglycemia or hypotension that required medical intervention.

- The pharmacist's MRR identified that medications were not being given as ordered (such as antiparkinsons or pain medications not given prior to physical therapy), which may have contributed to impaired function. The facility failed to take any action to adhere to the orders.

- **The physician and/or director of nursing failed to act in response to the pharmacist's MRR which identified the indefinite continuation of an antidepressant in a resident who had no history of depression, who had been placed on the antidepressant without an evaluation to confirm presence of depression, and whose function and mood were not monitored while getting the medication for months. The resident experienced clinically significant adverse consequences such as falls, constipation, or change in weight.**

- The pharmacist's MRR failed to identify and report the medication regimen as a possible cause of recurrent falling in a resident who was given increasing doses of anticonvulsants to treat behavioral symptoms related to dementia, resulting in serious injury.

- The pharmacist's MRR failed to identify and report clinically significant medication interactions in a resident who was started on warfarin, and who had also been receiving one or more of the following: digoxin, phenytoin, antibiotics, amiodarone, or an oral antifungal, resulting in a marked elevation in the INR with significant gastrointestinal bleeding or hematuria.

- Findings of noncompliance at Severity Level 3 at tag(s) F309, F329, F332, F333 that show evidence of process failures for conducting the MRR.

NOTE: If Severity Level 3 (actual harm that is not immediate jeopardy) has been ruled out based upon the evidence, then evaluate as to whether Severity Level 2 (no actual harm with the potential for more than minimal harm) exists.

Severity Level 2 Considerations: No Actual Harm with Potential for More Than Minimal Harm that is Not Immediate Jeopardy

Level 2 indicates noncompliance that resulted in a resident outcome of no more than minimal discomfort and/or has the potential to compromise the resident's ability to maintain or reach his or her highest practicable level of well-being. The potential exists for greater harm to occur if interventions are not provided. Examples include, but are not limited to:

- **The facility failed to respond to the pharmacist's notification that the resident was not receiving all the medications ordered; however, there was no change in the resident condition.**

- The pharmacist's MRR failed to identify and report a resident who is receiving multiple antihypertensive medications, but is not being monitored for postural hypotension, and who complains of lightheadedness especially while upright.

- The pharmacist's MRR failed to identify and report risks of hyperkalemia in a resident who has impaired renal function and is receiving an ACE inhibitor and potassium supplements.

- The pharmacist's MRR failed to evaluate and report on the potential adverse consequences of a medication known to cause anorexia for a resident with a recently decreased appetite, who had not yet experienced a significant unplanned weight loss.

- Findings of noncompliance at Severity Level 2 at tag(s) F309, F329, or F332, F333 that show evidence of process failures for conducting the MRR.

NOTE: If Severity Level 2 (no actual harm with potential for more than minimal harm that is not immediate jeopardy) has been ruled out based upon the evidence, then evaluate as to whether Severity Level 1 (no actual harm with the potential for minimal harm) exists.

Severity Level 1 Considerations: No Actual Harm with Potential for Minimal Harm

Level 1 indicates noncompliance that resulted in no harm to the resident, and the potential for no more than minimal harm. Examples may include, but are not limited to:

- The pharmacist conducted the medication review, identified an irregularity that has not resulted in a negative outcome and is of minimal consequence (such as a multi-vitamin not being given as ordered) and reported to the director of nursing and attending physician, but neither of them acted upon the report.

F431

(Rev. 22, Issued: 12-15-06, Effective/Implementation: 12-18-06)

§483.60(b) Service Consultation. The facility must employ or obtain the services of a licensed pharmacist who--

(2) Establishes a system of records of receipt and disposition of all controlled drugs in sufficient detail to enable an accurate reconciliation; and

(3) Determines that drug records are in order and that an account of all controlled drugs is maintained and periodically reconciled.

§483.60(d) Labeling of Drugs and Biologicals

Drugs and biologicals used in the facility must be labeled in accordance with currently accepted professional principles, and include the appropriate accessory and cautionary instructions, and the expiration date when applicable.

(e) Storage of Drugs and Biologicals

(1) In accordance with State and Federal laws, the facility must store all drugs and biologicals in locked compartments under proper temperature controls, and permit only authorized personnel to have access to the keys.

(2) The facility must provide separately locked, permanently affixed compartments for storage of controlled drugs listed in Schedule II of the Comprehensive Drug Abuse Prevention and Control Act of 1976 and other drugs subject to abuse, except

when the facility uses single unit package drug distribution systems in which the quantity stored is minimal and a missing dose can be readily detected.

INTENT (F431) 42 CFR 483.60(b)(2)(3)(d) Labeling of Drugs and Biologicals & (e) Storage of Drugs and Biologicals

The intent of this requirement is that the facility, in coordination with the licensed pharmacist, provides for:

- Safe and secure storage (including proper temperature controls, limited access, and mechanisms to minimize loss or diversion) and safe handling (including disposition) of all medication;

- Accurate labeling to facilitate consideration of precautions and safe administration of medications;

- A system of medication records that enables periodic accurate reconciliation and accounting of all controlled medications; and

- Identification of loss or diversion of controlled medications so as to minimize the time between actual loss or diversion and the detection and determination of the extent of loss or diversion.

NOTE: For purposes of this guidance, references to "the pharmacist" mean the licensed pharmacist, whether employed directly by the facility or through arrangement.

DEFINITIONS (refer to F425 and F428 for additional definitions)

- "Adverse consequence" refers to an unpleasant symptom or event that is due to or associated with a medication, such as impairment or decline in an individual's mental or physical condition or functional or psychosocial status. It may include various types of adverse drug reactions and interactions (e.g., medication-medication, medication-food, and medication-disease).

- "Clinically significant" refers to effects, results, or consequences that materially affect or are likely to affect an individual's physical, mental, or psychosocial well-being either positively by preventing, stabilizing, or improving a condition or reducing a risk, or negatively by exacerbating, causing, or contributing to a symptom, illness, or decline in status.

OVERVIEW

Due to the number and types of medications that may be used and the vulnerable populations being served, the regulations require a long term care facility to have formal mechanisms to safely handle and control medications, and to maintain accurate and timely medication records. These regulations also require the facility to use a pharmacist to help establish and evaluate these mechanisms or systems. This guidance addresses those portions of the facility's pharmaceutical services related to medication access and storage, appropriate security and safeguarding of controlled medications, and labeling of medications to assure that they are stored safely and are provided to the residents accurately and in accordance with the prescriber's instructions.

MEDICATION ACCESS AND STORAGE

A facility is required to secure all medications in a locked storage area and to limit access to authorized personnel (for example, pharmacy technicians or assistants who have been delegated access to medications by the facility's pharmacist as a function of their jobs) consistent with state or federal requirements and professional standards of practice.

Storage areas may include, but are not limited to, drawers, cabinets, medication rooms, refrigerators, and carts. Depending on how the facility locks and stores medications, access to a medication room may not necessarily provide access to the medications (for example, medications stored in a locked cart, locked cabinets, a locked refrigerator, or locked drawers within the medication room). When medications are not stored in separately locked compartments within a storage area, only appropriately authorized staff may have access to the storage area.

Access to medications can be controlled by keys, security codes or cards, or other technology such as fingerprints. Schedule II medications must be maintained in separately locked, permanently affixed compartments. The access system (e.g. key, security codes) used to lock Schedule II medications and other medications subject to abuse, cannot be the same access system used to obtain the non-scheduled medications. The facility must have a system to limit who has security access and when access is used. Exception: Controlled medications and those subject to abuse may be stored with non-controlled medications as part of a single unit package medication distribution system, if the supply of the medication(s) is minimal and a shortage is readily detectable.

During a medication pass, medications must be under the direct observation of the person administering the medications or locked in the medication storage area/cart. In addition, the facility should have procedures for the control and safe storage of medications for those residents who can self-administer medications.

Safe medication storage includes the provision of appropriate environmental controls. Because many medications can be altered by exposure to improper temperature, light, or humidity, it is important that the facility implement procedures that address and monitor the safe storage and handling of medications in accordance with manufacturers' specifications, State requirements and standards of practice (e.g., United States Pharmacopeia (USP) standards).

CONTROLLED MEDICATIONS

Regulations require that the facility have a system to account for the receipt, usage, disposition, and reconciliation of all controlled medications. This system includes, but is not limited to:

- **Record of receipt of all controlled medications with sufficient detail to allow reconciliation (e.g., specifying the name and strength of the medication, the quantity and date received, and the resident's name). However, in some delivery systems (e.g., single unit package medication delivery system or automated dispensing systems utilizing single-unit packages of medications that are not dispensed pursuant to a specific order), the resident's name may not be applicable;**

  NOTE: **The facility may store some controlled medications in an emergency medication supply in accordance with state requirements. The facility's policies and procedures must address the reconciliation and monitoring of this supply.**

- **Records of usage and disposition of all controlled medications with sufficient detail to allow reconciliation (e.g., the medication administration record [MAR], proof-of-use sheets, or declining inventory sheets), including destruction, wastage, return to the pharmacy/manufacturer, or disposal in accordance with applicable State requirements;**

- Periodic reconciliation of records of receipt, disposition and inventory for all controlled medications (monthly or more frequently as defined by facility procedures or when loss is identified). The reconciliation identifies loss or diversion of controlled medications so as to minimize the time between the actual loss or diversion and the time of detection and follow-up to determine the extent of loss. Because diversion can occur at any time, the reconciliation should be done often enough to identify problems. Some State or other federal requirements may specify the frequency of reconciliation.

  - If discrepancies are identified during the reconciliation, the pharmacist and the facility develop and implement recommendations for resolving them.

  - If the systems have not been effective in preventing or identifying diversion or loss, it is important that the pharmacist and the facility review and revise related controls and procedures, as necessary, such as increasing the frequency of monitoring or the amount of detail used to document controlled substances.

NOTE: The pharmacist is not required by these regulations to perform the reconciliation, but rather to evaluate and determine that the facility maintains an account of all controlled medications and completes the reconciliation according to its procedures, consistent with State and federal requirements.

LABELING OF MEDICATIONS AND BIOLOGICALS

This section requires facility compliance with currently accepted labeling requirements, even though the pharmacies are responsible for the actual labeling. Labeling of medications and biologicals dispensed by the pharmacy must be consistent with applicable federal and State requirements and currently accepted pharmaceutical principles and practices. Although medication delivery systems may vary, the medication label at a minimum includes the medication name (generic and/or brand) and strength, the expiration date when applicable, and typically includes the resident's name, route of administration, appropriate instructions and precautions (such as shake well, with meals, do not crush, special storage instructions).

For medications designed for multiple administrations (e.g., inhalers, eye drops), the label is affixed in a manner to promote administration to the resident for whom it was prescribed.

When medications are prepared or compounded for intravenous infusion, the label contains the name and volume of the solution, resident's name, infusion rate, name and quantity of each additive, date of preparation, initials of compounder, date and time of administration, initials of person administering medication if different than compounder, ancillary precautions as applicable, and date after which the mixture must not be used.

For over-the-counter (OTC) medications in bulk containers (e.g., in states that permit bulk OTC medications to be stocked in the facility), the label contains the original manufacturer's or pharmacy-applied label indicating the medication name, strength, quantity, accessory instructions, lot number, and expiration date when applicable. If supplies of bulk OTC medications are used for a specific resident, the container identifies that resident by name and must contain the original manufacturer's or pharmacy-applied label.

The facility ensures that medication labeling in response to order changes is accurate and consistent with applicable state requirements.

INVESTIGATIVE PROTOCOL

For investigating compliance with the requirement at 483.60(d) & (e), see State Operations Manual, Appendix P, II.B. The Traditional Standard Survey, Task 5, Sub-Task 5E Investigative Protocol: Medication Pass and Pharmacy Services.

DETERMINATION OF COMPLIANCE (Task 6, Appendix P)

Synopsis of regulation (F431)

This requirement has several aspects. The pharmaceutical services must:

- Provide for the safe and secure storage of medications, i.e., medications must be stored at proper temperatures and locked at all times (except when under direct staff observation);
- Limit access to medications only to authorized staff;
- Label medications in accordance with Federal and State labeling requirements and accepted standards of practice; and
- Have safeguards and systems in place to control, account for, and periodically reconcile controlled medications.

Criteria for Compliance

Compliance with 42 CFR 483.60(b)(2)(3)(d)(e), F431, Labeling, Storage, and Controlled Medications

The facility is in compliance if:

- The facility safeguards medications by locking the medications, limiting access, and disposing of medications appropriately;
- Medications are stored under proper temperature controls and in accordance with manufacturers' specifications;
- Medication labeling identifies, at a minimum, the medication's name, strength, expiration date when applicable, and lot number, and provides instructions as necessary for safe administration;
- Schedule II medications are stored in separately locked, permanently affixed compartments, except when the facility uses single unit medication distribution systems in which the quantity stored is minimal and a missing dose can be readily detected; and
- Controlled medications are reconciled accurately.

If not, cite F431.

Noncompliance for F431

After completing the investigation, determine whether compliance with the regulation exists. Noncompliance for F431 may include (but is not limited to) facility failure to:

- Store medications to preserve their integrity, for example allowing medications that should be stored between 40 and 86 degrees Fahrenheit to either reach temperatures below 32 degrees or above 100 degrees;

- Provide accurate labeling with appropriate accessory and cautionary instructions, thereby creating a potential for the wrong medication to be administered or for the correct medications to be given by the wrong route; and

- Accurately reconcile controlled medications.

IV. DEFICIENCY CATEGORIZATION (Part IV, Appendix P)

Once the survey team has completed its investigation, analyzed the data, reviewed the regulatory requirements, and determined that noncompliance exists, the team must determine the severity of each deficiency, based on the resultant harm or potential for harm to the resident.

The key elements for severity determination for F431 are as follows:

1. Presence of actual or potential harm/negative outcome(s) due to a facility failure related to storage, labeling, or reconciliation of controlled medications.

Identify actual or potential harm/negative outcomes for F431 which may include, but are not limited to:

- Accidental ingestion of medication(s) by a resident(s) as a result of failure to lock medications;

- One or more residents received (or had the potential to receive) the wrong medication or dose or the correct medication by the wrong route as a result of inaccurate or incomplete labeling; or

- Potential for a resident(s) to receive potentially ineffective medication(s) as a result of storing medications or vaccines at wrong temperatures, resulting in their potential inactivation.

2. Degree of actual or potential harm/negative outcome(s) due to a facility failure related to storage, labeling, or reconciliation of controlled medications.

Identify how the facility practices caused, resulted in, allowed, or contributed to the actual or potential for harm:

- If harm has occurred, determine if the harm is at the level of serious injury, impairment, death, compromise, or discomfort; or

- If harm has not yet occurred, determine the potential for serious injury, impairment, death, compromise, or discomfort to occur to the resident.

3. **The immediacy of correction required.**

Determine whether the noncompliance requires immediate correction in order to prevent serious injury, harm, impairment, or death to one or more residents.

The survey team must evaluate the harm or potential for harm based upon the following levels of severity for tag F431. First, the team must rule out whether Severity Level 4, Immediate Jeopardy, to a resident's health or safety, exists by evaluating the deficient practice in relation to immediacy, culpability, and severity. (Follow the guidance in Appendix Q, Guidelines for Determining Immediate Jeopardy.)

NOTE: The death or transfer of a resident who was harmed or injured as a result of facility noncompliance does not remove a finding of immediate jeopardy. The facility is required to implement specific actions to remove the jeopardy and correct the noncompliance which allowed or caused the immediate jeopardy.

Severity Level 4 Considerations: Immediate Jeopardy to Resident Health or Safety

Immediate Jeopardy is a situation in which the facility's noncompliance with one or more requirements of participation:

- Has caused/resulted in, or is likely to cause, serious injury, harm, impairment, or death to a resident; and

- Requires immediate correction as the facility either created the situation or allowed the situation to continue by failing to implement preventative or corrective measures.

Examples may include, but are not limited to:

- The facility failed to restrict access to medications resulting in serious injury or harm or death from ingestion of the medications (e.g., warfarin, digoxin, antibiotics, opioids, anticonvulsants, antipsychotics) or posed a significant risk to the health of the residents resulting in the potential for clinically significant adverse consequences such as kidney or liver failure, anaphylaxis, cardiac arrest, or death; or

- As a result of an incorrect label on the package, staff administered the wrong medication or wrong dose(s) of a medication (e.g., anticonvulsant, antihyperglycemic, benzodiazepine) with a potential for clinically significant adverse consequences, which resulted in or had the potential for serious harm or death (e.g., toxic levels of the medication, unresponsiveness, uncontrolled seizures).

NOTE: If immediate jeopardy has been ruled out based upon the evidence, then evaluate whether actual harm that is not immediate jeopardy exists at Severity Level 3.

Severity Level 3 Considerations: Actual Harm that is Not Immediate Jeopardy

Level 3 indicates noncompliance that resulted in actual harm, and can include but may not be limited to compromise, decline, or interference with the resident's ability to maintain and/or reach his/her highest practicable well-being. Examples may include, but are not limited to:

- Medication labeling was incomplete and lacked instructions that the medication was not to be given with specific foods (e.g., milk or milk-based products) resulting in altered effectiveness of the medication and worsening of the residents' symptoms, requiring medical intervention; or

- The facility failed to implement a system to reconcile controlled medications. As a result, medications were unavailable for residents for whom the medications were prescribed. Residents experienced moderate pain that compromised their ability to perform ADLs.

NOTE: If Severity Level 3 (actual harm that is not immediate jeopardy) has been ruled out based upon the evidence, then evaluate as to whether Severity Level 2 (no actual harm with the potential for more than minimal harm) exists.

Severity Level 2 Considerations: No Actual Harm with Potential for More Than Minimal Harm that is Not Immediate Jeopardy

Level 2 indicates noncompliance that resulted in a resident outcome of no more than minimal discomfort and/or the potential to compromise the resident's ability to maintain or reach his or her highest practicable level of well-being. The potential exists for greater harm to occur if interventions are not provided. Examples may include, but are not limited to:

- The facility's medication cart was not kept locked or under direct observation of authorized staff and a wandering resident with dementia ingested a medication that he/she had taken off the cart but did not suffer any adverse consequences; or

- As a result of inaccurate labeling, the resident received the wrong medication or dose or the correct medication by the wrong route and experienced discomfort but did not require any interventions.

NOTE: If Severity Level 2 (no actual harm with potential for more than minimal harm that is not immediate jeopardy) has been ruled out based upon the evidence, then evaluate as to whether Severity Level 1 (no actual harm with the potential for minimal harm) exists.

Severity Level 1 Considerations: No Actual Harm with Potential for Minimal Harm

Level 1 indicates noncompliance that resulted in no harm to the resident, and the potential for no more than minimal harm. Examples may include, but are not limited to:

- The facility failed to reconcile controlled medications but there was no negative resident outcome and no potential for more than minimal harm.

F441

§483.65 Infection Control

The facility must establish and maintain an infection control program designed to provide a safe, sanitary, and comfortable environment and to help prevent the development and transmission of disease and infection.

§483.65(a) Infection Control Program

The facility must establish an infection control program under which it--

(1) Investigates, controls, and prevents infections in the facility;

(2) Decides what procedures, such as isolation should be applied to an individual resident; and

(3) Maintains a record of incidents and corrective actions related to infections.

Intent §483.65(a)

The intent of this regulation is to assure that the facility has an infection control program which is effective for investigating, controlling, and preventing infections. If infection control has been identified as an area of concern during Phase 1 of the survey, investigate aspects of the program, as appropriate, during Phase 2.

Interpretive Guidelines §483.65(a)

The facility's infection control program must have a system to monitor and investigate causes of infection (nosocomial and community acquired) and manner of spread. A facility should, for example, maintain a separate record on infection that identifies each resident with an infection, states the date of infection, the causative agent, the origin or site of infection, and describes what cautionary measures were taken to prevent the spread of the infection within the facility. The system must enable the facility to analyze clusters, changes in prevalent organisms, or increases in the rate of infection in a timely manner.

Surveillance data should be routinely reviewed and recommendations made for the prevention and control of additional cases.

The written infection control program should be periodically reviewed by the facility and revised as indicated.

Current standards for infection control program address the following. The following are not regulatory requirements but provide guidance for evaluating the facility's program.

- Definition of nosocomial/facility acquired infections and communicable diseases.

- Risk assessment of occurrence of communicable diseases for both residents and staff that is reviewed annually, or more frequently if indicated.

- Methods for identifying, documenting and investigating nosocomial infections and communicable diseases. The infection control program should be able to identify new infections quickly, paying particular attention to residents at high risk of infection of infection (e.g. residents who are immobilized, have invasive devices or procedures, have pressure sores, have been recently discharged from a hospital to the long term care facility, have MI or MR, have decreased mental status, are nutritionally compromised or have altered immune systems).

- Early detection of residents who have signs and symptoms of TB and a referral protocol to a facility where TB can be evaluated and managed appropriately.

- Measures for prevention of infections, especially those associated with intravascular therapy, indwelling urinary catheters, tracheostomy care, stoma care, respiratory care, immunosuppression, pressures sores, bladder and bowel incontinence and any other factors which compromise a resident's resistance to infections.

- Measures for the prevention of communicable disease outbreaks, including tuberculosis, flu, hepatitis, scabies, MRSA.

- Procedures to inform and involve a local or State epidemiologist, as required by the State for non-sporadic, facility-wide infections that are difficult to control.

- Isolation procedures and requirements for infected and at risk or immunosuppressed nursing home residents.

- Use of and inservice education regarding standard precautions, (e.g., universal precautions/body substance isolation).

- Handwashing, respiratory protection, linen handling, housekeeping, needle and hazardous waste disposal, as well as other means for limiting the spread of communicable organisms.

- Authority, indications, and procedures for obtaining and acting upon microbiological cultures from residents and for isolating residents.

- Proper use of disinfectants, antiseptics and germicides in accordance with the manufacturers' instructions and EPA of FDA label specifications to avoid harm to staff, residents and visitors and to ensure its effectiveness.

- Orientation of all new facility personnel to the infection control program and periodic updates for all staff.

- Measures for the screening of the health care workers for communicable diseases, and for the evaluation of workers exposed to residents with communicable diseases including TB and Blood Borne Pathogens.

- Work restriction guidelines for an employee that is infected or ill with a communicable disease.

- Measures which address prevention of infection common to nursing home residents (e.g., vaccination for influenza and pneumococcal pneumonia as appropriate) TB screening and testing.

- Sanitization of tubs, whirlpools and multiple use equipment to be performed according to manufacturer's recommendations.

Observe whether staff including direct care, housekeeping, kitchen staff, use gloves in accord with aseptic principles.

Determine if there is consistent use of aseptic technique for dressing changes.

If breaks in technique are observed, verify that the facility has a system in place for routine monitoring of staff infection control practices.

Ask direct care giver staff what do they do and who do they notify when an infection is noted.

Procedures: §483.65(a)

Observe sanitation of tub, shower, multiple residents' whirlpool and care equipment, as necessary.

Identify all residents in the sample who are currently on antibiotic therapy and verify that these residents are reported on the facility's infection control logs/records to ensure that infections are being identified timely and that these residents are being adequately monitored for infection.

Review policies related to infection control if observation, record review, or staff interview indicate a problem with infection control.

Observe direct care staff routinely washing their hands according to facility written protocols.

Probes: §483.65(a)

- Are there unexplained and/or similar infections?
- For sampled residents at high risk of infection, what has staff done to reduce residents' risk of infection?
- Do surveillance data show a significant increase in the rate of infection from month to month? Over several months? How is this being addressed?
- What infection control policies does the facility use for persons with AIDS, TB, or hepatitis B? Do these policies conform with Occupational Safety and Health Administration's requirements for protecting employees and current accepted standards of practice recommended by Centers for Disease Control and Prevention (CDC)? Does the staff follow its own procedures?
- How does the facility define and dispose of its infectious waste?

F442

§483.65(b) Preventing Spread of Infection

(1) When the infection control program determines that a resident needs isolation to prevent the spread of infection, the facility must isolate the resident.

Intent §483.65(b)

The intent of this regulation is to assure that the facility isolates residents appropriately to prevent the spread of infection. If infection control has been identified as an area of concern during Phase 1 of the survey, investigate aspects of the program, as appropriate, during Phase 2.

Interpretive Guidelines: §483.65(b)

Procedures must be followed to prevent cross-contamination, including handwashing and/or changing gloves after providing personal care, or when performing tasks among individuals which provide the opportunity for cross-contamination to occur. Facilities for handwashing must exist and be available to staff. The facility should follow the CDC's "Guideline for Handwashing and Hospital Environmental Control," 1985 for handwashing.

The facility should isolate infected residents only to the degree needed to isolate the infecting organism. The method used should be the least restrictive possible, while maintaining the integrity of the process. For example, the HIV virus is present in blood and other body fluids. The facility should take universal or standard blood and body fluid precautions related to HIV contamination for the following:

- Blood;
- Semen;
- Vaginal secretions;
- Cerebrospinal fluid;
- Synovial fluid;
- Pleural fluid;
- Peritoneal fluid;
- Pericardial fluid;
- Amniotic fluid; and/or
- Fluids with visible blood.

Residents, visitors and employees should be protected from these fluids. Although the resident infected with HIV should not be isolated routinely, the resident should be isolated if he/she is in the communicable stages of an opportunistic infection, his/her body fluids cannot be contained or he/she has very poor hygiene and the likelihood of spillage is high.

NOTE: TB isolation rooms are not needed if the facility does not provide care to active TB patients/residents.

"Universal precautions" or "Standard blood and body fluid precautions" is an approach to infection control where all human blood and certain human body fluids are treated as if known to be infectious for HIV, HBV, and other bloodborne pathogens.

Probes: §483.65(b)

- For isolated residents, does the facility need to segregate them to control the infectious agent?

- For residents who have been isolated appropriately, does staff use correct procedures consistently? For example, if isolation procedures require wearing gowns, do **all** staff put on and dispose of the gown in a way that lessens the spread of infection?

- How does the facility control the spread of infection by persons who visit infectious residents? Is there a written protocol?

- Do persons with a communicable disease or infected skin lesions provide care to residents?

- Have any residents developed a communicable disease as defined by State law while in the facility? If so, have appropriate barrier or isolation precautions been followed to control further spread of infection?

Procedures: §483.65(b)(1)

Verify that all residents who require isolation as determined by the infection control program are isolated. Observe residents that have been isolated. Determine what level of isolation they are required to have. Evaluate isolation procedures utilized by staff members. Determine if the facility has isolated the resident in the least restrictive environment possible.

F443

§483.65(b)(2) The facility must prohibit employees with a communicable disease or infected skin lesions from direct contact with residents or their food, if direct contact will transmit the disease.

Intent: §483.65(b)(2)

The intent of this regulation is to prevent the spread of communicable diseases from employees to residents when the employee has a communicable disease or an infected skin lesion.

Skin lesions should be considered infected if they have purulent drainage, or are res, hot, indurated without purulent drainage.

Procedures: §483.65(b)(2)

Determine if the facility prohibits employees with diseases communicable through direct contact or infected skin lesions from having direct contact with residents. To make this determination, observe residents' condition and treatments provided, interview facility staff, and review relevant facility policies and procedures for preventing the spread of infection.

F444

§483.65(b)(3) The facility must require staff to wash their hands after each direct resident contact for which handwashing is indicated by accepted professional practice.

Intent: §483.65(b)(3)

The intent of this regulation is to assure that staff use appropriate handwashing techniques to prevent the spread of infection from one resident to another

Interpretive Guidelines: §483.65(b)(3)

Procedures must be followed to prevent cross-contamination, including handwashing or changing gloves after providing personal care, or when performing tasks among individuals which provide the opportunity for cross-contamination to occur. Facilities for handwashing must exist and be readily available to staff. The facility should follow the CDC's "Guideline for Handwashing and Hospital Environmental Control, 1985," for handwashing.

Procedures: §483.65(b)(3)

Verify that the facility has policy that requires staff to wash their hands after each direct resident contact when indicated. Observe hand washing by staff after direct contact with residents.

It is important for the surveyor to begin a thorough investigation of the facility's infection control program when poor resident outcomes and poor practices are observed.

Probes: §483.65(b)(3)

- Does the facility have a written protocol describing handwashing practices and is it consistent with the latest published standards?
- Do staff follow the facility policy and protocol for handwashing?

F445

§483.65(c) Linens

Personnel must handle, store, process, and transport linens so as to prevent the spread of infection

Intent: §483.65(c)

The intent of this regulation is to prevent the spread of infection through linens.

Interpretive Guidelines: §483.65(c)

Soiled linens should be handled to contain and to minimize aerosolization and exposure to any waste products. Soiled linen storage areas should be well ventilated and maintained under a relative negative air pressure. The laundry should be designed to eliminate crossing of soiled and clean linen.

Probes: §483.65(c)

- Do staff handle linens on the resident care floors and in the laundry area to prevent the spread of infection?
- Do staff follow the facility's protocols for handling linens?
- Are linens processed, transported, stored, and handled properly?

F454

§483.70 Physical Environment

The facility must be designed, constructed, equipped, and maintained to protect the health and safety of residents, personnel and the public.

§483.70(a) Life Safety From Fire

§483.70(a)(1) Except as otherwise provided in this section –

§483.70(a)(1)(i) the facility must meet the applicable provisions of the 2000 edition of the Life Safety Code of the National Fire Protection Association. The Director of the Office of the Federal Register has approved the NFPA 101® 2000 edition of the Life Safety Code, issued January 14, 2000, for incorporation by reference in accordance with 5 U.S.C. 552(a) and 1 CFR part 51. A copy of the Code is available for inspection at the CMS Information Resource Center, 7500 Security Boulevard, Baltimore, MD or at the National Archives and Records Administration (NARA). For information on the availability of this material at NARA, call 202-741-6030, or go to http://www.archives.gov/federal_register/code_of_federal_regulations/ibr_locations.html. Copies may be obtained from the National Fire Protection Association, 1 Batterymarch Park, Quincy, MA 02269. If any changes in this edition of the Code are incorporated by reference, CMS will publish notice in the FEDERAL REGISTER to announce the changes.

§483.70(a)(1)(ii) Chapter 19.3.6.3.2, exception number 2 of the adopted edition of the LSC does not apply to long-term care facilities.
§483.70(a)(2) After consideration of State survey agency findings, CMS may waive specific provisions of the Life Safety Code which, if rigidly applied, would result in unreasonable hardship upon the facility, but only if the waiver does not adversely affect the health and safety of the patients.

§483.70(a)(3) The provisions of the Life Safety Code do not apply in a State where CMS finds, in accordance with applicable provisions of sections 1819(d)(2)(B)(ii) and 1919(d)(2)(B)(ii) of the Act, that a fire and safety code imposed by State law adequately protects patients, residents and personnel in long term care facilities.

§483.70(a)(4) Beginning March 13, 2006, a long-term care facility must be in compliance with Chapter 19.2.9, Emergency Lighting.

§483.70(a)(5) Beginning March 13, 2006, Chapter 19.3.6.3.2, exception number 2 does not apply to long-term care facilities.

§483.70(a)(6) Notwithstanding any provisions of the 2000 edition of the Life Safety Code to the contrary, a long-term care facility may install alcohol-based hand rub dispensers in its facility if -

§483.70(a)(6)(i) Use of alcohol-based hand rub dispensers does not conflict with any State or local codes that prohibit or otherwise restrict the placement of alcohol-based hand rub dispensers in health care facilities;

§483.70(a)(6)(ii) The dispensers are installed in a manner that minimizes leaks and spills that could lead to falls;

§483.70(a)(6)(iii) The dispensers are installed in a manner that adequately protects against access by vulnerable populations; and

§483.70(a)(6)(iv) The dispensers are installed in accordance with chapter 18.3.2.7 or chapter 19.3.2.7 of the 2000 edition of the Life Safety Code, as amended by NFPA Temporary Interim Amendment 00-1(101), issued by the Standards Council of the National Fire Protection Association on April 15, 2004. The Director of the Office of the Federal Register has approved NFPA temporary interim Amendment 00-1(101) for incorporation by reference in accordance with 5 U.S.C. 552(a) and 1 CFR part 51. A copy of the amendment is available for inspection at CMS Information Resource Center, 7500 Security Boulevard, Baltimore, MD and at the Office of the Federal Register, 800 North Capitol Street NW, Suite 700, Washington, DC. Copies may be obtained from the National Fire Protection Association, 1 Battery March Partk, Quincy, MA 02269. If any additional changes are made to this amendment, CMS will publish notice in the Federal Register to announce the changes.

§483.70(a)(7) A long-term care facility must:

§483.70(a)(7)(i) Install battery-operated smoke detectors in resident sleeping rooms and public areas by May 24, 2006.

§483.70(a)(7)(ii) Have a program for testing, maintenance, and battery replacement to insure the reliability of the smoke detectors.

§483.70(a)(7)(iii) Exception:

§483.70(a)(7)(iii)(A) The facility has a hard-wired AC smoke detection system in patient rooms and public areas that is installed, tested, and maintained in accordance with NFPA 72, National Fire Alarm Code, for hard-wired AC systems; or

§483.70(a)(7)(iii)(B) The facility has a sprinkler system throughout that is installed, tested, and maintained in accordance with NFPA 13, Automatic Sprinklers.

Interpretive Guidelines: §483.70(a)

A waiver of specific provisions of the Life Safety Code is reviewed each time a facility is certified. The State fire authority will determine if the waiver continues to be justified, in that compliance with the requirement would result in an unreasonable hardship upon the facility and does not adversely affect the health and safety of residents or personnel. The State fire authority will forward its findings and recommendation as soon as possible to the State survey agency which will forward it to the CMS RO for a decision on granting a waiver.

Procedures: §483.70(a)

The survey for safety from fire is normally conducted by the designated State fire authority. The State agency must establish a procedure for the State fire authority to notify them whether the facility is or is not in compliance with the requirement. If the survey team observes fire hazards or possible deficiencies in life safety from fire, they must notify the designated State fire authority or the RO.

F455

§483.70(b) Emergency Power

(1) An emergency electrical power system must supply power adequate at least for lighting all entrances and exits; equipment to maintain the fire detection, alarm, and extinguishing systems; and life support systems in the event the normal electrical supply is interrupted.

Interpretive Guidelines: §483.70(b)(1)

"**Emergency electrical power system**" includes, at a minimum, battery-operated lighting for all entrances and exits, fire detection and alarm systems, and extinguishing systems.

An "**exit**" is defined as a means of egress which is lighted and has three components: an exit access (corridor leading to the exit), an exit (a door), and an exit discharge (door to the street or public way). We define an entrance as any door through which people enter the facility. Furthermore, when an entrance also serves as an exit, its components (exit access, exit, and exit discharge) must be lighted. A waiver of lighting required for both exits and entrances is not permitted.

Procedures: §483.70(b)(1)

Review results of inspections by the designated State fire safety authority that the emergency power system has been tested periodically and is functioning in accordance with the Life Safety Code.

Check placement of lighting system to ensure proper coverage of the listed areas. Test all batteries to ensure they work.

Probes: §483.70(b)(1)

Is emergency electrical service adequate?

Additional guidance is available in the National Fire Protection Association's Life Safety Code 99 and 101 (NFPA 99 and NFPA 101), 12-5.1.3 which is surveyed in Tags K105 and K106 of the Life Safety code survey.

§483.70(b)(2) When life support systems are used, the facility must provide emergency electrical power with an emergency generator (as defined in NFPA 99, Health Care Facilities) that is located on the premises

Interpretive Guidelines: §483.70(b)(2)

"**Life support systems**" is defined as one or more Electro-mechanical device(s) necessary to sustain life, without which the resident will have a likelihood of dying (e.g., ventilators suction machines if necessary to maintain an open airway). The determination of whether a piece of equipment is life support is a **medical determination** dependent upon the condition of the individual residents of the facility e.g. suction machine maybe required "life support equipment" in a facility, depending on the needs of its residents).

Procedures: §483.70(b)(2)

If life support systems are used determine if there is a working emergency generator at the facility, A generator is not required if a facility does not use life support systems. Check that the emergency generator starts and transfers power under load conditions within 10 seconds after interruption of normal power. Where residents are on life support equipment, **do not test** transfer switches by shutting off the power unless there is an uninterruptible power supply available.

Probes: §483.70(b)(2)

Is there a working generator if the facility is using life support systems?

---

§483.70(c) Space and Equipment

The facility must--

(1) Provide sufficient space and equipment in dining, health services, recreation, and program areas to enable staff to provide residents with needed services as required by these standards and as identified in each resident's plan of care; and

Intent: §483.70 (c)(1)

The intent of this regulation is to ensure that dining, health services, recreation, activities and programs areas are large enough to comfortably accommodate the needs of the residents who usually occupy this space.

Dining, health services, recreation, and program areas should be large enough to comfortably accommodate the persons who usually occupy that space, including the wheelchairs, walkers, and other ambulating aids used by the many residents who require more than standard movement spaces. "Sufficient space" means the resident can access the area, it is not functionally off-limits, and the resident's functioning is not restricted once access to the space is gained.

Program areas where resident groups engage in activities focused on manipulative skills and hand-eye coordination should have sufficient space for storage of their supplies and "works in progress."

Program areas where residents receive physical therapy should have sufficient space and equipment to meet the needs of the resident's therapy requirement.

Recreation/activities area means any area where residents can participate in those activities identified in their plan of care.

Procedures: §483.70(c)(1)

In the use of space, consider if available space allows residents to pursue activities and receive health services and programs as identified in their care plan.

F456

§483.70(c)(2) Maintain all essential mechanical, electrical, and patient care equipment in safe operating condition.

Probes: §483.70(c)(2)

Is essential equipment (e.g., boiler room equipment, nursing unit/medication room refrigerators, kitchen refrigerator/freezer and laundry equipment) in safe operating condition?

Is equipment maintained according to manufacturers recommendations.

---

§483.70(d) Resident Rooms

Resident rooms must be designed and equipped for adequate nursing care, comfort, and privacy of residents.

F457

§483.70(d)(1) Bedrooms must--

§483.70(d)(1)(i) Accommodate no more than four residents;

Interpretive Guidelines: §483.70(d)(1)(i)

See §483.70(d)(3) regarding variations.

Probes: §483.70(d)(1)(i)

Unless a variation has been applied for and approved under §483.70(d)(3), do the residents' bedrooms accommodate no more than four residents?

F458

§483.70(d)(1)(ii) Measure at least 80 square feet per resident in multiple resident bedrooms, and at least 100 square feet in single resident rooms;

Interpretive Guidelines: §483.70(d)(1)(ii)

See §483.70(d)(3) regarding variations.

The measurement of the square footage should be based upon the useable living space of the room. Therefore, the minimum square footage in resident rooms should be measured based upon the floor's measurements exclusive of toilets and bath areas, closets, lockers, wardrobes, alcoves, or vestibules. However, if the height of the alcoves or vestibules reasonably provides useful living area, then the corresponding floor area may be included in the calculation.

The space occupied by movable wardrobes should be excluded from the useable square footage in a room unless it is an item of the resident's own choice and it is in addition to the individual closet space in the resident's room. Non-permanent items of the resident's own choice should have no effect in the calculation of useable living space.

Protrusions such as columns, radiators, ventilation systems for heating and/or cooling should be ignored in computing the useable square footage of the room if the area involved is minimal (e.g., a baseboard heating or air conditioning system or ductwork that does not protrude more than 6 to 8 inches from the wall, or a column that is not more than 6 to 8 inches on each side) and does not have an adverse effect on the resident's health and safety or does not impede the ability of any resident in that room to attain his or her highest practicable well-being. If these protrusions are not minimal they would be deducted from useable square footage computed in determining compliance with this requirement.

The swing or arc of any door which opens directly into the resident's room should not be excluded from the calculations of useable square footage in a room.

Procedures: §483.70(d)(1)(ii)

The facility layout may give square footage measurements. Carry a tape measure and take measurements if the room appears small.

Probes: §483.70(d)(1)(ii)

Unless a variation has been applied for and approved under §483.70(d)(3), are there at least 80 square feet per resident in multiple resident rooms and at least 100 square feet for single resident rooms?

F459

§483.70(d)(1)(iii) Have direct access to an exit corridor;

Interpretive Guidelines: §483.70(d)(1)(iii)

There is no authority under current regulations to approve a variation to this requirement. Additional guidance is available in the National Fire Protection Association's Life Safety Code 101 (NFPA 101), 12-2.5.1, which is Tag K41 of the Life Safety Code Survey

---

F460

§483.70(d)(1)(iv) Be designed or equipped to assure full visual privacy for each resident;

Interpretive Guidelines: §483.70(d)(1)(iv)

"**Full visual privacy**" means that residents have a means of completely withdrawing from public view while occupying their bed (e.g., curtain, moveable screens, private room).

The guidelines do not intend to limit the provisions of privacy to solely one or more curtains, movable screens or a private room. Facility operators are free to use other means to provide full visual privacy, with those means varying according to the needs and requests of residents. However, the requirement explicitly states that bedrooms must "be designed or equipped to assure full visual privacy for each resident." For example, a resident with a bed by the window cannot be required to remain out of his or her room while his/her roommate is having a dressing change. Room design or equipment must provide privacy. Surveyors will assess whether the means the facility is using to assure full visual privacy meets this requirement without negatively affecting any other resident rights.

Procedures: §483.70(d)(1)(iv)

There are no provisions for physician statements to be used as a basis for variation of the requirements for full visual privacy.

Probes: §483.70(d)(1)(iv)

Observe whether each resident selected for a comprehensive or focused review has a means to achieve full visual privacy.

§483.70(d)(1)(v) In facilities initially certified after March 31, 1992, except in private rooms, each bed must have ceiling suspended curtains, which extend around the bed to provide total visual privacy in combination with adjacent walls and curtains;

Interpretive Guidelines: §483.70(d)(1)(v)

The term "**initially certified**" is defined as all newly certified nursing facilities (NFs) or SNFs as well as NFs and SNFs after March 31, 1992, which re-enter the Medicare or Medicaid programs, whether they voluntarily or involuntarily left the program.

It is not necessary for the bed to be accessible from both sides when the privacy curtain in pulled.

Additional guidance is available in the National Fire Protection Association's Life Safety Code 101 (NFPA 101), 31-1.4.1, 31-4.5, which is Tag K74 of the Life Safety Code Survey.

F461

§483.70(d)(1)(vi) Have at least one window to the outside; and

Interpretive Guidelines **§483.70(d)(1)(vi)**

A facility with resident room windows, as defined by section 13-3.8.1 of the 1985 edition of the Life Safety Code, that open to an atrium in accordance with Life Safety Code 6-2.2.3.5 can meet this requirement for a window to the outside.

In addition to conforming with the Life Safety Code, this requirement was included to assist the resident's orientation to day and night, weather, and general awareness of space outside the facility. The facility is required to provide for a "safe, clean, comfortable and homelike environment" by deemphasizing the institutional character of the setting, to the extent possible. Windows are an important aspect in assuring the homelike environment of a facility.

Probes: §483.70(d)(1)(vi)

Is there at least one window to the outside?

§483.70(d)(1)(vii) Have a floor at or above grade level.

Interpretive Guidelines **§483.70(d)(1)(vii)**

"**At or above grade level**" is defined as a room in which the floor is at or above ground level.

Probes: §483.70(d)(1)(vii)

Are the bedrooms at or above ground level?

Additional guidance is available in the National Fire Protection Association's Life Safety Code 101 (NFPA 101), 12-2.5.1, 12-2.5.7, which is Tag K41 of the Life Safety Code survey.

---

§483.70(d)(2) The facility must provide each resident with--

(i) A separate bed of proper size and height for the convenience of the resident;

(ii) A clean, comfortable mattress;

(iii) Bedding appropriate to the weather and climate; and

Probes: §483.70(d)(2)(i), (ii), and (iii)

Are mattresses clean and comfortable?

Is bedding appropriate to weather and climate?

§483.70(d)(2)(iv) Functional furniture appropriate to the resident's needs, and individual closet space in the resident's bedroom with clothes racks and shelves accessible to the resident.

Interpretive Guidelines §483.70(d)(2)(iv)

"Functional furniture appropriate to the residents' needs" means that the furniture in each resident's room contributes to the resident attaining or maintaining his or her highest practicable level of independence and well-being. In general, furnishings include a place to put clothing away in an organized manner that will let it remain clean, free of wrinkles, and accessible to the resident while protecting it from casual access by others; a place to put personal effects such as pictures and a bedside clock, and furniture suitable for the comfort of the resident and visitors (e.g., a chair).

There may be instances in which individual residents determine that certain items are not necessary or will impede their ability to maintain or attain their highest practicable well-being (e.g., Both the resident and spouse use wheelchairs. They visit more easily without another chair in the room.) In this case, the resident's wishes should determine the furniture needs.

"Shelves accessible to the resident" means that the resident, if able, or a staff person at the direction of the resident, can get to their clothes whenever they choose.

Probes: §483.70(d)(2)(iv)

Functional furniture: Is there functional furniture, appropriate to residents' needs?

Closet space: Is there individual closet space with accessible clothes racks and shelves?

§483.70(d)(3) CMS, or in the case of a nursing facility the survey agency, may permit variations in requirements specified in paragraphs (d)(1)(i) and (ii) of this section relating to rooms in individual cases when the facility demonstrates in writing that the variations--

(i) Are in accordance with the special needs of the residents; and

(ii) Will not adversely affect residents' health and safety.

Interpretive Guidelines: §483.70(d)(3)

A variation must be in accordance with the special needs of the residents and must not adversely affect the health or safety of residents. Facility hardship is not part of the basis for granting a variation. Since the special needs of residents may change periodically, or different residents may be transferred into a room that has been granted a variation, variations must be reviewed and considered for renewal whenever the facility is certified. If the needs of the residents within the room have not changed since the last annual inspection, the variance should continue if the facility so desires.

Interpretive Guidelines: §483.70(d)(1)(i):

As residents are transferred or discharged from rooms with more than four residents, beds should be removed from the variance until the number of residents occupying the room does not exceed four.

F462

§483.70(e) Toilet Facilities

Each resident room must be equipped with or located near toilet facilities.

Interpretive Guidelines: §483.70(e)

"**Toilet facilities**" is defined as a space that contains a lavatory and a toilet. If the resident's room is not equipped with an adjoining toilet facility, then "located near" means residents who are independent in the use of a toilet, including chairbound residents, can routinely use a toilet in the unit.

Probes: §483.70(e)

Are resident rooms equipped with or located near toilet and bathing facilities?

F463

§483.70(f) Resident Call System

The nurses' station must be equipped to receive resident calls through a communication system from--

(1) Resident rooms; and

(2) Toilet and bathing facilities.

Intent: §483.70(f)

The intent of this requirement is that residents, when in their rooms and toilet and bathing areas, have a means of directly contacting staff at the nurse's station. This communication may be through audible or visual signals and may include "wireless systems."

Interpretive Guidelines: §483.70(f)

This requirement is met only if all portions of the system are functioning (e.g., system is not turned off at the nurses' station, the volume too low to be heard, the light above a room or rooms is not working).

Probes: §483.70(f)

Is there a functioning communication system from rooms, toilets, and bathing facilities?

F464

§483.70(g) Dining and Resident Activities

The facility must provide one or more rooms designated for resident dining and activities.

These rooms must--

§483.70(g)(1) Be well lighted;

Interpretive Guidelines: §483.70(g)(1)

"**Well lighted**" is defined as levels of illumination that are suitable to tasks performed by a resident.

Probes: §483.70(g)(1)

Are there adequate and comfortable lighting levels?

Are illumination levels appropriate to tasks with little glare?

Does lighting support maintenance of independent functioning and task performance?

§483.70(g)(2) Be well ventilated, with nonsmoking areas identified;

Interpretive Guidelines: §483.70(g)(2)

"**Well ventilated**" is defined as good air circulation, avoidance of drafts at floor level, and adequate smoke exhaust removal.

"**Nonsmoking areas identified**" is defined as signs posted in accordance with State law regulating indoor smoking policy and facility policy.

Probes: §483.70(g)(2)

How well is the space ventilated?

Is there good air movement?

Are temperature, humidity, and odor levels all acceptable?

Are non-smoking areas identified?

§483.70(g)(3) Be adequately furnished; and

Interpretive Guidelines: §483.70(g)(3)

An "**adequately furnished**" dining area accommodates different residents' physical and social needs. An adequately furnished organized activities area accommodates the specific activities offered by the facility.

Probes: §483.70(g)(3)

How adequate are furnishings?

Are furnishings structurally sound and functional (e.g., chairs of varying sizes to meet varying needs of residents, wheelchairs can fit under the dining room table)?

§483.70(g)(4) Have sufficient space to accommodate all activities.

Interpretive Guidelines: §483.70(g)(4)

"**Sufficient space to accommodate all activities**" means that the space available is adaptable to a variety of uses and residents' needs.

Probes: §483.70(g)(4)

How sufficient is space in dining, health services, recreation and program areas to accommodate all activities?

Are spaces adaptable for all intended uses?

Is resident access to space limited?

Do residents and staff have maximum flexibility in arranging furniture to accommodate residents who use walkers, wheelchairs, and other mobility aids?

Is there resident crowding?

F465

§483.70(h) Other Environmental Conditions

The facility must provide a safe, functional, sanitary, and comfortable environment for residents, staff and the public.

F466

The facility must--

§483.70(h)(1) Establish procedures to ensure that water is available to essential areas when there is a loss of normal water supply;

Interpretive Guidelines: §483.70(h)(1)

The facility should have a written protocol which defines the source of water, provisions for storing the water, both potable and non-potable, a method for distributing water, and a method for estimating the volume of water required.

Procedures §483.70(h)(1)

During the entrance conference, ask the administrator the facility's procedure to ensure water availability.

F467

§483.70(h)(2) Have adequate outside ventilation by means of windows, or mechanical ventilation, or a combination of the two;

Probes: §483.70(h)(2)

How well is the space ventilated?

Is there good air movement?

Are temperature, humidity, and odor levels all acceptable?

F468

§483.70(h)(3) Equip corridors with firmly secured handrails on each side; and

Interpretive Guidelines §483.70(h)(3)

"**Secured handrails**" means handrails that are firmly affixed to the wall.

Probes: §483.70(h)(3)

Are handrails secure?

F469

§483.70(h)(4) Maintain an effective pest control program so that the facility is free of pests and rodents.

Interpretive Guidelines: §483.70(h)(4)

An "**effective pest control program**" is defined as measures to eradicate and contain common household pests (e.g., roaches, ants, mosquitoes, flies, mice, and rats).

Procedures: §483.70(h)(4)

As part of the overall review of the facility, look for signs of vermin. Evidence of pest infestation in a particular space is an indicator of noncompliance.

Probes: §483.70(h)(4)

Is area pest free?

F490

§483.75 Administration

A facility must be administered in a manner that enables it to use its resources effectively and efficiently to attain or maintain the highest practicable physical, mental, and psychosocial well-being of each resident.

Procedures: §483.75

If there is a deficiency in §483.13, Resident behavior and facility practices; §483.15, Quality of life; or §483.25, Quality of care, which has the scope and/or severity to be defined as substandard quality of care, fully review for compliance all the tags within this section (§483.75).

F491

§483.75(a) Licensure

A facility must be licensed under applicable State and local law.

Interpretive Guidelines:§483.75(a)

Applicable licenses, permits, and approvals must be available to you for inspection upon request.

Procedures: §483.75(a)

If there are problems with care provided or supervised by licensed personnel, verify applicable licenses, permits and approvals.

F492

§483.75(b) Compliance With Federal, State, and Local Laws and Professional Standards

The facility must operate and provide services in compliance with all applicable Federal, State, and local laws, regulations, and codes, and with accepted professional standards and principles that apply to professionals providing services in such a facility.

Intent: §483.75(b)

The intent of this regulation is to ensure that a facility is in compliance with Federal, State, and local laws, regulations, and codes relating to health, safety, and sanitation.

Interpretive Guidelines: §483.75(b)

The State is responsible for making decisions about whether there are violations of State laws and regulations. Licenses, permits and approvals of the facility must be available to you upon request. Current reports of inspections by State and/or local health authorities are on file, and notations are made of action taken by the facility to correct deficiencies.

§483.75(c) Relationship to Other HHS Regulations

In addition to compliance with the regulations set forth in this subpart, facilities are obliged to meet the applicable provisions of other HHS regulations, including but not limited to those pertaining to nondiscrimination on the basis of race, color, or

national origin (45 CFR part 80); nondiscrimination on the basis of handicap (45 CFR part 84); nondiscrimination on the basis of age (45 CFR part 91); protection of human subjects of research (45 CFR part 46); and fraud and abuse (42 CFR part 455). Although these regulations are not in themselves considered requirements under this part, their violation may result in the termination or suspension of, or the refusal to grant or continue payment with Federal funds.

Procedures: §483.75(b)

If resident/family interviews reveal possible problems with admission contracts, review these contracts for violations of requirements at §§483.10 and 483.12. As appropriate, refer problems to an ombudsman or other agencies, e.g., Office for Civil Rights.

Some State or local laws are more stringent than the Federal requirement on the same issue. Failure of the facility to meet a Federal, State or local law may be cited at this tag only when the authority having jurisdiction has **both** made a determination of noncompliance and has taken a final adverse action as a result.

Accepted professional standards and principles include the various practice acts and scope of practice regulations in each State, and current, commonly accepted health standards established by national organizations, boards and councils.

If interviews with residents suggest that the facility may have required deposits from Medicare residents at admission, review the facility's admissions documents.

Procedures: §483.75(c)

If during the survey you identify problems relating to one or more of these requirements, which are under the purview of another Federal agency, forward the information to the RO, who will forward it to the appropriate Federal agency.

F493

§483.75(d) Governing Body

(1) The facility must have a governing body, or designated persons functioning as a governing body, that is legally responsible for establishing and implementing policies regarding the management and operation of the facility; and

(2) The governing body appoints the administrator who is--

(i) Licensed by the State where licensing is required; and

(ii) Responsible for the management of the facility.

Interpretive Guidelines: §483.75(d)(2)(1)

The administrator must be licensed where required by the State.

§483.75(e) Required Training of Nursing Aides

(Rev. 26; Issued: 08-17-07; Effective/Implementation Dates: 08-17-07)

(1) Definitions

"Licensed health professional" means a physician; physician assistant; nurse practitioner; physical, speech, or occupational therapist; physical or occupational therapy assistant; registered professional nurse; licensed practical nurse; or licensed or certified social worker.

"Nurse aide" means any individual providing nursing or nursing-related services to residents in a facility who is not a licensed health professional, a registered dietitian, or someone who volunteers to provide such services without pay.

Nurse aides do not include those individuals who furnish services to residents only as paid feeding assistants as defined in §488.301 of this chapter.

F494

§483.75(e)(2) General rule

A facility must not use any individual working in the facility as a nurse aide for more than 4 months, on a full-time basis, unless:

(i) That individual is competent to provide nursing and nursing related services; and

(ii)(A) That individual has completed a training and competency evaluation program, or a competency evaluation program approved by the State as meeting the requirements of §§483.151-483.154 of this part; or

(B) That individual has been deemed or determined competent as provided in §483.150(a) and (b).

§483.75(e)(3) Non-permanent employees

A facility must not use on a temporary, per diem, leased, or any basis other than a permanent employee any individual who does not meet the requirements in paragraphs (e)(2)(i) and (ii) of this section.

(See Tag F495 for guidelines, probes, and procedures for §483.75(e)(2-4))

F495

(4) Competency

A facility must not use any individual who has worked less than 4 months as a nurse aide in that facility unless the individual--

(i) Is a full-time employee in a State-approved training and competency evaluation program;

(ii) Has demonstrated competence through satisfactory participation in a State-approved nurse aide training and competency evaluation program or competency evaluation program; or

(iii) Has been deemed or determined competent as provided in §483.150(a) and (b).

Interpretive Guidelines: §483.75(e)(2 - 4)

Facilities may use, as nurse aides, any individuals who have successfully completed either a nurse aide training and competency evaluation program or a competency evaluation program. However, if an individual has not completed a program at the time of employment, a facility may **only** use that individual as a nurse aide if the individual is in a nurse aide training and competency evaluation program (**not a competency evaluation program alone**) and that individual is a permanent employee in his or her first four months of employment in the facility.

Facilities may not use non-permanent employees as nurse aides unless they have either completed a training and competency evaluation program, or a competency evaluation program.

Probes: §483.75(e)(2 - 4)

During an extended or partial extended survey:

- Have all nurse aides completed a nurse aide training and competency evaluation program or a competency evaluation program? If not, are those nurse aides permanent employees enrolled in a training and competency evaluation program who have worked in the facility for 4 months or less?

- Ask nurse aides where they received their training, how long the training was and how long they have worked in the facility as a nurse aide.

During all surveys:

- If incorrect nurse aide work performance is observed during the survey, check to see if the nurse aide received training and licensed nurse supervision to correctly carry out the task.

A "**permanent employee**" is defined as any employee you expect to continue working on an ongoing basis.

Procedures: §483.75(e)(2-4)

Review competency requirements for nurse aides if you identify potential deficient care practices in quality of care, resident rights, resident behavior and facility practice or quality of life which may be related to nurse aide competency. Is there evidence that the nurse aide has successfully completed the competency evaluation program, or has the individual been grandfathered in by the State?

If you identify deficient care practices by nurse aides who do not have evidence of having successfully completed a competency evaluation program, determine:

- If the aide is currently receiving training an a State approved Nurse Aide Training Program;
- If the aide is under the supervision of a licensed nurse; and
- If the aide has been trained and determined to be proficient for the tasks to which he or she is assigned. See §483.152 for specific training that the aide is to receive. This training includes:
- At least 16 hours of training in the following subjects **before** any direct contact with the resident:
    - Communication and interpersonal skills;
    - Infection control;
    - Safety and emergency procedures, including the Heimlich Maneuver;
    - Promoting resident's independence; and
    - Respecting resident's rights.
- Basic nursing skills;

- Personal care skills;
- Mental health and social services of residents;
- Care of cognitively impaired residents;
- Basic restorative services; and
- Resident's rights.

F496

§483.75(e)(5) Registry verification

Before allowing an individual to serve as a nurse aide, a facility must receive registry verification that the individual has met competency evaluation requirements unless--

(i) The individual is a full-time employee in a training and competency evaluation program approved by the State; or

(ii)The individual can prove that he or she has recently successfully completed a training and competency evaluation program or competency evaluation program approved by the State and has not yet been included in the registry. Facilities must follow up to ensure that such an individual actually becomes registered.

§483.75(e)(6) Multi-State registry verification

Before allowing an individual to serve as a nurse aide, a facility must seek information from every State registry established under sections 1819(e)(2)(A) or 1919(e)(2)(A) of the Act the facility believes will include information on the individual.

§483.75(e)(7) Required retraining

If, since an individual's most recent completion of a training and competency evaluation program, there has been a continuous period of 24 consecutive months during none of which the individual provided nursing or nursing-related services for monetary compensation, the individual must complete a new training and competency evaluation program or a new competency evaluation program.

Interpretive Guidelines: §483.75(e)(7)

If an individual does not wish to be retrained, the individual must establish that he or she performed nursing or nursing-related services for monetary compensation for at least one documented day (i.e., 8 consecutive hours) during the previous 24 months. The State is required to remove the individual's name from the registry if the services are not provided for monetary compensation during the 24-month period. Thus, in the absence of any evidence to the contrary, you can assume that the retraining requirement does not apply to an individual whose name appears on the registry.

F497

§483.75(e)(8) Regular In-Service Education

The facility must complete a performance review of every nurse aide at least once every 12 months, and must provide regular in-service education based on the outcome of these reviews. The in-service training must--

> **(i) Be sufficient to ensure the continuing competence of nurse aides, but must be no less than 12 hours per year;**
>
> **(ii) Address areas of weakness as determined in nurse aides' performance reviews and may address the special needs of residents as determined by the facility staff; and**
>
> **(iii) For nurse aides providing services to individuals with cognitive impairments, also address the care of the cognitively impaired.**

Interpretive Guidelines: §483.75(e)(8)

The adequacy of the in-service education program is measured not only by documentation of hours of completed in-service education, but also by demonstrated competencies of nurse aide staff in consistently applying the interventions necessary to meet residents' needs.

If there has been deficient care practices identified during Phase 1 of the survey, review as appropriate training received by nurse aides in that corresponding subject area. For example, if the facility has deficiencies in infection control, review the infection control unit in the facility's inservice nurse aide training program.

Each nurse aide must have no less than twelve hours of in-service education per year. Calculate the date by which a nurse aide must receive annual in-service education by the employment date rather than the calendar year.

Probes: §483.75(e)(8)

During an extended or partial extended survey, or during any survey in which nurse aide performance is questioned. (See §483.75(f).)

- Does the facility review the performance of its nurse aides?

- How has in-service education addressed areas of weakness identified in performance reviews, special resident needs, and needs of residents with cognitive impairments?

- How has in-service education addressed quality of care problems including those of special care needs and resident rights?

F498

§483.75(f) Proficiency of Nurse Aides

The facility must ensure that nurse aides are able to demonstrate competency in skills and techniques necessary to care for residents' needs, as identified through resident assessments, and described in the plan of care.

Interpretive Guidelines: §483.75(f)

"Competency in skills and techniques necessary to care for residents' needs" includes competencies in areas such as communication and personal skills, basic nursing skills, personal care skills, mental health and social service needs, basic restorative services and resident rights.

Procedures: §483.75(f)

During the Resident Review, observe nurse aides.

Probes: §483.75(f)

Do nurse aides show competency in skills necessary to:

- Maintain or improve the resident's independent functioning, e.g.:
  - Performing range of motion exercises,
  - Assisting the resident to transfer from the bed to a wheelchair,
  - Reinforcing appropriate developmental behavior for persons with MR, or

  - o Psychotherapeutic behavior for persons with MI;

- Observe and describe resident behavior and status and report to charge nurse;
- Follow instructions; and
- Carry out appropriate infection control precautions and safety procedures.

F499

§483.75(g) Staff Qualifications

(1) The facility must employ on a full-time, part-time or consultant basis those professionals necessary to carry out the provisions of these requirements.

(2) Professional staff must be licensed, certified, or registered in accordance with applicable State laws.

Procedures: §483.75(g)

If there is reason to doubt the qualifications of temporary agency personnel working in the facility, check with the appropriate registry or professional licensing board.

F500

§483.75(h) Use of Outside Resources

(1) If the facility does not employ a qualified professional person to furnish a specific service to be provided by the facility, the facility must have that service furnished to residents by a person or agency outside the facility under an arrangement described in section 1861(w) of the Act or an agreement described in paragraph (h)(2) of this section.

(2) Arrangements as described in section 1861(w) of the Act or agreements pertaining to services furnished by outside resources must specify in writing that the facility assumes responsibility for--

(i) Obtaining services that meet professional standards and principles that apply to professionals providing services in such a facility; and

(ii) The timeliness of the services.

F501

§483.75(i) Medical Director

(1) The facility must designate a physician to serve as medical director.

(2) The medical director is responsible for –

(i) Implementation of resident care policies; and

(ii) The coordination of medical care in the facility.

INTENT:

The intent of this requirement is that:

- The facility has a licensed physician who serves as the medical director to coordinate medical care in the facility and provide clinical guidance and oversight regarding the implementation of resident care policies;
- The medical director collaborates with the facility leadership, staff, and other practitioners and consultants to help develop, implement and evaluate resident care policies and procedures that reflect current standards of practice; and
- The medical director helps the facility identify, evaluate, and address/resolve medical and clinical concerns and issues that:
  - Affect resident care, medical care or quality of life; or
  - Are related to the provision of services by physicians and other licensed health care practitioners.

NOTE: While many medical directors also serve as attending physicians, the roles and functions of a medical director are separate from those of an attending physician. The medical director's role involves the coordination of facility-wide medical care while the attending physician's role involves primary responsibility for the medical care of individual residents.[1]

DEFINITIONS

Definitions are provided to clarify terms related to the provision of medical director services.

- "Attending Physician" refers to the physician who has the primary responsibility for the medical care of a resident.

- "Current standards of practice" refers to approaches to care, procedures, techniques, treatments, etc., that are based on research and/or expert consensus and that are contained in current manuals, textbooks, or publications, or that are accepted, adopted or promulgated by recognized professional organizations or national accrediting bodies.

- "Medical care" refers to the practice of medicine as consistent with State laws and regulations.

- "Medical director" refers to a physician who oversees the medical care and other designated care and services in a health care organization or facility. Under these regulations, the medical director is responsible for coordinating medical care and helping to develop, implement and evaluate resident care policies and procedures that reflect current standards of practice.

- "Resident care policies and procedures" – Resident care policies are the facility's overall goals, directives, and governing Statements that direct the delivery of care and services to residents. Resident care procedures describe the processes by which the facility provides care to residents that is consistent with current standards of practice and facility policies.

OVERVIEW

The medical director has an important leadership role in actively helping long term care facilities provide quality care. The regulation requires each facility to have a medical director who is responsible for the implementation of resident care policies and the coordination of medical care. These two roles provide the basis for the functions and tasks discussed in this guidance. The medical director's roles and functions require the physician serving in that capacity to be knowledgeable about current standards of practice in caring for long term care residents, and about how to coordinate and oversee related practitioners. As a clinician, the medical director plays a pivotal role in providing clinical leadership regarding application of current standards of practice for resident care and new or proposed treatments, practices, and approaches to care. The medical director's input promotes the attainment of optimal resident outcomes which may also be influenced by many other factors, such as resident characteristics and preferences, individual attending physician actions, and facility support. The 2001 Institute of Medicine report, "Improving the Quality of Long Term Care," urged facilities to give medical directors greater authority for medical services and care. The report states, "nursing homes should develop structures and processes that enable and require a more focused and dedicated medical staff responsible for patient care."[2]

The medical director is in a position, because of his/her roles and functions, to provide input to surveyors on physician issues, individual resident's clinical issues, and the facility's clinical practices. The text "Medical Direction in Long Term Care"[3] asserts that:

> "The Medical Director has an important role in helping the facility deal with regulatory and survey issues…the medical director can help ensure that appropriate systems exist to facilitate good medical care, establish and apply good monitoring systems and effective documentation and follow up of findings, and help improve physician compliance with regulations, including required visits. During and after the survey process, the medical director can clarify for the surveyors clinical questions or information about the care of specific residents, request surveyor clarification of citations on clinical care, attend the exit conference to demonstrate physician interest and help in understanding the nature and scope of the facility's deficiencies, and help the facility draft corrective actions."

Nationally accepted statements concerning the roles, responsibilities and functions of a medical director can be found at the American Medical Directors Association Web site at www.amda.com.

> **NOTE:** References to non-CMS sources or sites on the Internet are provided as a service and do not constitute or imply endorsement of these organizations or their programs by CMS or the U.S. Department of Health and Human Services. CMS is not responsible for the content of pages found at these sites. URL addresses were current as of the date of this publication.

MEDICAL DIRECTION

The facility is responsible for designating a medical director, who is currently licensed as a physician in the State(s) in which the facility(ies) he/she serves is (are) located. The facility may provide for this service through any of several methods, such as direct employment, contractual arrangements, or another type of agreement. Whatever the arrangement or method employed, the facility and the medical director should identify the expectations for how the medical director will work with the facility to effectively implement resident care policies and coordinate medical care.

> **NOTE:** While the roles of medical directors who work for multi-facility organizations with corporate or regional offices may vary for policy development, the medical directors, nonetheless, should be involved in facility level issues such as application of those policies to the care of the facility's residents.

Implementation of Resident Care Policies and Procedures

The facility is responsible for obtaining the medical director's ongoing guidance in the development and implementation of resident care policies, including review and revision of existing policies. The medical director's role involves collaborating with the facility regarding the policies and protocols that guide clinical decision making (for example, interpretation of clinical information, treatment selection, and monitoring of risks and benefits of interventions) by any of the following: facility staff; licensed physicians; nurse practitioners; physician assistants; clinical nurse specialists; licensed, certified, or registered health care professionals such as nurses, therapists, dieticians, pharmacists, social workers, and other health care workers.

The medical director has a key role in helping the facility to incorporate current standards of practice into resident care policies and procedures/guidelines to help assure that they address the needs of the residents. Although regulations do not require the medical director to sign the policies or procedures, the facility should be able to show that its development, review, and approval of resident care policies included the medical director's input.

This requirement does not imply that the medical director must carry out the policies and procedures or supervise staff performance directly, but rather must guide, approve, and help oversee the implementation of the policies and procedures. Examples of resident care policies include, but are not limited to:

- Admission policies and care practices that address the types of residents that may be admitted and retained based upon the ability of the facility to provide the services and care to meet their needs;

- The integrated delivery of care and services, such as medical, nursing, pharmacy, social, rehabilitative and dietary services, which includes clinical assessments, analysis of assessment findings, care planning including preventive care, care plan monitoring and modification, infection control (including isolation or special care), transfers to other settings, and discharge planning;

- The use and availability of ancillary services such as x-ray and laboratory;

- The availability, qualifications, and clinical functions of staff necessary to meet resident care needs;

- Resident formulation and facility implementation of advance directives (in accordance with State law) and end-of-life care;

- Provisions that enhance resident decision making, including choice regarding medical care options;

- Mechanisms for communicating and resolving issues related to medical care;

- Conduct of research, if allowed, within the facility;

- Provision of physician services, including (but not limited to):
    - Availability of physician services 24 hours a day in case of emergency;
    - Review of the resident's overall condition and program of care at each visit, including medications and treatments;
    - Documentation of progress notes with signatures;
    - Frequency of visits, as required;
    - Signing and dating all orders, such as medications, admission orders, and re-admission orders; and
    - Review of and response to consultant recommendations.
- Systems to ensure that other licensed practitioners (e.g., nurse practitioners) who may perform physician-delegated tasks act within the regulatory requirements and within the scope of practice as defined by State law; and
- Procedures and general clinical guidance for facility staff regarding when to contact a practitioner, including information that should be gathered prior to contacting the practitioner regarding a clinical issue/question or change in condition.

Coordination of Medical Care

The medical director is responsible for the coordination of medical care in the facility. The coordination of medical care means that the medical director helps the facility obtain and maintain timely and appropriate medical care that supports the healthcare needs of the residents, is consistent with current standards of practice, and helps the facility meet its regulatory requirements. In light of the extensive medical needs of the long term care population, physicians have an important role both in providing direct care and in influencing care quality. The medical director helps coordinate and evaluate the medical care within the facility by reviewing and evaluating aspects of physician care and practitioner services, and helping the facility identify, evaluate, and address health care issues related to the quality of care and quality of life of residents. "A medical director should establish a framework for physician participation, and physicians should believe that they are accountable for their actions and their care."[4]

The medical director addresses issues related to the coordination of medical care identified through the facility's quality assessment and assurance committee and quality assurance program, and other activities related to the coordination of care. This includes, but is not limited to, helping the facility:

- Ensure that residents have primary attending and backup physician coverage;

- Ensure that physician and health care practitioner services are available to help residents attain and maintain their highest practicable level of functioning, consistent with regulatory requirements;
- Develop a process to review basic physician and health care practitioner credentials (e.g., licensure and pertinent background);
- Address and resolve concerns and issues between the physicians, health care practitioners and facility staff; and
- Resolve issues related to continuity of care and transfer of medical information between the facility and other care settings.

Throughout this guidance, a response from a physician implies appropriate communication, review, and resident management, but does not imply that the physician must necessarily order tests or treatments recommended or requested by the staff, unless the physician agrees that those are medically valid and indicated.

In addition, other areas for medical director input to the facility may include:

- Facilitating feedback to physicians and other health care practitioners about their performance and practices;
- Reviewing individual resident cases as requested or as indicated;
- Reviewing consultant recommendations;
- Discussing and intervening (as appropriate) with a health care practitioner about medical care that is inconsistent with applicable current standards of care;
- Assuring that a system exists to monitor the performance of the health care practitioners;
- Guiding physicians regarding specific performance expectations;
- Identifying facility or practitioner educational and informational needs;
- Providing information to the facility practitioners from sources such as nationally recognized medical care societies and organizations where current clinical information can be obtained; and
- Helping educate and provide information to staff, practitioners, residents, families and others.

NOTE: This does not imply that the medical director must personally present educational programs.

REFERENCES

[1] Pattee JJ, Otteson OJ. (1991). Medical direction in the nursing home (p.5). Minneapolis, MN: Northridge Press.

[2] Institute of Medicine (2001). Improving The Quality Of Long-Term Care (pp. 201). Washington, DC: National Academy Press.

[3] Levenson, S. A. (1993). Medical Direction In Long-Term Care. A Guidebook For The Future (2nd ed., pp. 135). Durham, NC: Carolina Academic Press.

[4] Levenson, SA. Medical Director and Attending Physicians Policy and Procedure Manual for Long-term Care. Dayton, Ohio: MedPass. 2005.

INVESTIGATIVE PROTOCOL

MEDICAL DIRECTOR

Objective

- To determine whether the facility has designated a licensed physician to serve as medical director; and
- To determine whether the medical director, in collaboration with the facility, coordinates medical care and the implementation of resident care policies.

Use

Use this protocol for all initial and extended surveys or, as indicated, during any other type of survey. Use this protocol if the survey team has identified:

- That the facility does not have a licensed physician serving as medical director; and/or
- That the facility has designated a licensed physician to serve as medical director; however, concerns or noncompliance identified indicate that:
    - The facility has failed to involve the medical director in his/her roles and functions related to coordination of medical care and/or the implementation of resident care policies; and/or
    - The medical director may not have performed his/her roles and functions related to coordination of medical care and/or the implementation of resident care policies.

Procedures

The investigation involves interviews, review of pertinent policies and procedures, and may involve additional review of resident care.

Provision of a Medical Director

Determine whether the medical director is available during the survey to respond to surveyor questions about resident care policies, medical care, and physician issues.

Interview the facility leadership (e.g., Administrator, Director of Nursing [DON], others as appropriate) about how it has identified and reviewed with the medical director his/her roles and functions as a medical director, including those related to coordination of medical care and the facility's clinical practices and care.

Interview the medical director about his/her understanding and performance of the medical director roles and functions, and about the extent of facility support for performing his/her roles and functions.

If the survey team has identified that the facility lacks a medical director, collect information from the facility administrator to:

- Determine the duration and possible reasons for this problem; and
- Identify what the facility has been doing to try to retain a medical director.

Facility/Medical Director Responsibility for Resident Care Policies

After identifying actual or potential noncompliance with the provision of resident care or medical care:

- Review related policies/procedures;
- Interview facility leadership (e.g., Administrator, DON) to determine how or if they involved the medical director in developing, reviewing, and implementing policies and procedures regarding clinical care of residents (especially where these involve medical and clinical issues; for example, management of causes of delirium, falling, and weight loss) to ensure that they are clinically valid and consistent with current standards of care;
- Interview the medical director regarding his/her input into:
    - Scope of services the facility has chosen to provide;
    - The facility's capacity to care for its residents with complex or special care needs, such as dialysis, hospice or end-of-life care, respiratory support with ventilators, intravenous medications/fluids, dementia and/or related conditions, or problematic behaviors or complex mood disorders;
    - The following areas of concern:
        - Appropriateness of care as it relates to clinical services (for example, following orders correctly, communicating important information to physicians in a timely fashion, etc.);
        - Processes for accurate assessment, care planning, treatment implementation, and monitoring of care and services to meet resident needs; and

- The review and update of policies and procedures to reflect current standards of practice for resident care (e.g., pressure ulcer prevention and treatment and management of incontinence, pain, fall risk, restraint reduction, and hydration risks) and quality of life.

Coordination of Medical Care/Physician Leadership

If the survey team has identified issues or concerns related to the provision of medical care:

- Interview appropriate facility staff and management as well as the medical director to determine what happens when a physician (or other healthcare practitioner) has a pattern of inadequate or inappropriate performance or acts contrary to established rules and procedures of the facility; for example, repeatedly late in making visits, fails to take time to discuss resident problems with staff, does not adequately address or document key medical issues when making resident visits, etc;

- If concerns are identified for any of the following physician services, determine how the facility obtained the medical director's input in evaluating and coordinating the provision of medical care:

    - Assuring that provisions are in place for physician services 24 hours a day and in case of emergency (§483.40(b));

    - Assuring that physicians visit residents, provide medical orders, and review a resident's medical condition as required (§483.40(b)&(c));

    - Assuring that other practitioners who may perform physician delegated tasks, act within the regulatory requirements and within their scope of practice as defined by State law (§483.40(e)&(f));

    - Clarifying that staff know when to contact the medical director; for example, if an attending or covering physician fails to respond to a facility's request to evaluate or discuss a resident with an acute change of condition;

    - Clarifying how the medical director is expected to respond when informed that the staff is having difficulty obtaining needed consultations or other medical services; or

    - Addressing other concerns between the attending physician and the facility, such as issues identified on medication regimen review, or the problematic use of restraints.

In addition, determine how the facility and medical director assure that physicians are informed of expectations and facility policies, and how the medical director reviews the medical care and provides guidance and feedback regarding practitioner performance, as necessary.

Regardless of whether the medical director is the physician member of the quality assurance committee, determine how the facility and medical director exchange information regarding the quality of resident care, medical care, and how the facility disseminates information from the committee to the medical director and attending physicians regarding clinical aspects of care and quality such as infection control, medication and pharmacy issues, incidents and accidents, and other emergency medical issues (§483.75(o)).

DETERMINATION OF COMPLIANCE (Task 6, Appendix P)

Synopsis of Regulation (F501)

This requirement has 3 aspects: Having a physician to serve as medical director, implementing resident care policies, and coordinating medical care. As with all other long term care requirements, the citation of a deficiency at F501, Medical Director, is a deficiency regarding the facility's failure to comply with this regulation. The facility is responsible for designating a physician to serve as medical director and is responsible for oversight of, and collaboration with, the medical director to implement resident care policies and to coordinate medical care.

Criteria for Compliance

The facility is in compliance if:

- They have designated a medical director who is a licensed physician;
- The physician is performing the functions of the position;
- The medical director provides input and helps the facility develop, review and implement resident care policies, based on current clinical standards; and
- The medical director assists the facility in the coordination of medical care and services in the facility.

If not, cite F501.

Noncompliance for F501

After completing the Investigative Protocol, analyze the data in order to determine whether or not noncompliance with the regulation exists. The survey team must identify whether the noncompliance cited at other tags relates to the medical director's roles and responsibilities. In order to cite at F501 when noncompliance has been identified at another tag, the team must demonstrate an association between the identified deficiency and a failure of medical direction. Noncompliance for F501 may include (but is not limited to) the **facility's** failure to:

- Designate a licensed physician to serve as medical director; or
- Obtain the medical director's input for timely and ongoing development, review and approval of resident care policies;

Noncompliance for F501 may also include (but is not limited to) the **facility** and **medical director** failure to:

- Coordinate and evaluate the medical care within the facility, including the review and evaluation of aspects of physician care and practitioner services;
- Identify, evaluate, and address health care issues related to the quality of care and quality of life of residents;
- Assure that residents have primary attending and backup physician coverage;
- Assure that physician and health care practitioner services reflect current standards of care and are consistent with regulatory requirements;
- Address and resolve concerns and issues between the physicians, health care practitioners and facility staff;
- Resolve issues related to continuity of care and transfer of medical information between the facility and other care settings;
- Review individual resident cases, as warranted, to evaluate quality of care or quality of life concerns or other problematic situations and take appropriate steps to resolve the situation as necessary and as requested;
- Review, consider and/or act upon consultant recommendations that affect the facility's resident care policies and procedures or the care of an individual resident, when appropriate;
- Discuss and intervene (as appropriate) with the health care practitioner about medical care that is inconsistent with applicable current standards of care; or
- Assure that a system exists to monitor the performance and practices of the health care practitioners.

This does not presume that a facility's noncompliance with the requirements for the delivery of care necessarily reflects on the performance of the medical director.

V. DEFICIENCY CATEGORIZATION (Part V, Appendix P)

Once the survey team has completed its investigation, analyzed the data, reviewed the regulatory requirements, and determined that noncompliance exists, the team must determine the severity of each deficiency, based on the resultant effect or potential for harm to the resident.

The key elements for severity determination for F501 are as follows:

1. Presence of harm/negative outcome(s) or potential for negative outcomes because of lack of resident care policies and/or medical care.

Deficient practices related to actual or potential harm/negative outcome for F501 may include but are not limited to:

- Lack of medical director involvement in the development, review and/or implementation of resident care policies that address the types of residents receiving care and services, such as a resident with end-stage renal disease, pressure ulcers, dementia, or that address practices such as restraint use;
- Lack of medical director involvement in coordinating medical care regarding problems with physician coverage or availability; or
- Lack of medical director response when the facility requests intervention with an attending physician regarding medical care of a resident.

2. Degree of harm (actual or potential) related to the noncompliance.

Identify how the facility practices caused, resulted in, allowed or contributed to the actual or potential for harm:

- If harm has occurred, determine if the harm is at the level of serious injury, impairment, death, compromise, or discomfort; and
- If harm has not yet occurred, determine the potential for serious injury, impairment, death, compromise, or discomfort to occur to the resident.

3. The immediacy of correction required.

Determine whether the noncompliance requires immediate correction in order to prevent serious injury, harm, impairment, or death to one or more residents.

The survey team must evaluate the harm or potential for harm based upon the following levels of severity for F501. First, the team must rule out whether Severity Level 4, Immediate Jeopardy, to a resident's health or safety exists by evaluating the deficient practice in relation to immediacy, culpability, and severity. (Follow the guidance in Appendix Q.)

Severity Level 4 Considerations: Immediate Jeopardy to Resident Health or Safety

Immediate Jeopardy is a situation in which the facility's noncompliance with one or more requirements of participation:

- Has allowed/caused/resulted in, or is likely to allow/cause /result in serious injury, harm, impairment, or death to a resident; and
- Requires immediate correction, as the facility either created the situation or allowed the situation to continue by failing to implement preventative or corrective measures.

NOTE: The death or transfer of a resident who was harmed or injured as a result of facility noncompliance does not remove a finding of immediate jeopardy. The facility is required to implement specific actions to correct the noncompliance which allowed or caused the immediate jeopardy.

In order to cite immediate jeopardy at this tag, the surveyor must be able to identify the relationship between noncompliance cited as immediate jeopardy at other regulatory tags, and the failure of the medical care and systems associated with the roles and responsibilities of the medical director. **In order to select severity level 4 at F501, both of the following must be present:**

1. Findings of noncompliance at Severity Level 4 at another tag:
    - Must have allowed, caused or resulted in, or is likely to allow, cause or result in serious injury, harm, impairment or death and require immediate correction. The findings of noncompliance associated with immediate jeopardy are written at tags that also show evidence of process failures with respect to the medical director's responsibilities; and
2. There is no medical director or the facility failed to involve the medical director in resident care policies or resident care or medical care as appropriate, or the medical director had knowledge of a problem with care, or physician services, or lack of resident care policies and practices that meet current standards of practice and failed:

- To get involved or to intercede with the attending physician in order to facilitate and/or coordinate medical care; and/or
- To provide guidance and/or oversight for relevant resident care policies.

NOTE: If immediate jeopardy has been ruled out based upon the evidence, then evaluate whether actual harm that is not immediate jeopardy exists at Severity Level 3.

Severity Level 3 Considerations: Actual Harm that is not Immediate Jeopardy

Level 3 indicates noncompliance that results in actual harm, and may include, but is not limited to, clinical compromise, decline, or the resident's inability to maintain and/or reach his/her highest practicable well-being.

In order to cite actual harm at this tag, the surveyor must be able to identify a relationship between noncompliance cited at other regulatory tags and failure of medical care or processes and practices associated with roles and responsibilities of the medical director, such as:

1. Findings of noncompliance at Severity Level 3 at another tag must have caused actual harm:

    - The findings of noncompliance associated with actual harm are written at tags that show evidence of process failures with respect to the medical director's responsibilities; and

2. There is no medical director or the facility failed to involve the medical director in resident care policies or resident care or medical care as appropriate or the medical director had knowledge of a problem with care, or physician services, or lack of resident care policies and practices that meet current standards of practice and failed:

    - To get involved or intercede with the attending physician in order to facilitate and/or coordinate medical care (medical care and systems associated with roles and responsibilities of the medical director show evidence of breakdown); or

    - To provide guidance and/or oversight for resident care policies.

NOTE: If Severity Level 3 (actual harm that is not immediate jeopardy) has been ruled out based upon the evidence, then evaluate as to whether Level 2 (no actual harm with the potential for more than minimal harm) exists.

Severity Level 2 Considerations: No Actual Harm with Potential for More than Minimal Harm that is not Immediate Jeopardy

In order to cite no actual harm with potential for more than minimal harm at this tag, the surveyor must be able to identify a relationship between noncompliance cited at other regulatory tags and the failure of medical care, processes and practices associated with roles and responsibilities of the medical director, such as:

1. Findings of noncompliance at Severity Level 2 at another tag:

- Must have caused no actual harm with potential for more than minimal harm (Level 2). Level 2 indicates noncompliance that results in a resident outcome of no more than minimal discomfort and/or has the potential to compromise the resident's ability to maintain or reach his or her highest practicable level of well being. The potential exists for greater harm to occur if interventions are not provided; and

2. There is no medical director or the facility failed to involve the medical director in resident care policies or resident care as appropriate or the medical director had knowledge of an issue with care or physician services, and failed:

- To get involved with or intercede with attending physicians in order to facilitate and/or coordinate medical care; or

- To provide guidance and/or oversight for resident care policies.

Severity Level 1 Considerations: No Actual Harm with Potential for Minimal Harm

In order to cite no actual harm with potential for minimal harm at this tag, the survey team must have identified that:

- There is no medical director; and
    - There are no negative resident outcomes that are the result of deficient practice; and
    - Medical care and systems associated with roles and responsibilities of the medical director are in place; and
    - There has been a relatively short duration of time without a medical director; and
    - The facility is actively seeking a new medical director.

F502

§483.75(j) Laboratory Services

(1) The facility must provide or obtain laboratory services to meet the needs of its residents. The facility is responsible for the quality and timeliness of the services.

Intent: §483.75(j)(1)

The intent of this regulation is to assure that laboratory services are accurate and timely so that the utility of laboratory testing for diagnosis, treatment, prevention or assessment is maximized. The facility is responsible for quality and timely laboratory services whether or not services are provided by the facility or an outside agency.

Interpretive Guidelines: §483.75(j)(1)

A "**laboratory service or test**" is defined as any examination or analysis of materials derived from the human body for purposes of providing information for the diagnosis, prevention, or treatment of any disease or impairment of, or the assessment of the health of human beings.

Services provided must be both accurate and timely. Timely means that laboratory tests are completed and results are provided to the facility (or resident's physician) within timeframes normal for appropriate intervention. All laboratories providing services for facility residents must meet applicable requirements of 42 CFR Part 493. The purpose of this requirement is to assist in assuring quality of laboratory services.

Procedures: §483.75(j)(1)

Verify that laboratory services are provided to meet the needs of the residents. If a problem in quality of care leads you to suspect a problem in laboratory services, timeliness or quality, refer to the interpretive guidelines for laboratory testing found in Appendix C.

Probes: §483.75(j)(1)

Are problems attributable to:

- An inability to order laboratory tests in a timely manner, including delays in transporting the resident to and from the source of service, if needed?
- A delay of treatment due to untimely receipt of lab results?
- A large lag time between an order for a test and the recording of the results that may have resulted in poor care?

F503

§483.75(j)(1)(i) If the facility provides its own laboratory services, the services must meet the applicable requirements for laboratories specified in part 493 of this chapter.

§483.75(j)(1)(ii) If the facility provides blood bank and transfusion services, it must meet the applicable requirements for laboratories specified in Part 493 of this chapter.

§483.75(j)(1)(iii) If the laboratory chooses to refer specimens for testing to another laboratory, the referral laboratory must be certified in the appropriate specialties and subspecialties of services in accordance with the requirements of part 493 of this chapter.

§483.75(j)(1)(iv) If the facility does not provide laboratory services on site, it must have an agreement to obtain these services from a laboratory that meets the applicable requirements of part 493 of this chapter.

Intent: §483.75(j)(1)(i) - (iv)

The intent of this regulation is to assure that laboratory services, blood bank and transfusion services are obtained from an entity that meets the requirements of 42 CFR Part 493 in order to provide a standard of quality for laboratory and transfusion services. If the long term care facility does not provide laboratory services on site, there must be an agreement to obtain these services from a laboratory that meets the same requirements.

Interpretive Guidelines: §483.75(j)(1)(i) - (iv)

If a facility provides its own laboratory services, the provisions of 42 CFR Part 493 apply.

The facility must have a Clinical Laboratory Improvement Amendments (CLIA) certificate appropriate for the level of testing performed. An application for a certificate of waiver may be made if the facility performs only those tests categorized as waived under CLIA.

Direct questions concerning the application of these requirements to your State laboratory consultant or the CMS RO.

Procedures: §483.75(j)(1)(i) - (iv)

Determine if all laboratory services provided for the facility are provided by a laboratory that meets the requirements of 42 CFR Part 493.

The surveyor should determine if the facility has an arrangement in writing to assume responsibility for (a) obtaining services that meet professional standards and principles that apply to professionals providing services in such a facility; and (b) the timeliness of the services.

Probes: §483.75(j)(1)(i) - (iv)

Are problems attributable to:

- Lack of an arrangement to provide or obtain clinical laboratory services from a source that meets the applicable conditions for coverage of the services?
- Delays in interpreting the results of laboratory tests?

F504

§483.75(j)(2) The facility must--

§483.75(j)(2)(i) Provide or obtain laboratory services only when ordered by the attending physician;

Intent §483.75(j)(2)(i)

The intent of this regulation is to assure that only medically necessary laboratory services are ordered.

Procedures §483.75(j)(2)(i)

Verify that all laboratory services received were ordered by the attending physician.

F505

§483.75(j)(2)(ii) Promptly notify the attending physician of the findings;

Intent §483.75(j)(2)(ii)

The intent of this regulation is to assure that the physician is notified of all lab results so that prompt, appropriate action may be taken if indicated for the resident's care.

Procedures §483.75(j)(2)(ii)

If you have reason to believe that a physician(s) may not have been notified of laboratory results in a timely manner, determine if the facility has a policy/procedure for routine notification of physician and if the procedure is implemented.

Probes: §483.75(j)(2)(ii)

- Are any problems identified as relating to lack of prompt notification of the attending physician, contributing to delays in changing the course of treatment or care plan?

F506

§483.75(j)(2)(iii) Assist the resident in making transportation arrangements to and from the source of service, if the resident needs assistance; and

Intent §483.75(j)(2)(iii)

The intent of this regulation is to assure that residents are able to get to and receive necessary laboratory testing when the testing is conducted outside of the facility.

Probes: §483.75(j)(2)(iii)

- Does the resident ever have to cancel lab service appointments due to difficulties with transportation?

F507

§483.75(j)(2)(iv) File in the resident's clinical record laboratory reports that are dated and contain the name and address of the testing laboratory.

Intent §483.75(j)(2)(iv)

The intent of this regulation is to assure that the laboratory performing the tests is Medicare approved, and that test results are accurate and are available for clinical management.

F508

§483.75(k) Radiology and Other Diagnostic Services

(1) The facility must provide or obtain radiology and other diagnostic services to meet the needs of its residents. The facility is responsible for the quality and timeliness of the services.

Intent §483.75(k)(1)

The intent of this regulation is to assure that the resident receives quality radiologic and diagnostic services in a timely manner to meet his/her needs for diagnosis, treatment, and prevention.

Probes: §483.75(k)(1)

If problems are identified in radiology or other diagnostic services, are problems attributable to:

- An inability to order radiological and diagnostic services in a timely manner, including delays in transporting the resident for these services?
- Delays in interpreting the results of x-rays and other tests?
- Lack of prompt notification, in writing, of test results to the attending physician, contributing to delays in changing care plans or the course of treatment?

F509

§483.75(k)(1)(i) If the facility provides its own diagnostic services, the services must meet the applicable conditions of participation for hospitals contained in §482.26 of this subchapter.

§483.75(k)(1)(ii) If the facility does not provide it's own diagnostic services, it must have an agreement to obtain these services from a provider or supplier that is approved to provide these services under Medicare.

F510

§483.75(k)(2) The Facility must---

(i) Provide or obtain radiology and other diagnostic services only when ordered by the attending physician;

F511

§483.75(k)(2)(ii) Promptly notify the attending physician of the findings;

F512

§483.75(k)(2)(iii) Assist the resident in making transportation arrangements to and from the source of service, if the resident needs assistance; and

---

F513

§483.75(k)(2)(iv) File in the resident's clinical record signed and dated reports of x-ray and other diagnostic services.

F514

§483.75(l) Clinical Records

(1) The facility must maintain clinical records on each resident in accordance with accepted professional standards and practices that are--

(i) Complete;

(ii) Accurately documented;

(iii) Readily accessible; and

(iv) Systematically organized.

Intent §483.75(l)(1)

To assure that the facility maintains accurate, complete and organized clinical information about each resident that is readily accessible for resident care.

Interpretive Guidelines **§483.75(l)(1)**

A complete clinical record contains an accurate and functional representation of the actual experience of the individual in the facility. It must contain enough information to show that the facility knows the status of the individual, has adequate plans of care, and provides sufficient evidence of the effects of the care provided. Documentation should provide a picture of the resident's progress, including response to treatment, change in condition, and changes in treatment.

The facility determines how frequently documentation of an individual's progress takes place apart from the annual comprehensive assessment, periodic reassessments when a significant change in status occurs, and quarterly monitoring assessments. Good practice indicates that for functional and behavioral objectives, the clinical record should document change toward achieving care plan goals. Thus, while there is no "right" frequency or format for "reporting" progress, there is a unique reporting schedule to chart each resident's progress in maintaining or improving functional abilities and mental and psychosocial status. Be more concerned with whether the staff has sufficient progress information to work with the resident and less with how often that information is gathered.

In cases in which facilities have created the option for an individual's record to be maintained by computer, rather than hard copy, electronic signatures are acceptable. In cases when such attestation is done on computer records, safeguards to prevent unauthorized access, and reconstruction of information must be in place. The following guideline is an example of how such a system may be set up:

- There is a written policy, at the health care facility, describing the attestation policy(ies) in force at the facility.
- The computer has built-in safeguards to minimize the possibility of fraud.
- Each person responsible for an attestation has an individualized identifier.
- The date and time is recorded from the computer's internal clock at the time of entry
- An entry is not to be changed after it has been recorded.
- The computer program controls what sections/areas any individual can access or enter data, based on the individual's personal identifier (and, therefore his/her level of professional qualifications).

Procedures §483.75(l)(1)

In reviewing sampled residents' clinical records:

- Is there enough record documentation for staff to conduct care programs and to revise the program, as necessary, to respond to the changing status of the resident as a result of interventions?
- How is the clinical record used in managing the resident's progress in maintaining or improving functional abilities and mental and psychosocial status?

§483.75(l)(5) the clinical record must contain--

(i) Sufficient information to identify the resident;

(ii) A record of the resident's assessments;

(iii) the plan of care and services provided;

(iv) The results of any preadmission screening conducted by the State; and

(v) progress notes.

F515

§483.75(l)(2) Clinical records must be retained for--

(i) The period of time required by State law; or

(ii) Five years from the date of discharge when there is no requirement in State law; or,

(iii) For a minor, three years after a resident reaches legal age under State law.

F516

§483.20(f)(5)

(5) Resident-identifiable information.

(i) A facility may not release information that is resident-identifiable to the public.

(ii) The facility may release information that is resident-identifiable to an agent only in accordance with a contract under which the agent agrees not to use or disclose the information except to the extent the facility itself is permitted to do so.

Interpretive Guidelines §483.20(f)(5):

Automated RAI data are part of a resident's clinical record and as such are protected from improper disclosure by facilities under current law. Facilities are required by §§1819(c)(1)(A)(iv) and 1919(c)(1)(A)(iv) of the Act and 42 CFR Part 483.75(l)(3) and (l)(4), to keep confidential all information contained in the resident's record and to maintain safeguards against the unauthorized use of a resident's clinical record information, regardless of the storage method of the records.

§483.75(l) (3) The facility must safeguard clinical record information against loss, destruction, or unauthorized use;

Intent §483.75(l)(3)

To maintain the safety and confidentiality of the resident's record.

Procedures §483.75(l)(3)

Determine through observations and interviews with staff, the policy and implementation of that policy, for maintaining confidentiality of residents' records.

Probes: §483.75(1)(3)

- How does the facility ensure confidentiality of resident records/
- If there is a problem with confidentiality, is it systematic, that is, does the problem lie in the recordkeeping system, or with a staff person's use of records, e.g., leaving records in a place easily accessible to residents, visitors, or other unauthorized persons?

Intent: §483.75(l)(3)

To maintain the safety and confidentiality of the resident's record.

Procedures: §483.75(l)(3)

Determine through observations and interviews with staff, the policy and implementation of that policy, for maintaining confidentiality of residents' records.

Probes: §483.75(1)(3)

- How does the facility ensure confidentiality of resident records/
- If there is a problem with confidentiality, is it systematic, that is, does the problem lie in the recordkeeping system, or with a staff person's use of records, e.g., leaving records in a place easily accessible to residents, visitors, or other unauthorized persons?

---

§483.75(m) Disaster and Emergency Preparedness

F517

§483.75(m)(1) The facility must have detailed written plans and procedures to meet all potential emergencies and disasters, such as fire, severe weather, and missing residents.

F518

§483.75(m)(2) The facilities must train all employees in emergency procedures when they begin to work in the facility, periodically review the procedures with existing staff, and carry out unannounced staff drills using those procedures.

Interpretive Guidelines §483.75(m)

The facility should tailor its disaster plan to its geographic location and the types of residents it serves. "Periodic review" is a judgment made by the facility based on its unique circumstances changes in physical plant or changes external to the facility can cause a review of the disaster review plan

The purpose of a "staff drill" is to test the efficiency, knowledge, and response of institutional personnel in the event of an emergency. Unannounced staff drills are directed at the responsiveness of staff, and care should be taken not to disturb or excite residents.

Procedures; §483.75(m)

Review and disaster and emergence preparedness plan, including plans for natural or man made disasters

Probes: §483.75(m)

Ask two staff persons separately (e.g., nurse aide, housekeeper, maintenance person) and the charge nurse:

- If the fire alarm goes off, what do you do?
- If you discover that a resident missing, what do you do?
- What would you do if you discovered a fire in a resident's room?
- Where are fire alarms and fire extinguisher(s) located on this unit?
- How do you use the fire extinguisher?

NOTE: Also, construct probes relevant to a geographically specific natural emergencies (e.g., for areas prone to hurricanes, tornadoes, earthquakes, or floods, each of which may require a different response).

Are the answers to these questions correct (staff answers predict competency in assuring resident safety)?

F519

§483.75(n) Transfer Agreement

(1) In accordance with section 1861(1) of the Act, the facility (other than a nursing facility which is located in a State on an Indian reservation) must have in effect a written transfer agreement with one or more hospitals approved for participation under the Medicare and Medicaid programs that reasonably assures that—

> **(i) Residents will be transferred from the facility to the hospital, and ensured of timely admission to the hospital when transfer is medically appropriate, as determined by the attending physician; and**
>
> **(ii) Medical and other information needed for care and treatment of residents, and , when the transferring facility deems it appropriate, for determining whether such residents can be adequately cared for in a less expensive setting than either the facility or the hospital, will be exchanged between the institutions**

(2) The facility is considered to have a transfer agreement in effect if the facility has attempted in good faith to enter into an agreement with a hospital sufficiently close to the facility to make transfer feasible.

F520

483.75(o) Quality Assessment and Assurance

(1) A facility must maintain a quality assessment and assurance committee consisting of –

- **(i) The director of nursing services;**
- **(ii) A physician designated by the facility; and**
- **(iii) At least 3 other members of the facility's staff.**

(2) The quality assessment and assurance committee –

> **(i) Meets at least quarterly to identify issues with respect to which quality assessment and assurance activities are necessary; and**
>
> **(ii) Develops and implements appropriate plans of action to correct identified quality deficiencies.**

(3) State or the Secretary may not require disclosure of the records of such committee except insofar as such disclosure is related to the compliance of such committee with the requirements of this section.

(4) Good faith attempts by the committee to identify and correct quality deficiencies will not be used as a basis for sanctions.

Intent: 483.75(o) Quality Assurance and Assessment

The intent of this requirement is that:

- The facility has an ongoing quality assessment and assurance (QAA) committee that includes designated key members and that meets at least quarterly; and

- The committee identifies quality deficiencies and develops and implements plans of action to correct these quality deficiencies, including monitoring the effect of implemented changes and making needed revisions to the action plans.

Definitions

Definitions are provided to clarify terms related to the requirement for a quality assessment and assurance committee.

- "Quality Assessment" is an evaluation of a process and/or outcomes of a process to determine if a defined standard of quality is being achieved.

- "Quality Assurance" is the organizational structure, processes, and procedures designed to ensure that care practices are consistently applied and the facility meets or exceeds an expected standard of quality. Quality assurance includes the implementation of principles of continuous quality improvement.

- "Quality Deficiencies" are potential markers of quality that the facility considers to be in need of investigating and which, after investigation, may or may not represent a deviation from quality that results in a potential or actual undesirable outcome. The term "quality deficiency" in this regulation is meant to describe a deficit or an area for improvement. This term is not synonymous with a deficiency cited by surveyors.
- "Quality Improvement (QI)" is an ongoing interdisciplinary process that is designed to improve the delivery of services and resident outcomes.

NOTE: Many facilities have changed their terminology for the QAA processes to "quality improvement (QI)." However, in these guidelines, we will continue to use the designation of QAA, as specified in the requirement. The elements are comparable regardless of the terminology.

Overview

QAA is a management process that is ongoing, multi-level, and facility-wide. It encompasses all managerial, administrative, clinical, and environmental services, as well as the performance of outside (contracted or arranged) providers and suppliers of care and services. Its purpose is continuous evaluation of facility systems with the objectives of:

- Keeping systems functioning satisfactorily and consistently including maintaining current practice standards;
- Preventing deviation from care processes from arising, to the extent possible;
- Discerning issues and concerns, if any, with facility systems and determining if issues/concerns are identified; and
- Correcting inappropriate care processes.

Several studies conducted under the auspices of the U.S. Department of Health and Human Services have examined quality of care and quality of life in nursing homes.[1,2] These studies have concluded that QAA committees provide an important point of accountability for ensuring both quality of care and quality of life in nursing homes. The QAA committees represent key internal mechanisms that allow nursing homes opportunities to deal with quality deficiencies in a confidential manner.

Resources are available that recommend processes and standards to develop and enhance quality improvement programs. Some Web site resources include:

- American Medical Directors Association (www.amda.com);
- American Health Care Association (www.ahca.org);
- American College of Physicians Quality Indicators for Assessing Care of Vulnerable Elders (www.acponline.org/sci-policy/acove/);
- American Geriatric Society (www.americangeriatrics.org);
- Agency for Healthcare Research and Quality (www.ahrq.gov);
- Medicare Quality Improvement Community (www.Medqic.org);

- American Association of Homes and Services for the Aging (www.aahsa.org); and

- The American Health Quality Association (www.ahqa.org).

NOTE: References to non-CMS sources or sites on the Internet are provided as a service and do not constitute or imply endorsement of these organizations or their programs by CMS or the U.S. Department of Health and Human Services. CMS is not responsible for the content of pages found at these sites. The URL addresses were current as of the date of this publication.

The guidance below includes sections that describe facility responsibilities to meet the various aspects of the QAA requirement, including:

- The composition of the QAA committee and the minimum frequency of committee meetings;

- The committee's monitoring of systems and identification of concerns with the quality of facility systems; and

- Modification and correction of facility systems, when needed, including monitoring the effect of action plans.

QAA COMMITTEE FUNCTIONS

Key aspects of the QAA requirements include the specifications that the facility must have a QAA committee, that this committee must include certain staff members, and that the committee must meet at least quarterly. The QAA committee is responsible for identifying whether quality deficiencies are present (potential or actual deviations from appropriate care processes or facility procedures) that require action. If there are quality deficiencies, the committee is responsible for developing plans of action to correct them and for monitoring the effect of these corrections. These functions of the QAA committee are described below.

Committee Composition and Frequency of Meetings

The regulation states that the QAA committee must include the director of nursing, a physician, and three other staff. These additional members may include:

- The administrator (facilities with effective QAA committees include members who have knowledge of facility systems and the authority to change those systems, including the administrator or assistant administrator due to their responsibility to manage the facility, and make changes to facility systems);

- The medical director (part of the medical director's responsibility (see F501)) is to guide the facility's development and implementation of resident care policies and coordination of medical care. If the medical director is not a committee member, exchange of information with the medical director enhances the functioning of the QAA committee);

- Staff with responsibility for direct resident care and services, such as nursing aides, therapists, staff nurses, social workers, activities staff members; and

- Staff with responsibility for the physical plant, such as maintenance, housekeeping, and laundry staff.

NOTE: Facilities may have a larger committee than required by the regulation. Consideration should be given as to how committee information is provided to consultants who may not be members of the committee, but whose responsibilities include oversight of departments or services.

Meetings of the QAA committee must be held at least quarterly or more often as the facility deems necessary to fulfill committee functions and operate effectively. The Committee should maintain a record of the dates of all meetings and the names/titles of those attending each meeting.

Identification of Quality Deficiencies

Facilities can collect and analyze data about their performance from various sources that may help them to identify quality deficiencies. These may include information from reports such as open and closed record audits, facility logs and tracking forms, incident reports, consultants' reports, and other reports as part of the QAA function. Quality deficiencies related to facility operations and practices are not only related to those that cause negative outcomes, but also may be directed toward enhancing quality of care and quality of life for residents. The committee responds to quality deficiencies and serves a preventative function by reviewing and improving systems.

Records of the committee meetings identifying quality deficiencies, by statute, may not be reviewed by surveyors unless the facility chooses to provide them. However, the documents the committee used to determine quality deficiencies are subject to review by the surveyors.

NOTE: A State or the Secretary may not require disclosure of the records of the QAA committee except insofar as such disclosure is related to the compliance of the QAA committee with the regulations.

If concerns, especially repeat survey deficiencies, have not been identified by the facility's QAA committee, this may be an indication that the committee is not performing the functions required by this regulation.

Development of Action Plans

In order to fulfill the regulatory mandate, the facility's QAA committee, having identified the root causes which led to their confirmed quality deficiencies, must develop appropriate corrective plans of action. Action plans may include, but are not limited to, the development or revision of clinical protocols based on current standards of practice, revision of policies and procedures, training for staff concerning changes, plans to purchase or repair equipment and/or improve the physical plant, and standards for evaluating staff performance.

Implementation of Action Plans and Correction of Identified Quality Deficiencies

The facility's action plans to address quality deficiencies may be implemented in a variety of ways, including: staff training and deployment of changes to procedures; monitoring and feedback mechanisms; and processes to revise plans that are not achieving or sustaining desired outcomes. The committee may delegate the implementation of action plans to various facility staff and/or outside consultants.

ENDNOTES

[1] Institute of Medicine (2001). Improving the Quality of Long-Term Care. Washington, DC: National Academy Press.

[2] Office of Inspector General (2003) Quality Assurance Committees in Nursing Homes, Baltimore, MD: U.S. Department of Health and Human Services (OEI-01-01-00090).

INVESTIGATIVE PROTOCOL

QUALITY ASSESSMENT AND ASSURANCE

Objectives

- To determine if the facility has a QAA committee consisting of the director of nursing, a physician designated by the facility, and at least three other staff members; and

- To determine if the QAA committee:

    - Meets at least quarterly (or more often, as necessary);

    - Identifies quality deficiencies; and

    - Develops and implements appropriate plans of action to address identified quality deficiencies.

Use

Use this protocol for all initial and standard surveys. Also, use it as necessary on revisits and abbreviated standard surveys (complaint investigations).

Procedures

During Offsite Survey Preparation (see Appendix P, Task 1), the survey team must review information about the facility prior to the survey. Sources include, at a minimum:

- Quality Measure/Quality Indicator Reports;

- The OSCAR 3 Report (includes a 4-year history of the facility's deficiencies from standard surveys, revisits, and complaint surveys). The survey team should determine if the facility has had repeat deficiencies as well as recent serious deficiencies (Levels F and H and above); and

- Information from the State ombudsman.

The regulation states that good faith attempts by the committee to identify and correct quality deficiencies will not be used as a basis for sanctions. The facility is not required to release the records of the QAA committee to the surveyors to review, and the facility is not required to disclose records of the QAA committee beyond those that demonstrate compliance with the regulation (F520). However the facility may choose such disclosure if it is the facility's only means of showing the composition and functioning of the QAA committee. If the facility has provided the records for surveyor review, this information may not be used to cite deficiencies unrelated to the QAA committee requirement. It is recommended that surveyors not review QAA records (if provided) until after they complete their investigations of other tags.

If the survey team's review of the QAA committee records reveals that the committee is making good faith efforts to identify quality deficiencies and to develop action plans to correct quality deficiencies, this requirement (F520) should not be cited. However, if the survey team had already independently (not through use of the records) identified noncompliance in the same areas as those that have been selected by the QAA committee, the team is expected to cite the noncompliance for the other requirements.

Throughout the survey, the survey team may become aware of other concerns regarding the delivery of care and services that may reflect that the QAA committee is not functioning in identifying ongoing and current quality deficiencies.

During the daily meetings, the team discusses concerns about facility compliance that they are identifying through observations, interviews, and record reviews. The information from the entrance conference about the composition and meetings of the QAA committee is reviewed and relayed to the team.

The team coordinator assigns a surveyor to obtain information from the person the facility has designated as responsible for the QAA committee. The surveyor should interview this designated person to determine:

- How the committee identifies current and ongoing issues for committee action. This could include how they monitor the provision of care and services on an ongoing basis, and how they ascertain from residents and/or their families information regarding the facility's provision of care and services, in addition to facility staff throughout the various departments, and outside consultants and/or suppliers and providers of care;

- The methods the committee uses to develop action plans; and

- How current action plans are being implemented, including: staff training; deployment of changes to procedures; monitoring and feedback mechanisms that have been established; and, for any plans that are not achieving or sustaining desired outcomes to correct the deficiencies, the process underway for revision to these plans.

The assigned surveyor should interview staff in various departments to determine if they know how to bring an issue to the attention of the QAA committee.

If, during the course of the survey, the survey team identifies noncompliance at a particular requirement, the assigned surveyor should interview the designated person responsible for the QAA committee to determine whether the committee knew of or should have known of the issues related to the noncompliance. The assigned surveyor should determine if the committee had considered the quality deficiency and if it was determined that an action plan was needed. If so, the surveyor determines whether the committee developed and implemented any action plans to address these concerns. The survey team should verify that the action plans that are described are actually implemented, and that staff are providing care and services according to the directives of these action plans.

DETERMINATION OF COMPLIANCE (Task 6, Appendix P)

NOTE: Although the literature of QAA and QI provides various definitions of the facility's achievement of quality, surveyors will need to determine the facility's compliance based on the language of this regulation.

Synopsis of Regulation (F520)

This requirement has two aspects: the facility must have a committee composed of certain key members that meets at least quarterly (or more often, as necessary); and the committee functions to develop and implement appropriate plans of actions to correct identified quality deficiencies.

Criteria for Compliance

The facility is in compliance if:

- It has a functioning QAA committee, consisting of the director of nursing, a physician, and at least three other staff members, that meets at least quarterly; and
- The committee:
  - Identifies quality deficiencies; and
  - **Develops and implements appropriate plans of actions.**

If not, cite F520.

Noncompliance for F520

After completing the investigative protocol, the survey team determines whether or not compliance with the regulation exists. Examples of noncompliance may include, but are not limited to, the following:

- Lack of a physician member of the committee;
- The committee met only twice during the previous year;
- The action plan to correct a quality deficiency regarding food temperatures was not being followed by staff in the dietary department, and food was not being served at proper temperatures; or
- An action plan was developed to correct a problem with inadequate assessment of root causes of falls. Staff did not implement the plan, and residents continued to experience serious falls.
- An action plan that was developed to correct the issue of resident falls did not take account of the root cause of the falls being overuse of sedative type medications. The plan was to increase the use of restraints which was an inappropriate action plan.

DEFICIENCY CATEGORIZATION (Part V, Appendix P)

Once the survey team has determined that noncompliance exists, the team will select the appropriate level of severity for the deficiency using the guidance below.

The survey team must identify a relationship between noncompliance at other regulatory requirements and the facility's failure to have a functional QAA committee. The key elements for severity determination for F520 are as follows:

1. Presence of harm/negative outcome(s) or potential for negative outcomes because of a failure of the QAA committee structure or function

   Actual or potential harm/negative outcome for F520 may include, but is not limited to:

   - Failure of the QAA committee to identify and implement an action plan to reduce of medication errors committed by agency staff, resulting in the noncompliance for medication errors based on the resident receiving the wrong medication, which resulted in the resident experiencing insulin shock; or

- Failure of the QAA committee to develop an action plan to address assessment of the cause of a pattern of recent falls of several residents, resulting in noncompliance at the accident requirement based on several residents sustaining avoidable falls with bruises but no fractures.

2. Degree of harm (actual or potential) related to the noncompliance

Identify how the facility practices caused, resulted in, allowed, or contributed to the actual or potential for harm:

- If harm has occurred, determine if the harm is at the level of serious injury, impairment, death, compromise, or discomfort; and

- If harm has not yet occurred, determine how likely is the potential for serious injury, impairment, death, compromise, or discomfort to occur to the resident.

3. The immediacy of correction required

Determine whether the noncompliance requires immediate correction in order to prevent serious injury, harm, impairment, or death to one or more residents.

The survey team must evaluate the harm or potential for harm based upon the following levels of severity for Tag F520. First, the team must rule out whether Severity Level 4, Immediate Jeopardy to a resident's health or safety, exists by evaluating the deficient practice in relation to immediacy, culpability, and severity. (Follow the guidance in Appendix Q.)

Severity Level 4 Considerations: Immediate Jeopardy to Resident Health or Safety

Immediate Jeopardy is a situation in which the facility's noncompliance with one or more requirements of participation:

- Has caused, or is likely to cause, serious injury, harm, impairment, or death to a resident; and

- Requires immediate correction, as the facility either created the situation or allowed the situation to continue by failing to implement preventive or corrective measures.

NOTE: The death or transfer of a resident who was harmed or injured as a result of facility noncompliance does not remove a finding of immediate jeopardy. The facility is required to implement specific actions to correct the noncompliance which allowed or caused the immediate jeopardy.

In order to select Severity Level 4 for this regulation, the surveyor must be able to identify the relationship between the facility's noncompliance cited at Severity Level 4 at other regulatory tags, and the failure of the QAA Committee to function effectively. In order to select Severity Level 4 at F520, both of the following must be present:

- Deficiency(ies) has been cited at Severity Level 4 in other tags that are related to QAA committee failure; and
- The facility does not have a QAA committee, or the facility's QAA committee failed to develop and implement appropriate plans of action to correct identified quality deficiencies.

Severity Level 3: Actual Harm that is Not Immediate Jeopardy

In order to select Severity Level 3 for this regulation, the surveyor must be able to identify the relationship between the facility's noncompliance cited at Severity Level 3 at other regulatory tags, and the failure of the QAA Committee to function effectively. In order to select Severity Level 3 at F520, both of the following must be present:

- Deficiency(ies) has been cited at Severity Level 3 in other tags that are related to QAA committee failure; and
- The facility does not have a QAA committee, or the facility's QAA committee failed to develop and implement appropriate plans of action to correct identified quality deficiencies.

Severity Level 2: No Actual Harm with Potential for More than Minimal Harm that is Not Immediate Jeopardy

In order to select Severity Level 2 for this regulation, the surveyor must be able to identify the relationship between the facility's noncompliance cited at Severity Level 2 at other regulatory tags, and the failure of the QAA Committee to function effectively. In order to select Severity Level 2 at F520, both of the following must be present:

- Deficiency(ies) has been cited at Severity Level 2 in other tags that are related to QAA committee failure; and
- The facility does not have a QAA committee, or the facility's QAA committee failed to develop and implement appropriate plans of action to correct identified quality deficiencies.

Severity Level 1: No Actual Harm with Potential for Minimal Harm

Severity Level 1 should be selected if any of the following circumstances are present:

- The facility does not have a QAA committee, and there have been no other deficiencies cited above Severity Level 1; or

- The facility has a QAA committee that has failed to meet the regulatory specifications for the composition of the committee and/or the frequency of committee meetings, and there have been no deficiencies cited above Severity Level 1; or

- The facility's QAA committee meets regulatory specifications for committee membership and frequency of meetings, and deficiencies have been cited at Severity Level 1 in other tags. In order to select Severity Level 1 in this case, the surveyor must be able to identify the relationship between the facility's noncompliance cited at Severity Level 1 at other tags, and the failure of the QAA committee to function effectively.

F522

§483.75(p) Disclosure of Ownership

(1) The facility must comply with the disclosure requirements of §§420.206 and 455.104 of this chapter.

(2) The facility must provide written notice to the State agency responsible for licensing the facility at the time of change, if a change occurs in--

(i) Persons with an ownership or control interest, as defined in §§420.201 and 455.101 of this chapter;

(ii) The officers, directors, agents, or managing employees;

(iii) The corporation, association, or other company responsible for the management of the facility; or

(iv) The facility's administrator or director of nursing.

(3) The notice specified in the paragraph (p)(2) of this section must include the identity of each new individual or company.

ENDNOTES

[63] Gurwitz, J.H., Field, T.S., Avorn, J., McCormick, D., Jain, S., Eckler, M., Benser, M., Edmondson, A.C., & Bates, D.W. (2000). Incidence and preventability of adverse drug events in nursing homes. American Journal of Medicine, 109, pp. 87-94.

[64] Gurwitz, J.H., Field, T.S., Judge, J., Rochon, P., Harrold, L.R., Cadoret, C., Lee, M., White, K., LaPrino, J., Erramuspe-Mainard, J., DeFlorio, M., Gavendo, L., Auger, J., & Bates, D.W. (2005). Incidence of adverse drug consequences in two large academic long-term care facilities. American Journal of Medicine, 118, pp. 251-258.

ENDNOTES

[65] Adapted from American Society of Consultant Pharmacists (ASCP) Guidelines for Assessing the Quality of Drug Regimen Review in Long-Term Care Facilities.

[66] Adapted from Hepler, C.D., & Strand, L.M., (1990). Opportunities and responsibilities in pharmaceutical care. American Journal of Hospital Pharmacy, 47, pp.533-543.

[67] Adapted from Top 10 Dangerous Drug Interactions in Long-Term Care presented by the Multidisciplinary Medication Management Project, a collaborative initiative of the American Society of Consultant Pharmacists (ASCP) and the American Medical Directors Association (AMDA).

§483.75(q) Required Training of Feeding Assistants

(Rev. 26; Issued: 08-17-07; Effective/Implementation Dates: 08-17-07)

A facility must not use any individual working in the facility as a paid feeding assistant unless that individual has successfully completed a State-approved training program for feeding assistants, as specified in §483.160 of this part.

Guidelines: §483.75(q)

Note: Refer to F373

Transmittals Issued for this Appendix

Rev #	Issue Date	Subject	Impl Date	CR#
R26SOM	08/17/2007	Revised Appendix P and Appendix PP-New Tag F373	08/17/2007	N/A
R22SOM	12/105/2006	Revisions to Appendix P and PP	12/18/2006	N/A
R21SOM	10/20/2006	Revised Appendix P &Appendix PP-New Tag F334	10/15/2006	N/A
R19SOM	06/01/2006	Revisions to Appendix PP	06/01/2006	N/A
R15SOM	11/28/2005	Medical Director Guidance	11/25/2005	N/A
R14SOM	11/25/2005	Medical Director Guidance – Replaced by Transmittal 15	11/25/2005	N/A
R12SOM	10/14/2005	Appendix PP Technical Corrections	10/14/2005	N/A
R08SOM	06/28/2008	Revision of Appendix PP-Section 483.25(d)-Urinary Incontinence, Tags F315 and F316	06/27/2005	N/A
R07SOM	06/27/2005	Revision of Appendix PP-Section 483.25(d)-Urinary Incontinence, Tags F315 and F316 – Replaced by Transmittal 8	06/28/2005	N/A
R05SOM	11/19/2004	Revisions to Appendix P and Appendix PP	11/19/2004	N/A
R04SOM	11/12/2004	Guidance to Surveyors for Long Term Care Facilities	11/12/2004	N/A
R01SOM	05/21/2004	Initial Release of Pub 100-07	N/A	N/A

PART 3

IMMEDIATE JEOPARDY

State Operations Manual

Appendix Q - Guidelines for Determining Immediate Jeopardy - (Rev. 1, 05-21-04)

PREAMBLE

Changes made to Appendix Q – Guidelines for Determining Immediate Jeopardy, reflect CMS' concern that crisis situations in which the health and safety of individuals are at risk, are accurately identified, thoroughly investigated and resolved as quickly as possible. In the interest of consistency, the new Guidelines standardize the definitions of Immediate Jeopardy, abuse and neglect across all certified Medicare/Medicaid entities (excluding CLIA), and describe the process surveyors use in making a determination of Immediate Jeopardy. The Guidelines provide a detailed analysis of the steps surveyors should follow to assist them in accurately identifying those circumstances which constitute Immediate Jeopardy: preparation, investigation, decision-making and implementation. "Triggers" alert surveyors that some circumstances may have the potential to be identified as Immediate Jeopardy situations and therefore require further investigation before any determination is made. A detailed review of three sample cases "walk" surveyors through the steps necessary to carefully analyze and accurately determine whether or not an Immediate Jeopardy situation exists. To provide further guidance to surveyors, Attachment B uses actual examples of situations in which Immediate Jeopardy has been cited.

In the interest of reducing or eliminating abuse and neglect to all beneficiaries, the Guidelines caution surveyors that when abuse or neglect has been identified, the circumstances must be thoroughly evaluated to determine if Immediate Jeopardy exists.

The Guidelines also clarify that actual harm, as well as the **potential** for harm, to one or to more than one individual may constitute Immediate Jeopardy.

I - Introduction

Immediate Jeopardy is interpreted as a crisis situation in which the health and safety of individual(s) are at risk (see SOM §3010). These guidelines are for use in determining if circumstances pose an Immediate Jeopardy to an individual's health and safety. These guidelines will assist Federal and State Survey and Certification personnel and Complaint Investigators in recognizing situations that may cause or permit Immediate Jeopardy.

These guidelines apply to all certified Medicare/Medicaid entities (excluding CLIA) and to all types of surveys and investigations: certifications, recertifications, revisits, and complaint investigations. In these guidelines, "entity" applies to all Medicare/Medicaid certified providers, suppliers, and facilities. "Surveyor" represents both surveyors and complaint investigators. "Team" represents either a single surveyor or multiple surveyors. The term "Immediate Jeopardy" replaces the terms "Immediate and Serious Threat" and "Serious and Immediate Threat" for all certified Medicare/Medicaid entities.

NOTE: The primary goals of these Immediate Jeopardy guidelines are to identify and to prevent serious injury, harm, impairment, or death.

II - Definitions

The following definitions apply to all certified Medicare/Medicaid entities:

Immediate Jeopardy - "A situation in which the provider's noncompliance with one or more requirements of participation has caused, or is likely to cause, serious injury, harm, impairment, or death to a resident." (See 42 CFR Part 489.3.)

Abuse - "The willful infliction of injury, unreasonable confinement, intimidation, or punishment with resulting physical harm, pain, or mental anguish." (See 42 CFR Part 488.301.)

Neglect - "Failure to provide goods and services necessary to avoid physical harm, mental anguish, or mental illness." (See 42 CFR Part 488.301.)

III - Principles

The goal of the survey process is to ensure the provision of quality care to all individuals receiving care or services from a certified Medicare/Medicaid entity. The identification and removal of Immediate Jeopardy, either psychological or physical, are essential to prevent serious harm, injury, impairment, or death for individuals.

- Only **ONE INDIVIDUAL** needs to be at risk. Identification of Immediate Jeopardy for one individual will prevent risk to other individuals in similar situations.

- **Serious harm, injury, impairment, or death** does **NOT** have to occur before considering Immediate Jeopardy. The high potential for these outcomes to occur in the very near future also constitutes Immediate Jeopardy.

- Individuals must not be subjected to abuse by **anyone** including, but not limited to, entity staff, consultants or volunteers, family members or visitors.

- Serious harm can result from both abuse and neglect.

- Psychological harm is as serious as physical harm.

- When a surveyor has established through investigation that a cognitively impaired individual harmed an individual receiving care and services from the entity due to the entity's failure to provide care and services to avoid physical harm, mental anguish, or mental illness, this should be considered neglect.

- Any time a team cites abuse or neglect, it should consider Immediate.

Upon recognizing a situation that may constitute Immediate Jeopardy, the investigation process must proceed until it confirms or rules out Immediate. The serious harm, injury, impairment or death may have occurred in the past, may be occurring at present, or may be likely to occur in the very near future as a result of the jeopardy situation. After determining that the harm meets the definition of Immediate Jeopardy, consider the following points regarding entity compliance:

- The entity either created a situation or allowed a situation to continue which resulted in serious harm or a potential for serious harm, injury, impairment or death to individuals.

- The entity had an opportunity to implement corrective or preventive measures.

After recognizing Immediate Jeopardy and completing the investigation, the team will then choose the specific Federal regulation(s) to address the deficient practice. Although a specific Federal regulation may not be found for each situation, all Medicare/Medicaid entities have a responsibility to provide quality care. The principles of Immediate Jeopardy apply to all certified entities and need to be followed for all individuals receiving care and services in those entities. The team should determine which Federal regulation(s) to document the deficient practices(s).

NOTE: The key factor in the use of Immediate Jeopardy termination authority is, as the name implies, limited to **Immediate Jeopardy**. Immediate Jeopardy procedures must not be used to enforce compliance quickly on more routine deficiencies.

IV - Immediate Jeopardy Triggers

This guide lists issues with associated triggers. The issues include general statements of practices such as "Failure to protect from abuse." The guide includes situations that most likely create jeopardy to an individual's psychological and/or physical health and safety.

Triggers that will assist the surveyor in considering Immediate Jeopardy accompany each issue. Triggers describe situations that will cause the surveyor to consider if further investigation is needed to determine the presence of Immediate Jeopardy. The listed triggers do not automatically equal Immediate Jeopardy. The team must investigate and use professional judgment to determine if the situation has caused or is likely to cause serious harm, injury, impairment or death. These triggers are general examples and are not all-inclusive. Many triggers may apply to more than one issue. A trigger for an issue such as C, "Failure to Protect from Psychological Harm," could well be an example of A, "Failure to Prevent Abuse," or B, "Failure to Prevent Neglect." The team must rely on professional judgment and utilize the resources of the State survey agency, the Regional Office and/or, in the case of Medicaid-only facilities, the State Medicaid Agency to determine the presence of Immediate Jeopardy.

NOTE: **Harm** does **NOT** have to occur before considering Immediate Jeopardy. Consider both potential and actual harm when reviewing the triggers in the table.

Triggers	
Issue	**Triggers**
A Failure to protect from abuse.	1. Serious injuries such as head trauma or fractures; 2. Non-consensual sexual interactions; e.g., sexual harassment, sexual coercion or sexual assault; 3. Unexplained serious injuries that have not been investigated; 4. Staff striking or roughly handling an individual; 5. Staff yelling, swearing, gesturing or calling an individual derogatory names; 6. Bruises around the breast or genital area; or Suspicious injuries; e.g., black eyes, rope marks, cigarette burns, unexplained bruising.
B Failure to Prevent Neglect	1. Lack of timely assessment of individuals after injury; 2. Lack of supervision for individual with known special needs; 3. Failure to carry out doctor's orders; 4. Repeated occurrences such as falls which place the individual at risk of harm without intervention; 5. Access to chemical and physical hazards by individuals who are at risk; 6. Access to hot water of sufficient temperature to cause tissue injury; 7. Non-functioning call system without compensatory measures; 8. Unsupervised smoking by an individual with a known safety risk; 9. Lack of supervision of cognitively impaired individuals with known elopement risk; 10. Failure to adequately monitor individuals with known severe self-injurious behavior; 11. Failure to adequately monitor and intervene for serious medical/surgical conditions; 12. Use of chemical/physical restraints without adequate monitoring; 13. Lack of security to prevent abduction of infants; 14. Improper feeding/positioning of individual with known aspiration risk; or 15. Inadequate supervision to prevent physical altercations.
C Failure to protect from psychological harm	1. Application of chemical/physical restraints without clinical indications; 2. Presence of behaviors by staff such as threatening or demeaning, resulting in displays of fear, unwillingness to communicate, and recent or sudden changes in behavior by individuals; or 3. Lack of intervention to prevent individuals from creating an environment of fear.

Triggers	
Issue	**Triggers**
D Failure to protect from undue adverse medication consequences and/or failure to provide medications as prescribed.	1. Administration of medication to an individual with a known history of allergic reaction to that medication; 2. Lack of monitoring and identification of potential serious drug interaction, side effects, and adverse reactions; 3. Administration of contraindicated medications; 4. Pattern of repeated medication errors without intervention; 5. Lack of diabetic monitoring resulting or likely to result in serious hypoglycemic or hyperglycemic reaction; or 6. Lack of timely and appropriate monitoring required for drug titration.
E Failure to provide adequate nutrition and hydration to support and maintain health.	1. Food supply inadequate to meet the nutritional needs of the individual; 2. Failure to provide adequate nutrition and hydration resulting in malnutrition; e.g., severe weight loss, abnormal laboratory values; 3. Withholding nutrition and hydration without advance directive; or 4. Lack of potable water supply.
F Failure to protect from widespread nosocomial infections; e.g., failure to practice standard precautions, failure to maintain sterile techniques during invasive procedures and/or failure to identify and treat nosocomial infections	1. Pervasive improper handling of body fluids or substances from an individual with an infectious disease; 2. High number of infections or contagious diseases without appropriate reporting, intervention and care; 3. Pattern of ineffective infection control precautions; or 4. High number of nosocomial infections caused by cross contamination from staff and/or equipment/supplies.
G Failure to correctly identify individuals.	1. Blood products given to wrong individual; 2. Surgical procedure/treatment performed on wrong individual or wrong body part; 3. Administration of medication or treatments to wrong individual; or 4. Discharge of an infant to the wrong individual.

Triggers	
Issue	**Triggers**
H Failure to safely administer blood products and safely monitor organ transplantation.	1. Wrong blood type transfused; 2. Improper storage of blood products; 3. High number of serious blood reactions; 4. Incorrect cross match and utilization of blood products or transplantation organs; or 5. Lack of monitoring for reactions during transfusions.
I Failure to provide safety from fire, smoke and environment hazards and/or failure to educate staff in handling emergency situations.	1. Nonfunctioning or lack of emergency equipment and/or power source; 2. Smoking in high risk areas; 3. Incidents such as electrical shock, fires; 4. Ungrounded/unsafe electrical equipment; 5. Widespread lack of knowledge of emergency procedures by staff; 6. Widespread infestation by insects/rodents; 7. Lack of functioning ventilation, heating or cooling system placing individuals at risk; 8. Use of non-approved space heaters, such as kerosene, electrical, in resident or patient areas; 9. Improper handling/disposal of hazardous materials, chemicals and waste; 10. Locking exit doors in a manner that does not comply with NFPA 101; 11. Obstructed hallways and exits preventing egress; 12. Lack of maintenance of fire or life safety systems; or 13. Unsafe dietary practices resulting in high potential for food borne illnesses.

Triggers	
Issue	**Triggers**
J Failure to provide initial medical screening, stabilization of emergency medical conditions and safe transfer for individuals and women in active labor seeking emergency treatment (Emergency Medical Treatment and Active Labor Act).	1. Individuals turned away from ER without medical screening exam; 2. Women with contractions not medically screened for status of labor; 3. Absence of ER and OB medical screening records; 4. Failure to stabilize emergency medical condition; or 5. Failure to appropriately transfer an individual with an unstabilized emergency medical condition.

Guidelines for Determining Immediate Jeopardy

V - Procedures

A - Preparation

The team should be familiar with the contents of Appendix Q. The guidelines should be foremost in the team's mind to decrease the potential for missing Immediate Jeopardy. The team should also be familiar with the recommended Key Components of an entity's systemic approach to prevent abuse and neglect. The seven Key Components include: screening, training, prevention, identification, investigation, protection, and reporting/response. (Refer to Attachment C.) Both Appendix Q and the Key Components apply to all certified Medicare/Medicaid entities.

B - Investigation

The investigation must be conducted in an impartial, objective manner to obtain accurate data sufficient to support a reasonable conclusion.

1. Observation is a key component of any investigation. All observations need to be thoroughly documented. Be specific in noting time, location and exact observations.

2. The interview notes must be clear and detailed. The documentation should include the full name of the person interviewed. The time and date of the interview should be documented. Any witnesses present should be indicated.

3. Record review is used to support observations and interviews. Obtain copies of relevant documentation supporting the Immediate Jeopardy as you investigate (e.g., nurses' notes, and investigation reports).

4. If the case involves a potential criminal action, the surveyor should be aware that any physical evidence must be preserved for law enforcement agencies.

5. Team Actions

    a. Notify the team leader immediately when an Immediate Jeopardy situation is suspected. The team leader will then coordinate the investigative efforts.

    b. Contact the State survey agency (SA) per the SA protocol.

    c. Gather information to address who, what, when, where and why, such as:

WHO: Who was involved in the Immediate Jeopardy situation: staff, individuals receiving care and services, and others?

Does the individual(s) at risk have special needs? Has this happened to other individuals? If yes, how many? Are there others to whom this is likely to occur? If so, how many and who? Which entity staff knew or should have known about the situation?

WHAT: What harm has occurred, is occurring, or most likely will occur?

How serious is the potential/actual harm? How did the situation occur? What was the sequence of events? What attempts did the entity make to assess, plan, correct, and re-evaluate regarding the potential/actual harm? What did the entity do to prevent any further occurrences of the same nature?

WHEN: When did the situation first occur?

How long has the situation existed? Has a similar occurrence happened before? Has the entity had an opportunity to correct the situation? Did the entity thoroughly investigate the event? Did you agree with the facility's conclusion after their investigation? Did the entity implement corrective measures to prevent any further similar situations? Did they follow up and evaluate the effectiveness of their measures?

WHERE: Where did the potential/actual harm occur? Is this an isolated incident or an entity wide problem?

WHY: Why did the potential/actual harm occur?

Was the Immediate Jeopardy preventable? Is there a system in place to prevent further occurrences? Is this a repeat deficient practice? Is there a pattern of similar deficient practices?

The team then needs to proceed to **validate** the gathered information with facility staff.

Following are two examples of teams gathering information during the investigation to answer the questions: who, what, when, where and why. Refer to C – Decision Making for the completion of the examples.

Example Case #1: The resident was admitted following a hospitalization for psychiatric care. The resident had a history of exiting behavior, impulsiveness and impaired cognition and judgment. Diagnoses included dementia with psychosis and delusion, psychomotor agitation, acute behavioral disturbances, and possible right cerebral vascular accident (CVA). Documented behavior of standing by the facility door waiting for someone to open the door and then sneaking out very fast was included in the chart.

TRIGGER: Lack of supervision of cognitively impaired individuals with known elopement risk.

Investigation:

WHO: Who is the resident? Is the resident cognitively impaired with poor decision-making skills? Is the resident's diagnosis pertinent in this case? Is the resident physically impaired? What is the resident's ambulatory status? Was the resident identified by the facility as a wanderer oblivious to physical and safety needs? Does the resident have a history of leaving the facility without informing the staff? Does the resident's care plan address wandering and risk for elopement? Does the resident wear a safety alarm device? Is there a history of elopement from this facility? How many residents were/are at risk for elopement?

WHAT: What happened? What was the resident's physical, mental, and emotional status prior to elopement? Was the resident injured? Did the facility seek outside medical treatment for the resident? If so, what did the reports from the ER physician's exam include regarding the resident's condition when examined?

WHEN: When was the resident last seen? When did the resident leave the facility? When did the facility take action? When was the resident found? Who found the resident? Was the potential for injury present? Was the outdoor temperature excessively hot or cold? Was it raining, snowing, or storming, etc.? If excessively cold temperatures were present, what was the wind chill factor? How was the resident dressed? What areas of the skin were exposed and for how long?

WHERE: Where did the resident reside? Was the resident on a special unit with extra elopement precautions? Where did this happen? How did the resident exit the facility? Describe the exact location of exit. Where is the facility located (urban or rural)? What hazards were present in the vicinity of the facility (railroad, high motor vehicle traffic, construction zones, farm fields, lakes, ponds, etc.)?

WHY: Why did this happen? Was the care plan followed? Were door alarms working properly? Were exit doors visible at all times? If so, by whom? What was the facility's plan to supervise the resident? Was it followed? If so, why did it fail? What was the physician's version of the cause for harm? Were crucial medications involving therapeutic blood/serum levels involved in the elopement (i.e., insulin, psychotropic, antihypertensives, etc.)? What other contributing factors, such as diagnosis, should be considered?

Example Case #2: Confused, debilitated 75 year old female admitted as an inpatient to the hospital has orders to discontinue all nutrition and hydration support.

TRIGGER: Withholding nutrition and hydration without sufficient documentation of advance directives could be an Immediate Jeopardy situation.

Investigation:

WHO: Who wrote the order? Is this the patient's primary care physician? Who has the authority to make the medical care decisions? Does the patient have a living will? Does the patient have a durable power of attorney? Who has spoken with the person designated to make health care decisions for the patient; e.g., social worker, primary care physician, specialist, hospice nurse, or chaplain?

WHAT: What is the patient's diagnosis? Is documentation of a terminal disease process by the attending physician contained in the progress notes? What does the progress note contain about risks and benefits of discontinuation of hydration and nutrition? What alternative treatment options have been considered and discussed with the person responsible for making health care decisions for this patient? What events precipitated the decision to discontinue hydration and nutrition? What care and services have been planned during the absence of nutrition and hydration? What steps have been taken to ascertain the patient's wishes? What is State law regarding advance directives and end of life issues?

WHEN: When did the hospital obtain evidence of the patient's wishes regarding end of life treatment? When did the physician discuss end of life issues, diagnosis, prognosis and the patient's wishes with the person designated by the patient or by law to make health care decisions?

WHERE: If the patient has an advance directive, how easy/difficult is it to find in the chart to verify the patient's wishes? If the advance directive is not in the chart, does the chart indicate where the advance directive is kept? If the patient does not have an advance directive, where is the documentation in the chart to support the patient's wishes to discontinue nutrition and hydration at the end of life? Where is the documentation to support that the person making the health care decisions is fully informed of the risks and benefits and is making the decisions the patient would have made? If the patient does not have an advance directive, does the patient's chart reflect compliance with the State law and the legal representative's decision-making authority concerning withdrawal of hydration and nutrition? Has the person with decision-making authority been fully informed of all options, including home care, hospice and long term care placement?

WHY: If the physician wrote an order to discontinue nutrition and hydration, does the progress note contain documentation of the rationale? Is there clear documentation to support the decision?

C - Decision-Making

The information gathered is used to evaluate the provision of related care and services, occurrence frequency, and the likelihood of repetition. The team needs to have gathered and validated sufficient information to address the three components of Immediate Jeopardy (listed below) to begin the decision process.

Components of Immediate Jeopardy

1. **Harm**

    a. **Actual -** Was there an outcome of harm? Does the harm meet the definition of Immediate Jeopardy, e.g., has the provider's noncompliance caused serious injury, harm, impairment, or death to an individual?

    b. **Potential -** Is there a likelihood of potential harm? Does the potential harm meet the definition of Immediate Jeopardy; e.g., is the provider's noncompliance likely to cause serious injury, harm, impairment, or death to an individual?

2. **Immediacy** - Is the harm or potential harm likely to occur in the very near future to this individual or others in the entity, if immediate action is not taken? (Refer to the SOM §3010(B)(6) for timelines during normal termination.)

3. **Culpability**

    a. Did the entity know about the situation? If so when did the entity first become aware?

    b. Should the entity have known about the situation?

    c. Did the entity thoroughly investigate the circumstances?

    d. Did the entity implement corrective measures?

    e. Has the entity re-evaluated the measures to ensure the situation was corrected?

Note: The team must consider the entity's response to any harm or potential harm that meets the definition of Immediate Jeopardy. The stated lack of knowledge by the entity about a particular situation does not excuse an entity from knowing and preventing Immediate Jeopardy. The team should use knowledge and experience to determine if the circumstances could have been predicted. The Immediate Jeopardy investigation should proceed until the team has gathered enough information to evaluate any prior indications or warnings regarding the jeopardy situation and the entity's response. The crisis situations in which an entity did not have any prior indications or warnings, and could not have predicted a potential serious harm, are very rare.

Team Actions:

- Meet as a team;

- Follow Appendix Q;
- Share collected data;
- Identify the three components of Immediate Jeopardy;
- Decide if you have enough information to make a decision. If not, continue the investigation;
- Identify any inconsistencies or contradictions between interviews, observations and record reviews;
- Clarify any inconsistencies or contradictions;
- Determine the specific Federal regulation for the situation; and
- Consult with the SA, as necessary.

The following are examples of decision-making as the team analyzes the information obtained during the investigation. Example #1 and 2 are continuations from B-Investigation.

Example Case #1 (Continued): (Refer to B - Investigation) During the survey, the resident was observed to enter the code and exit the unit without assistance 5 times in 30 minutes and was brought back by nursing staff from the unit, nursing staff from other units and administrative staff. The front door to the facility had a broken alarm and did not latch properly and was easily accessible after exiting the locked unit. The facility was aware of the broken alarm and latch. The chart contained documentation that the facility was aware of the resident's ability to operate the door keypads for at least 60 days. The facility was located in an urban area on a busy street. A row of trees prevented anyone in the facility from viewing a resident exiting the property and crossing the street.

The record included documentation of the resident exiting the building successfully without notice. The documentation included only a brief description of the incident. After a search, the resident was located in an area emergency room being treated for a minor laceration of the lip. Police notified the facility that bystanders who had called 911 had found the resident lying down with blood on her face. The chart included subsequent reports of repeated frequent attempts to elope 25-40 times per shift, and the statement, "Patient requires 1:1, care not safe on this unit secondary to continuous exit seeking." A review of the facility investigations revealed that the facility had not completed any investigations for this resident.

Decision Making:

- Has actual harm occurred? Yes.
- Does the actual harm that occurred meet the definition of Immediate Jeopardy? No.
- Is there a likelihood of potential serious harm? Yes.
- Does the potential harm meet the definition of Immediate Jeopardy? Yes.
- Is the harm likely to recur in the very near future, if immediate action is not taken? Yes.
- Did the facility have knowledge of the situation? Yes. If so when did they first become aware? Before admission when notified of history.
- Did they thoroughly investigate the circumstances? No.
- Did they implement corrective measures? No.
- Does this meet the definition of Immediate Jeopardy? Yes.
- Which is the most appropriate tag to define the failed practice?

Outcome:

- The team identifies the most appropriate regulation that applies to the situation.
- The team proceeds with documentation of the Immediate Jeopardy deficient practice.
- The SA proceeds with the termination procedures per the SOM.
- Except in the case of Medicaid-only facilities, the RO proceeds with termination actions.

Example Case #2 (Continued): (Refer to <u>B - Investigation</u>) During the investigation, the surveyor finds that the chart does not include a copy of the patient's advance directive. The progress note does not contain any documentation of the patient ever stating a wish to have nutrition and hydration withdrawn at the end of life. The patient has a diagnosis of advance dementia with a documented history of refusal to eat in a long-term care facility. The patient had been admitted because of continued weight loss and dehydration related to the refusal to eat or drink. The patient has a daughter who actively participates in her mother's care, is identified as the legal representative, and is identified in the social service notes as the closest living family member. The primary care physician documented a discussion with the daughter concerning the patient's poor prognosis for meaningful recovery. While death is not imminent as a result of the dementia, death is the expected result at some unknown time in the future. The chart does not include any documentation that the daughter expressed a wish to have nutrition and hydration support withdrawn. The social worker was unable to confirm that the daughter had expressed a wish to have all support withdrawn. The social worker is uncertain why the nutrition and hydration were discontinued. When contacted, the daughter is unaware that support has been withdrawn and is very upset. The surveyor copies the order sheet, the progress notes and the social service notes. The surveyor clearly documents the interviews with the social worker and the daughter. There is a discrepancy between the written order for withdrawal of support and the daughter's and the social worker's knowledge of the situation. The surveyor decides to present the information to the team prior to contacting the physician.

Decision Making:

- Has actual harm occurred? No.
- Is there a likelihood of potential serious harm? Yes.
- Does the potential serious harm meet the definition of Immediate Jeopardy, e.g., serious injury, harm, impairment, or death? Yes.
- Is the potential serious harm likely to occur in the very near future, if immediate action is not taken? Yes.
- Did the facility have knowledge of the situation? Yes.
- If so, when did they first become aware? After the doctor's order was written?
- Did they thoroughly investigate the circumstances? No.
- Did they implement corrective measures? No.
- Does this meet the definition of Immediate Jeopardy? Yes.
- Which is the most appropriate tag to define the failed practice?

Outcome:

- The team identifies the most appropriate regulation that applies to the situation.
- The team proceeds with documentation of the Immediate Jeopardy deficient practice.

- The SA proceeds with the termination procedures per the SOM.
- The RO proceeds with termination actions.

Example Case #3: An outside intruder entered a resident's room by cutting through the screen. A resident with a diagnosis of advanced dementia was raped. The resident did not notify staff at the time of the incident. The intruder was not observed entering the facility by any facility staff. However, nightshift staff immediately called the police after noticing a stranger in the courtyard at the back of the facility. The police came and were unable to locate anyone. The police checked the grounds without incident and then encouraged the staff to check the locks on the doors and windows and obtain services to monitor the premises for increased security. The police indicated that no prior intruders had been reported in the neighborhood.

The facility immediately contacted a local security service and hired a security guard to monitor the outside grounds. The security guard arrived within 45 minutes and began patrolling the grounds. The facility staff checked all the doors and windows to ensure security. They checked on all of the residents and did not observe any problems. During morning rounds, the resident reported that someone had hurt her during the night. The staff noted that the screen had been damaged and immediately contacted the police and the SA. The police came and had the resident transported to the nearest emergency room for a rape assessment. The emergency room confirmed that the resident had been raped.

Decision-Making:

- Has actual harm occurred? Yes.
- Does the harm meet the definition of Immediate Jeopardy, e.g., serious injury, harm, impairment, or death to an individual? Yes.
- Is the harm likely to recur in the very near future, if immediate action is not taken? Yes.
- Did the entity have knowledge of the situation? Yes.
- If so when did they first become aware? In the morning when the resident reported she had been hurt.
- Did they thoroughly investigate the circumstances? Yes.
- Did they implement corrective measures? Yes.
- Does this meet the definition of Immediate Jeopardy? No. The facility reacted appropriately and followed the recommendations of the law enforcement experts

to protect all residents. The harm to the resident had already occurred before the facility had any indications or warnings, and could not have been predicted or prevented.

Outcome:

- The team gathered sufficient data to reach the conclusion that the facility had no predictable way of knowing that residents were at risk for harm from an intruder.
- The team also gathered sufficient data to reach a decision that the facility reacted immediately to protect residents when they had knowledge of a potential risk.
- The team concludes that there was no failed practice.
- The team concludes their investigation of this complaint.

VI - Implementation

A - Team Actions

If the team reaches a consensus concerning the presence of Immediate Jeopardy, the team leader then contacts the SA per the protocol established by the SA. The SA review should be expedited. If the team is unable to follow the SA protocol for administrative consultation, actions to proceed with implementation of Immediate Jeopardy must continue. Decide if any other agencies need to be notified, e.g., Law Enforcement Agency, Nurses Aide Registration Board.

NOTE: Any criminal act needs to be reported to the local law enforcement agency. The entity should be encouraged to make the report, if needed. The surveyor should only assume this responsibility if the entity refuses.

B - SA Actions

Upon review of the findings, if the SA concurs with the team's consensus of Immediate Jeopardy, the SA will inform the RO for all Medicare and dually certified entities. For Medicaid-only facilities, the SA will notify the State Medicaid Agency. For Immediate Jeopardy in Medicaid-only facilities, contact the RO per the protocol established between the SA and the RO.

C - Team Action

Once the team has decided that Immediate Jeopardy exists, the team should notify the administration of the Immediate Jeopardy. A verbal notice should be given with the specific details, including the individuals at risk, before the survey team leaves the premises of the entity. **The entity should begin immediate removal of the risk to**

individuals, and immediately implement corrective measures to prevent repeat Jeopardy situations. The team should encourage the entity to provide evidence of their implementation of corrective measures.

The notice describing the Immediate Jeopardy must be delivered to the entity no later than 2 days (refer to specific SOM reference) of the end of the survey. If official notification of **all** deficiencies, i.e., Form CMS-2567, was not given on the second day, a completed Form CMS-2567 must be sent to the entity on the tenth working day.

VII - Documentation

A - Skilled Nursing Facilities/Nursing Facilities (SNF/NF)

1 - Confirmation of Removal of Immediate Jeopardy

Only onsite confirmation of implementation of the facility's corrective actions justifies a determination that the Immediate Jeopardy has been removed.

2 - Immediate Jeopardy Removed, Deficient Practice Corrected

If the facility is able to remove the Immediate Jeopardy before the survey team leaves the facility and to correct associated deficient practices, cite the Immediate Jeopardy at the Immediate Jeopardy severity and scope (J, K or L). Document evidence of the facility's actions, including dates that indicate that the facility has removed the Immediate Jeopardy and corrected the deficient practice. The date of full correction will be shown on the Form CMS-2567B, a copy of which can be found at http://cms.hhs.gov/forms/cms2567b.pdf

3 - Immediate Jeopardy Removed, Deficient Practice Present

If the facility is able to employ immediate corrective measures that remove the Immediate Jeopardy, but an associated deficient practice still exists at a lesser severity and scope, cite the Immediate Jeopardy at the Immediate Jeopardy severity and scope. Include the documentation to support the remaining deficient practice. Document the level of harm and the identified residents in the Statement of Deficiencies. Attach the corrective measures submitted by the facility as an immediate plan of correction.

4 - Immediate Jeopardy Not Removed

If the facility is unable or unwilling to remove the Immediate Jeopardy before the end of the survey, inform the administration that the RO will be notified of the Immediate Jeopardy and termination procedures will be initiated. Use the appropriate SOM reference to define the end of the survey.

B - All Entities Not Noted Above

Immediate Jeopardy is always cited at the **Condition** level on the Form CMS-2567, a copy of which can be found at http://www.cms.hhs.gov/forms/cms2567.pdf.

1 - Confirmation of Removal of Immediate Jeopardy

Only onsite confirmation of implementation of the facility's corrective action justifies a determination that the Immediate Jeopardy has been removed.

2 - Immediate Jeopardy Removed, Deficient Practice Corrected

If the entity is able to remove the Immediate Jeopardy and correct associated deficient practices before the team exits, cite the Immediate Jeopardy at the Condition level on the Form CMS-2567. Corrective actions taken by the provider/supplier will be included in the Form CMS-2567 documentation. The date of full correction will be shown on the Form CMS-2567B.

3 - Immediate Jeopardy Removed, Deficient Practice Present at Condition Level

If the entity is able to employ immediate corrective measures that remove the Immediate Jeopardy, but an associated deficient practice still remains at the condition level for the same Condition of Participation, cite the Condition of Participation as not met and proceed with 90-day termination procedures. Include documentation of both the Immediate Jeopardy with subsequent removal, and the remaining deficient practice in this citation.

4 - Immediate Jeopardy Removed, Deficient Practice Present at Standard or Elemental Level

If the entity is able to employ immediate corrective measures, which remove the Immediate Jeopardy but an associated deficient practice still remains at the standard or elemental level, cite the Immediate Jeopardy at the Condition of Participation level on Form CMS-2567. Cite the remaining deficiency at the most appropriate standard or elemental tag. The date of removal of the Immediate Jeopardy will be shown on the Form CMS-2567B.

5 - Immediate Jeopardy Not Removed

If the entity is unable or unwilling to remove the Immediate Jeopardy before the team's exit, inform the administration that the RO will be notified of the Immediate Jeopardy situation and termination procedures will be initiated. In the case of a Medicaid-only facility, the State Medicaid Agency will be notified of the Immediate Jeopardy.

VIII - Enforcement

A - Termination for Title XIX-Only NFs, ICFs/MR

Refer to SOM §3005 E for specific instructions.

B - Enforcement for SNF/NF

Refer to SOM §§7307-7309 for specific instructions.

C - Termination for all other Medicare Entities

Refer to SOM §3010.

IX - References

- SOM Appendices (Excluding Appendix C, CLIA)
- Principles of Documentation
- SOM §3005 E
- SOM §§3010-3012
- SOM §§7307-7309

Attachment A

The jeopardy situations that follow are actual citations that have been upheld.

IMMEDIATE JEOPARDY NOT REMOVED BEFORE EXIT

ICF/MR Failed Practice

Condition of Participation - The facility failed to assure medical services were provided to a client with an emergency medical condition.

Summary - At 4:30 a.m. on x/x/x, the nursing staff was notified that Client #1 had not slept during their shift and had three to four liquid stools that night. Nursing staff assessed the client, found his bed smeared with feces (color and consistency not described), his color slightly pale, abdomen slightly distended, and dried blood around his mouth. Assessed vital signs were blood pressure 100/60, heart rate 70 beats per minute, temperature 100.5 degrees Fahrenheit. His treatment consisted of Tylenol (given orally) at 5:10 a.m.

At approximately 5:45 a.m., Client #1 became unsteady while exiting the bathroom and was lowered to the floor with staff assistance. At 6:00 a.m., the client was described as, "skin cold, clammy - color pale." His blood pressure had dropped to 88/50, heart rate 85 beats per minute, oxygen saturation 93%. The client was placed on oxygen at 5 liters per minute and preparations were initiated to transfer the client to the infirmary.

At 6:25 a.m., Client #1 was still on the floor outside of the bathroom and the records indicated he was unresponsive. His blood pressure was 80/50, and his heart rate dropped to 67 beats per minute. The client tried to remove the nasal cannula that supplied him with oxygen and "insisted on sitting up." After sitting up, his skin was documented as decreased in color and "sallow." He had coffee ground drooling coming from both corners of his mouth.

At 6:40 a.m., the community emergency response number (911) was called. At 6:45 a.m., Client #1 was documented as being unresponsive with absent blood pressure, pulse, and respirations. Cardiopulmonary Resuscitation (CPR) was initiated. At 6:49 a.m., the community 911-response team arrived and took over CPR. The client expired at 7:00 a.m..

The Superintendent stated that staff were expected to use their own judgment as to when to access 911 emergency services. Review of facility Procedure #X revealed a lack of clear guidelines to facility staff on when to call for community 911 emergency response.

Issue - Failure to protect from neglect.

Trigger - Failure to adequately monitor and intervene for serious medical/surgical conditions.

Decision Making:

- Has actual harm occurred? Yes
- Does the harm meet the definition of Immediate Jeopardy, e.g., serious injury, harm, impairment, or death to an individual? Yes
- Is the harm likely to recur in the very near future, if no immediate action is taken? Yes
- Did the entity have knowledge of the situation? Yes If so, when did the entity first become aware? On the night shift.
- Did they thoroughly investigate the circumstances? No
- Did they implement corrective measures? No
- Does this meet the definition of Immediate Jeopardy? Yes
- Which is the most appropriate tag to define the failed practice? Cite the most appropriate tag at the Condition of Participation level for Immediate Jeopardy.

Outcome - The team cited the Condition of Participation, Health Care Services (Tag W318). The facility implemented a corrective action plan after receiving written notice. Onsite revisit confirmed correction.

IMMEDIATE JEOPARDY NOT REMOVED PRIOR TO EXIT

Home Health Agency Failed Practice

Condition of Participation - The agency failed to assure medications were provided to patients in accordance with physician's orders and the patient's plans of care.

Summary - Patient #1: The patient was admitted on x/x/x with a diagnosis of Insulin Dependent Diabetes Mellitus. Orders were: Humulin Insulin N 2 units and Regular (Reg) Insulin 3 units subcutaneously every morning and evening plus sliding scale Regular insulin coverage for blood sugar ranges of: 200-299=2 units Reg. Insulin, 300-399=4 units Reg. Insulin, 400+=6 units Reg. Insulin. The frequency of the sliding scale coverage was not included in the physician's orders, nor was the frequency of blood glucose testing. A subsequent physician's order for NPH 3u BID was transcribed as NPH 3 units every evening.

The Director of Professional Services made an assumption that the blood glucose testing and sliding scale insulin coverage was two times a day. Because of missing documentation, it was unclear when the patient actually received the correct dose of insulin. On 11 occasions, the patient's blood glucose levels were between 200-299 or 300-399. There was no documentation that the sliding scale was followed. On 6 occasions, the patient's blood glucose levels were below 200 and regular insulin was giving contrary to the sliding scale. On x/x/x, the patient's blood glucose was 431 and 4 units of regular insulin were given, rather than 6 units per the sliding scale.

Patient #2 - The patient had a diagnosis of Insulin Dependent Diabetes Mellitus and orders for routine insulin coverage BID. The plan of care included teaching the patient's caregiver diabetes management. There were no orders for blood glucose testing in the plan of care. The nurse directed the caregiver to perform blood glucose levels twice a day. Subsequent nursing notes indicated the caregiver was performing the blood glucose levels four times a day. On x/x/x, new orders for sliding scale insulin were received and implemented by the nurse without a frequency for administration. The nurse did not address the sliding scale insulin coverage or the caregiver's ability to carry out the insulin administration during subsequent visits. There was no documentation of the sliding scale insulin being administered to the patient.

Issue - Failure to protect from undue adverse medication consequences and/or failure to provide medications as prescribed.

Trigger - Pattern of repeated medication errors without intervention, lack of diabetic monitoring resulting or likely to result in serious hypoglycemic or hyperglycemic reaction.

Issue - Failure to prevent neglect

Trigger - Failure to carry out doctor's orders

Decision Making;

- Has actual harm occurred? No
- Is there a likelihood of potential serious harm? Yes
- Does the potential serious harm meet the definition of Immediate Jeopardy, e.g., serious injury, harm, impairment, or death to an individual? Yes
- Is the potential outcome likely to occur in the very near future, if no action is taken? Yes.
- Did the entity have knowledge of the situation? Yes

- If so, when did they first become aware? When an incomplete doctor's order was received.
- Did they thoroughly investigate the circumstances? No
- Did they implement corrective measures? No
- Does this meet the definition of Immediate Jeopardy? Yes
- Which is the most appropriate tag to define the failed practice? Cite the most appropriate tag at the Condition of Participation level for Immediate Jeopardy.

Outcome - The State Agency attempted to hand deliver the completed Form CMS-2567. The HHA was closed with a sign posted on the door indicating the agency was moving and the administrative staff was in the field making discharge plans for the patients. An on-call number was given. The on-call nurse stated that all of the agency's patients had been discharged. The agency submitted a written notice of closure upon request. State Agency completed a referral to the Board of Nursing regarding the Director of Nursing.

IMMEDIATE JEOPARDY REMOVED, DEFICIENT PRACTICE STILL REMAINS

SNF/NF Failed Practice

Severity - Level 4, Scope - Isolated--The facility failed to prevent neglect, failed to provide appropriate emergency care, and failed to provide supervision to prevent accidents.

Summary - The resident had a diagnosis of Alzheimer's dementia with a history of falls and wandering. The resident ambulated with a special walker. The resident was found lying at the base of a flight of stairs, in a pool of blood, bleeding from the nose and ears with a large laceration on his head. The alarm on the door leading to the stairs had not been reset after a fire alarm. Following the resident's fall down the flight of stairs, the nurse talked to the resident, helped him to his walker and asked an aide to take him back to his room. The resident was not transported to his room, but was requested to ambulate using his walker with the stand-by assistance of an aide. The nurse returned to the unit, completed pending tasks and then called the doctor who directed her to call an ambulance. The resident was taken to the hospital and returned to the facility after a decision not to perform neurosurgery. The resident died 36 hours after the injury.

The resident fell while the nurse was off the unit in the boarding home giving medication. This was a regular part of the assigned duties for the nurse.

Issue - Failure to prevent neglect.

Trigger - Lack of timely assessment of individuals after injury and lack of supervision for individual with known special needs.

Decision-Making:

- Has as actual harm occurred? Yes
- Does the harm meet the definition of Immediate Jeopardy, e.g., serious injury, harm, impairment, or death to an individual? Yes
- Is the harm likely to recur in the very near future to this individual or others in the entity, if immediate action is not taken? Yes
- Did the entity have knowledge of the situation? Yes. If so, when did they first become aware? Prior to the fall, when a history of falls and wandering was documented.
- Did they thoroughly investigate the circumstances? Yes
- Did they implement corrective measures? No
- Does this meet the definition of Immediate Jeopardy? Yes
- Which is the most appropriate tag to define the failed practice? Cite the Immediate Jeopardy at the appropriate tag. Also document the remaining deficient practice under the same tag. Define the level of harm for the residents in the failed practice statement (e.g., the facility failed to prevent neglect for 1 of 10 residents (#8) which resulted in Immediate Jeopardy, and for 2 of 10 residents (#4 and #5) which resulted in harm).

Outcome - Revisit confirmed the removal of the Immediate Jeopardy; however, during revisit, another Immediate Jeopardy was recognized. A subsequent revisit confirmed the removal of the second Immediate Jeopardy identified. A deficient practice still remained. Termination stopped. Substantial compliance was reached 30 days later.

Attachment B

Documentation for Immediate Jeopardy should follow the Principles of Documentation. The following are examples of Forms CMS-2567 documenting Immediate Jeopardy.

Example for LTC: Failure to Prevent Abuse

F223

483(b) Requirements: Abuse

Scope and Severity B Level is J - The resident has the right to be free from verbal, sexual, physical and mental abuse, corporal punishment, and involuntary seclusion.

This requirement is not met as evidenced by the following:

Based on interview, and record reviews, it was determined the facility failed to assure that the female residents on the North Wing had an environment that was free from sexual abuse. The findings constituted an Immediate Jeopardy situation. Facility staff had knowledge of the inappropriate sexual behaviors of two male residents (Residents #12 and 27). The facility had not consistently identified the victims, had not conducted investigations, and had not implemented effective preventive measures to protect the female residents on North Wing from actual and potential sexual abuse. There were multiple incidents of actual harm with three identified sample residents (Residents #3, 14, and 25). There were three incidents of potential harm for three unidentified residents.

Findings include:

1. A review of Resident #12's record revealed a nurse's note dated xx/xx/xx, at 1:30 a.m., the resident was found sitting next to Resident #3 in the common area. Resident #12 had "one hand on [Resident #3's] buttock and one hand on the breast. [Resident #3] was attempting to push Resident #12's hand away." At 4:00 a.m., the same day, Resident #12 was found in the hallway with hands on an unidentified, nude female resident.

2. Resident #12 record revealed that on xx/xx/xx, at 11:30 p.m., the resident was found in an unidentified female resident's bed with both side rails up. Resident #12 had one hand directly on the female's labia. The female resident was unable to respond. The nurses notes dated xx/xx/xx, stated, "Resident #12 was sexually inappropriate with a female resident who could not give consent."

3. On xx/xx/xx, at 7:15 p.m., a nurses note in Resident #12's record stated that the resident was found standing in the hall, behind Resident #14, who was sitting in a

wheelchair. Resident #12's hands were on Resident #14's breast. Resident #14 stated, "I am going to call the police."

4. Interview with the Administrator and DON on xx/xx/xx, confirmed that none of the incidents involving Resident #12 had been reported to the State per the State's complaint protocol.

5. On xx/xx/xx at 3:30 a.m., Resident #27's record revealed the resident was found in the room of Resident #25 (a severely cognitively impaired resident, who was unable to communicate) standing by the bed, with pajama bottoms down and hands in Resident #25's genital area. An incident report, dated xx/xx/xx revealed Resident #25 "looked frightened, with widened eyes, unable to defend self or call for help."

6. Nurses notes dated xx/xx/xx, at 10:30 p.m., revealed Resident #27 was found in an unidentified resident's room, with the covers pulled back, and hands in the resident's genital area.

7. There were no incident reports for xx/xx/xx or xx/xx/xx for Resident #27. Interview with the charge nurse on xx/xx/xx, revealed that she had no knowledge of the incidents, whether an investigation of the incidents had been conducted, or if efforts had been made to protect female residents.

Example for All Other Entities with Conditions of Participation or Conditions of Coverage: Failure to provide safety from fire, smoke and environmental hazards and/or failure to educate staff in handling emergency situations

---

I 117

485.723 Condition: Physical Environment

The building housing the organization is constructed, equipped, and maintained to protect the health and safety of patients, personnel, and the public and provides a functional, sanitary, and comfortable environment.

This Condition is not met as evidenced by the following:

Based on observation, interview and review of policies and procedures, the agency failed to assure patients were protected from fire hazards, failed to provide adequate egress for emergencies (refer to I-118) and failed to provide adequate protection from hazardous chemicals (refer to I-158). These deficiencies resulted in potential harm for 20 of 20 sample patients (#1-20) and the 90 additional patients receiving care at the agency. An Immediate Jeopardy to the patients and the public was created by these deficiencies.

I-118

485.723(a) Standard Safety of Patients

The organization satisfies the following requirements:

1. It complies with all applicable State and local building, fire, and safety codes.

2. Permanently attached automatic fire-extinguishing systems of adequate capacity are installed in all areas of the organization considered to have special fire hazards. Fire extinguishers are conveniently located on each floor of the premises. Fire regulations are prominently posted.

3. Doorways, passageways, and stairwells negotiated by patients are:

   a. Of adequate width to allow for easy movement of all patients (including those on stretchers or in wheelchairs);

   b. Free from obstruction at all times;

   c. In the case of stairwells, equipped with firmly attached handrails on at least one side;

   d. Lights are placed at exits and in corridors used by patients and are to be supported by an emergency power source;

   e. A fire alarm system with local alarm capability and, where applicable, an emergency power source is functional;

   f.. At least two persons are on duty on the premises of the organization whenever a patient is being treated; and

   g. No occupancies or activities undesirable or injurious to the health and safety of patients are located in the building.

This Standard is not met as evidenced by the following:

Based on an observation and interview, the agency failed to provide unobstructed hallways and exits for 1 of 2 exit doors and hallways; failed to provide adequate maintenance of exit lighting for 1 of 2 exits and 2 of 4 emergency lights; and failed to provide a fire alarm system; resulting in the potential harm for all the agency's current patients including 20 of 20 sample patients (#1-20). This resulted in an Immediate Jeopardy.

Findings Include:

1. Observation of the passageway on xx/xx/xx at 3 p.m. and on xx/xx/xx at 10 a.m., revealed that the east hallway was partially obstructed with several items of furniture and other obstacles. During interview, at 11 a.m. on xx/xx/xx, the administrator stated that the building manager was temporarily storing these items in the hallway. The administrator was unable to provide a date when the items might be relocated.

2. Observation at 12 noon on xx/xx/xx, revealed that the exercise pool for the agency was located in the basement in a windowless room. The room had two exit doors, located at opposite ends of the pool with narrow walkways on each side of the pool. One of the emergency exit signs above the door was not illuminated. The other exit door, with the illuminated emergency light, was locked. Four small battery powered flashlights had been placed throughout the room. Two of the four lights failed to illuminate when activated. The two remaining lights, when activated, failed to provide adequate lighting to allow visibility for egress.

3. Review of the agency's policies and procedures indicated that, in case of fire, employees were to pull the manual alarm. Interview with staff during the survey revealed that seven of the seven staff members on duty were unable to identify where the pull alarm was located. Observation on xx/xx/xx at 10 a.m. failed to provide any evidence of a fire alarm. During interview with the administrator on xx/xx/xx at 12 noon, the absence of a fire alarm was confirmed.

I 158

485.723(b) Standard: Maintenance of Equipment/Buildings/Grounds

The organization establishes a written preventive maintenance program to ensure that:

1. The equipment is operative and is properly calibrated; and

2. The interior and exterior of the building are clean and orderly and maintained free of any defects that are a potential hazard to patients, personnel, and the public.

This Standard is not met as evidenced by the following:

Based on observation and review of the policies and procedures, the agency failed to provide preventative maintenance of the clothes dryer resulting in a potential fire hazard, and failed to properly store pool supplies resulting in a potential chemical hazard for 20 of 20 sample residents (#1-20) and all of the current patients. This resulted in Immediate Jeopardy.

Findings Include:

1. Observation of the laundry room on xx/xx/xx at 12:50 a.m., revealed a large amount of dryer lint on top of the dryer and the water heater, behind the washer, dryers, and water heater, and covering the ceiling and the ceiling roof vent. The washing machine repairman, during interview on xx/xx/xx at 1 p.m., related the extent of the lint accumulation to a plugged dryer exhaust vent and stated that this was an "extreme fire hazard." The administrator was notified of the potential fire hazard on xx/xx/xx at 1:30 p.m.. The vent had not been cleaned, nor had the lint been removed by xx/xx/xx, even though the administrator had been notified of the potential hazard 2 days prior.

2. Observation of the storage area for pool supplies and equipment on xx/xx/xx at 2 p.m., revealed that the chlorine powder was stored in barrels with damaged lids which did not close properly. The chlorine powder had been spilled on the floor and had been tracked out into the pool area. Neither the storage area nor the pool area contained any hazardous chemical warnings. An interview with the pool maintenance staff on xx/xx/xx at 2:15 p.m., did not provide any evidence that the staff had been educated regarding the precautions for hazardous chemicals. The staff was unable to locate any policies or procedures regarding how employees should respond to a chemical spill.

Attachment C - Overview - Recommended Key Components of Systemic Approach to Prevent Abuse and Neglect

Examples--Key Components applied to the following provider types:

Key Components Applicable To All Providers

1. Prevent

The facility or system has the capacity to prevent the occurrence of abuse and neglect and reviews specific incidents for "lessons learned" which form a feedback loop for necessary policy changes.

Nursing Homes

Regulation Authority: 483.13(b), 483.13(c), 483.13(c)(3)

Survey Guidance - Surveyors determine if:

The facility must develop and implement written policies and procedures that include the seven key components: screening, training, prevention, identification, investigation, protection and reporting/response; the facility identifies, corrects and intervenes in situations in which abuse or neglect is more likely to occur, and the facility identifies characteristics of physical environment and deployment of staff and residents (e.g., those with aggressive behaviors) likely to precipitate abuse or neglect.

ICFs/MR

Regulation Authority: 483.420(a)(5), 483.420(d)(1), 483.420(d)(1)(I)

Survey Guidance - Surveyors determine if:

The facility has and implements abuse prevention policies and procedures; and the facility organizes itself in such a manner that individuals are free from threat to their health and safety.

2. Screen

The facility or system provides evidence and maintains efforts to determine if persons hired have records of abuse or neglect.

Nursing Homes

Regulation Authority - 483.13(c)(1)(ii) (A)&(B)

Survey Guidance - Surveyors determine if: The facility screens potential employees for a history of abuse, neglect, or mistreating residents as defined by the applicable requirements.

ICFs/MR

Regulation Authority - 483.420(c)(1)(iii)

Survey Guidance - Surveyors determine if: The facility screens potential employees to prohibit the employment of individuals with a conviction or prior employment history of child or client abuse, neglect, or mistreatment.

3. Identify

The facility or system creates and maintains a proactive approach to identify events and occurrences that may constitute or contribute to abuse and neglect.

Nursing Homes

Regulation Authority - 483.13(c)(2)

Survey Guidance - Surveyors determine if: The facility identifies events such as suspicious bruising of residents, occurrences, patterns and trends that may constitute abuse; and determine the direction of the investigation.

ICFs/MR

Regulation Authority - 483.420(a)(5)

Survey Guidance - Surveyors determine if: The facility identifies patterns or isolated incidents of unexplained functional regression, or other evidence of physical, verbal, sexual or psychological abuse or punishment posing a serious and immediate threat to individuals.

4. Train

The facility or system, during its orientation program, and through an ongoing trainng program, provides all employees with information regarding abuse and neglect and related reporting requirements, including prevention, intervention and detection.

Nursing Homes

Regulation Authority - 483.74(e)

Survey Guidance - Surveyors determine if: The facility has procedures to train employees, through orientation and on-going sessions, on issues related to abuse prohibition practices.

ICFs/MR

Regulation Authority - 483.420(d)(1), 483.430(e)(1)

Survey Guidance - Surveyors determine if: Facility ensures that staff can define what constitutes abuse and punishment and actively promotes respect for individuals; and facility assures that staff have received training, both upon hiring and on an ongoing basis, which results in the competencies needed to do their job.

5. Protect

The facility or system must protect individuals from abuse and neglect during investigation of any allegations of abuse or neglect.

Nursing Homes

Regulation Authority - 483.13(c)(3)

Survey Guidance - Surveyors determine if: The facility has procedures to protect residents from harm during an investigation.

ICFs/MR

Regulation Authority - 483.430(d)(3)

Survey Guidance - Surveyors determine if: The facility prevents further potential abuse while the investigation is in progress.

6. Investigate

The facility or system ensures, in a timely and thorough manner, objective investigation of all allegations of abuse, neglect, or mistreatment.

Nursing Homes

Regulation Authority - 483.13(c)(2)(3)&(4)

Survey Guidance - Surveyors determine if: The facility has procedures to investigate different types of abuse; and identify staff member responsible for the initial reporting of results to the proper authorities.

ICFs/MR

Regulation Authority - 483.420(d)(3)

Survey Guidance - Surveyors determine if: The facility investigates all injuries of unknown origin and allegations of mistreatment, neglect, or abuse.

7. Report/ Respond

The facility or system must assure that any incidents of substantiated abuse and neglect are reported and analyzed, and the appropriate corrective, remedial or disciplinary action occurs, in accordance with applicable local, State or Federal law.

Nursing Homes

Regulation Authority - 483.13(c)(1)(iii), 483.13(c)(2), 483.13(c)(4)

Survey Guidance - Surveyors determine if: The facility has procedures to report all alleged violations and substantiated incidents to the State agency and to all other agencies, as required, and to take all necessary corrective actions, depending on the results of the investigation; report to State nurse aide registry or licensing authorities any knowledge it has of any action by a court of law which would indicate an employee is unfit for service, and analyze the occurrences to determine what changes are needed, if any, to policies and procedures to prevent further occurrences.

ICFs/MR

Regulation Authority - 483.420(1)(6), 483.420(d)(2), 483.420(d)(4)

Survey Guidance - Surveyors determine if: The results of all investigations are reported to the administrator or designated representative or to other officials in accordance with State law within 5 working days of the incident and, if the alleged violation is verified, appropriate corrective action is taken.